Congenital Diseases in the Right Heart

Andrew N. Redington · Glen S. Van Arsdell
Robert H. Anderson

Editors

Congenital Diseases in the Right Heart

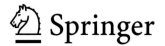 Springer

Editors

Andrew N. Redington, MD, FRCP
(Canada and UK)
The Labatt Family Heart Centre
The Hospital for Sick Children
Toronto
Canada
andrew.redington@sickkids.ca

Glen S. Van Arsdell, MD
The Labatt Family Heart Centre
The Hospital for Sick Children
Toronto
Canada
glen.vanarsdell@sickkids.ca

Robert H. Anderson, MD, FRCPath
Cardiac Unit
Institute of Child Health
University College London
London
UK
r.anderson@ ich.ucl.ac.uk

ISBN: 978-1-84800-377-4   e-ISBN: 978-1-84800-378-1
DOI 10.1007/978-1-84800-378-1

British Library Cataloguing in Publication Data
A catalogue record for this book is available from the British Library
Congenital diseases in the right heart
    1. Congenital heart disease 2. Heart – Right ventricle – Diseases
    I. Redington, Andrew II. Van Arsdell, Glen III. Anderson, Robert Henry
    616.1'2043

Library of Congress Control Number: 2008937583

Printed on acid-free paper

Springer Science+Business Media
springer.com

Preface

Ten years ago it was fashionable, and largely correct, to say that the right heart had been ignored in terms of its functional contribution to the circulation in acquired and congenital heart disease. While it remains a popular characterization, our understanding of right heart hemodynamics, pathophysiology, and its contribution to cardiac disease has matured immensely. It seems timely then to revisit this increasingly important area in cardiovascular disease.

Similar to our first contribution on the topic (*The Right Heart in Congenital Heart Disease*, ISBN 1 900 151 847) this book represents the written narrative from an international symposium, bringing together experts in the field of right heart disease from all over the world. More than simply a *proceedings* document, the mandate for each of the authors was to produce a state-of-the-art contribution for a standalone textbook that we hope to be definitive in the field. Consequently, this book leads us from the most recent findings regarding embryologic origins of the right heart to the most practical aspects of management of right heart disease in acquired and congenital heart anomalies.

In putting this book together, we, the editors, would like to thank each of the authors for their excellent contributions. This text comes at a cost of many evenings and weekends of extracurricular work, but hopefully such a distillation of thought and expertise will provide the reader with a comprehensive resource. Indeed, we believe this edition remains unique in its focus. That having been said, we do not discuss the right heart to the exclusion of its left-sided counterpart. Indeed, the last 10 years have taught us that the right heart, just as with the left, cannot be described in isolation. There is virtually no aspect of cardiac anatomy, physiology, or disease that is not influenced by biventricular interactions. The understanding and therapeutic modification of such interactions will be a challenge for scientists and clinicians over the next 10 years. In the meantime, we do hope you find this text a valuable contribution to your library.

Andrew Redington
Glen S. Van Arsdell
Robert H. Anderson

Contents

Contributors

Claudia L. Almedia, MD Department of Pediatric Cardiology, Instituto Nacional De Cardiologia, Rio De Janeiro, Brazil

Osman O. Al-Radi, MBBS, MSc, FRCSC Department of Surgery, Hospital for Sick Children, Toronto, ON, Canada

Robert H. Anderson, MD Department of Cardiac Services, Great Ormond Street Hospital for Children, London, UK

Lee Benson, MD, FRCP(C), FACC, FSCAI, Department of Paediatrics, Hospital for Sick Children, Toronto, ON, Canada

Desmond J. Bohn, MB, BCh, FFARCS, MRCP, FRCPC Department of Critical Care Medicine, Hospital for Sick Children, Toronto, ON, Canada

Edward L. Bove, MD Department of Surgery, University of Michigan, Ann Arbor, MI, USA

Benoit G. Bruneau, PhD Department of Paediatrics, Gladstone Institute of Cardiovascular Disease , and University of California, San Francisco, CA, USA

Tiscar Cavalle-Garido Department of Paediatrics, Hospital for Sick Children, Toronto, ON, Canada

Rajiv Chaturvedi, MD Department of Paediatrics, Hospital for Sick Children, Toronto, ON, Canada

Michael Cheung, MD Department of Paediatrics, Hospital for Sick Children, Toronto, ON, Canada

Nicholas Collins, BMed, FRACP Toronto General Cardiac Centre for Adults, University Health Network, Toronto, ON, Canada

Andrew C. Cook, PhD Department of Cardiac Services, Great Ormond Street Hospital for Children, London, UK

Anne Dipchand, MD Department of Paediatrics, Hospital for Sick Children, Toronto, ON, Canada

Annie Dore, MD, FRCP (C) Department of Medicine, Montreal Heart Institute, Montreal, QC, Canada

Jeffrey R. Fineman, MD Cardiovascular Research Institute, University of California, San Francisco, CA, USA

Gil J. Gross, MD Department of Paediatrics, Hospital for Sick Children, Toronto, ON, Canada

Lars Grosse-Wortmann Department of Paediatrics, Hospital for Sick Children, Toronto, ON, Canada

Robert M. Hamilton, MD, FRCP(C), MHSc Department of Pediatrics, Hospital for Sick Children, Toronto, ON, Canada

Louise Harris, MB, ChB Division of Cardiology, University Health Network, Toronto, ON, Canada

Jennifer C. Hirsch, MD, MS Department of Surgery, University of Michigan, Ann Arbor, MI, USA

Eric M. Horlick, MDCM, FRCPC Division of Cardiology, Toronto General Hospital, Toronto, ON, Canada

Tilman Humpl, MD, PhD Department of Critical Care Medicine, Hospital for Sick Children, Toronto, ON, Canada

Edgar Jaeggi, MD, FRCPC Department of Paediatrics, Hospital for Sick Children, Toronto, ON, Canada

Paul F. Kantor, MBBCh, FRCPC Department of Paediatrics, Hospital for Sick Children, Toronto, ON, Canada

Andrea Kassner, PhD Department of Medical Imaging, Hospital for Sick Children, Toronto, ON, Canada

Paul Khairy, MD, PhD, FRCP (C) Department of Medicine, Montreal Heart Institute, Montreal, QC, Canada

Philip J. Kilner, MB, BS, MD, PhD CMR Unit, Royal Brompton Hospital, London, UK

Siho Kim Department of Pediatrics, Hospital for Sick Children, Toronto, ON, Canada

Kyong-Jin Lee, MD, FRCPC Department of Paediatrics, Hospital for Sick Children, Toronto, ON, Canada

Christopher K. Macgowan, PhD Department of Medical Biophysics & Medical Imaging, Hospital for Sick Children, Toronto, ON, Canada

Andrew S. Mackie, MD MAUDE Unit, McGill University Health Center, , Montreal, QC, Canada

Giuseppe Martucci MAUDE Unit, McGill University Health Center, , Montreal, QC, Canada

Brian W. McCrindle, MD, MPH Department of Paediatrics, Hospital for Sick Children, Toronto, ON, Canada

Sandra Merklinger, RN, MN, PhD Department of Surgery, Hospital for Sick Children, Toronto, ON, Canada

Michael E. Mitchell, MD Department of Cardiothoracic Surgery, Children's Hospital of Wisconsin, Milwaukee, WI, USA

William J McKenna, MD, DSc, FRCP Inherited Cardiovascular Disease Group, University College London, London, UK

Peter Oishi, MD Department of Pediatrics, University of California, San Francisco, CA, USA

Giovanni Quarta, MD Inherited Cardiovascular Disease Group, University College London, London, UK

Andrew N. Redington, MD, FRCP (UK & Canada) Department of Paediatrics, Hospital for Sick Children, Toronto, ON, Canada

Shubhayan Sanatani, BSc, MD British Columbia Children's Hospital, Vancouver, BC, Canada

Steven M. Schwartz, MD Department of Critical Care Medicine, Hospital for Sick Children, Toronto, ON, Canada

Srijita Sen-Chowdhry, MA, MBBS, MRCP, MD Inherited Cardiovascular Disease Group, University College London, London, UK

Norman H. Silverman, MD, DSc Department of Paediatric Cardiology, Stanford University, Stanford, CA, USA

Elizabeth A. Stephenson, MD, MSc Department of Paediatrics, Hospital for Sick Children, Toronto, ON, Canada

Duncan J. Stewart, MD Department of Medicine, Ottawa Health Research Institute, Ottawa, ON, Canada

Paul E. Szmitko, MD Department of Internal Medicine, St Michael's Hospital, University of Toronto, Toronto, ON, Canada

Dr. Glenn P. Taylor, MD, FRCPC Department of Paediatric Laboratory Medicine, Hospital for Sick Children, Toronto, ON, Canada

Judith Therrien, MD MAUDE Unit, McGill University Health Center, Montreal, QC, Canada

Maria Teresa Tomé Esteban, PhD Inherited Cardiovascular Disease Group, University College London, London, UK

James S. Tweddell, MD Department of Cardiothoracic Surgery, Children's Hospital of Wisconsin, Milwaukee, WI, USA

Glen S. Van Arsdell, MD Department of Surgery, Hospital for Sick Children, Toronto, ON, Canada

Michael F. Vogel, MD, PhD Department of Congenital Heart Disease, Deutsches Herzzentrum Kinderherzpraxis, München, Germany

Dr Manfred Vogt, MD Department of Congenital Heart Disease, Deutsches Herzzentrum Kinderherzpraxis, München, Germany

Mark A. Walsh, MD Department of Paediatrics, Hospital for Sick Children, Toronto, ON, Canada

Deirdre J. Ward, Mb, BCh, BAO, MRCPI Inherited Cardiovascular Disease Group, University College London, London, UK

Shi-Joon Yoo, MD, PhD Department of Diagnostic Imaging, Hospital for Sick Children, Toronto, ON, Canada

Tae Jin Yun, MD, PhD Department of Pediatric Cardiac Surgery, Asan Medical Centre, Seoul, Republic of Korea

Section I
Basic Topics

Origin and Identity of the Right Heart

1

Benoit G. Bruneau

Great beauty, great strength, and
great riches are really and truly of no
great use; a right heart exceeds all.
Benjamin Franklin

The heart is the first functional organ formed during embryogenesis, and its normal function is critical for survival of the mammalian embryo. Defects in embryonic patterning of the heart are the root cause of human congenital heart defects (CHDs) [1, 2]. The major building blocks of the heart are its two atria, two ventricles, and the outflow tract that gives rise to the great vessels. Each pair of chambers, the atria and the ventricles, is thought to arise initially from a shared primordial chamber that then separated into left and right components [3]. This division of the chambers has evolved to permit the adaptation of vertebrates to life on land by allowing distinct systemic and pulmonary circulations. Indeed, fish have a single atrium and a single ventricle, frogs have paired atria but a single ventricle, and mammals have the fully evolved four-chambered heart. Not surprisingly, many CHDs disrupt this division of left and right sides, thus leading to impaired heart function. Several CHDs affect very specifically the right heart, in such instances as hypoplastic right heart, tetralogy of Fallot, Ebstein's anomaly, and tricuspid atresia, to name a few.

Recent evidence has contradicted the view that the left and right ventricles come from a single embryonic chamber that separates into left and right components. In fact, the right heart arises from a completely distinct lineage of cells, termed the anterior, or second heart field [4–7]. This finding has caused a profound reevaluation of how the heart forms, and has provided some welcome insight into the etiology of human CHDs such as those found in

22q11 microdeletion (DiGeorge) syndrome, among others [8, 9].

1.1 The Second Heart Field and the Origins of the Right Heart

As with several important findings in biology, the discovery of the origins of the right heart was as a result of a combination of careful investigation and fortuitous observation. Three papers appeared simultaneously describing the embryonic origin of the outflow tract as separate from the rest of the heart [5–7]. The first two papers utilized classic embryology techniques such as gene expression analysis, lineage tracing, explant culture, and cell ablation to show that a population of cells that did not express heart markers, but was immediately adjacent to the developing heart, gave rise to a portion of the developing outflow tract [6, 7]. The third paper was based on the fortuitous expression in the outflow of the heart of a randomly integrated lacZ transgene, showing the typical blue staining that lacZ confers in the outflow tract of the embryonic heart [5]. Most intriguing was the finding that prior to outflow tract formation, the lacZ staining was observed in a discrete population of cells medial to and posterior from the field of heart cells that were thought to give rise to the entire heart. The transgene had integrated into a gene called *Fgf10*, and indeed *Fgf10* expression could be found in the outflow tract.

Two definitive experiments followed that showed that the outflow tract and right ventricle were added from this new field of heart cells, dubbed the "secondary heart field" or "anterior heart field". The first was again a fortuitous find: mice lacking a gene called *Isl1*, which was mostly studied in the context of neural development, had very malformed hearts [4]. Indeed, mice lacking *Isl1* had no outflow tract or right ventricle, and were missing most of their atria. Further study showed that *Isl1* is not expressed in the heart, instead it is expressed in a field of

B.G. Bruneau (✉)
Gladstone Institute of Cardiovascular Disease, Department of Pediatrics, University of California, 1650 Owens St, San Francisco, CA, 94158, USA
e-mail: bbruneau@gladstone.ucsf.edu

A.N. Redington et al. (eds.), *Congenital Diseases in the Right Heart*, DOI 10.1007/978-1-84800-378-1_1,
© Springer-Verlag London Limited 2009

embryonic cells that appeared to correspond to the newly defined anterior heart field [4]. Using a clever genetic labeling technique, Cai et al. were able to show that *Isl1*-expressing cells contribute to the heart by migrating into the developing heart, and that in the absence of *Isl1* these precursors were "stuck" and unable to provide new cells to the heart. This proved the existence of a second heart field. The finding of *Isl1*-expressing precursors indicated that the cells could be fated, or poised, to become cardiac myocytes. It was discovered subsequently that some of these precursor cells persist postnatally, thus providing a potential source of regenerating heart cells [10]. The second set of experiments that proved the existence of a second heart field was a series of lineage-tracing experiments performed using clonal cell analysis [11, 12]. These difficult experiments showed that while all heart cells are related from a very early time point during embryogenesis, several lineages arise during development, including a clear distinction between a lineage that contributes largely to the left ventricle (the first lineage) and one that contributes to the outflow tract, right ventricle, and atria (the second lineage). This was further confirmed by additional lineage tracing, combined with explant culture of mice expressing chamber-specific transgenes [13].

It should be noted that the right heart as defined from a ventricle-centric perspective is in fact the anterior pole of the heart. Thus, an initially anteroposterior arrangement becomes left–right. The atria are the exception to this as they arise from a common chamber that separates into left and right auricles early in development. Very few markers distinguish the left and right atria; the only evident marker of one side of the atria during development is *Pitx2*, which is expressed primarily in the left atrium [14]. Mice lacking *Pitx2* display right atrial isomerism, indicating a critical role for this gene in the left–right identity of the atrial chambers [15].

1.2 Genes That Control Formation of the Right Heart

Several genes have been identified that specifically control the formation of the right side of the heart, especially the right ventricle and outflow tract. These include *Hand2*, *mBop*, *Tbx20*, *Mef2c*, and *FoxH1*. Several of these, as detailed below, function in an interacting genetic cascade.

The first gene shown to affect a specific chamber of the heart was *Hand2*, formerly known as *dHand* [16]. A mouse lacking *Hand2* was shown to lack the right ventricle specifically and completely. *Hand2* is a transcription factor expressed largely in the right ventricle [17], and its major role in right ventricle formation is to promote survival of

the myocardial cells of this chamber [18]. These observations were of considerable importance in understanding the modular assembly of the developing heart. The related gene *Hand1* is also thought to be important for the formation the left ventricle, as it is expressed specifically in the left ventricle [17, 19, 20]. However, genetic deletion of *Hand1* has not shown that it confers the same chamber-specific properties that *Hand2* has [19, 21, 22]. Interestingly, expression of *Hand1* throughout the developing heart leads to the loss of the interventricular septum and of most distinctions between left and right ventricles, suggesting that the left-sided expression of *Hand1* helps set up the location of the interventricular septum [23]. More recently, a chromatin-modifying protein called mBop was shown to be expressed specifically in heart and muscle, and in mice lacking *mBop*, similar loss of the right ventricle was observed [24]. This could be attributed in part to the regulation of *Hand2* by *mBop*.

Mef2c, another transcription factor gene, was also found to be important for right ventricle formation [25]. The basis for the loss of the right ventricle in *Mef2c* knockout mice was not clear until detailed analysis of the expression and regulation of *Mef2c* was performed, which showed that as for *Hand2*, *Mef2c* was expressed at its highest level in the right ventricle, and prior to this it was expressed in the anterior heart field [26]. It is still not clear what gene expression program *Mef2c* regulates that is critical for right ventricular formation, but this may include mBop, as *Mef2c* is essential for the regulation of mBop in the right ventricle, acting directly on an enhancer element that directs expression to this chamber [27]. Yet another transcription factor gene, *FoxH1*, was found to be important for formation of the outflow tract and right ventricle [28], in large part via regulation of *Mef2c*.

The T-box transcription factor gene *Tbx20* has also been found to be a critical dose-sensitive factor in the morphogenesis of the right ventricle. Mice completely lacking *Tbx20* have a severely deformed heart [29–31], but those with only a partial reduction in *Tbx20* have specific defects in the morphogenesis of the right heart (Fig. 1.1). Specifically, partial reduction in *Tbx20* levels results in hypoplastic right ventricle, tricuspid atresia, and persistent truncus arteriosus [31]. The precise reason for the sensitivity of the right ventricle to decreased *Tbx20* dosage is not clear, but it is likely to be related to *Tbx20*'s preferential expression in the right ventricle primordia. The mechanisms underlying the defects observed are yet to be determined.

Finally, the *Gata4* transcription factor is critical for heart formation and differentiation, but its most pronounced role is in the formation of the right ventricle [32]. Again, *Hand2* expression was decreased in *Gata4* knockout mice, suggesting that *Gata4*-mediated regulation of *Hand2* could account for the defective right

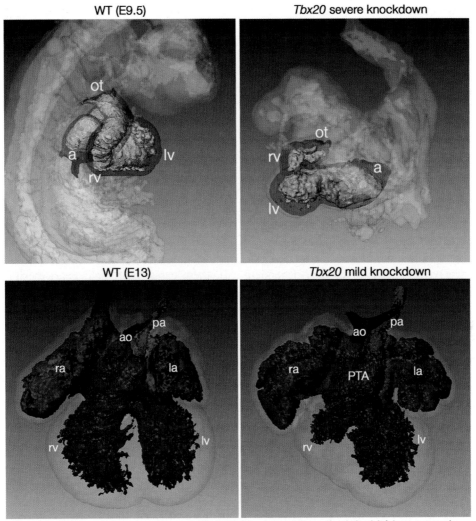

WT (E9.5)   Tbx20 severe knockdown

WT (E13)   Tbx20 mild knockdown

Top: Tbx20 knockdown embryo at E9.5 (right, viewed from the left side) has severely hypoplastic right ventricle, and absent outflow tract. Compare to WT embryo viewed from the right side (left). Embryo body is in translucent white, heart tissue in translucent red, and heart chamber fill in solid yellow.

Bottom: Tbx20 partial knockdown results in hypoplastic right ventricle (rv), and persistent truncus arteriosus (PTA; compare to crisscrossing outflow of WT).

a: atrium, ao: aorta, la: left atrium, lv: left ventricle, ot: outflow tract, pa: pulmonary artery, ra: right atrium, rv: right ventricle

Fig. 1.1 *Tbx20* regulates formation of the right heart. Top: *Tbx20* knockdown embryo at embryonic day (E) 9.5 (right, viewed from the left side) has severely hypoplastic right ventricle, and absent outflow tract. Compare to wild-type (WT) embryo viewed from the right side (left). Embryo body is translucent white, heart tissue in translucent red, and heart chamber filled in solid yellow. Bottom: *Tbx20* partial knockdown results at E13 in hypoplastic right ventricle (rv) and persistent truncus arteriosus (PTA; compare to crisscrossing outflow of WT) Adapted with permission from Ref. [42]

ventricle formation downstream of *Gata4*. It also interacts with *Isl1* to activate *Mef2c* in the primary heart field [33]. As *Gata4*, *Isl1*, and *Tbx20* also interact to activate gene expression [31, 33, 34], one can envisage a tight regulation of multiple genes that are critical for activation of gene expression in the right heart progenitors.

Thus, an intricate intersecting network of transcription factors is clearly essential for the formation of the right ventricle and outflow tract.

1.3 *Tbx1* and the Etiology of Outflow Tract Defects

An evidence that is immediately relevant to clinical pathogenesis came from the study of *Tbx1* in the second heart field. Advanced mouse engineering experiments had revealed that *Tbx1* was the most likely gene responsible for the cardiac and thymic defects in human 22q11.2 microdeletion syndrome, also known as DiGeorge syndrome [35–37]. Indeed, discrete mutations in *TBX1* were identified in patients with 22q11.2 microdeletion syndrome lacking any chromosomal microdeletion [38]. However, the expression pattern of *Tbx1* in embryogenesis did not directly correlate with the defects observed, especially the outflow tract anomalies seen in *Tbx1* mutant mice.

It was a lineage analysis similar to that performed with the *Isl1* gene that gave an answer. The *Tbx1*-dependent cell lineage contributes to the outflow tract and the distal portion of the right ventricle, and in mice lacking functional *Tbx1*, this contribution is abrogated [9]. Gain of function experiments in which the field of *Tbx1* was expanded led to an expansion of the outflow tract, showing that *Tbx1* is both necessary and sufficient for growth of the outflow tract [8].

How then does *Tbx1* regulate the expansion and differentiation of the outflow tract? It may be partly via the regulation of fibroblast growth factor (FGF) genes, including the *Fgf10* gene that initially led to the identification of the second heart field. Both *Fgf10* and the related gene *Fgf8* appear to be regulated by *Tbx1* in the mouse [8, 9]. In fact, a potential role for *Fgf8* had been already presumed from investigating mice that lacked the *Fgf8* gene, in which outflow tract and aortic arch defects strikingly similar to those in *Tbx1* mutant mice were observed [39–41]. Indeed, *Tbx1* and *Fgf8* genetically interact in the formation of the outflow tract [42].

1.4 The Right Ventricle Has a Distinct Gene Expression Program

Besides its obviously distinct morphology, the right ventricle expresses a genetic program that is distinct from that of the left ventricle. In this most comprehensive assay, microarray analysis of the main cardiac chambers was performed to gain a global view of chamber-specific gene expression [43, 44]. Not surprisingly, more differences were seen between atria and ventricles, but several genes were found to be differentially expressed between left and right ventricles. Interestingly, the response of the left and right ventricles to remodeling postinfarction was significantly different, for example, for such genes as the

Ca^{2+} ATPase gene *Serca2a* and other calcium-handling protein-encoding genes [43]. In another important example, the distribution of repolarizing ion channels is markedly distinct between the right and left ventricles [45–47], presumably imparting important features to the right ventricular myocardium.

Several studies aimed at delineating the cardiac-specific regulatory elements of several genes have uncovered surprising modularity in the control of chamber-specific gene expression. For example, the regulatory elements of the *Nkx2-5* gene, which is ubiquitously expressed throughout the heart at all stages of development, including adulthood [48], can be isolated as modular elements, several of which drive expression specifically in the right ventricle [49]. Modularity of enhancer function has also been shown with those controlling several cardiac contractile proteins. In these cases, both right heart-specific enhancers have been identified, as well as enhancers that are actively excluded from the right heart, indicating perhaps both positive and negative regulation of chamber-specific gene expression [13, 50–52]. Other enhancers that can confer specific right ventricular expression include the *mBop*, *Hand2*, and *Mef2c* enhancers, conforming with their predominant expression in this chamber [27, 28, 33, 53].

1.5 Conclusions

The distinct identities and morphologies of the chambers of the heart have their origins in the earliest glimpses of cardiac differentiation. The recent evidence obtained from embryological studies has provided a complete reevaluation of the origin of the right side of the heart, and this important set of findings will set the stage for our understanding of the basis of right-sided congenital heart defects, as well as the different adaptive physiology of the right heart. Further challenges await, but at least it is now for the heart, unlike in politics, clear where the right and left come from, and where they stand on the issues!

References

1. Bruneau, B. G. 2003. The developing heart and congenital heart defects: a make or break situation. Clin Genet **63**:252–61.
2. Clark, K. L., K. E. Yutzey, and D. W. Benson. 2005. Transcription Factors and Congenital Heart Defects. Annu Rev Physiol.
3. Srivastava, D., and E. N. Olson. 2000. A genetic blueprint for cardiac development. Nature **407**:221–6.
4. Cai, C. L., X. Liang, Y. Shi, P. H. Chu, S. L. Pfaff, J. Chen, and S. Evans. 2003. Isl1 Identifies a Cardiac Progenitor Population

that Proliferates Prior to Differentiation and Contributes a Majority of Cells to the Heart. Dev Cell **5**:877–89.

5. Kelly, R. G., N. A. Brown, and M. E. Buckingham. 2001. The arterial pole of the mouse heart forms from Fgf10-expressing cells in pharyngeal mesoderm. Developmental Cell **1**:435–440.

6. Mjaatvedt, C. H., T. Nakaoka, R. Moreno-Rodriguez, R. A. Norris, M. J. Kern, C. A. Eisenberg, D. Turner, and R. R. Markwald. 2001. The outflow tract of the heart is recruited from a novel heart-forming field. Dev Biol **238**:97–109.

7. Waldo, K. L., D. H. Kumiski, K. T. Wallis, H. A. Stadt, M. R. Hutson, D. H. Platt, and M. L. Kirby. 2001. Conotruncal myocardium arises from a secondary heart field. Development **128**:3179–3188.

8. Hu, T., H. Yamagishi, J. Maeda, J. McAnally, C. Yamagishi, and D. Srivastava. 2004. Tbx1 regulates fibroblast growth factors in the anterior heart field through a reinforcing autoregulatory loop involving forkhead transcription factors. Development **131**:5491–502.

9. Xu, H., M. Morishima, J. N. Wylie, R. J. Schwartz, B. G. Bruneau, E. A. Lindsay, and A. Baldini. 2004. Tbx1 has a dual role in the morphogenesis of the cardiac outflow tract. Development:3217–3227.

10. Laugwitz, K. L., A. Moretti, J. Lam, P. Gruber, Y. Chen, S. Woodard, L. Z. Lin, C. L. Cai, M. M. Lu, M. Reth, O. Platoshyn, J. X. Yuan, S. Evans, and K. R. Chien. 2005. Postnatal isl1+ cardioblasts enter fully differentiated cardiomyocyte lineages. Nature **433**:647–53.

11. Meilhac, S. M., M. Esner, R. G. Kelly, J. F. Nicolas, and M. E. Buckingham. 2004. The clonal origin of myocardial cells in different regions of the embryonic mouse heart. Dev Cell **6**:685–98.

12. Meilhac, S. M., R. G. Kelly, D. Rocancourt, S. Eloy-Trinquet, J. F. Nicolas, and M. E. Buckingham. 2003. A retrospective clonal analysis of the myocardium reveals two phases of clonal growth in the developing mouse heart. Development **130**:3877–89.

13. Zaffran, S., R. G. Kelly, S. M. Meilhac, M. E. Buckingham, and N. A. Brown. 2004. Right ventricular myocardium derives from the anterior heart field. Circ Res **95**:261–8.

14. Franco, D., M. Campione, R. Kelly, P. S. Zammit, M. Buckingham, W. H. Lamers, and A. F. Moorman. 2000. Multiple transcriptional domains, with distinct left and right components, in the atrial chambers of the developing heart. Circ Res **87**:984–91.

15. Franco, D., and M. Campione. 2003. The role of Pitx2 during cardiac development. Linking left-right signaling and congenital heart diseases. Trends Cardiovasc Med **13**: 157–63.

16. Srivastava, D., T. Thomas, Q. Lin, M. L. Kirby, D. Brown, and E. N. Olson. 1997. Regulation of cardiac mesodermal and neural crest development by the bHLH transcription factor, dHAND. Nat Genet **16**:154–60.

17. Thomas, T., H. Yamagishi, P. A. Overbeek, E. N. Olson, and D. Srivastava. 1998. The bHLH factors, dHAND and eHAND, specify pulmonary and systemic cardiac ventricles independent of left-right sidedness. Dev. Biol. **196**:228–236.

18. Yamagishi, H., C. Yamagishi, O. Nakagawa, R. P. Harvey, E. N. Olson, and D. Srivastava. 2001. The combinatorial activities of Nkx2.5 and dHAND are essential for cardiac ventricle formation. Dev Biol **239**:190–203, doi:10.1006.

19. Firulli, A. B., D. G. McFadden, Q. Lin, D. Srivastava, and E. N. Olson. 1998. Heart and extra-embryonic mesodermal defects in mouse embryos lacking the bHLH transcription factor Hand 1. Nat. Genet. **18**:266–270.

20. Riley, P. R., M. Gertenstein, K. Dawson, and J. C. Cross. 2000. Early exclusion of Hand1-deficient cells from distinct regions of the left ventricular myocardium in chimeric mouse embryos. Dev Biol **227**:156–168.

21. McFadden, D. G., A. C. Barbosa, J. A. Richardson, M. D. Schneider, D. Srivastava, and E. N. Olson. 2004. The Hand1 and Hand2 transcription factors regulate expansion of the embryonic cardiac ventricles in a gene dosage–dependent manner. Development.

22. Riley, P., L. Anson-Cartwright, and J. C. Cross. 1998. The Hand1 bHLH transcription factor is essential for placentation and cardiac morphogenesis. Nat. Genet. **18**:271–275.

23. Togi, K., T. Kawamoto, R. Yamauchi, Y. Yoshida, T. Kita, and M. Tanaka. 2004. Role of Hand1/eHAND in the dorsoventral patterning and interventricular septum formation in the embryonic heart. Mol Cell Biol **24**:4627–35.

24. Gottlieb, P. D., S. A. Pierce, R. J. Sims, H. Yamagishi, E. K. Weihe, J. V. Harriss, S. D. Maika, W. A. Kuziel, H. L. King, E. N. Olson, O. Nakagawa, and D. Srivastava. 2002. Bop encodes a muscle-restricted protein containing MYND and SET domains and is essential for cardiac differentiation and morphogenesis. Nat Genet **31**:25–32.

25. Lin, Q., J. Schwarz, C. Bucana, and E. N. Olson. 1997. Control of mouse cardiac morphogenesis and myogenesis by transcription factor MEF2C. Science **276**:1404–7.

26. Verzi, M. P., D. J. McCulley, S. De Val, E. Dodou, and B. L. Black. 2005. The right ventricle, outflow tract, and ventricular septum comprise a restricted expression domain within the secondary/anterior heart field. Dev Biol **in press**.

27. Phan, D., T. L. Rasmussen, O. Nakagawa, J. McAnally, P. D. Gottlieb, P. W. Tucker, J. A. Richardson, R. Bassel-Duby, and E. N. Olson. 2005. BOP, a regulator of right ventricular heart development, is a direct transcriptional target of MEF2C in the developing heart. Development **132**:2669–78.

28. von Both, I., C. Silvestri, T. Erdemir, H. Lickert, J. Walls, R. M. Henkelman, J. Rossant, R. P. Harvey, L. Attisano, and J. L. Wrana. 2004. Foxh1 is essential for development of the anterior heart field. Dev Cell **7**:331–345.

29. Cai, C. L., W. Zhou, L. Yang, L. Bu, Y. Qyang, X. Zhang, X. Li, M. G. Rosenfeld, J. Chen, and S. Evans. 2005. T-box genes coordinate regional rates of proliferation and regional specification during cardiogenesis. Development **132**:2475–87.

30. Stennard, F. A., M. W. Costa, D. Lai, C. Biben, M. B. Furtado, M. J. Solloway, D. J. McCulley, C. Leimena, J. I. Preis, S. L. Dunwoodie, D. E. Elliott, O. W. Prall, B. L. Black, D. Fatkin, and R. P. Harvey. 2005. Murine T-box transcription factor Tbx20 acts as a repressor during heart development, and is essential for adult heart integrity, function and adaptation. Development **132**:2451–62.

31. Takeuchi, J. K., M. Mileikovskaia, K. Koshiba-Takeuchi, A. B. Heidt, A. D. Mori, E. P. Arruda, M. Gertsenstein, R. Georges, L. Davidson, R. Mo, C. C. Hui, R. M. Henkelman, M. Nemer, B. L. Black, A. Nagy, and B. G. Bruneau. 2005. Tbx20 dose-dependently regulates transcription factor networks required for mouse heart and motoneuron development. Development **132**:2463–74.

32. Zeisberg, E. M., Q. Ma, A. L. Juraszek, K. Moses, R. J. Schwartz, S. Izumo, and W. T. Pu. 2005. Morphogenesis of the right ventricle requires myocardial expression of Gata 4. J Clin Invest **115**:1522–31.

33. Dodou, E., M. P. Verzi, J. P. Anderson, S. M. Xu, and B. L. Black. 2004. Mef2c is a direct transcriptional target of ISL1 and GATA factors in the anterior heart field during mouse embryonic development. Development **131**:3931–42.

34. Stennard, F. A., M. W. Costa, D. A. Elliott, S. Rankin, S. J. Haast, D. Lai, L. P. McDonald, K. Niederreither, P. Dolle, B. G. Bruneau, A. M. Zorn, and R. P. Harvey. 2003. Cardiac T-box factor Tbx20 directly interacts with Nkx2-5, GATA4, and GATA5 in regulation of gene expression in the developing heart. Dev Biol **262**:206–24.

35. Jerome, L. A., and V. E. Papaioannou. 2001. Di George syndrome phenotype in mice mutant for the T-box gene, *Tbx1*. Nat Genet **27**:286–291.

36. Lindsay, E. A., F. Vitelli, H. Su, M. Morishima, T. Huynh, T. Pramparo, V. Jurecic, G. Ogunrinu, H. F. Sutherland, P. J. Scambler, A. Bradley, and A. Baldini. 2001. *Tbx1* haploinsufficiency in the DiGeorge syndrome region causes aortic arch defects in mice. Nature **410**:97–101.

37. Merscher, S., B. Funke, J. A. Epstein, J. Heyer, A. Puech, M. M. Lu, R. J. Xavier, M. B. Demay, R. G. Russell, S. Factor, K. Tokooya, B. St. Jore, M. Lopez, R. K. Pandita, M. Lia, D. Carrion, H. Xu, H. Schorle, J. B. Kobler, P. J. Scambler, A. Wynshaw-Boris, A. I. Skoultchi, B. E. Morrow, and R. Kucherlapati. 2001. *TBX1* is responsible for cardiovascular defects in velo-cardio-facial/DiGeorge syndrome. Cell **104**:619–629.

38. Yagi, H., Y. Furutani, H. Hamada, T. Sasaki, S. Asakawa, S. Minoshima, F. Ichida, K. Joo, M. Kimura, S. Imamura, N. Kamatani, K. Momma, A. Takao, M. Nakazawa, N. Shimizu, and R. Matsuoka. 2003. Role of TBX1 in human del22q11.2 syndrome. Lancet **362**:1366–73.

39. Abu-Issa, R., G. Smyth, I. Smoak, K. Yamamura, and E. N. Meyers. 2002. Fgf8 is required for pharyngeal arch and cardiovascular development in the mouse. Development **129**:4613–25.

40. Frank, D. U., L. K. Fotheringham, J. A. Brewer, L. J. Muglia, M. Tristani-Firouzi, M. R. Capecchi, and A. M. Moon. 2002. An Fgf8 mouse mutant phenocopies human 22q11 deletion syndrome. Development **129**:4591–603.

41. Park, E. J., L. A. Ogden, A. Talbot, S. Evans, C. L. Cai, B. L. Black, D. U. Frank, and A. M. Moon. 2006. Required, tissue-specific roles for Fgf8 in outflow tract formation and remodeling. Development **133**:2419–33.

42. Vitelli, F., I. Taddei, M. Morishima, E. N. Meyers, E. A. Lindsay, and A. Baldini. 2002. A genetic link between Tbx1 and fibroblast growth factor signaling. Development **129**:4605–11.

43. Chugh, S. S., S. Whitesel, M. Turner, C. T. Roberts, Jr., and S. R. Nagalla. 2003. Genetic basis for chamber-specific ventricular phenotypes in the rat infarct model. Cardiovasc Res **57**:477–85.

44. Tabibiazar, R., R. A. Wagner, A. Liao, and T. Quertermous. 2003. Transcriptional profiling of the heart reveals chamber-specific gene expression patterns. Circ Res **93**:1193–201.

45. Brunet, S., F. Aimond, W. Guo, H. Li, J. Eldstrom, D. Fedida, K. A. Yamada, and J. M. Nerbonne. 2004. Heterogeneous Expression of Repolarizing, Voltage-Gated K+ Currents in Adult Mouse Ventricles. J Physiol **559**:103–120.

46. Nerbonne, J. M., and W. Guo. 2002. Heterogeneous expression of voltage-gated potassium channels in the heart: roles in normal excitation and arrhythmias. J Cardiovasc Electrophysiol **13**:406–9.

47. Oudit, G. Y., Z. Kassiri, R. Sah, R. J. Ramirez, C. Zobel, and P. H. Backx. 2001. The molecular physiology of the cardiac transient outward potassium current (I(to)) in normal and diseased myocardium. J Mol Cell Cardiol **33**:851–72.

48. Lints, T. J., L. M. Parsons, L. Hartley, I. Lyons, and R. P. Harvey. 1993. Nkx-2.5: a novel murine homeobox gene expressed in early heart progenitor cells and their myogenic descendants. Development **119**:419–31.

49. Schwartz, R. J., and E. N. Olson. 1999. Building the heart piece by piece: modularity of cis-elements regulating Nkx2-5 transcription. Development **126**:4187–92.

50. Franco, D., R. Kelly, W. H. Lamers, M. Buckingham, and A. F. Moorman. 1997. Regionalized transcriptional domains of myosin light chain 3f transgenes in the embryonic mouse heart: morphogenetic implications. Dev Biol **188**:17–33.

51. Kelly, R., S. Alonso, S. Tajbakhsh, G. Cossu, and M. Buckingham. 1995. Myosin light chain 3F regulatory sequences confer regionalized cardiac and skeletal muscle expression in transgenic mice. J Cell Biol **129**:383–96.

52. Kelly, R. G., P. S. Zammit, V. Mouly, G. Butler-Browne, and M. E. Buckingham. 1998. Dynamic left/right regionalisation of endogenous myosin light chain 3F transcripts in the developing mouse heart. J Mol Cell Cardiol **30**:1067–81.

53. McFadden, D. G., J. Charite, J. A. Richardson, D. Srivastava, A. B. Firulli, and E. N. Olson. 2000. A GATA-dependent right ventricular enhancer controls dHAND transcription in the developing heart. Development **127**:5331–41.

How Much of the Right Heart Belongs to the Left?

Andrew C. Cook and Robert H. Anderson

2.1 Introduction

In the preceding chapter, we have seen how from the outset of development the right heart has very separate origins from the left. We have learned how the cells from the secondary heart field are responsible for the formation of the right ventricle and outflow tract, and how they are added to the initial linear heart tube slightly later in development compared to the part that gives rise to the left ventricle [1–5]. We now know that the apical components of the ventricles balloon from the linear heart tube, which is made up of primary myocardium, and that the molecular characteristics of the working myocardium of the right and left ventricles thus formed differ markedly from the primary variant [6]. In this chapter, we explore how these embryonic features are carried over into the structure of the heart subsequent to the completion of septation. In an effort to describe just how much, in morphological terms, of the right heart belongs to the left, we begin by emphasizing the current gaps in our understanding of the mechanics of early myocardial organization. We then define our approach to analysis of the ventricular component of the heart. We put this into the historical perspective of myocardial structure and contrast this traditional approach, based on centuries of investigation, and which is in keeping with our own observations, with recent spurious suggestions that the myocardium making up the ventricular mass can be *unwrapped* in the form of a unique band, which takes its origin in the fashion of skeletal muscle from the pulmonary trunk, and inserts at the aorta [7]. In terms of this latter concept, we show that, despite its apparent attraction to those seeking to explain the helical movements of the ventricular mass during contraction and relaxation, it is fatally flawed due to the total lack of supporting scientific evidence.

2.2 Organization of the Ventricular Myocardium

Recent work on the molecular biology of the embryonic myocardium has provided new insights into the origins of the populations of cells that give rise to the walls of the morphologically right and left ventricles. There is now little doubt that a second migration of cells from the initial heart-forming field is crucial for the formation of the morphologically right ventricle, the outflow tract, and the arterial trunks [1–5]. Marking experiments [5], as well as immunohistochemical labeling [1–4], have shown that this population of cells is added to the initial linear heart tube, the latter primordium giving rise almost exclusively to the morphologically left ventricle (Fig. 2.1). In mouse mutants, subsequent to knock-out of the gene *d-hand*, there is a virtual absence of the morphologically right ventricle [8, 9]. Similarly, experiments in the chick, in which parts of the secondary heart-forming field are ablated, produce abnormalities of the right heart, including tetralogy of Fallot [10]. The studies of Moorman and colleagues showed how expansion from the myocardium forming the linear heart tube, so-called primary myocardium, was responsible for formation of the atrial appendages and the apical components of the ventricles [6]. They also showed that the apical part of the left ventricle ballooned from the initial linear heart tube, while the apical part of the right ventricle ballooned from the part of the tube derived from the second migration from the heart-forming fields (Fig. 2.2). This *ballooning* model provides strong evidence to support the concept that, from the outset, the ventricles are modifications of a primitive blood vessel. The evidence at molecular level to support this notion is equally convincing, with the chamber myocardium of both ventricles having a distinctive phenotype when compared with the characteristics of the primary myocardium [6].

All of these experiments, however, have been performed at the very early stages of development, well before the ventricular myocardium becomes organized

A.C. Cook (✉)
Department of Cardiac Services, Great Ormond Street Hospital for Children, London, UK

A.N. Redington et al. (eds.), *Congenital Diseases in the Right Heart*, DOI 10.1007/978-1-84800-378-1_2,

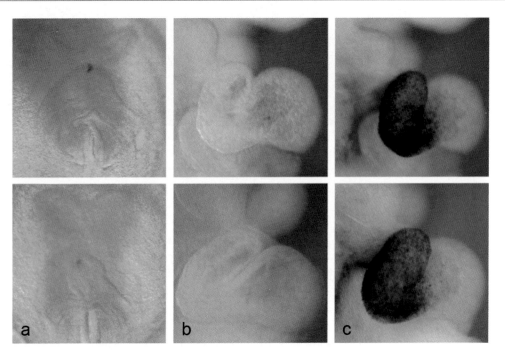

Fig. 2.1 Two sets of mouse embryos (upper and lower panels) have been marked either with the label DiI (panels a and b) or stained to show expression of fibroblast growth factor 8 (*fgf8*). In the left hand panel (a), the DiI (red dot) marks the cranial border of the forming heart crescent. The middle panel shows the same two embryos following further culture. In both, the DiI label is now located between the developing left (LV) and right ventricles (RV). This demonstrates that the right ventricle has been added onto the part of the heart derived initially from the myocardial crescent. The content that has been added is highlighted by the beta-galactosidase expression in panel c Figure courtesy: Prof Nigel Brown, St. George's Medical School, London, UK, who conducted the experiments

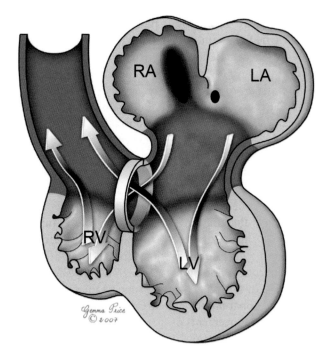

Fig. 2.2 The ballooning model of development of the atrial (RA, LA) and ventricular (RV, LV) chambers as promulgated by Moorman and his colleagues, with the artwork modified with their permission from their initial illustrations. The *arrows* show the direction of flow of blood. The artwork illustrates the expansion of the chamber myocardium (*yellow*) from the primary myocardium of the initial heart tube (coloured in *grey*). Note that it is the atrial appendages, and the apical components of the ventricles, that are the components produced by ballooning
Modified and reproduced with kind permission of Prof Anton Moorman, Academic Medical Centre, Amsterdam, The Netherlands

into the three-dimensional network of aggregated myocytes set in their supporting fibrous matrix typical of the postnatal heart. While the structure of the ventricular walls has been extensively studied since the time of Senac in the eighteenth century, very little is known about the timing and mechanism for the transformation from early stages, with primarily trabeculated myocardial walls, to the definitive situation in which the large component of the wall is made up of compacted myocardium. Unraveling the mechanics of these changes will not only provide answers to the understanding of basic myocardial organization in the normal heart, but also to the processes underscoring ventricular noncompaction, particularly the association between noncompaction and various forms of congenital cardiac disease. What little evidence that exists currently suggests that, in the frame of developmental evolution, myocardial organization is a relatively late event, and one which occurs subsequent to the completion of cardiac septation, in other words, in the period following the end of the eighth week of fetal gestation. There have been hardly any studies of the three-dimensional changes occurring during the early organization of the fetal ventricular myocardium, the notable exception being the careful study of Jouk and his colleagues [11]. In their most recent study, these authors confirm that, in the developing human heart, there is no evidence to support the notion of a *unique myocardial band*, although they have hesitated to extrapolate concerning the structure of the postnatal heart. With regard to the developing heart, additional information can

be gleaned indirectly from studies of the organization of the fetal myocardium at a cellular level, particularly in terms of the organization of intercellular contacts. It is intuitive to suggest that any aggregated collections of myocytes cannot achieve an axial orientation, be it tangential or radial, until the myocytes themselves have developed their own specific axes. The axis of an individual myocyte is determined by the presence of intercalated discs at its *poles*, which themselves depend on the formation and organization of tight junctions between adjacent myocytes. Several investigators have now shown that the development of intercalated discs is progressive throughout fetal development. Initially, tight junctions and gap junctions are both arranged in circumferential manner around each myocyte [12, 13]. Work from our laboratory using human fetal myocardium shows that, even at 14 weeks of gestation, tight junctions, as demonstrated using antibodies for cadherins, are arranged around the periphery of each myocyte (Fig. 2.3a). It is not possible at this early stage of development, therefore, to discern the orientation of specific myocytes. Only between 14 and 20 weeks of gestation do we see the gradual coalescence of the tight junctions, as marked by pan-cadherin, at the poles of the myocytes, and the subsequent appearance of stepped, and then more linear, intercalated discs (Fig. 2.3b–d). To our mind, it is only from this time of development that the three-dimensional organization of the myocardium can be ascertained. During the same period, our gross observations show that the myocardial walls undergo the process of compaction. Over this period, the structure of the walls of both ventricles changes from an

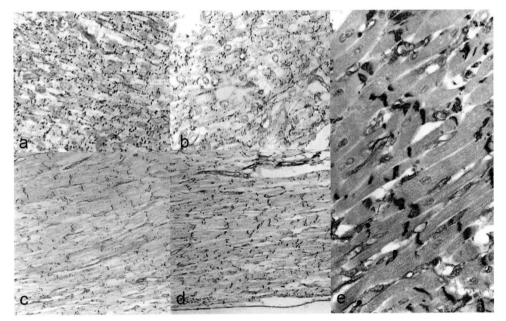

Fig. 2.3 Sections from human fetuses ranging in gestation from 14(a), 16(b), 18(c), 20(d), 24(e) weeks gestation compared to a heart seen on the first day of postnatal life (e).They are stained to show the tight junctions between the maturing myocytes using antibodies to Cadherin, and show the progressive development of the intercalated discs, and therefore polarity of the myocytes. Initially, the junctions are located around the entire periphery of the cells. It is only beyond 24 weeks that these line up at the ends of the cells. Only once the polarity of the myocytes has been achieved can the 'grain' of the myocardium can be determined

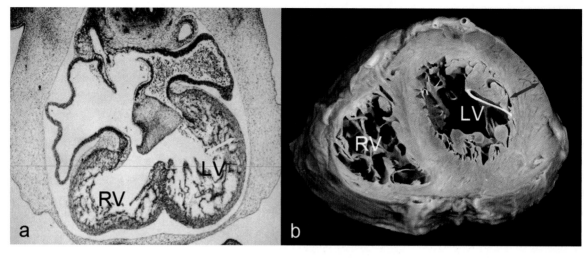

Fig. 2.4 Changes in proportion of the trabecular as opposed to compact myocardium in the walls of the ventricles of the early human embryo (panel a) and the adult heart. In the embryo (a), the trabeculations within the left ventricle (LV) are thick (*yellow arrow*), whereas the extent of the wall formed by compact myocardial is minimal. The reverse is true of the adult heart, in which most the trabecular layer in the left ventricle has been lost, with the compact myocardium predominating (blue arrow). RV – right ventricle

arrangement in which the greater part of the mural thickness is made up of a trabecular network, with deep recesses extending from endocardium close to the epicardium (Fig. 2.4a) into the more typical postnatal pattern, with discrete compact and noncompact layers, the compact layer then predominating (Fig. 2.4b). At this stage, we are unable to state whether the extensive columns of cells that initially made up the initial trabecular layer themselves coalesced to form the compacted part of the wall, or whether the lace-like layer effectively disappeared, perhaps by the process of apoptosis. Further analysis of the changes is required at a gross level, not only to aid our understanding of normal myocardial organization, but also to permit us to understand the pathological changes seen in individuals with noncompaction. There is now evidence that, even among populations of healthy individuals, there is variation in the normal degree of myocardial compaction [14]. Rather than being a distinct pathology, this suggests that those with noncompaction, as defined by current echocardiographic criterions, form the tail of a normal distribution of compaction found among the general population. If this is the case, it will be crucial to understand whether there is a cut-off in terms of proportions of trabecular and compacted layers, at which a normal distributional variant becomes a distinct pathological entity.

2.3 Analysis of the Ventricular Segment of the Heart

Leaving these unresolved questions aside, we can now provide reasonable recommendations as how best to approach the structure of the ventricular mass in the fully

formed heart, and how to analyze this part when the heart is congenitally malformed. We can then ask how this knowledge of the basic structure of the ventricles permits us to determine how much of the morphologically right ventricle belongs to the left? Examination of congenitally malformed hearts shows that the most consistent means of describing normal and abnormal ventricles is to take note of their three functional components, namely, the inlet, the apical trabecular portion, and the outlet (Figs. 2.5 and 2.6). While both the morphologically right and left ventricles contain all of these three components in the normal situation, there are major differences in the relationship of the components within the two ventricles. These differences are relevant to the overall organization of the myocardium. On both the right and left sides, the ventricular mass extends from the atrioventricular to the ventriculoarterial junctions (Figs. 2.5 and 2.6). The junctions themselves are discrete and obvious anatomic entities, albeit that the anatomic ventriculoarterial junctions are crossed by the semilunar attachments of the leaflets of the arterial valves, with these latter structures marking the hemodynamic junctions. On the left side of the heart, the valves guarding the ventricular inlet and outlet components are positioned directly adjacent to one another, with fibrous continuity present between their leaflets, thus permitting the two valves to fit within the circular profile of the left ventricle (Fig. 2.7). Within the right ventricle, the situation is markedly different. The atrioventricular and ventriculoarterial junctions are well separated from one another by the muscular supraventricular crest, being positioned at either end of a banana-shaped right ventricular cavity. Hence, the pulmonary valve lacks any fibrous continuity with any of the other three cardiac valves, being elevated from the

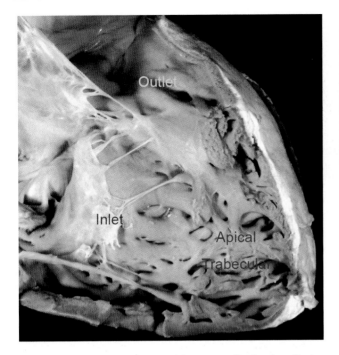

Fig. 2.5 The normal right ventricle can readily be described as possessing inlet, apical trabecular, and outlet components. Note that the supraventricular crest, incorporating the subpulmonary infundibulum, interposes between the attachments of the leaflets of the valves guarding the inlet and outlet components

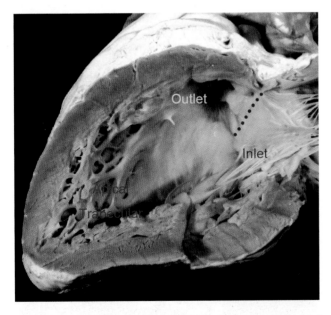

Fig. 2.6 As with the right ventricle (Fig. 2.5), the normal left ventricle can also be described in terms of its inlet, apical trabecular, and outlet components. In the left ventricle, however, there is fibrous continuity in the ventricular roof between the leaflets of the arterial and atrioventricular valves (*dashed red line*)

ventricular base by the free-standing muscular sleeve which forms the subpulmonary infundibulum (Fig. 2.7). Indeed, it is this extension to the right ventricular cavity, provided by the free-standing subpulmonary infundibulum which

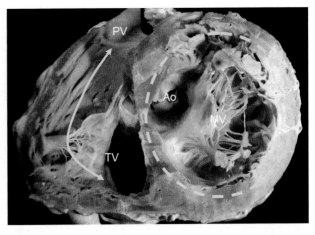

Fig. 2.7 A short axis section of the ventricular mass demonstrates well the difference in shape between the right and left sides of the heart, and the relationships between inlet and outlet ventricular components. The left ventricle has a circular profile, with the ventricular septum forming the anterior border. Contained within this profile are both the aortic (Ao) and mitral valves (MV). In contrast, the right heart curves around the left ventricle, with the inlet (TV) and outlet (PV) separated by the musculature of the supraventricular crest and subpulmonary infundibulum

allows the pulmonary valve to sit to the left side of the aortic root when the heart is viewed in attitudinally appropriate position. This free-standing nature of the subpulmonary infundibulum also shows that the outlet component of the right ventricle has no relationship to the left ventricle, in keeping with its initial embryonic origins (Fig. 2.8). Proof of its individuality is provided by the Ross procedure, when the surgeon excises the entire infundibulum and the pulmonary valve, cutting obliquely across its base in order to avoid the septal-perforating arteries, but not entering the left ventricle in so doing. The myocytes forming the

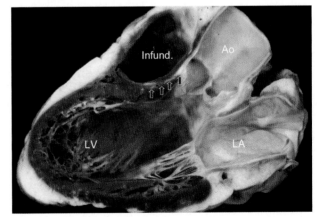

Fig. 2.8 A parasternal long axis section of an adult heart shows how the outflow tract of the right ventricle overlies the aortic (Ao) root. A fibrofatty tissue plane (*arrows*), containing the septal-perforating arteries, can be seen separating the aortic root and septum from the free-standing muscular subpulmonary infundibulum (infund). LV – left ventricle; LA – left atrium

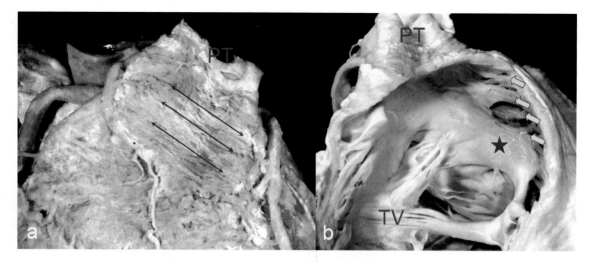

Fig. 2.9 The dissection shows the orientation of the aggregated myocytes within the right ventricular outflow tract. The myocytes within this region of the heart are aggregated together in oblique fashion, and encircle the infundibulum (*arrows*) on the epicardial surface (a). Internally (b), the outflow is lined by a series of muscular bundles, including the septo-parietal trabeculations (*arrows*) and the septomarginal trabeculation (*star*). PT – pulmonary trunk; TV – tricuspid valve

infundibular sleeve are aggregated primarily in circumferential fashion, with their long axes encircling the outflow tract (Fig. 2.9). At the base of the infundibulum, there are inner, longitudinally aligned myocytes, these forming the series of septoparietal trabeculations that branch laterally from the prominent septomarginal trabeculation, or septal band (Fig. 2.9).

It is only the inlet and apical trabecular portions of the right ventricle, therefore, which are directly related to their left-sided counterparts. It is then only the apical trabecular components of the two ventricles that are arranged in directly apposing manner, such that, for instance, a defect within the apical component of the right ventricle passes into the apical component of the left. This is not the case with the inlet component of the right ventricle. In the normal heart, due to the deeply wedged location of the subaortic outflow tract, the right ventricular inlet is adjacent to the outlet, rather than the inlet, of the left ventricle. A defect opening from the inlet of the right ventricle looks directly into the outlet of the left ventricle (Fig. 2.10). This relationship of the ventricular components means that the part of the ventricular septum related to the inlet of the right ventricle is, for its larger part, an inlet–outlet septum. Indeed, there is very little true *inlet septum* in the normally constructed heart.

In the normally constructed heart, as well seen in short axis (Fig. 2.7), the greater part of the muscular septum is an integral part of the left, rather than the right, ventricle. Indeed, as shown in the next section, the majority of the myocytes making up the septum are aligned in circular fashion around the left ventricle. Of late, questions have been raised concerning a *line* seen by echocardiographers

within the ventricular septum. It has been suggested that this represents the *plane of cleavage* between the right and left sides of the septum [15]. It is certainly the case that such a plane of cleavage can be found at the ventricular base, with the branches of the septal-perforating arteries passing down through this plane between the back of the subpulmonary infundibulum and the aortic root

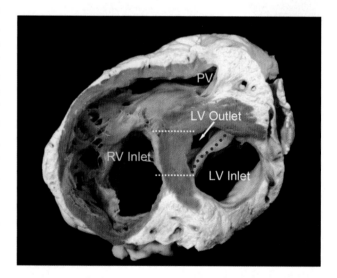

Fig. 2.10 The image shows the relationship between the inlet component of the right ventricle (**RV**) and the outlet of the left ventricle (**LV**). A short axis section has been taken across an adult heart, near its base, to show how the inlet of the right ventricle, guarded by the septal leaflet of the tricuspid valve, is directly opposite the outlet of the left ventricle (*dotted lines on septum*). This relationship exists because of the wedged location of the outlet of the left ventricle between the left side of the ventricular septum and the aortic leaflet of the mitral valve (*dashed red line*). PV – pulmonary valve

(Fig. 2.8). When assessed in the long axis planes, none-theless, the plane is also seen to be positioned so as to place the larger part of the septum with the left ventricle, with only a minor part of its thickness having a right ventricular identity. It remains to be established, therefore, whether it is this plane of cleavage providing the entrance for the septal-perforating arteries (Fig. 2.8) that also represents the *line* identified by echocardiographers.

That the muscular ventricular septum *belongs* primarily to the left ventricle is also supported by its structure when the heart is congenitally malformed. In the setting of hypoplasia of the left ventricle, the size of the left ventricular cavity has a marked influence on the support provided for the tension apparatus of the tricuspid valve (Fig. 2.11). In hypoplasia of the right ventricle, in contrast, the thickened septum seen when the apical and outlet components are obliterated by mural hypertrophy protrudes into the outlet of the left ventricle, showing again the importance of the relationship of the inlet of the right to the outlet of the left ventricle. And when the inlet of the right ventricle is totally absent, as in univentricular connection to a dominant left ventricle, the incomplete right ventricle is positioned either to the right or the left, but on the anterosuperior shoulders of the dominant left ventricle (Fig. 2.12).

2.4 The Myocardium as a Three-Dimensional Network

The importance of providing a correct description for the basic anatomic plan of the ventricular mass becomes more apparent when we then examine closely the arrangement of the myocytes that are aggregated within the ventricular mass. It has long been known that, at a histologic level, and after the end of the first trimester, myocytes possess a long axis, with intercalated discs at their poles (Fig. 2.4), enabling them to join together in chains.

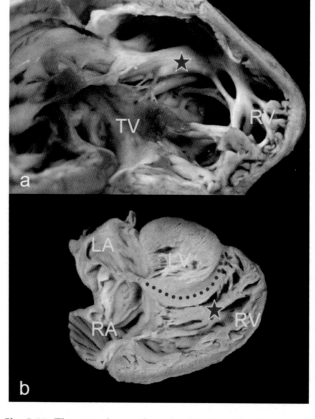

Fig. 2.11 These two hearts show the close interplay between the right and left ventricles (RV, LV), demonstrating the changes in the conformation of the right ventricle and its trabeculations that result from deformation of the left ventricle due to hypoplastic left heart with aortic atresia and patent mitral valve and intact ventricular septum. In both panels, the septomarginal trabeculation (*starred*) is not attached to the right side of the ventricular septum, as it usually is in the normal heart, but has become a free-standing structure within the right ventricle. In the lower panel (b), the ventricular septum (*red dashed line*) bows to the left, and encroaches on the inlet of the right ventricle. TV – tricuspid valve; RA – right atrium; LA – left atrium

Fig. 2.12 The relationship of a hypoplastic and incomplete right ventricle to the dominant left ventricle when there is double inlet left ventricle. The incomplete right ventricle (MRV) can be located either to the left (*panel a*), or right (panel b) of the dominant left ventricle (*dom LV*), but is always situated anterosuperiorly with respect to the ventricular septum, the ventricular septum itself interposing between the apical trabecular parts of the ventricles

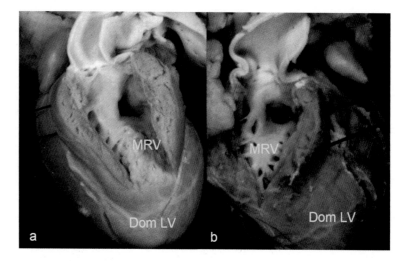

Each myocyte also possesses side branches, which form side-to-side connections with their neighbors, the overall arrangement forming a three-dimensional meshwork supported by a fibrous matrix. It is this arrangement that allows for the coordinated conduction of the cardiac impulse, and also for contraction of the myocardium. Therefore, to explain the thickening of the ventricular walls occurring during ventricular systole, it is best to consider the myocytes to be arranged so that they can slip among each other within the mesh. This is because the myocytes thicken by no more that 5% as they shorten, whereas the ventricular walls thicken by at least 40% during systole [16]. This rearrangement of the myocytes within the thickness of the ventricular wall is made possible because of the organization of the matrix of connective tissue. This is arranged as epimysial, perimysial, and endomysial networks (Fig. 2.13). Although the perimysial layers surround individual groups of myocytes, the arrangement is not sufficiently uniform to permit the aggregates to be described as *fibers*, nor is the perimysial component of the fibrous matrix arranged in such a fashion as to permit discrete layers, or sheets, of myocytes to be recognized within the thickness of the ventricular walls. Instead, the matrix provides an elastic scaffold that supports the intermingling myocytes, permitting their probable realignment across the ventricular wall during the process of systolic thickening. Despite this lack of fascial sheaths traversing the ventricular walls in radial direction, and the known absence of discrete muscular bands within the ventricular mass, it has long been recognized that a prevailing *grain* can be discerned within the various depths of the walls. The orientation of this grain varies markedly relative to the equatorial plane of the atrioventricular junctions, depending on the depth within the walls (Fig. 2.14). Already by the middle of the nineteenth century, this change in grain had been illustrated by Pettigrew [17], although his illustrations do give the marked, albeit unjustified, impression of discrete layers within the wall (Fig. 2.15). He summarized at the beginning of the twentieth century that such layers were no more than artifacts of dissection, stating that "unlike the generality of voluntary muscles, the fibres of the ventricles, as a rule, have neither origin nor insertion, that is, they are continuous alike at the apex of the ventricles and at the base" [17]. During the course of the twentieth century, many others showed that it was possible to dissect the ventricular mass by a process of progressive peeling, thus revealing the orientation of the long axes of the aggregated myocytes. In two important reviews, first Lev and Simkins [18], and then Grant [19], pointed to the essential artifactual nature of such dissections, which of necessity are destructive, parts of the wall having to be removed to reveal the deeper constituents.

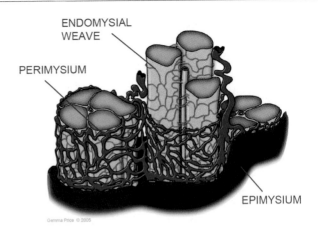

Fig. 2.13 The fibrous matrix supporting the ventricular myocytes in the normal heart differs markedly from the fibrous sheaths that demarcate different skeletal muscles. In the heart, the fibrous matrix takes the form of a three-dimensional supporting mesh that can be described on the basis of an endomysial weave surrounding individual myocytes, and joining them via struts. Bundles of myocytes are then encased in markedly anisotropic fashion by the perimysial weave, with the entire ventricular walls encased in the thicker epimysial layers, which form the endocardium and the epicardium

Due to the subjective nature of such dissections, and the difficulty in providing accurate three-dimensional reconstruction of the histologic arrangement, it is hardly surprising that current interpretations of the three-dimensional pattern of the myocytes continue to vary markedly. Some have suggested that the ventricular walls are uniformly compartmentalized by *laminar sheets*, which extend in a radial fashion from epicardium to endocardium [20]. This is despite the fact that even the most cursory examination of a full-thickness section of ventricular myocardium shows the absence of any such uniform fibrous structures (Fig. 2.16). Jouk and his colleagues [11] have described a system of *nested warped pretzels* within the cone of left ventricular myocardium, albeit there is great difficulty in understanding their concept. Throughout the latter part of the twentieth century, however, an even more radical suggestion was made, namely, that the ventricular mass could be unwrapped in the form of a *unique myocardial band* [7]. This concept has now been enthusiastically championed by a group of surgeons, who not only propose that surgical maneuvers should be designed according to the concept, but also advance new theories of embryogenesis on the basis of the purported anatomic findings [21–23]. These surgeons also choose to ignore totally the corpus of existing anatomic evidence, not least that the septum *belongs* to the left ventricle, arguing, again in the total lack of evidence, that the septum is the *lion of the right ventricle*.

The caveats involved in demonstrating the structure of the ventricular mass, therefore, are worthy of further

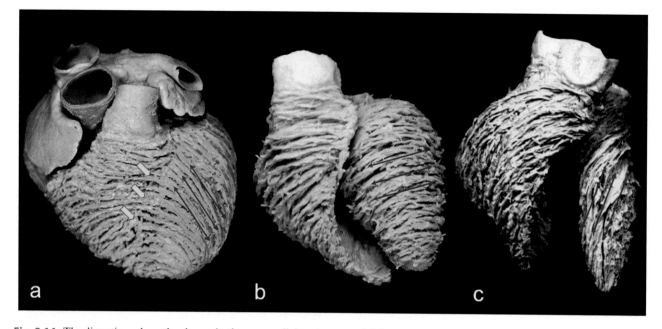

Fig. 2.14 The dissections show the change in the myocardial *grain*, representing the overall orientation of the aggregated myocytes, in the superficial, middle, and deep layers of the ventricular walls. Within the left ventricle, there is a prominent middle layer (*panel b*), which is circumferential, and represents the *triebwerkzeug* described by Krehl. This layer is absent or minimal within the normal right ventricle. The superficial (epicardial, *panel a*) and deep (endocardial, *panel c*) layers run obliquely and at right angles to each other. Note that there is continuity between the superficial fibres of the right and left heart (*yellow arrows*). The nature of the overlapping fibers, as well as other intruding fibers, is ignored completely when the heart is unwrapped using the method of Torrent-Guasp
Dissections prepared by Prof. Damian Sanchez-Quintana, University of Badajoz, Spain, and reproduced with his permission

emphasis. As pointed out by Lev and Simkins [18], and Grant [19], the patterns produced by dissection are very much at the whim of the prosector. It is important, therefore, to validate any dissections with histological studies, and equally important to reconstruct the histological findings themselves so as to provide an accurate three-dimensional model of ventricular mural architecture. Previous investigations made by both dissection and histological studies have shown that within the walls of the left ventricle the orientation of the long axis of the

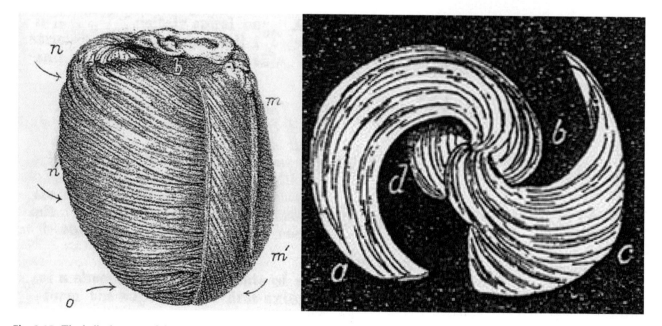

Fig. 2.15 The helical nature of the myocardial grain has long been recognized, albeit often misinterpreted. These two etchings show early descriptions of myocardial grain found within the left heart as produced by Pettigrew in the nineteenth century

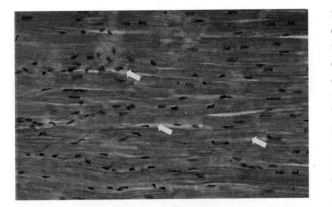

Fig. 2.16 The section of myocardium from the ventricular wall of a porcine heart shows that, while there are fibrous strands between collections of adjacent myocytes (*arrows*), these do exist as a laminar sheets. There is marked anisotropy in the arrangement of these thickened perimysial strands
Original section prepared by Professor Paul Lunkenheimer, University of Munster, Germany, and modified with his permission

aggregated myocytes relative to the equatorial plane, known as the helical angle, changes from values of 60°–80° superficially, through arrays of myocytes with their long axes parallel to the Equator, and then to deeper arrays, which again move closer to longitudinal orientations, but with angles opposite to those forming the superficial parts of the walls (Fig. 2.17). Most of these investigations presume that all the myocytes are also oriented with their long axes parallel to the epicardial and endocardial surfaces, that is, oriented in

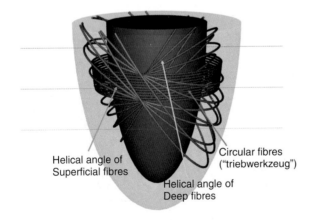

Helical angle of
Superficial fibres

Circular fibres
("triebwerkzeug")

Helical angle of
Deep fibres

Fig. 2.17 This schematic summarizes the orientation of the aggregated myocytes within the ventricular walls as shown by the dissection illustrated in Fig. 2.14. The so-called helical angle within the left ventricle changes from the epicardium (superficial layer) to the endocardium (deep layer). Note the myocytes aggregated together in circular fashion to form the middle layer of the left, but not right ventricle. Note also that the helical angles of the myocytes making up the superficial and deep layers of the wall are perpendicular to one another
Original artwork prepared by Professor Paul Lunkenheimer, University of Munster, Germany, and modified with his permission

tangential fashion. When careful studies are made to examine the precise angle of these myocytes relative to the transmural plane, which is possible when the myocytes themselves are cut along their long axis, a significant proportion is found to intrude within the wall, running from the epicardium toward the endocardium. These histological studies showing the presence of intruding myocytes have now been confirmed by resonance imaging studies in porcine hearts, and a solitary human heart [24]. The three-dimensional mesh, with change not only of the helical angle, but also of the angle of intrusion, the latter varying in relation to both remaining orthogonal planes, permits a better explanation to be provided for the different forces that can be recorded within the depths of the left ventricular wall. The larger part of these forces aids ventricular emptying, and hence is described as *unloading*. The smaller part, in contrast, still further augments the contraction, and therefore, these forces are auxotonic [16]. Both forces act in an antagonistic fashion to permit normal systolic contraction, followed by diastolic thinning of the ventricular walls.

There is also a change in orientation of the myocytes aggregated within the depths of the walls of the right ventricle. Unlike the situation in the left ventricle, very few myocytes, other than those forming the subpulmonary infundibulum, are seen with a circular orientation for their long axes. The myocytes orientated in circular fashion within the left ventricle had previously been termed by Krehl [25] as the *triebwerkzeug*, being recognized by him as providing the activating force for ventricular emptying. In this respect, therefore, it is surely significant that substantial arrays of myocytes oriented in circumferential fashion are found in the hypertrophied walls of the right ventricle of patients with tetralogy of Fallot (Fig. 2.18). Their functional correlate remains to be determined.

2.5 Unraveling the Unique Myocardial Band

As already discussed, it is the ability of individual dissectors to impose their own will on the ventricular mass by following the grain within the myocardium that has led currently to one of the most popular, and yet most flawed, concepts of myocardial organization, namely, that of the *unique myocardial band*. Although promoted as providing a *revolution in understanding*, there is no scientific evidence supporting these claims. It is certainly possible to recognize helical configurations within the ventricular walls, but these exist globally within the three-dimensional mesh, although the precise angulation of the helices varies from site to site. As we have discussed, such helical

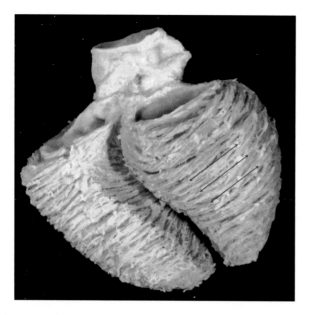

Fig. 2.18 Change in the orientation of the aggregated myocytes in patients with tetralogy of Fallot and right ventricular hypertrophy. In this situation, there is a third, prominent, circular middle layer within the right ventricle, which is not seen in the normal heart. Dissection prepared by Prof. Damian Sanchez-Quintana, University of Badajoz, Spain, and reproduced with his permission

configurations have long been recognized [17]. They are readily explained simply by the change in radial axis of the aggregated myocytes within the depth of the ventricular walls. It is impossible to unwrap the ventricular walls uniformly to produce the solitary muscular strip purported to have its origin at the pulmonary trunk, and its insertion at the aortic root. Not only does such unraveling take no notice of the basic anatomic arrangement of the ventricular mass but the very process of dissection entails the production of artifactual cleavage planes within the myocardium (Fig. 2.14a). If it were possible to dissect the myocardium as a solitary band, and if it acted like a pulley rope as proposed by Torrent-Guasp [7], fibrous sheaths separating the various components of the band would be required as they wrap around each other, as is the case with skeletal muscles. If the dissectors were following the long axis of the aggregated myocytes, then cells within the unraveled band would require to be aligned in uniformly parallel fashion to its long axis. Neither of these anatomical features has been demonstrated by the supporters of the unique myocardial band. Furthermore, a recent investigation of the alignment of the myocytes aggregated within the unwrapped myocardial band shows no evidence of the necessary parallel arrangement [26]. Instead, there is marked disarray along the length of the band, and at different depths within the band. Thus, there is no evidence whatsoever to support the concept of the unique myocardial band. In contrast, the evidence continues

to emerge, from dissection, histology, and now three-dimensional reconstruction, to show that the ventricular walls take the form of a three-dimensional meshwork of myocytes set within a supporting matrix of fibrous tissue.

2.6 Conclusions

Much of the previous work related to the ventricular mass has concentrated on the left ventricle, with relatively few attempting to describe the relationship between the two ventricles. As we have shown, there is a close anatomic relationship between two of the three components of the right and left ventricles, specifically their apical trabecular portions, and the part of the ventricular septum that separates the inlet of the right ventricle from the outlet of left. How the myocardium becomes organized into a three-dimensional meshwork, encased in a fibrous matrix extending from one ventricle to the other, is uncertain. Finding the link between the known separate embryonic origins of the morphologically right and left ventricles and their known mature spatial organization will be the key to future understanding of the interplay between the right and left ventricles.

References

1. Kelly RG. Molecular inroads into the anterior heart field. Trends Cardiovasc Med. 2005;15(2):51–6.
2. Waldo KL, Kumiski DH, Wallis KT, Stadt HA, Hutson MR, Platt DH, et al. Conotruncal myocardium arises from a secondary heart field. Development. 2001;128:3179–3188.
3. Mjaatvedt CH, Nakaoka T, Moreno-Rodriguez R, Norris RA, Kern MJ, Eisenberg CA, et al. The outflow tract of the heart is recruited from a novel heart-forming field. Dev Biol. 2001;238: 97–109.
4. Kelly RG, Brown NA, Buckingham ME. The arterial pole of the mouse heart forms from Fgf10-expressing cells in pharyngeal mesoderm. Dev Cell. 2001;1:435–440.
5. Zaffran S, Kelly RG, Meilhac SM, Buckingham ME, Brown NA. Right ventricular myocardium derives from the anterior heart field. Circ Res. 2004;95(3):261–8.
6. Moorman AF, Christoffels VM. Cardiac chamber formation: development, genes, and evolution. Physiol Rev. 2003;83(4): 1223–67.
7. Torrent-Guasp F. La estructuration macroscopica del miocardio ventricular. Rev Esp Cardiol. 1980;33:265–287.
8. McFadden DG, Barbosa AC, Richardson JA, Schneider MD, Srivastava D, Olson EN. The Hand1 and Hand2 transcription factors regulate expansion of the embryonic cardiac ventricles in a gene dosage-dependent manner. Development. 2005;132(1): 189–201.

9. Srivastava D, Thomas T, Lin Q, Kirby ML, Brown D, Olson EN. Regulation of cardiac mesodermal and neural crest development by the bHLH transcription factor, dHAND. Nat Genet. 1997;16(2):154–60.

10. Ward CW, Stadt H, Hutson M, Kirby ML. Ablation of the secondary heart field leads to tetralogy of Fallot and pulmonary atresia. Dev Biol. 2005;284:72–83.

11. Jouk PS, Usson Y, Michalowicz G, Grossi L. Three-dimensional cartography of the pattern of the myofibres in the second trimester fetal human heart. Anat Embryol (Berl). 2000;202(2):103–18.

12. Hirschy A, Schatzmann F, Ehler E, Perriard JC. Establishment of cardiac cytoarchitecture in the developing mouse heart. Dev Biol. 2006;289(2):430–41.

13. Luo Y, Radice GL. Cadherin-mediated adhesion is essential for myofibril continuity across the plasma membrane but not for assembly of the contractile apparatus. J Cell Sci. 2003;116(Pt 8):1471–9.

14. Petersen SE, Selvanayagam JB, Wiesmann F, Robson MD, Francis JM, Anderson RH, et al. Left ventricular non-compaction: insights from cardiovascular magnetic resonance imaging. J Am Coll Cardiol. 2005;46(1):101–5.

15. Boettler P, Claus P, Herbots L, McLaughlin M, D'hooge J, Bijnens B, et al. New aspects of the ventricular septum and its function: an echocardiographic study. Heart. 2005;91(10):1343–8.

16. Lunkenheimer PP, Redmann K, Florek J, Fassnacht U, Cryer CW, Wubbeling F, et al. The forces generated within the musculature of the left ventricular wall. Heart. 2004;90(2):200–7.

17. Pettigrew JB. On the arrangement of the musclar fibres in the ventricular portion of the heart of the mammal (Croonian lecture). Proc R Soc. 1860;10:433–440.

18. Lev M, Simkins CS. Architecture of the human ventricular myocardium. Lab Invest. 1956; 5:398–409.

19. Grant RP. Notes on the muscular architecture of the left ventricle. Circulation. 1965;32:301–8.

20. LeGrice IJ, Smaill BH, Chai LZ, Edgar SG, Gavin JB, Hunter PJ. Laminar structure of the heart: ventricular myocyte arrangement and connective tissue architecture in the dog. Am J Physiol. 1995;269(2 Pt 2):H571–82.

21. Suma H, Isomura T, Horii T, Buckberg G; RESTORE Group. Role of site selection for left ventriculoplasty to treat idiopathic dilated cardiomyopathy. Heart Fail Rev. 2004;9(4):329–36.

22. Buckberg GD, Coghlan HC, Torrent-Guasp F. The structure and function of the helical heart and its buttress wrapping. VI. Geometric concepts of heart failure and use for structural correction. Semin Thorac Cardiovasc Surg. 2001;13(4):386–401.

23. Buckberg GD. The structure and function of the helical heart and its buttress wrapping. II. Interface between unfolded myocardial band and evolution of primitive heart. Semin Thorac Cardiovasc Surg. 2001;13(4):320–32.

24. Lunkenheimer PP, Redmann K, Kling N, Jiang X, Rothaus K, Cryer CW, et al. Three-dimensional architecture of the left ventricular myocardium. Anat Rec A. Discov Mol Cell Evol Biol. 2006;288(6):565–78.

25. Krehl L. Beiträge zur Kenntnis der Füllung und Enterleerung des Herzens. Abhandlungen d. math.-physischen Classe d. Königl. Säches. Ges. d. Wiss., Hirzel, Lepizig 1891;17:341–383.

26. Lunkenheimer PP, Redmann K, Westermann P, Rothaus K, Cryer CW, Niederer P, et al. The myocardium and its fibrous matrix working in concert as a spatially netted mesh: a critical review of the purported tertiary structure of the ventricular mass. Eur J Cardiothorac Surg. 2006;29 Suppl 1:S41–9.

Andrew N. Redington

In Chapters 1 and 2, the unique embryonic and anatomic features of the right ventricle were discussed. In this chapter, the physiology of the normal and abnormal right ventricle will be discussed, with particular emphasis on the relationship between the right ventricle and the pulmonary vascular bed (heart–lung interactions) and its relationship with the left ventricle (ventriculo-ventricular interactions).

3.1 The Normal Right Ventricle

Given the anatomic discussions in Chapter 2, it is perhaps spurious to discuss right ventricular physiology as an independent phenomenon. This concept will be further explored in the section regarding ventriculo-ventricular interactions. Nonetheless, the right ventricle has a unique physiology, largely dependent upon the low hydraulic impedance characteristics of the pulmonary vascular bed. While there are some data to suggest that the myocardium itself is intrinsically different than the left (e.g., a faster twitch velocity in isolated right ventricular muscle bundles greater than the left [1]), the characteristics of right ventricular contraction are primarily dependent on its loading conditions. Right ventricular output approximates that of the left, but the right ventricular cardiac output is achieved with a myocardial energy cost of approximately one-fifth of that of the left. Not only is this because of the low-pressure pulmonary system, but also because of the unique characteristics of the right ventricular pressure–volume relationship. It was Shaver et al. in 1971 [2], who first suggested that the "isovolumic" periods of the right ventricle may be markedly different than that of the left. Using simultaneous micromanometer pressure recordings in humans undergoing cardiac catheterization, he described the so called "hangout period"—the time difference between pulmonary arterial dichrotic notch and simultaneous right ventricular pressure measurement. The hangout period was absent on the left side of the heart (the left ventricular pressure and aortic pressure were identical and synchronous at the time of the aortic dichrotic notch), whereas pulmonary valve closure was occurring well after the onset of right ventricular pressure decline in the normal right heart (Fig. 3.1). Furthermore, this hangout period shortened with increasing right ventricular afterload. The implication of this hangout period was that pulmonary blood flow continued in the presence of right ventricular pressure decline. It was not until 1988 that human right ventricular pressure–volume relationships were defined [3]. Using biplane angiograms with simultaneous pressure measurements, the normal right ventricular pressure–volume relationship was defined as a triangular or trapezoidal form, with ill-defined periods of isovolumic contraction, and particularly isovolumic relaxation. This pattern has subsequently been confirmed by many other authors [4, 5]. Interestingly, despite the lack of an obvious "end systolic" shoulder, the elastance model of ventricular performance appears to be valid for that of the right ventricle. In an important study performed by Burkhoff et al. [6], appropriate changes in maximal elastance, defined as maximal pressure/volume (Emax) rather than end-systolic elastance (Ees), were noted with changes in inotropy, with the slope of maximum pressure/volume being linear over a wide range of boundary conditions.

Thus, unlike the square-wave pump of the left ventricle, the right ventricle is an energetically efficient pump. As mentioned above, however, this efficiency is almost entirely predicated by the low pulmonary hydraulic impedance. Interestingly, when the morphologic left ventricle is anatomically sited beneath the normal pulmonary artery (e.g., in the setting of congenitally corrected transposition), its pressure–volume characteristics are identical to those of the normal right ventricle [7]. Furthermore, small changes in afterload lead to major changes in right

A.N. Redington (✉)
Department of Paediatrics, Hospital for Sick Children, Toronto, ON, Canada

A.N. Redington et al. (eds.), *Congenital Diseases in the Right Heart*, DOI 10.1007/978-1-84800-378-1_3,
© Springer-Verlag London Limited 2009

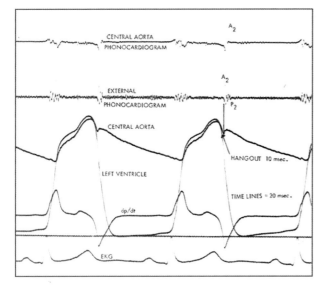

Fig. 3.1 The left hand panel shows the relationship between left ventricular pressure and aortic dichrotic notch pressure and timing. The hangout period is 10 ms. The right hand panel shows similar micromanometer recordings made in the right ventricle (RV) and pulmonary artery. Note how the RV pressure has fallen to low levels by the time of pulmonary valve closure, marked at its dichrotic notch. See text for details

ventricular pressure–volume relationships and its performance [7]. With a slowly progressive rise in pulmonary arterial impedance, there is a progressive change toward a "left ventricular" pattern of the pressure–volume loop. However, it is well known that acute changes in acute pulmonary impedance (e.g., acute massive pulmonary embolism) are poorly tolerated by the right ventricle. Consequently, it has been suggested that the afterload reserve of the normal right ventricle is approximately one-third of that of the left ventricle.

3.2 Heart–Lung Interactions

While the pressure–volume relationships of the normal right ventricle are a manifestation of one form of heart–lung interaction, there is clearly another important factor that must be taken into account when assessing both the normal and abnormal right heart circulation. The influence of the mechanical work of breathing has a major impact on beat-by-beat and breath-by-breath right heart hemodynamics [8]. With each inspiration, the small (2–5 cm/H_2O) change in intrapleural pressure leads to a significant increase in venous return and right ventricular preload. This accounts for the waxing and waning of right ventricular stroke volume during the respiratory cycle. The converse, that is, a fall in right ventricular stroke volume as mean airway pressure increases, is, in part, due to changes in preload, but not entirely. In a fascinating study by Henning [9], the original concept developed

by the classical experiments of Cornand [10] was challenged. Cournand had shown, in experiments involving healthy young volunteers, that facemask positive pressure ventilation led to a fall in cardiac output, and postulated that this was a consequence of decreased preload because of decreased venous return consequent upon increased intrathoracic pressure. In Henning's later experimental canine study, the typical fall in cardiac output was observed with a modest increase in mean airway pressure during positive pressure ventilation. However, restoration of preload with volume infusions (back to the baseline levels) failed to restore right ventricular stroke volume to baseline. This important study confirms the afterload dependency of right ventricular contractile performance. Even relatively modest changes in total pulmonary resistance (in this case, imposed by a small change in mean airway pressure) leads to decreased contractile performance and a worse cardiac output. This reduction in cardiac output of approximately 10–15% with positive pressure ventilation has been confirmed in subsequent studies [11], both in children and adults with normal right ventricular physiology. In the congenitally malformed right heart circulation, these heart–lung interactions can be even more profound. The Fontan procedure is an ideal natural model of beneficial heart–lung interactions. In the absence of a subpulmonary right ventricle, and increasingly nowadays, in the absence of a subpulmonary blood reservoir (right atrium), the pulmonary hemodynamics are markedly dependent on the work of breathing. This concept will be explored in more detail in chapter 23 and will not be explored in any greater detail here. Suffice it to say, that these heart–lung interactions have a major impact on postoperative management and progress in patients with complex congenital heart disease, and cardiac output can frequently be manipulated by changes in ventilatory strategy.

3.3 Ventriculo-ventricular Interactions

While it has been traditional to consider ventricular physiology as independent entities pertaining to either the left or the right ventricle, this concept is clearly flawed. Not only do the ventricles share the same visceral cavity (the pericardium), but also share common myofibers (See chapter 2), particularly in their superficial layers [12]. Consequently, it is impossible to consider abnormalities of the right ventricle in isolation, and vice versa.

It is now well known that normal right ventricular contractile performance is markedly dependent on that of the left. In a classical physiological experiment published in 1994, Damiano and colleagues [13] beautifully demonstrated this ventricular interdependence. By electrically isolating the two ventricles, in the otherwise intact heart, they were able to demonstrate the effect of contralateral ventricular contraction. Right ventricular contraction, in the presence of an otherwise inert left ventricle, led to very little contribution to left ventricular pressure developments. However, left ventricular contraction led to marked pressure generation in the electrically isolated right ventricle. This suggests that the normal geometry of the right ventricle, wrapped around the left ventricle in its short axis, produces right ventricular shortening, as well as a "trans-septal" contribution to right ventricular pressure generation. Indeed, the authors suggested that approximately 30% of the contractile energy of the right ventricle was generated by that of the left. A further illustration of the left ventricular contribution to right ventricular contraction is demonstrated by Hoffman and co-workers [14]. In their experiments, the whole of the right ventricular free wall was replaced by a noncontractile material. Remarkably, right ventricular pressure generation was virtually normal, despite the lack of a contractile element to the right ventricular free wall. Interestingly, enlargement of the artificial right ventricle markedly undermined the ability of the "right ventricle" to generate pressure. The author suggested that intact ventricular geometry was required for this beneficial ventriculo-ventricular interaction. There was tentative evidence that a dilated right ventricle in and of itself generated adverse ventriculo-ventricular interactions, however. As the right ventricular cavity was enlarged in this experiment, left ventricular pressure generation also fell. Whether this was a series effect (reflecting reduced right ventricular cardiac output and therefore leading to reduced left ventricular preload) or a parallel effect (changes in right ventricular geometry adversely affecting left ventricular contractile performance) could not be answered in this experiment. In a follow-up to this experiment, the question as to whether this interaction is a series or parallel effect was examined using simultaneous conductance catheter-derived pressure–volume analysis in the right and left ventricles as right ventricular dilatation is induced. This study, performed by Brooks and co-workers [15], generated right ventricular dilatation by right coronary artery ischemia. Load-independent indices of ventricular contractile performance were measured during this acute geometric change, in order to tease out the fundamental mechanisms of ventriculo-ventricular interactions. Furthermore, the experiments were performed with an open and intact pericardium, to better understand the influence of pericardial constraint on this phenomenon. The results of this study were clear. In the presence of an intact pericardium, acute right ventricular dilatation interferes with left ventricular contractile performance in a parallel fashion. Intrinsic left ventricular contractility was reduced with right ventricular dilatation, presumably reflecting adverse geometry and abnormal function of shared myofibers. Figure 3.2a shows right ventricular pressure–volume relationships under these circumstances. There is a marked fall in both left ventricular volumes, as well as end-systolic pressure. Figure 3.2b shows the effect of releasing pericardial constraint. Under these circumstances, there is virtually no change in left ventricular size, but a similar fall in left ventricular end-systolic pressure, again reflecting decreased contractility. Albeit an experiment in pigs, this latter study suggests that any disease that leads to acute right heart dilatation may manifest itself in terms of not only adverse right ventricular, but also left ventricular contractile performance. The results of the experiment suggest that modification of right ventricular contractile performance could be mediated by changes in left ventricular contractility [16, 17], an area hitherto unexplored clinically. In experimental studies of right ventricular failure, acute aortic constriction to abruptly increase left ventricular afterload and pressure generation, led to increased right ventricular stroke volume and pressure generation. If a similar effect were demonstrable clinically, then efforts to increase left ventricular function might have beneficial secondary effects on right ventricular dysfunction, and vice versa.

These ventriculo-ventricular interactions are clearly important in congenital heart disease where both acute and chronic abnormalities of right ventricular function and volume are frequently encountered. In tetralogy of Fallot, for example, there is a loose, but linear, relationship between right ventricular and left ventricular ejection

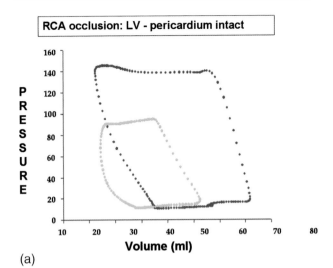

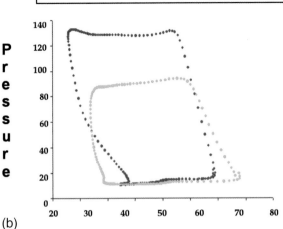

(a)

(b)

Fig. 3.2 a (*left panel*). The effect of acute right ventricular dilation on left ventricular pressure–volume relations. Note how the end diastolic volume and end-systolic pressure both fall. In Fig. 3.2b, the effect of opening the pericardium is demonstrated. Note how the end-systolic pressure and volume remains similar, but the end-diastolic volume increases. See text for details

fraction, as the right ventricle dilates [18]. Furthermore, when present, abnormal left ventricular function (in the presence of chronic pulmonary regurgitation and right ventricular dilatation) predicts a worse outcome in terms of survival [19]. Other direct geometric implications of ventriculo-ventricular interactions are increasingly understood. For example, in congenitally corrected transposition, tricuspid valve competency can be related directly to septal position. It is now well established that modification of septal position by increasing subpulmonary morphologic left ventricular pressure can modify the degree of tricuspid incompetence by its effect on septal leaflet apposition to the anterosuperior and mural leaflets [20]. This is discussed in more detail in Chapter 11. Finally, the whole area of ventriculo-ventricular interactions, particularly with the advent of biventricular pacing, has become increasingly relevant in congenital heart disease and represents a fruitful area of potential research in the future.

3.4 Summary and Conclusion

Physiologically, the normal right ventricle is very different from its left ventricular counterpart. The impact of congenital heart disease, and its modification by surgery, provide for natural models of both abnormal right ventricular physiology, and in particular, heart–lung and ventriculo-ventricular interactions. With increasing understanding of the relevance of these issues, more applicable therapeutic interventions will be developed.

References

1. Rouleau JL, Paradis P, Shenasa H, Juneau C. Faster time to peak tension and velocity of shortening in right versus left ventricular trabeculae and papillary muscles of dogs. Circ Res. Nov 1986;59(5):556–61.
2. Shaver JA. Clinical implications of the hangout interval. Int J Cardiol. Mar 1984;5(3):391–8.
3. Redington AN, Gray HH, Hodson ME, Rigby ML, Oldershaw PJ. Characterisation of the normal right ventricular pressure-volume relation by biplane angiography and simultaneous micromanometer pressure measurements. Br Heart J. Jan 1988;59(1):23–30.
4. Gaynor SL, Maniar HS, Bloch JB, Steendijk P, Moon MR. Right atrial and ventricular adaptation to chronic right ventricular pressure overload. Circulation. Aug 30 2005;112 Suppl 9:I212–8.
5. Belenkie I, Horne SG, Dani R, Smith ER, Tyberg JV. Effects of aortic constriction during experimental acute right ventricular pressure loading. Further insights into diastolic and systolic ventricular interaction. Circulation. Aug 1 1995;92(3):546–54.
6. Dickstein ML, Yano O, Spotnitz HM, Burkhoff D. Assessment of right ventricular contractile state with the conductance catheter technique in the pig. Cardiovasc Res. Jun 1995;29(6):820–6.
7. Redington AN, Rigby ML, Shinebourne EA, Oldershaw PJ. Changes in the pressure-volume relation of the right ventricle when its loading conditions are modified. Br Heart J. Jan 1990;63(1):45–9.
8. Pinsky MR. Determinants of pulmonary arterial flow variation during respiration. J Appl Physiol. May 1984;56(5):1237–45.
9. Henning RJ. Effects of positive end-expiratory pressure on the right ventricle. J Appl Physiol. Sep 1986;61(3):819–26.
10. Cournand A. A discussion of the concept of cardiac failure in the light of recent physiologic studies in man. Ann Intern Med. Oct 1952;37(4):649–63.
11. Shekerdemian LS, Bush A, Lincoln C, Shore DF, Petros AJ, Redington AN. Cardiopulmonary interactions in healthy children and children after simple cardiac surgery: the effects of positive and negative pressure ventilation. Heart. Dec 1997;78(6):587–93.

12. Sanchez-Quintana D, Anderson RH, Ho SY. Ventricular myo-architecture in tetralogy of Fallot. Heart. Sep 1996;76(3):280–6.

13. Damiano RJ Jr, La Follette P Jr, Cox JL, Lowe JE, Santamore WP. Significant left ventricular contribution to right ventricular systolic function. Am J Physiol. Nov 1991;261(5 Pt 2):H1514–24.

14. Hoffman D, Sisto D, Frater RW, Nikolic SD. Left-to-right ventricular interaction with a noncontracting right ventricle. J Thorac Cardiovasc Surg. Jun 1994;107(6):1496–502.

15. Brookes C, Ravn H, White P, Moeldrup U, Oldershaw P, Redington A. Acute right ventricular dilatation in response to ischemia significantly impairs left ventricular systolic performance. Circulation. Aug 17 1999;100(7):761–7.

16. Yamashita H, Onodera S, Imamoto T, Obara A, Tanazawa S, Takashio T, et al. Functional and geometrical interference and interdependency between the right and left ventricle in cor pulmonale: an experimental study on simultaneous measurement of biventricular geometry of acute right ventricular pressure overload. Jpn Circ J. Oct 1989;53(10):1237–44.

17. Ghignone M, Girling L, Prewitt RM. Volume expansion versus norepinephrine in treatment of a low cardiac output complicating an acute increase in right ventricular afterload in dogs. Anesthesiology. Feb 1984;60(2):132–5.

18. Davlouros PA, Kilner PJ, Hornung TS, Li W, Francis JM, Moon JC, et al. Right ventricular function in adults with repaired tetralogy of Fallot assessed with cardiovascular magnetic resonance imaging: detrimental role of right ventricular outflow aneurysms or akinesia and adverse right-to-left ventricular interaction. J Am Coll Cardiol. Dec 4 2002;40(11):2044–52.

19. Ghai A, Silversides C, Harris L, Webb GD, Siu SC, Therrien J. Left ventricular dysfunction is a risk factor for sudden cardiac death in adults late after repair of tetralogy of Fallot. J Am Coll Cardiol. Nov 6 2002;40(9):1675–80.

20. van Son JA, Reddy VM, Silverman NH, Hanley FL. Regression of tricuspid regurgitation after two-stage arterial switch operation for failing systemic ventricle after atrial inversion operation. J Thorac Cardiovasc Surg. Feb 1996;111(2):342–7.

Section 2
The Pulmonary Vascular Bed

Peter Oishi and Jeffrey R. Fineman

4.1 Introduction

The development of pulmonary hypertension and its associated altered vascular reactivity commonly accompany congenital cardiac disease. The risk and timing of the development of advanced pulmonary arterial hypertension are dependent upon the type of cardiac defect, and likely a presently uncharacterized genetic predisposition. The cardiac defects associated with the greatest risk are those that cause increased pulmonary blood flow and/or pulmonary venous pressure, which subject the pulmonary vasculature to pathologic mechanical forces. Overtime, these abnormal hemodynamics lead to progressive functional and morphologic abnormalities, including altered pulmonary vascular reactivity, increased pulmonary vascular resistance, and structural alterations, or remodeling, of the pulmonary vasculature [1–4]. Early surgical repair of these congenital cardiac malformations has decreased the incidence of irreversible pulmonary vascular disease. Even children with reversible vascular changes, nonetheless, suffer significant morbidity and mortality in the peri- and postoperative periods secondary to both chronic and acute elevations in pulmonary vascular resistance. In addition, mild elevations in pulmonary vascular resistance in infants with functionally univentricular physiology may eliminate certain surgical options, such as caval-pulmonary anastomoses and the Fontan procedures. The state of the pulmonary vasculature, therefore, is often the principal determinant of the clinical course and feasibility of surgical treatment.

Although the pathophysiology of pulmonary arterial hypertension associated with congenitally malformed hearts is still incompletely understood, increasing evidence suggests that early pathological changes result from pulmonary vascular endothelial dysfunction that develops as a consequence of its exposure to abnormal mechanical forces, such as increased pressure and flow. In particular, a broad body of evidence indicates that aberrations in the nitric oxide and endothelin systems are intimately involved in the development of altered vascular reactivity and pulmonary arterial remodeling.

In the remaining sections, we present an initial overview of the cascades of nitric oxide and endothelin, with a focus on the pulmonary circulation. Thereafter, the pathophysiologic role of abnormal pulmonary vascular endothelial function in pulmonary arterial hypertension in the setting of congenital cardiac disease will be reviewed, with an emphasis of the therapeutic implications.

4.2 Biosynthesis and Regulation of Nitric Oxide

Nitric oxide is a labile humoral factor produced by nitric oxide synthase from l-arginine in the vascular endothelial cell [5–7] (Fig. 4.1). Three isoforms of the synthase have been identified. Constitutive forms are present in endothelial cells and neurons, and a third inducible isoform is present in macrophages [8–10]. The predominant vascular source of nitric oxide arises from stimulation of endothelial nitric oxide synthase (eNOS). Once produced, nitric oxide diffuses into the smooth muscle cell, resulting in vascular relaxation by increasing concentrations of guanosine $3'5'$-monophosphate (cGMP), via the activation of soluble guanylate cyclase [11, 12]. Nitric oxide is released in response to a variety of factors, including the shear stress produced by flow, and the binding of certain endothelial-dependent vasodilators, such as acetylcholine, ATP, and bradykinin, to receptors on the endothelial cell [13, 14].

Although initially considered to be a constitutively expressed enzyme, a large and increasing literature demonstrates that eNOS is dynamically regulated at the transcriptional, post-transcriptional, and post-translational levels

J.R. Fineman (✉)
Department of Pediatrics and The Cardiovascular Research Institute, University of California, San Francisco, USA

A.N. Redington et al. (eds.), *Congenital Diseases in the Right Heart*, DOI 10.1007/978-1-84800-378-1_4,
© Springer-Verlag London Limited 2009

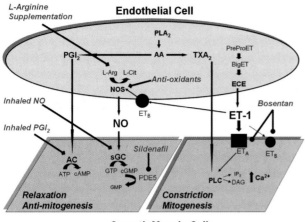

Fig. 4.1 Schematic of NO-cGMP, ET-1, and arachidonic acid cascades, with the pharmacologic site of action of the current and experimental endothelial-based pulmonary hypertension therapies Both l-arginine and antioxidants may increase bioavailable NO by improving NOS production; inhaled NO and inhaled PGI$_2$ are endothelium independent and selective vasodilators secondary to rapid inactivation. They induce vascular relaxation by increasing cGMP and cAMP, respectively. Sildenafil acts by inhibiting PDE5 and thereby preventing the breakdown of cGMP, and bosentan is a combined ET receptor anatogonist.

PGI$_2$ = prostaglandin I$_2$, PLA$_2$ = phospholipase A$_2$, AA = arachidonic acid, TXA$_2$= thromboxane A$_2$, L-Arg = l-arginine, L-Cit = L-citrulline, NOS = nitric oxide synthase, ET-1 = endothelin-1, ET$_A$ = endothelin A receptor, ET$_B$ = endothelin B receptor, NO = nitric oxide, sGC = soluble guanylate cyclase, GTP = guanosine-5'-triphosphate, cGMP = guanosine-3'-5'cyclic monophosphate, , GMP = guanosine monophosphate, AC = adenylate cyclase, ATP = adenosine-5'-triphosphate, cAMP = adenosine-3'-5'-monophosphate, AMP = adenosine monophosphate, PDE5 = phosphodiesterase type 5.

[15–18]. For example, laminar shear stress increases transcription, while stimuli such as growth of cells increase expression by prolonging the half-life of the eNOS mRNA [19, 20]. In addition, factors such as intracellular location, interactions with other proteins such as calmodulin, caveolin, and heat shock protein 90, phosphorylation, and the availability of the substrate and co-factors, may all dynamically regulate eNOS activity [15–18, 21–23]. The regulation of eNOS by mechanical forces is complex and incompletely understood. A variety of systems tested experimentally have clearly been shown to demonstrate that fluid shear stress upregulates expression of the eNOS gene by activation of the 5'-promotor region [19]. Similarly, during life, increases in flow secondary to exercise are associated with increased expression of both eNOS mRNA and protein [24]. Fluid shear stress has also been demonstrated to increase eNOS activity experimentally [15–18]. This appears to be regulated, in part, by potassium channels and serine phosphorylation [25, 26]. The potential effects of pressure on

eNOS transcription are less well delineated, but the majority of experimental studies suggest that pressure alone does not upregulate expression [19, 27]. In addition to these biomechanical forces, other factors that are particularly relevant to congenital heart disease, and that are known to regulate eNOS, include growth factors, changes in oxygen tension, and vasoactive factors such as endothelin-1.

Basal release of nitric oxide is an important mediator of both resting pulmonary and systemic vascular tone in the fetus, newborn, and adult, as well as a mediator of the normal fall in pulmonary vascular resistance that occurs immediately after birth [6, 28, 29]. Interestingly, in addition to its effect on vascular tone, nitric oxide is a potent inhibitor of platelet aggregation and smooth muscle mitogenesis. Given these properties, it is not surprising that increasing data demonstrate that aberrant NO-cGMP signaling is integral to the pathophysiology of pulmonary hypertension, as well as a number of other vascular disorders [30–37].

4.3 Biosynthesis and Regulation of Endothelin-1

Endothelin-1, a 21-amino acid polypeptide produced by vascular endothelial cells, has potent vasoactive properties [38]. The gene for human endothelin-1 is located on chromosome 6, and is translated to a 203-amino acid peptide precursor, abbreviated to preproET-1, which is then cleaved to form proendothelin-1. Proendothelin, so-called "big" endothelin-1, is then cleaved by a membrane-bound metalloprotein-converting enzyme, or ECE-1, into its functional form (Fig. 4.1). ECE-1 exists in two isoforms, ECE-1α and ECE-1β, with ECE-1α considered to be the most important biologically [39]. The vasoactive properties of endothelin-1 are complex, and studies have shown varying hemodynamic effects on different vascular beds [40–44]. Its most striking property is its sustained hypertensive action. The hemodynamic effects are mediated by at least two distinct receptor populations, ET$_A$ and ET$_B$, the densities of which depend on the vascular bed studied. ET$_A$ receptors are located on vascular smooth muscle cells and mediate vasoconstriction, whereas ET$_B$ receptors are located on endothelial cells and mediate vasodilation [45, 46]. In addition, a second subpopulation of ET$_B$ receptors are located on smooth muscle cells and mediate vasoconstriction [47]. The vasodilating effects of endothelin-1 are associated with the release of nitric oxide and activation of potassium channels [40–42, 48]. Its vasoconstricting effects are associated with phospholipase activation, the hydrolysis of phosphoinositol to inositol 1,4,5-triphosphate and diacylglycerol, and the subsequent release of calcium ions [49]. Experimental studies on the pulmonary circulation from our laboratory, and others, have demonstrated that exogenous endothelin-1 can produce sustained vasoconstriction, transient vasodilation, or a biphasic response of transient vasodilation followed by sustained vasoconstriction [40–42, 48]. In the clinical situation, vasoconstriction induced by endothelin-1 occurs in both isolated pulmonary arteries and veins [50, 51]. The varied hemodynamic responses to exogenous endothelin-1 are dependent upon a variety of factors, including species, baseline pulmonary vascular tone, integrity of the vascular endothelium, alterations in receptor densities and receptor binding, and age. Endothelin-1 is produced by a variety of cells within the lung, including vascular endothelial cells, vascular and airway smooth muscle cells, and airway epithelial cells [52].

Although not completely delineated, the regulation of its production appears to occur at the transcriptional level of both preproET-1 and ECE-1. Experimental studies demonstrate that expression of preproET-1 mRNA is increased in endothelial cells exposed to various stimulations, which include growth factors, cytokines, and vasoactive substances [53–56]. In addition, levels of ECE-1 mRNA may be increased by exposure to growth factors and vascular injury [57–59]. Other potential regulators of levels of endothelin-1 in plasma and the tissues include rapid release from intracellular secretory granules, alterations in ECE-1 activity, and alterations in clearance, which appear to be mediated in part by ET_B receptors [60–63]. The regulation of endothelin-1 by mechanical forces is incompletely understood. Experimental data suggests that it is regulated by shear stress, but its effect is dependent upon a variety of factors, including the level and duration of the stimulus, and the cell type investigated [62, 64–67]. The majority of these studies suggest that laminar shear stress decreases expression of the preproET-1 and ECE-1 genes, as well as release of endothelin itself [62, 64–66]. The limited data in pulmonary vascular endothelial cells, however, suggest that laminar shear stress does not alter expression of the endothelin gene [68]. Similarly, increases in flow of blood to the lungs seen in the clinical situation secondary to exercise or pneumonectomy are not associated with significant changes in pulmonary levels of endothelin-1 [69–72]. Information on the effect of mechanical stretch and pressure on regulation is even sparser, but very limited data does suggest that stretch and pressure upregulate expression and release of endothelin-1. For example, cultured vascular endothelial cells exposed to either increases in chamber pressure or mechanical stretch demonstrate increased preproET-1 and ECE-1 mRNA, and rapid release of endothelin-1 [63, 67, 68, 73].

As opposed to nitric oxide, basal activity of endothelin-1 does not appear to have a major role in regulating normal pulmonary vascular tone, but rather appears much more prominent when activated in disease states. In addition to its vasoactive properties, endothelin-1 promotes platelet aggregation, superoxide generation, and smooth muscle cell mitogenesis, and therefore may participate in vascular remodeling [74].

4.4 Endothelial Dysfunction in Congenital Cardiac Disease

Over the last 2 decades, evidence has mounted to suggest that endothelial dysfunction is present in patients with congenitally malformed hearts and pulmonary hypertension. For example, lung biopsies from children with pulmonary hypertension secondary to congenital cardiac disease demonstrate both altered anatomic and metabolic endothelial abnormalities as displayed by altered endothelial structure and alignment and altered production of von Willebrand factor. In addition, patients with primary or secondary advanced pulmonary hypertension have alterations in endothelially produced prostanoids, with elevated excretion over 24 h of a thromboxane A_2 metabolite, which promotes vasoconstriction, and reduced excretion of a prostacyclin metabolite, which promotes vasodilation [75].

Given the integral role of nitric oxide and endothelin-1 in the mechanisms that affect vascular tone, mitogenesis, inflammation, and fibrosis, it is not surprising that a growing number of investigations have focused on a potential pathogenic role of these factors in the development of pulmonary vascular disease. For example, Giaid et al. [30] demonstrated that, in patients with primary or secondary forms of pulmonary arterial hypertension, expression of nitric oxide synthase is significantly reduced in endothelial cells of pulmonary arteries with medial thickening and intimal fibrosis [30]. Conversely, endothelin-1 immunoreactivity is abundant in these vessels, and a strong correlation was observed between the intensity of immunoreactivity and pulmonary vascular resistance [76]. Since most patients who undergo histologic evaluation have advanced pulmonary hypertension, it has been difficult to document endothelial injury as a precursor of pulmonary hypertension in the setting of congenital cardiac disease. Interestingly, Celemejar et al. [77] demonstrated an early selective impairment of endothelium-dependent pulmonary relaxation in infants and children with increased pulmonary blood flow prior to the development of pulmonary hypertension, suggesting an early decrease in bioavailable nitric oxide [77]. In addition, elevated levels of endothelin-1 have been detected in both children and adults with congenitally malformed hearts and increased pulmonary blood flow, and those with pulmonary hypertension have a gradient of concentrations of endothelin-1 in the plasma across the pulmonary circulation, suggesting production in the lungs [78–81]. Interestingly, in adults with congestive heart failure secondary to congenital cardiac disease, levels of endothelin-1 in the plasma significantly correlated with functional class in the categorization of the New York Heart Association, and ventricular impairment, independent of the original cardiac defect, suggesting an important role for endothelin-1 in the cardiac failure found in association with congenitally malformed hearts [79].

4.5 Animal Models Supporting a Role for Nitric Oxide and Endothelin in the Development of Pulmonary Arterial Hypertension

The use of animal models has greatly enhanced the ability to investigate the pathogenic role of the cascades in the early development of pulmonary vascular alterations secondary to congenital cardiac disease. To model congenital heart disease with increased pulmonary blood flow, we created aortopulmonary shunts in fetal lambs. Following spontaneous delivery, these lambs had hemodynamic and morphologic alterations that mimicked the human disease. Subsequently, we have used this model extensively to characterize early endothelial dysfunction, and its potential role in the development of pulmonary hypertension and its associated altered vascular reactivity secondary to congenital cardiac disease [82].

At 1 week of life, nitric oxide signaling is intact, as demonstrated by preserved endothelium-dependent vasodilation and normal tissue levels of NOx, an indirect measure of bioavailable nitric oxide, eNOS protein, and eNOS activity. Over the ensuing 8 weeks, endothelium-dependent pulmonary vasodilation becomes impaired, and there is a decrease in levels of NOx, suggestive of decreasing bioavailable nitric oxide, despite unchanged expression of the eNOS gene. Interestingly, this is associated with an increase in superoxide production, which can actively scavenge nitric oxide and form peroxynitrite. Peroxynitrite can further decrease production of nitric oxide by NOS via NOS nitration. The increase in superoxide is likely secondary to an upregulation of NADPH oxidase, which increases superoxide production [83]. In addition, recent data demonstrate that eNOS itself is a source of superoxide production in these lambs (Fig. 4.2) [83]. Under certain conditions, such as decreased precursor

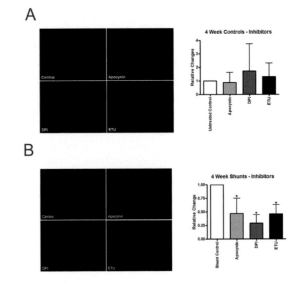

Adapted from Grobe AC, et al. Am J Physiol, 290:L1069-1077, 2006.

Fig. 4.2 Both NADPH oxidase and endothelial NO synthase contribute to the increased superoxide generation in lambs with aortopulmonary shunts
Panel A. Unfixed frozen sections (5 μm) of peripheral lung were prepared from 4-week-old lambs: Control, and after a pulmonary–aorta communication was established *in utero* (Shunt) were incubated pretreated with inhibitors of NADPH oxidase (Apocynin), eNOS (ETU) or both (DPI) then the effects on DHE oxidation visualized by fluorescent microscopy. Under identical imaging conditions, DHE oxidation was significantly decreased by pretreatment apoycin, ETU and DPI in the pulmonary vessels of the Shunt lambs while DHE oxidation was unchanged by all treatments in control lambs. These data suggest that both NADPH oxidase and eNOS are sources of superoxide production in shunt lambs.
B. Average changes in DHE oxidation from images in A were determined. Values are means ± SD; $N = 6$. *$P<0.05$ versus untreated.
Adapted from Grobe AC, et al. Am J Physiol, 290:L1069–1077, 2006

and/or cofactor availability, eNOS can become *uncoupled* and make superoxide anions instead of nitric oxide. The progressive decrease in bioavailable nitric oxide under conditions of increased pulmonary blood flow in these lambs is likely secondary to a combination of increased scavenging by superoxide, and decreased production by eNOS.

In contrast to nitric oxide, endothelin signaling is altered within the first week of life, with increased concentrations of endothelin-1 in the tissues, increased protein levels of ECE-1, and decreased protein and function of the endothelial, vasodilating ET_B receptor [82]. After 4 weeks, an upregulation of the ET_A receptor and its associated pulmonary vasoconstriction develops in addition to the above derangements [84]. After 8 weeks, increased pulmonary blood flow and/or pressure results in the emergence of ET_B-mediated vasoconstriction, which coincides with the upregulation of ET_B receptors on

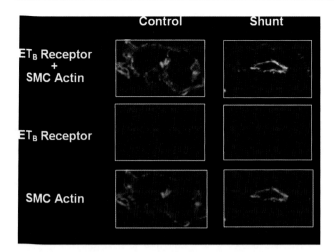

Fig. 4.3 Immunohistochemial localization of ET_A and ET_B protein expression in the lung *in vivo* from 8-week-old lambs. In both shunt and control lambs, ET_A receptors localize to smooth muscle cells. In 8-week control lambs, ET_B receptors localize to endothelial cells and smooth muscle cells
Polyclonal rabbit ET_A and ET_B receptor antibodies and monoclonal mouse anti-SMC–actin antibodies were used to localize expression. ET_A and ET_B protein expression is shown in red while SMC–actin expression is shown in green. Co-localization is shown in yellow. Magnification is 800×
Adapted from Black SM, et al. Circulation, 108:1646–1654, 2003

smooth muscle cells (Fig. 4.3) [84]. Interestingly, a report in humans with advanced pulmonary hypertension secondary to thromboembolism recently demonstrated a similar upregulation of smooth muscle cell ET_B receptors, while ET_A receptors were not increased [85]. These data suggest an important role for both the ET_A and ET_B receptors in the pathophysiology of pulmonary arterial hypertension.

4.6 Endothelial-Based Therapeutic Strategies

One of the most intriguing aspects of the investigation of endothelial abnormalities in the pathobiology of pulmonary hypertension is the ability to modulate these cascades pharmacologically. Figure 4.1 outlines the current approved or investigational therapies based on nitric oxide and endothelin-1, and their point of action within the cascades. To date, the treatment with the greatest impact has been the use of inhaled nitric oxide for children with pulmonary hypertensive disorders [86–98]. When administered to the lung in its natural gaseous form, nitric oxide diffuses through the alveolar wall to reach small pulmonary arteries. It then enters vascular smooth muscle cells, initiating a cascade that results in pulmonary vasodilation via increases in cGMP. After

entering the lumens of the blood vessels, nitric oxide is rapidly inactivated by hemoglobin, which confines its effects to the pulmonary vasculature. Because of these properties, inhaled nitric oxide has several advantages over other vasodilators, which include selective pulmonary vasodilation, rapid onset and elimination, and an improvement in ventilation–perfusion matching, due to the exclusive delivery of the gas to ventilated lung regions. Accordingly, inhaled nitric oxide has become a mainstay of treatment for acute pulmonary hypertensive disorders and the assessment of pulmonary vascular reactivity.

Clearly, the use of intravenous prostacyclin has been the mainstay of chronic treatment for adults with advanced forms of pulmonary vascular disease over the past 15 years. Its limitations include the need for chronic vascular access and its nonselective vascular effects. Inhaled prostacyclin has similar pulmonary selectivity to inhaled nitric oxide secondary to rapid inactivation by hemoglobin. It produces vasodilation by increasing cAMP concentrations. Currently, studies on the use of inhaled prostacyclin for children with pulmonary hypertension are sparse, and comparison studies between inhaled nitric oxide and inhaled prostacyclin are lacking [99–109].

Inhibitors of phosphodiesterases, a family of enzymes that hydrolyze the cyclic nucleotides cAMP and cGMP, are a relatively new class of cardiovascular agents [110]. There are several different phosphodisterase subtypes, which have preferential activity for cAMP or cGMP, and differing tissue distributions. PDE5 is the predominant subtype in the lung, and is relatively selective for cGMP [110–112]. Sildenafil is an inhibitor of PDE5 that has potent pulmonary vasodilating effects secondary to increasing cGMP concentrations [113]. The oral formulation was recently approved for adults with chronic pulmonary vascular disease, and recent short-term studies demonstrate beneficial effects in children with advanced pulmonary vascular disease [114]. The intravenous formulation is currently being investigated for acute pediatric pulmonary hypertensive disorders [115, 116].

As a result of the increasing data implicating alterations in endothelin-1 in the pathophysiology of pulmonary hypertension, as discussed above, ET-receptor antagonism has emerged as a potential therapeutic strategy [36, 76, 117–119]. Bosentan, an oral combined ET_A and ET_B receptor antagonist, has demonstrated efficacy as a chronic therapy for advanced pulmonary vascular disease [120, 121]. To date, there have been no large studies on the use of such receptor antagonists for acute pulmonary hypertensive disorders. Their use when given intravenously is under investigation, but has not yet reached clinical trials.

As extensions of the newer experimental data, both l-arginine supplementation and antioxidant treatment are under investigation for children with pulmonary hypertension. NOS uncoupling may occur in the setting of altered l-arginine metabolism and/or availability. In these situations, l-arginine supplementation may increase bioavailable nitric oxide. Children with pulmonary vasculopathy associated with sickle cell disease are known to have altered arginine metabolism, and recent studies demonstrate that l-arginine supplementation decreases pulmonary arterial pressure in these patients [122–127]. Similarly, scavenging superoxide anions may increase production of nitric oxide by decreasing scavenging and peroxynitrite production, and improving NOS activity. Preliminary data suggest that administration of superoxide dismutase improves pulmonary hemodynamics in animal models [128].

4.7 Conclusions

A strong body of evidence indicates that endothelial dysfunction is a key mediator in the pathogenesis of pulmonary vascular alterations that develop secondary to congenital heart disease. Endothelial-based therapies, such as intravenous prostacyclin, and oral bosentan and sildenafil, have proven to be efficacious for the chronic treatment of adults with advanced pulmonary hypertension. Other endothelial-based treatment strategies, such as l-arginine supplementation to augment endogenous production of nitric oxide, and antioxidant treatments to increase its bioavailability, are currently under investigation. These strategies may have therapeutic potential in a variety of disorders associated with congenital cardiac disease. These may include functional improvement in children and adults who suffer from pulmonary hypertension and low cardiac output syndrome following surgical repair of congenitally malformed hearts, infants and children with functionally univentricular disease with modest vascular remodeling that limits surgical options, and adults with Eisenmenger physiology. Clinical trials are warranted for these exciting potential endothelial-based therapies.

References

1. Rabinovitch M, Haworth SG, Castaneda AR, et al. Lung biopsy in congenital heart disease: a morphometric approach to pulmonary vascular disease. Circulation. Dec 1978;58(6):1107–22.
2. Burrows FA, Klinck JR, Rabinovitch M, et al. Pulmonary hypertension in children: perioperative management. Can Anaesth Soc J. Sep 1986;33(5):606–28.
3. Hoffman JI, Rudolph AM, Heymann MA. Pulmonary vascular disease with congenital heart lesions: pathologic features and causes. Circulation. Nov 1981;64(5):873–7.
4. Wheller J, George BL, Mulder DG, et al. Diagnosis and management of postoperative pulmonary hypertensive crisis. Circulation. Dec 1979;60(7):1640–44.
5. Bush PA, Gonzalez NE, Ignarro LJ. Biosynthesis of nitric oxide and citrulline from l-arginine by constitutive nitric oxide synthase present in rabbit corpus cavernosum. Biochem Biophys Res Commun. Jul 15 1992;186(1):308–14.
6. Ignarro LJ, Byrns RE, Buga GM, et al. Endothelium-derived relaxing factor from pulmonary artery and vein possesses pharmacologic and chemical properties identical to those of nitric oxide radical. Circ Res. Dec 1987;61(6):866–79.
7. Ignarro LJ, Ross G, Tillisch J. Pharmacology of endothelium-derived nitric oxide and nitrovasodilators. West J Med. Jan 1991;154(1):51–62.
8. Sessa WC, Harrison JK, Luthin DR, et al. Genomic analysis and expression patterns reveal distinct genes for endothelial and brain nitric oxide synthase. Hypertension. Jun 1993;21(6 Pt 2):934–38.
9. Lamas S, Marsden PA, Li GK, et al. Endothelial nitric oxide synthase: molecular cloning and characterization of a distinct constitutive enzyme isoform. Proc Natl Acad Sci U S A. Jul 15 1992;89(14):6348–52.
10. Lyons CR, Orloff GJ, Cunningham JM. Molecular cloning and functional expression of an inducible nitric oxide synthase from a murine macrophage cell line. J Biol Chem. Mar 25 1992;267(9):6370–74.
11. Ignarro LJ, Harbison RG, Wood KS, et al. Activation of purified soluble guanylate cyclase by endothelium-derived relaxing factor from intrapulmonary artery and vein: stimulation by acetylcholine, bradykinin and arachidonic acid. J Pharmacol Exp Ther. Jun 1986;237(3):893–900.
12. Murad F. Cyclic guanosine monophosphate as a mediator of vasodilation. J Clin Invest. Jul 1986;78(1):1–5.
13. Mulsch A, Bassenge E, Busse R. Nitric oxide synthesis in endothelial cytosol: evidence for a calcium-dependent and a calcium-independent mechanism. Naunyn Schmiedebergs Arch Pharmacol. Dec 1989;340(6 Pt 2):767–70.
14. Rubanyi GM, Romero JC, Vanhoutte PM. Flow-induced release of endothelium-derived relaxing factor. Am J Physiol. Jun 1986;250(6 Pt 2):H1145–49.
15. Papapetropoulos A, Rudic RD, Sessa WC. Molecular control of nitric oxide synthases in the cardiovascular system. Cardiovasc Res. Aug 15 1999;43(3):509–20.
16. Fleming I, Busse R. Signal transduction of eNOS activation. Cardiovasc Res. Aug 15 1999;43(3):532–41.
17. Andrew PJ, Mayer B. Enzymatic function of nitric oxide synthases. Cardiovasc Res. Aug 15 1999;43(3):521–31.
18. Govers R, Rabelink TJ. Cellular regulation of endothelial nitric oxide synthase. Am J Physiol Renal Physiol. Feb 2001;280(2):F193–206.
19. Ziegler T, Silacci P, Harrison VJ, et al. Nitric oxide synthase expression in endothelial cells exposed to mechanical forces. Hypertension. Aug 1998;32(2):351–55.
20. Searles CD, Miwa Y, Harrison DG, et al. Posttranscriptional regulation of endothelial nitric oxide synthase during cell growth. Circ Res. Oct 1 1999;85(7):588–95.
21. Shaul PW. Regulation of endothelial nitric oxide synthase: location, location, location. Annu Rev Physiol. 2002;64:749–74.
22. Fulton D, Gratton JP, Sessa WC. Post-translational control of endothelial nitric oxide synthase: why isn't calcium/calmodulin enough? J Pharmacol Exp Ther. Dec 2001;299(3):818–24.
23. Pritchard KA Jr, Ackerman AW, Gross ER, et al. Heat shock protein 90 mediates the balance of nitric oxide and superoxide

anion from endothelial nitric-oxide synthase. J Biol Chem. May 25 2001;276(21):17621–24.

24. Johnson LR, Rush JW, Turk JR, et al. Short-term exercise training increases ACh-induced relaxation and eNOS protein in porcine pulmonary arteries. J Appl Physiol. Mar 2001;90(3):1102–10.

25. Ohno M, Gibbons GH, Dzau VJ, et al. Shear stress elevates endothelial cGMP. Role of a potassium channel and G protein coupling. Circulation. 1993;88(1):193–97.

26. Corson MA, James NL, Latta SE, et al. Phosphorylation of endothelial nitric oxide synthase in response to fluid shear stress. Circ Res. 1996;79(5):984–91.

27. Malek AM, Izumo S, Alper SL. Modulation by pathophysiological stimuli of the shear stress-induced up-regulation of endothelial nitric oxide synthase expression in endothelial cells. Neurosurgery. 1999;45(2):334–44; discussion 344–35.

28. Brashers VL, Peach MJ, Rose CE Jr. Augmentation of hypoxic pulmonary vasoconstriction in the isolated perfused rat lung by in vitro antagonists of endothelium-dependent relaxation. J Clin Invest. Nov 1988;82(5):1495–502.

29. Fineman JR, Soifer SJ, Heymann MA. Regulation of pulmonary vascular tone in the perinatal period. Annu Rev Physiol. 1995;57:115–34.

30. Giaid A, Saleh D. Reduced expression of endothelial nitric oxide synthase in the lungs of patients with pulmonary hypertension. N Engl J Med. Jul 27 1995;333(4):214–21.

31. Black SM, Bekker JM, McMullan DM, et al. Alterations in nitric oxide production in 8-week-old lambs with increased pulmonary blood flow. Pediatr Res. Aug 2002;52(2):233–44.

32. Black SM, Fineman JR, Steinhorn RH, et al. Increased endothelial NOS in lambs with increased pulmonary blood flow and pulmonary hypertension. Am J Physiol. Nov 1998;275(5 Pt 2):H1643–51.

33. Fineman JR, Chang R, Soifer SJ. EDRF inhibition augments pulmonary hypertension in intact newborn lambs. Am J Physiol. May 1992;262(5 Pt 2):H1365–71.

34. Fineman JR, Crowley MR, Heymann MA, et al. In vivo attenuation of endothelium-dependent pulmonary vasodilation by methylene blue. J Appl Physiol. Aug 1991;71(2):735–41.

35. Fineman JR, Wong J, Mikhailov T, et al. Altered endothelial function in lambs with pulmonary hypertension and acute lung injury. Pediatr Pulmonol. Mar 1999;27(3):147–56.

36. Reddy VM, Wong J, Liddicoat JR, et al. Altered endothelium-dependent responses in lambs with pulmonary hypertension and increased pulmonary blood flow. Am J Physiol. Aug 1996;271(2 Pt 2):H562–70.

37. Steinhorn RH, Fineman JR. The pathophysiology of pulmonary hypertension in congenital heart disease. Artif Organs. Nov 1999;23(11):970–74.

38. Yanagisawa M, Kurihara H, Kimura S, et al. A novel potent vasoconstrictor peptide produced by vascular endothelial cells. Nature. Mar 31 1988;332(6163):411–15.

39. Shimada K, Takahashi M, Ikeda M, et al. Identification and characterization of two isoforms of an endothelin-converting enzyme-1. FEBS Lett. Sep 4 1995;371(2):140–4.

40. Bradley LM, Czaja JF, Goldstein RE. Circulatory effects of endothelin in newborn piglets. Am J Physiol. Nov 1990;259(5 Pt 2):H1613–17.

41. Cassin S, Kristova V, Davis T, et al. Tone-dependent responses to endothelin in the isolated perfused fetal sheep pulmonary circulation in situ. J Appl Physiol. Mar 1991;70(3):1228–34.

42. Wong J, Vanderford PA, Fineman JR, et al. Endothelin-1 produces pulmonary vasodilation in the intact newborn lamb. Am J Physiol. Oct 1993;265(4 Pt 2):H1318–25.

43. Wong J, Vanderford PA, Fineman JR, et al. Developmental effects of endothelin-1 on the pulmonary circulation in sheep. Pediatr Res. Sep 1994;36(3):394–401.

44. Perreault T, De Marte J. Maturational changes in endothelium-derived relaxations in newborn piglet pulmonary circulation. Am J Physiol. Feb 1993;264(2 Pt 2):H302–309.

45. Arai H, Hori S, Aramori I, et al. Cloning and expression of a cDNA encoding an endothelin receptor. Nature. Dec 20–27 1990;348(6303):730–32.

46. Sakurai T, Yanagisawa M, Takuwa Y, et al. Cloning of a cDNA encoding a non-isopeptide-selective subtype of the endothelin receptor. Nature. Dec 20–27 1990;348(6303):732–35.

47. Shetty SS, Okada T, Webb RL, et al. Functionally distinct endothelin B receptors in vascular endothelium and smooth muscle. Biochem Biophys Res Commun. Mar 15 1993;191(2):459–64.

48. Wong J, Vanderford PA, Winters J, et al. Endothelinb receptor agonists produce pulmonary vasodilation in intact newborn lambs with pulmonary hypertension. J Cardiovasc Pharmacol. Feb 1995;25(2):207–15.

49. La M, Reid JJ. Endothelin-1 and the regulation of vascular tone. Clin Exp Pharmacol Physiol. May 1995;22(5):315–23.

50. Steffan M, Russell JA. Signal transduction in endothelin-induced contraction of rabbit pulmonary vein. Pulm Pharmacol. 1990;3(1):1–7.

51. Russell JA, Roberts JM. Functional antagonism in rabbit pulmonary veins contracted by endothelin. Pulm Pharmacol. 1991;4(2):67–72.

52. Fagan KA, McMurtry IF, Rodman DM. Role of endothelin-1 in lung disease. Respir Res. 2001;2(2):90–101.

53. Kurihara H, Yoshizumi M, Sugiyama T, et al. Transforming growth factor-beta stimulates the expression of endothelin mRNA by vascular endothelial cells. Biochem Biophys Res Commun. Mar 31 1989;159(3):1435–40.

54. Imai T, Hirata Y, Emori T, et al. Induction of endothelin-1 gene by angiotensin and vasopressin in endothelial cells. Hypertension. Jun 1992;19(6 Pt 2):753–7.

55. Marsden PA, Brenner BM. Transcriptional regulation of the endothelin-1 gene by TNF-alpha. Am J Physiol. Apr 1992;262(4 Pt 1):C854–61.

56. Miyauchi T, Masaki T. Pathophysiology of endothelin in the cardiovascular system. Annu Rev Physiol. 1999;61:391–415.

57. Matsuura A, Kawashima S, Yamochi W, et al. Vascular endothelial growth factor increases endothelin-converting enzyme expression in vascular endothelial cells. Biochem Biophys Res Commun. Jun 27 1997;235(3):713–6.

58. Minamino T, Kurihara H, Takahashi M, et al. Endothelin-converting enzyme expression in the rat vascular injury model and human coronary atherosclerosis. Circulation. Jan 7 1997;95(1):221–30.

59. Teerlink JR, Loffler BM, Hess P, et al. Role of endothelin in the maintenance of blood pressure in conscious rats with chronic heart failure. Acute effects of the endothelin receptor antagonist Ro 47-0203 (bosentan). Circulation. Nov 1994;90(5):2510–18.

60. Mitsutomi N, Akashi C, Odagiri J, et al. Effects of endogenous and exogenous nitric oxide on endothelin-1 production in cultured vascular endothelial cells. Eur J Pharmacol. Jan 1 1999;364(1):65–73.

61. Fukuroda T, Fujikawa T, Ozaki S, et al. Clearance of circulating endothelin-1 by ETB receptors in rats. Biochem Biophys Res Commun. Mar 30 1994;199(3):1461–65.

62. Kuchan MJ, Frangos JA. Shear stress regulates endothelin-1 release via protein kinase C and cGMP in cultured endothelial cells. Am J Physiol. Jan 1993;264(1 Pt 2):H150–56.

63. Macarthur H, Warner TD, Wood EG, et al. Endothelin-1 release from endothelial cells in culture is elevated both acutely and chronically by short periods of mechanical stretch. Biochem Biophys Res Commun. Apr 15 1994;200(1):395–400.

64. Morawietz H, Talanow R, Szibor M, et al. Regulation of the endothelin system by shear stress in human endothelial cells. J Physiol. Jun 15 2000;525 Pt 3:761–70.

65. Harrison VJ, Ziegler T, Bouzourene K, et al. Endothelin-1 and endothelin-converting enzyme-1 gene regulation by shear stress and flow-induced pressure. J Cardiovasc Pharmacol. 1998;31 Suppl 1:S38–41.

66. Masatsugu K, Itoh H, Chun TH, et al. Physiologic shear stress suppresses endothelin-converting enzyme-1 expression in vascular endothelial cells. J Cardiovasc Pharmacol. 1998;31 Suppl 1:S42–5.

67. Ziegler T, Bouzourene K, Harrison VJ, et al. Influence of oscillatory and unidirectional flow environments on the expression of endothelin and nitric oxide synthase in cultured endothelial cells. Arterioscler Thromb Vasc Biol. May 1998;18(5):686–92.

68. Dschietzig T, Richter C, Bartsch C, et al. Flow-induced pressure differentially regulates endothelin-1, urotensin II, adrenomedullin, and relaxin in pulmonary vascular endothelium. Biochem Biophys Res Commun. Nov 23 2001;289(1):245–51.

69. Ohtsuka S. Changes of vasoactive peptides and effects of inhaled nitric oxide after pneumonectomy. Kurume Med J. 1996;43(4):295–304.

70. Cruden NL, Newby DE, Ross JA, et al. Effect of cold exposure, exercise and high altitude on plasma endothelin-1 and endothelial cell markers in man. Scott Med J. Oct 1999;44(5):143–6.

71. Lenz T, Nadansky M, Gossmann J, et al. Exhaustive exercise-induced tissue hypoxia does not change endothelin and big endothelin plasma levels in normal volunteers. Am J Hypertens. Aug 1998;11(8 Pt 1):1028–31.

72. Maeda S, Miyauchi T, Sakai S, et al. Prolonged exercise causes an increase in endothelin-1 production in the heart in rats. Am J Physiol. Dec 1998;275(6 Pt 2):H2105–112.

73. Lauth M, Berger MM, Cattaruzza M, et al. Elevated perfusion pressure upregulates endothelin-1 and endothelin B receptor expression in the rabbit carotid artery. Hypertension. Feb 2000;35(2):648–54.

74. Wedgwood S, Dettman R, Black S. ET-1 stimulates pulmonary arterial smooth muscle cell proliferation via induction of reactive oxygen species. Am J Physiol Lung Cell Mol Physiol. 2001;281:L1058–67.

75. Christman BW, McPherson CD, Newman JH, et al. An imbalance between the excretion of thromboxane and prostacyclin metabolites in pulmonary hypertension. N Engl J Med. Jul 9 1992;327(2):70–5.

76. Giaid A, Yanagisawa M, Langleben D, et al. Expression of endothelin-1 in the lungs of patients with pulmonary hypertension. N Engl J Med. Jun 17 1993;328(24):1732–39.

77. Celermajer DS, Cullen S, Deanfield JE. Impairment of endothelium-dependent pulmonary artery relaxation in children with congenital heart disease and abnormal pulmonary hemodynamics. Circulation. Feb 1993;87(2):440–6.

78. Cacoub P, Dorent R, Nataf P, et al. Plasma endothelin and pulmonary pressures in patients with congestive heart failure. Am Heart J. Dec 1993;126(6):1484–8.

79. Bolger AP, Sharma R, Li W, et al. Neurohormonal activation and the chronic heart failure syndrome in adults with congenital heart disease. Circulation. Jul 2 2002;106(1):92–9.

80. Yoshibayashi M, Nishioka K, Nakao K, et al. Plasma endothelin concentrations in patients with pulmonary hypertension associated with congenital heart defects. Evidence for increased production of endothelin in pulmonary circulation. Circulation. Dec 1991;84(6):2280–5.

81. Cacoub P, Dorent R, Nataf P, et al. Endothelin-1 in pulmonary hypertension. N Engl J Med. Dec 23 1993;329(26):1967–8.

82. Ovadia B, Reinhartz O, Fitzgerald R, et al. Alterations in ET-1, not nitric oxide, in 1-week-old lambs with increased pulmonary blood flow. Am J Physiol Heart Circ Physiol. Feb 2003;284(2):H480–90.

83. Grobe AC, Wells SM, Benavidez E, et al. Increased oxidative stress in lambs with increased pulmonary blood flow and pulmonary hypertension: role of NADPH oxidase and endothelial NO synthase. Am J Physiol Lung Cell Mol Physiol. Jun 2006;290(6):L1069–77.

84. Black SM, Mata-Greenwood E, Dettman RW, et al. Emergence of smooth muscle cell endothelin B-mediated vasoconstriction in lambs with experimental congenital heart disease and increased pulmonary blood flow. Circulation. Sep 30 2003;108(13):1646–54.

85. Bauer M, Wilkens H, Langer F, et al. Selective upregulation of endothelin B receptor gene expression in severe pulmonary hypertension. Circulation. Mar 5 2002;105(9):1034–36.

86. Day RW, Allen EM, Witte MK. A randomized, controlled study of the 1-hour and 24-hour effects of inhaled nitric oxide therapy in children with acute hypoxemic respiratory failure. Chest. Nov 5 1997;112(5):1324–31.

87. Inhaled nitric oxide in full-term and nearly full-term infants with hypoxic respiratory failure. The Neonatal Inhaled Nitric Oxide Study Group. N Engl J Med. Feb 27 1997;336(9):597–604.

88. Atz AM, Wessel DL. Inhaled nitric oxide in the neonate with cardiac disease. Semin Perinatol. Oct 1997;21(5):441–55.

89. Clark RH, Kueser TJ, Walker MW, et al. Low-dose nitric oxide therapy for persistent pulmonary hypertension of the newborn. Clinical Inhaled Nitric Oxide Research Group. N Engl J Med. Feb 17 2000;342(7):469–74.

90. Dellinger RP, Zimmerman JL, Taylor RW, et al. Effects of inhaled nitric oxide in patients with acute respiratory distress syndrome: results of a randomized phase II trial. Inhaled Nitric Oxide in ARDS Study Group. Crit Care Med. Jan 1998;26(1):15–23.

91. Dobyns EL, Cornfield DN, Anas NG, et al. Multicenter randomized controlled trial of the effects of inhaled nitric oxide therapy on gas exchange in children with acute hypoxemic respiratory failure. J Pediatr. Apr 1999;134(4):406–12.

92. Fineman JR, Zwass MS. Inhaled nitric oxide therapy for persistent pulmonary hypertension of the newborn. Acta Paediatr Jpn. Aug 1995;37(4):425–30.

93. Karamanoukian HL, Glick PL, Zayek M, et al. Inhaled nitric oxide in congenital hypoplasia of the lungs due to diaphragmatic hernia or oligohydramnios. Pediatrics. Nov 1994;94(5):715–18.

94. Kinsella JP, Truog WE, Walsh WF, et al. Randomized, multicenter trial of inhaled nitric oxide and high-frequency oscillatory ventilation in severe, persistent pulmonary hypertension of the newborn. J Pediatr. Jul 1997;131(1 Pt 1):55–62.

95. Lunn RJ. Inhaled nitric oxide therapy. Mayo Clin Proc. Mar 1995;70(3):247–55.

96. Roberts JD, Jr., Fineman JR, Morin FC, 3rd, et al. Inhaled nitric oxide and persistent pulmonary hypertension of the newborn. The Inhaled Nitric Oxide Study Group. N Engl J Med. Feb 27 1997;336(9):605–610.

97. Russell IA, Zwass MS, Fineman JR, et al. The effects of inhaled nitric oxide on postoperative pulmonary hypertension in infants and children undergoing surgical repair of congenital heart disease. Anesth Analg. Jul 1998;87(1):46–51.

98. Schreiber MD, Gin-Mestan K, Marks JD, et al. Inhaled nitric oxide in premature infants with the respiratory distress syndrome. N Engl J Med. Nov 27 2003;349(22):2099–107.

99. De Wet CJ, Affleck DG, Jacobsohn E, et al. Inhaled prostacyclin is safe, effective, and affordable in patients with pulmonary hypertension, right heart dysfunction, and refractory hypoxemia after cardiothoracic surgery. J Thorac Cardiovasc Surg. Apr 2004;127(4):1058–67.

100. Hache M, Denault A, Belisle S, et al. Inhaled epoprostenol (prostacyclin) and pulmonary hypertension before cardiac surgery. J Thorac Cardiovasc Surg. Mar 2003;125(3):642–9.

101. Kelly LK, Porta NF, Goodman DM, et al. Inhaled prostacyclin for term infants with persistent pulmonary hypertension refractory to inhaled nitric oxide. J Pediatr. Dec 2002;141(6):830–32.

102. Weston MW, Isaac BF, Crain C. The use of inhaled prostacyclin in nitroprusside-resistant pulmonary artery hypertension. J Heart Lung Transplant. Dec 2001;20(12):1340–44.

103. Hache M, Denault AY, Belisle S, et al. Inhaled prostacyclin (PGI2) is an effective addition to the treatment of pulmonary hypertension and hypoxia in the operating room and intensive care unit. Can J Anaesth. Oct 2001;48(9):924–9.

104. Fiser SM, Cope JT, Kron IL, et al. Aerosolized prostacyclin (epoprostenol) as an alternative to inhaled nitric oxide for patients with reperfusion injury after lung transplantation. J Thorac Cardiovasc Surg. May 2001;121(5):981–2.

105. Della Rocca G, Coccia C, Costa MG, et al. Inhaled areosolized prostacyclin and pulmonary hypertension during anesthesia for lung transplantation. Transplant Proc. Feb–Mar 2001;33(1–2):1634–36.

106. Abe Y, Tatsumi K, Sugito K, et al. Effects of inhaled prostacyclin analogue on chronic hypoxic pulmonary hypertension. J Cardiovasc Pharmacol. Mar 2001;37(3):239–51.

107. van Heerden PV, Barden A, Michalopoulos N, et al. Dose-response to inhaled aerosolized prostacyclin for hypoxemia due to ARDS. Chest. Mar 2000;117(3):819–27.

108. Max M, Rossaint R. Inhaled prostacyclin in the treatment of pulmonary hypertension. Eur J Pediatr. Dec 1999;158 Suppl 1:S23–26.

109. Olschewski H, Ghofrani HA, Walmrath D, et al. Inhaled prostacyclin and iloprost in severe pulmonary hypertension secondary to lung fibrosis. Am J Respir Crit Care Med. Aug 1999;160(2):600–607.

110. Beavo JA. Cyclic nucleotide phosphodiesterases: functional implications of multiple isoforms. Physiol Rev. Oct 1995;75(4):725–48.

111. Torphy TJ, Zhou HL, Burman M, et al. Role of cyclic nucleotide phosphodiesterase isozymes in intact canine trachealis. Mol Pharmacol. Mar 1991;39(3):376–84.

112. Thomas MK, Francis SH, Corbin JD. Characterization of a purified bovine lung cGMP-binding cGMP phosphodiesterase. J Biol Chem. Sep 5 1990;265(25):14964–70.

113. Watanabe H, Ohashi K, Takeuchi K, et al. Sildenafil for primary and secondary pulmonary hypertension. Clin Pharmacol Ther. May 2002;71(5):398–402.

114. Humpl T, Reyes JT, Holtby H, et al. Beneficial effect of oral sildenafil therapy on childhood pulmonary arterial hypertension: twelve-month clinical trial of a single-drug, open-label, pilot study. Circulation. Jun 21 2005;111(24):3274–30.

115. Shekerdemian LS, Ravn HB, Penny DJ. Interaction between inhaled nitric oxide and intravenous sildenafil in a porcine model of meconium aspiration syndrome. Pediatr Res. Mar 2004;55(3):413–18.

116. Stocker C, Penny DJ, Brizard CP, et al. Intravenous sildenafil and inhaled nitric oxide: a randomised trial in infants after cardiac surgery. Intensive Care Med. Nov 2003;29(11):1996–2003.

117. Faraci FM, Heistad DD. Regulation of the cerebral circulation: role of endothelium and potassium channels. Physiol Rev. Jan 1998;78(1):53–97.

118. Rosenberg AA, Kennaugh J, Koppenhafer SL, et al. Elevated immunoreactive endothelin-1 levels in newborn infants with persistent pulmonary hypertension. J Pediatr. Jul 1993;123(1):109–14.

119. Wong J, Reddy VM, Hendricks-Munoz K, et al. Endothelin-1 vasoactive responses in lambs with pulmonary hypertension and increased pulmonary blood flow. Am J Physiol. Dec 1995;269(6 Pt 2):H1965–72.

120. Channick RN, Simonneau G, Sitbon O, et al. Effects of the dual endothelin-receptor antagonist bosentan in patients with pulmonary hypertension: a randomised placebo-controlled study. Lancet. Oct 6 2001;358(9288):1119–23.

121. Rubin LJ, Badesch DB, Barst RJ, et al. Bosentan therapy for pulmonary arterial hypertension. N Engl J Med. Mar 21 2002;346(12):896–903.

122. Morris CR, Morris SM, Jr., Hagar W, et al. Arginine therapy: a new treatment for pulmonary hypertension in sickle cell disease? Am J Respir Crit Care Med. Jul 1 2003;168(1):63–9.

123. Morris CR. New strategies for the treatment of pulmonary hypertension in sickle cell disease : the rationale for arginine tTherapy. Treat Respir Med. 2006;5(1):31–45.

124. Morris CR, Kato GJ, Poljakovic M, et al. Dysregulated arginine metabolism, hemolysis-associated pulmonary hypertension, and mortality in sickle cell disease. Jama. Jul 6 2005;294(1):81–90.

125. Lopez BL, Kreshak AA, Morris CR, et al. L-arginine levels are diminished in adult acute vaso-occlusive sickle cell crisis in the emergency department. Br J Haematol. Feb 2003;120(3):532–34.

126. Morris CR, Kuypers FA, Larkin S, et al. Patterns of arginine and nitric oxide in patients with sickle cell disease with vaso-occlusive crisis and acute chest syndrome. J Pediatr Hematol Oncol. Nov–Dec 2000;22(6):515–20.

127. Morris CR, Kuypers FA, Larkin S, et al. Arginine therapy: a novel strategy to induce nitric oxide production in sickle cell disease. Br J Haematol. Nov 2000;111(2):498–500.

128. Steinhorn RH, Albert G, Swartz DD, et al. Recombinant human superoxide dismutase enhances the effect of inhaled nitric oxide in persistent pulmonary hypertension. Am J Respir Crit Care Med. Sep 1 2001;164(5):834–39.

The Pathobiology of Pulmonary Hypertension: Lessons from Experimental Studies

Sandra Merklinger

5.1 Introduction

Pulmonary arterial hypertension (PAH), a chronic and potentially devastating disorder of the pulmonary circulation, arises from multiple and diverse etiologies. Regardless of the initiating event, PAH is characterized by progressive structural remodeling of the pulmonary vascular bed, leading to increased pulmonary artery pressure (PAP) and pulmonary vascular resistance (PVR) and ultimately, to right-sided heart failure (reviewed in [1]).

5.2 Pathobiology of Pulmonary Hypertension

The pulmonary circulation is a normally high-flow, low-resistance, low-pressure system that plays a pivotal role in gas exchange and oxygen transport. To achieve these essential functions, the walls of the pulmonary vessels are thin and subsequently vulnerable to injury from developmental or acquired disorders affecting the heart or lungs as well as conditions that may affect the systemic vasculature. In the healthy individual, transient elevations in PAP, such as during exercise, are accommodated by a compensatory increase in the cross-sectional area of the pulmonary vascular bed owing to recruitment of previously unperfused vessels. In diseased states, however, vascular remodeling and vessel occlusion and loss lead to reduced compliance and progressive elevations in PAP and PVR.

Despite varying etiologic factors causing PAH, there are similar structural abnormalities observed during the progression of this disease. Quantitative analysis of lung tissue sections from infants and children with congenital heart disease (CHD) revealed a direct correlation between severity of altered growth and development of the pulmonary vascular bed and the hemodynamic state of the pulmonary circulation [2]. The first feature observed was extension of muscle into normally nonmuscular peripheral arteries. This process was initiated by an increase in pulmonary blood flow and is related to differentiation of smooth muscle cells (SMCs) from precursor cells, pericytes, and intermediate cells to mature SMCs [3]. Combined with a mild increase (< 1.5 times normal) in the wall thickness of normally muscular arteries, this initial structural alteration is consistent with morphometric grade A changes as established by Rabinovitch et al. [2].

Grade B vascular changes include greater extension of muscle along normally nonmuscular PAs in conjunction with medial hypertrophy of the normally muscular proximal arteries (> 1.5 times normal). A distinction of mild grade B is assigned when medial hypertrophy remains less than 2 times normal, while more severe hypertrophy (< 2 times normal wall thickness) denotes severe grade B changes (reviewed in [4]). The increase in medial wall thickness has been attributed to both hypertrophy and hyperplasia of resident SMCs and increased deposition of extracellular matrix (ECM) components and intercellular connective tissue, which ultimately manifest as an increase in mean PAP.

The highest morphometric grade, grade C, is attributed to conditions of vascular remodeling in which the medial hypertrophy of grade B is exacerbated by a reduced arterial concentration. Patients with this feature exhibit an increase in PVR. When the number of arteries becomes less than half of normal, severe grade C is assigned. The decrease in artery number is presumably due to the failure of normal vascularization, although resorption and loss of existing vessels, especially distal to occluded arteries with severe neointimal formation may also occur.

Morphometric grades A and B are refinements of Heath-Edwards grade I, an earlier nomenclature designed to classify pulmonary vascular changes [5]. This grading

S. MerklingerS. Merklinger (✉)
Department of Surgery, Hospital for Sick Children, Toronto.

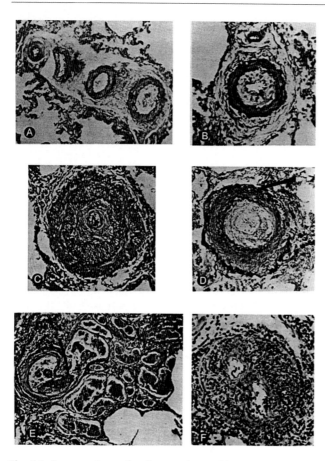

Fig. 5.1 Lung sections taken from patients with varying degrees of pulmonary vascular disease (panels A–F) demonstrating. Heath-Edwards classification of pulmonary vascular changes. **(A)** Grade I: medial hypertrophy. Elastin-van Giesen (EVG) stain, X150. **(B)** Grade II: cellular intimal proliferation in an abnormally muscular artery. EVG, X250. **(C)** Grade III: occlusive changes. Media is thickened due to fasciculi of longitudinal muscle and vessel is all but occluded by fibroelastic tissue. EVG, X150. **(D)** Grade IV: dilation. Vessel is dilated and muscular media is abnormally thin. Lumen is occluded by fibrous tissue. EVG, X150. **(E)** Grade V: plexiform lesion. There is cellular intimal proliferation and clusters of thin-walled vessels that terminate as capillaries in the alveolar wall. EVG, X95. **(F)** Grade VI: acute necrotizing arteritis. A severe, reactive inflammatory exudates is seen through all layers of the vessel. Hematoxylin eosin stain, X250. [reproduced from [4]]

system categorizes the progression of arterial changes (Fig. 5.1) where grade I represents medial hypertrophy. The remodeling attributed to grade C of the morphometric taxonomy may be found in Heath-Edwards grade I but is more commonly associated with grade II (cellular neointimal formation) and invariably with grade III (occlusive neointimal formation with fibrosis). Grade IV is identified by early to advanced arterial dilation, while grades V and VI are consistent with angiomatoid formation and fibrinoid necrosis, respectively. Plexiform lesions are seen in grades IV–VI and were classically thought to represent remodeling or recanalization of occluded vessels, that is, multiple endothelial channels are seen

associated with a dilated media. Although these grading systems were conceived to describe pulmonary vascular changes during diseased states, similar pathological features, specifically medial hypertrophy and occlusive neointimal formation, are seen with many systemic vascular diseases, including atherosclerosis and post-cardiac transplant coronary arteriopathy [6–8].

5.3 The Hypertensive Vessel

In 1986, Rabinovitch et al. applied scanning and transmission electron microscopy to lung biopsy specimens from patients with CHD to analyze the PA endothelium for alterations in surface characteristics and intracytoplasmic composition, which might reflect abnormal function [9]. These studies addressed the hypothesis that heightened pulmonary vascular reactivity resulted from endothelial dysfunction and that this dysfunction was related to the progression of pulmonary vascular disease (PVD) [9]. These studies revealed that the normal *corduroy* pattern of the endothelium was altered in patients with PAH, becoming tortuous, in that the endothelial cells formed winding ridges and deep gorges. This abnormally contoured endothelial surface is thought to be predisposed to altered interactions with marginating blood cells, possibly slowing their flow or trapping them and triggering the release of vasoconstrictive substances, such as thromboxane A2 and B2, both of which have been described as elevated in PAH patients [10, 11]. Platelet aggregates could also form blocking small blood vessels. In addition, alterations in shear stress leads to abnormal endothelial expression of genes associated with proliferation of SMCs (e.g., PDGF) [12] and enhanced connective tissue deposition (TGF-β family) [13]. Indeed, further studies revealed that the morphologically abnormal endothelial cells were also functionally altered in that they produced elevated amounts of a high-molecular weight form of vonWillibrand factor (vWF) and decreased antithrombin III, which promotes platelet aggregation and thrombus formation [14, 15]. More recent studies have identified a loss of production of the vasodilators, endothelial-derived relaxing factor (EDRF) and NO in PAH patients [16, 17], the effects of which may be further exacerbated by heightened circulating levels of the vasoconstrictor, endothelin-1 [18, 19].

The earlier electron microscopic study also described alterations in the internal structure of the endothelium, noting cytoskeletal reorganization in the form of an increased density of microfilament bundles and a heightened metabolic capacity, suggested by the abundant rough endoplasmic reticulum [9]. In addition, these ultrastructural studies revealed that the underlying sub-endothelium was markedly transformed, with the internal elastic lamina showing evidence of degradation and areas of neosynthesis. Although modulation of the ECM content has been related to elevated procollagen synthesis [20] and the expression of tropoelastin [21] and fibronectin [22], the mechanism of elastin degradation would subsequently be investigated using experimental models of PVD where it would prove to be pivotal to disease progression.

A widely accepted toxin-induced model of PAH is the monocrotaline model used in rats. The lung toxicity, for which this model is used, is associated with PA changes that can be correlated with hemodynamic evidence of progressive PAH and increased PVR [23–26]. Upon morphologic examination, the initiation of malignant pulmonary vascular changes in adult monocrotaline rats was associated with the apparent fragmentation of the internal elastic lamina [25]. This degradation was evident by day 4 following injection and suggested rapid activation of an enzyme that could proteolyze elastin and potentially, other ECM components as well. In fact, an early twofold rise in elastolytic activity 2 days after monocrotaline injection, with a second peak in activity between day 16 and 28 that correlated with the progression of structural and functional vascular alterations in the adult animals has been shown [25].

The concept that this progressive elastolytic activity was related to the development of malignant abnormalities is consistent with the observation that reversible hypoxia-induced PAH is associated with only a transient rise in elastase activity [27]. Characterization of the elastase enzyme has shown it to be a $\sim 20\,kD$ serine proteinase, related to the serine proteinase adipsin, and localized to vascular SMCs [28]. Indeed, serine elastase inhibitors, administered for 1 week beginning at the time of monocrotaline injection, suppress the rise in elastolytic activity and reduce the sequelae of vascular changes [29, 30]. Elastase inhibition was also shown to protect the endothelium from monocrotaline, likely by preventing the rise in PAP that contributes to progressive subendothelial edema [30].

5.4 Cell Biology of Pulmonary Hypertension

5.4.1 The Role of Elastase

Insights into the cellular processes underlying pulmonary vascular remodeling have been derived from analysis of clinical material, cultured cells, and studies in experimental animals. As discussed above, the increased activity of

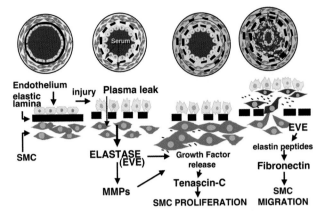

Fig. 5.2 Schematic summary of the putative mechanism involved in the initiation and progression of pulmonary vascular disease. In response to a stimulus, such as high flow and pressure, a disruption in the endothelial barrier permits extravasation of plasma factors into the subendothelium that subsequently induce SMC production of an endogenous vascular elastase. The proteolytic action of elastase, which is further enhanced by MMPs, leads to the release of SMC mitogens from storage sites in the ECM and to the upregulation of the ECM glycoprotein tenascin-C, which amplify the SMC proliferative response. Continued elastase activity is associated with SMC migration through the breakdown products of elastin, the elastin peptides. Elastin peptides stimulate the production of fibronectin, a glycoprotein that is pivotal in altering SMC shape, changing it from a contractile to a motile phenotype

an endogenous vascular elastase in clinical tissues and in experimental models of PVD has been correlated with the degree of vascular remodeling (Fig. 5.2) [25]. Elastases can be serine, cysteine, or metallo proteinases that share the ability to solubilize elastin fibers and other ECM proteins [31], particularly in tissues that exhibit regular matrix turnover. Although serine elastases can be produced locally by vascular SMCs [28, 32], potent serine elastases such as human leukocyte elastase, released by neutrophils, have been causally related to endothelial cell damage in the development of peripheral atherosclerosis [33, 34]. Regulatory control of serine elastase activity is accomplished by the concomitant production of endogenous inhibitors like α_1-proteinase inhibitor and α_2-macroglobulin [35] and elafin [36]. However, in a variety of pulmonary and systemic vascular disease states, a proteinase/antiproteinase imbalance ensues, generating an excess of serine elastolytic activity related to disease progression [34, 37–40].

Creation of a transgenic mouse that overexpresses the serine elastase inhibitor elafin [41] demonstrated a link between heightened elastase-inhibitory activity and reduced pulmonary and systemic vascular disease, that is, intimal formation and inflammatory cell infiltrate in a model of carotid artery wire injury [42]. Similarly, during the arterialization of vein grafts in rabbits, transfection with an expression vector encoding elafin resulted in reduced intimal formation and atherosclerotic degeneration in association with decreased macrophage and T-cell infiltration and suppressed vascular SMC proliferation [43].

It has been established that in response to an injury (e.g., high flow and pressure of a CHD), the endothelial cell layer is compromised and permits the extravasation of plasma factors into the subendothelium [32]. These factors, which include apolipoprotein A1, stimulate the production of SMC elastase activity through a signal transduction cascade involving phosphorylation of focal adhesion kinase and extracellular-regulated kinase (ERK)-1 [44]. Nuclear translocation of phosphorylated ERK-1 subsequently phosphorylates acute myelogenous leukemia (AML)-1, the transcription factor for neutrophil elastase [45] and therefore, a candidate transcription factor for vascular elastase [46]. In fact, antisense studies suppressing AML-1 production also reduces endogenous vascular elastase activity [46].

5.4.2 The Role of Matrix Metalloproteinases

The proteolytic action of serine elastase is further enhanced by the activation of matrix metalloproteinases (MMPs) found at sites of vascular remodeling [reviewed in [47]]. That is, elastase can convert MMPs from pro to active form and can inactivate tissue inhibitors of metalloproteinases (TIMPs). Of the approximately 19 identified MMP family members, the gelatinases (MMP-2 and MMP-9) are recognized for their ability to degrade type IV collagen in basement membranes, and gelatins, which are cleavage products of fibrillar collagens type I, II, and III. Recent evidence has demonstrated that gelatinases, formerly thought to have substrate specificity for denatured collagens (gelatins) only, are able to cleave interstitial collagens as well [48, 49]. It was suggested, therefore, that due to their ability to initiate and maintain the degradation of fibrillar collagens, gelatinases might play a more important role in the remodeling of collagenous ECM than has been previously thought [50].

Proteolytic degradation of the ECM is an essential feature of repair and remodeling during wound healing in various tissues (e.g., skin, vessel, heart). The role of MMPs in vascular pathologies has also been well documented [51–54]. Upregulation of MMP-1, -2, -3 and -9 by lipid-laden macrophages and vascular SMCs [55] has been related to atherosclerotic plaque instability including ulceration and rupture of aneurysms [56–59]. Furthermore, Strauss and colleagues [60–62] have

shown that experimentally induced restenotic lesions are characterized by serine elastase as well as MMP activity and excessive deposition of ECM components. Heightened MMP-2 and MMP-9 expression have been identified following balloon injury [63–65] and MMP inhibition has resulted in partial reduction in lesion size due to both a decrease in ECM accumulation and in inhibition of vascular SMC migration [53, 61, 66, 67]. The precise mechanism whereby excessive or inappropriate expression of MMPs may contribute to the pathogenesis of lung disease remains unknown, but these and other studies suggest a probable role for MMP-induced SMC migration and ECM synthesis.

5.4.3 The Role of Tenascin-C and Fibronectin

It has been determined that serine elastases can degrade the ECM and consequently release mitogenically active SMC growth factors, such as bFGF [68]. This function could be amplified via activation of MMPs. For cells to respond optimally to growth factors, however, their receptors must be available for ligand binding. Jones et al. demonstrated that this occurs when SMCs attach to the specific ECM glycoprotein tenascin-C, which is also upregulated in response to proteolytic matrix degradation [69]. This group identified a correlation between tenascin-C expression and severity of vascular lesions, and confirmed that tenascin-C co-localizes both temporally and spatially with proliferating SMCs, and promotes cell growth in response to bFGF and epidermal growth factor (EGF) [70].

The mechanism whereby tenascin-C promotes SMC proliferation was investigated in cell culture. Experiments using rat PA SMCs [71], where cell shape was altered by culturing cells on either attached or floating collagen gels, revealed an increase in tenascin-C expression when cells were cultured on attached gels. To offer further support of the relationship between cell shape and tenascin-C expression, microarray analysis identified tenascin-C as a gene upregulated in SMCs exposed to cyclic strain [72]. On attached collagen, deposition of endogenous tenascin-C is enhanced and acts as a pro-proliferative factor in that it further increases SMC number in response to bFGF and is a prerequisite for EGF-dependent SMC proliferation (Fig. 5.3) [71]. This process involves tenascin-C induced clustering of $\alpha v \beta 3$ integrins, which leads to rearrangement of actin filaments into focal contacts, and to concomitant aggregation of growth factor receptors [71]. Specifically, EGF receptors are clustered and when ligation with EGF occurs, a tyrosine phosphorylation cascade is set into motion that culminates in a nuclear

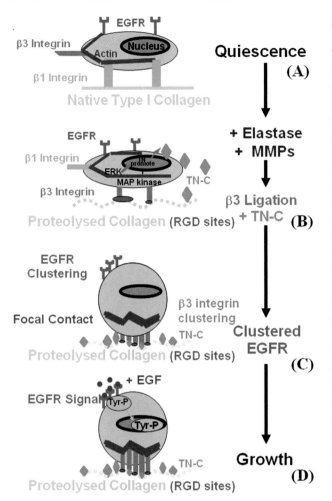

Fig. 5.3 Schematic model of the regulation and function of tenascin-C and its role in smooth muscle cell proliferation. (A) Vascular SMCs attach and spread on native type I collagen using β1 integrins. Under serum-free conditions, the cells withdraw from the cell cycle and become quiescent. (B) Degradation of native type I collagen by elastase and MMPs leads to exposure of cryptic RGD (Arg-Gly-Asp) sites that preferentially bind β3 subunit-containing integrins. In turn, occupancy and activation of β3 integrins signal the production of tenascin-C. (C) Incorporation of multivalent tenascin-C protein into the underlying substrate leads to further aggregation and activation of β3-containing integrins (αvβ3), and to the accumulation of tyrosine-phosphorylated (Tyr-P) signaling molecules and actin into a focal adhesion complex. The tenascin-C-dependent reorganization of the cytoskeleton leads to clustering of EGF receptors (EGFR). (D) Addition of the EGF ligand to clustered EGFRs results in rapid and substantial tyrosine phosphorylation of the EGFR and activation of downstream pathways culminating in the generation of nuclear signals leading to cell proliferation. Adapted from [71]

signal associated with cell growth. The collaboration of tenascin-C with growth factor receptors to induce proliferation has also been reported in other cell types [73–75]. Indeed, in lung biopsy tissue from patients with PAH, increased expression of tenascin-C co-distributes with increased immunoreactivity for EGF [69].

5.4.4 The Role of Elastin and Fibulin-5

The continued proteolytic action of elastase is also related to SMC migration associated with neointimal formation and occlusive PVD [reviewed in [76]]. The mechanism involved in this process has been related to expression of the matrix glycoprotein fibronectin, which is enhanced in pulmonary artery lesions with evidence of neointimal formation in patients with PAH [69]. By studying the ductus arteriosus, a fetal vessel in which abnormally assembled elastin is associated with the development of obstructive intimal cushions, Zhu et al. determined that neointimal formation is mediated by elastin peptides [77]. Further investigation revealed that elastin peptides are capable of upregulating fibronectin production, not only in the ductus arteriosus [78], but also in coronary arteries post-transplantion [76]. In the latter, selective elastase inhibition with elafin prevented neointimal formation by suppressing fibronectin-dependent SMC migration [79].

Recently, another elastin-binding protein was identified. Fibulin-5 (also known as DANCE or EVEC), a calcium-dependent ECM protein has been shown to localize to the surface of elastic fibers in vivo where it acts as a scaffold protein anchoring the elastic fibers to cells [80, 81]. The mechanism involved was related to its role as an integrin ligand, capable of binding to cell surface integrins (eg., αvβ3, αvβ5, and α9β1) through an RGD motif, and to elastin by its Ca^{2+}-binding EGF-like repeats [82]. Fibulin-5 is expressed abundantly in great vessels and cardiac valves during embryogenesis and in many adult tissues that contain elastic fibers. Mechanical injury has been shown to increase expression of fibulin-5 in vascular endothelial and SMCs [82, 83] suggesting a regulatory role for fibulin-5 in vasculogenesis and endothelial cell function. In fact, deletion of the fibulin-5 gene in mice produces profound elastinopathy (eg., disorganization of elastic fibers) in the skin, lung, and vasculature [80, 81]. Fibulin-5, by providing anchorage of the elastic fibers to cells is thought to facilitate stabilization and organization of the fibres [81] potentially augmenting their resistance to degradation.

5.5 Insights into Regression of Pulmonary Hypertension

5.5.1 Induction of Apoptosis

Based on our knowledge of the pathogenesis of PAH, attempts to prevent progression or to induce regression of advanced disease have targeted methods that inhibit vascular cell proliferation and migration. Apoptosis is a process of programmed cell death induced by the loss of cell/matrix interactions that is critical in embryonic development and tissue homeostasis [84, 85]. Adhesion of cells to the matrix predominantly through integrin binding [86] is necessary for survival of differentiated cells in the cardiopulmonary system including, but not limited to, endothelial and SMCs and is also crucial for mesenchymal stem cell differentiation [87]. This adhesion provides a *tensional integrity* that mediates cell behavior by mechanical forces [86], such as sheer stress for endothelial cells [88] and tensile stress for vascular SMCs [89]. Loss of this cellular tensional integrity results in apoptosis of adherent cells and has been related to intracellular and extracellular-mediated events.

In vascular pathology, apoptosis has been observed in primary atherosclerotic lesions [90, 91], in restenosis after percutaneous atherectomy [91], and in saphenous vein aorto-coronary grafts following occlusion [92]. In the rat model of balloon catheter vascular injury, apoptosis of SMCs is integral to neointimal formation [93]. Following injury, there is a rapid induction of SMC apoptosis (within 30 min) [94], resulting in a temporary loss of SMCs [95]. A temporal overlap of proliferating and apoptotic SMCs is later observed peaking at 20 days postinjury and ceasing with reendothelialization of the vessel at about 45 days [90, 93, 96]. Low levels of apoptosis, occurring in conjunction with continued cell proliferation, therefore, are involved in a chronic remodeling process.

In clinical disease, apoptosis has also been implicated in atherosclerotic plaque instability [51], thrombus formation [97, 98], induction of unstable angina, and may increase the risk of acute myocardial infarction [99]. The ability to control vascular SMC apoptosis, therefore, may offer tremendous potential to alter the structure and properties of the vessel wall.

5.5.2 Organ Culture Studies

Studies in PA organ culture have permitted investigation of the SMC response in the whole vessel in situations of stress unloading and in response to various inhibitors. In comparison to cultures on attached collagen gels, floating of cultures resulted in repression of elastase and tenascin-C expression, leading to SMC apoptosis, resorption of excess ECM, and regression of disease [100]. Treatment of hypertensive PAs in adherent collagen gels with elastase, MMP, or $\alpha v \beta 3$ integrin inhibitors similarly induced regression of PA hypertrophy directly.

5.5.3 Intact Animal Studies

Extrapolating the findings from organ culture studies to the intact rat with experimentally induced PAH has led to investigations into the potential reversibility of established PVD. Transplantation of a hypertensive lung harvested from a rat following monocrotaline injection into a normal rat effectively offloaded the pressure in the affected lung, and resulted in progressive normalization of medial hypertrophy and extension of muscle into distal vessels [101]. In a monocrotaline rat model of advanced PAH, the efficacy of orally available elastase inhibitors and epidermal growth factor receptor blockers has been demonstrated by the induction of disease regression [102, 103]. In both studies, survival was associated with SMC apoptosis in the abnormally muscularized and hypertrophied PAs and regression of medial wall thickening accompanied by PAP normalization.

With a focus on the microcirculation, cell-based gene therapy was applied successfully in the monocrotaline rat model. Campbell et al. [104] used cell-based methods of gene transfer to deliver SMCs transfected with either NOS or the angiogenic growth factor VEGF, and found, in both instances, reduced development of monocrotaline-induced PAH and attenuation of pulmonary vascular and RV remodeling.

Statins, the HMG-CoA reductase inhibitors, confer antiproliferative benefits by suppressing endothelial and vascular SMC responses to vascular injury in animal models. Nishimura and colleagues [105, 106] demonstrated in a monocrotaline rat model that treatment with simvastatin could reduce RVH and increase SMC apoptosis in the neointima and medial walls of PAs. Additionally, statins have been shown to induce upregulation of eNOS leading to vasodilation [107], and Akt kinase [108], which may contribute to vessel repair by increasing circulating endothelial progenitor cells.

Future Directions

Despite vast improvements in our knowledge of the pathophysiology of PAH, it remains a disease where medical treatment is limited and largely supportive. Pulmonary hypertension is a multifactorial disease involving both genetic and environmental factors and elucidating mechanisms that might protect against progression or that induce regression of disease may help in the future development of new treatment strategies. Since oral elastase inhibitors are not currently available, investigation of alternative strategies (e.g., EGF receptor blockade and cell-based gene therapy) to induce regression of pulmonary vascular remodeling need to be intensively evaluated. In addition, the search for new biomarkers of PAH and mechanisms that might protect against susceptibility to PVD need to be pursued and the translation of these and other emerging therapies to the patient population need to be of paramount importance.

References

1. Rabinovitch, M., *Pathology of Pulmonary Hypertension*. Progress in Pediatric Cardiology, 2001. **12**: p. 223–247.
2. Rabinovitch, M., et al., *Lung biopsy in congenital heart disease: a morphometric approach to pulmonary vascular disease*. Circulation, 1978. **58**(6): p. 1107–22.
3. Meyrick, B. and L. Reid, *Ultrastructural findings in lung biopsy material from children with congenital heart defects*. Am J Pathol, 1980. **101**(3): p. 527–42.
4. Rabinovitch, M., *Diseases of the Pulmonary Vasculature*, in *Comprehensive Cardiovascular Medicine*, T. EJ, Editor. 1998, Lippincott-Raven Publishers: Philadelphia. p. 3001–3029.
5. Heath, D. and J.E. Edwards, *The pathology of hypertensive pulmonary vascular disease; a description of six grades of structural changes in the pulmonary arteries with special reference to congenital cardiac septal defects*. Circulation, 1958. **18**(4 Part 1): p. 533–47.
6. Billingham, M.E., *Histopathology of graft coronary disease*. J Heart Lung Transplant, 1992. **11**(3 Pt 2): p. S38–44.
7. Ip, J.H., et al., *Syndromes of accelerated atherosclerosis: role of vascular injury and smooth muscle cell proliferation*. J Am Coll Cardiol, 1990. **15**(7): p. 1667–87.
8. Ross, R., *The pathogenesis of atherosclerosis-an update*. N Engl J Med, 1986. **314**(8): p. 488–500.
9. Rabinovitch, M., et al., *Pulmonary artery endothelial abnormalities in patients with congenital heart defects and pulmonary hypertension. A correlation of light with scanning electron microscopy and transmission electron microscopy*. Lab Invest, 1986. **55**(6): p. 632–53.
10. Fuse, S. and T. Kamiya, *Plasma thromboxane B2 concentration in pulmonary hypertension associated with congenital heart disease*. Circulation, 1994. **90**(6): p. 2952–5.
11. Christman, B.W., et al., *An imbalance between the excretion of thromboxane and prostacyclin metabolites in pulmonary hypertension*. N Engl J Med, 1992. **327**(2): p. 70–5.
12. Resnick, N. and M.A. Gimbrone, Jr., *Hemodynamic forces are complex regulators of endothelial gene expression*. Faseb J, 1995. **9**(10): p. 874–82.
13. Topper, J.N., et al., *Identification of vascular endothelial genes differentially responsive to fluid mechanical stimuli: cyclooxygenase-2, manganese superoxide dismutase, and endothelial cell nitric oxide synthase are selectively up-regulated by steady laminar shear stress*. Proc Natl Acad Sci U S A, 1996. **93**(19): p. 10417–22.
14. Turner-Gomes, S.O., et al., *Abnormalities in von Willebrand factor and antithrombin III after cardiopulmonary bypass operations for congenital heart disease*. J Thorac Cardiovasc Surg, 1992. **103**(1): p. 87–97.
15. Rabinovitch, M., et al., *Abnormal endothelial factor VIII associated with pulmonary hypertension and congenital heart defects*. Circulation, 1987. **76**(5): p. 1043–52.
16. Celermajer, D.S., S. Cullen, and J.E. Deanfield, *Impairment of endothelium-dependent pulmonary artery relaxation in children with congenital heart disease and abnormal pulmonary hemodynamics*. Circulation, 1993. **87**(2): p. 440–6.
17. Dinh Xuan, A.T., et al., *Impairment of pulmonary endothelium-dependent relaxation in patients with Eisenmenger's syndrome*. Br J Pharmacol, 1990. **99**(1): p. 9–10.
18. Adatia, I. and S.G. Haworth, *Circulating endothelin in children with congenital heart disease*. Br Heart J, 1993. **69**(3): p. 233–6.
19. Yoshibayashi, M., et al., *Plasma endothelin concentrations in patients with pulmonary hypertension associated with congenital heart defects. Evidence for increased production of endothelin in pulmonary circulation*. Circulation, 1991. **84**(6): p. 2280–5.
20. Botney, M.D., et al., *Active collagen synthesis by pulmonary arteries in human primary pulmonary hypertension*. Am J Pathol, 1993. **143**(1): p. 121–9.
21. Prosser, I.W., et al., *Regional heterogeneity of elastin and collagen gene expression in intralobar arteries in response to hypoxic pulmonary hypertension as demonstrated by in situ hybridization*. Am J Pathol, 1989. **135**(6): p. 1073–88.
22. Botney, M.D., et al., *Extracellular matrix protein gene expression in atherosclerotic hypertensive pulmonary arteries*. Am J Pathol, 1992. **140**(2): p. 357–64.
23. Plestina, R. and H.B. Stoner, *Pulmonary oedema in rats given monocrotaline pyrrole*. J Pathol, 1972. **106**(4): p. 235–49.
24. Hislop, A. and L. Reid, *Arterial changes in Crotalaria spectabilis-induced pulmonary hypertension in rats*. Br J Exp Pathol, 1974. **55**(2): p. 153–63.
25. Todorovich-Hunter, L., et al., *Increased pulmonary artery elastolytic activity in adult rats with monocrotaline-induced progressive hypertensive pulmonary vascular disease compared with infant rats with nonprogressive disease*. Am Rev Respir Dis, 1992. **146**(1): p. 213–23.
26. Wilson, D.W., et al., *Mechanisms and pathology of monocrotaline pulmonary toxicity*. Crit Rev Toxicol, 1992. **22**(5–6): p. 307–25.
27. Maruyama, K., et al., *Chronic hypoxic pulmonary hypertension in rats and increased elastolytic activity*. Am J Physiol, 1991. **261**(6 Pt 2): p. H1716–26.
28. Zhu, L., et al., *The endogenous vascular elastase that governs development and progression of monocrotaline-induced pulmonary hypertension in rats is a novel enzyme related to the serine proteinase adipsin*. J Clin Invest, 1994. **94**(3): p. 1163–71.
29. Ilkiw, R., et al., *SC-39026, a serine elastase inhibitor, prevents muscularization of peripheral arteries, suggesting a mechanism of monocrotaline-induced pulmonary hypertension in rats*. Circ Res, 1989. **64**(4): p. 814–25.
30. Ye, C.L. and M. Rabinovitch, *Inhibition of elastolysis by SC-37698 reduces development and progression of monocrotaline pulmonary hypertension*. Am J Physiol, 1991. **261**(4 Pt 2): p. H1255–67.
31. Bieth, J.G., *Mechanism of action of elastases.*, in *Elastin and elastases*. 1989, CRC Press Inc.: Boca Raton.
32. Kobayashi, J., et al., *Serum-induced vascular smooth muscle cell elastolytic activity through tyrosine kinase intracellular signalling*. J Cell Physiol, 1994. **160**(1): p. 121–31.
33. Mohacsi, A., et al., *[Serum elastin peptide concentration and human leukocyte elastase/antiproteinase balance in peripheral obstructive atherosclerosis]*. Orv Hetil, 1996. **137**(1): p. 15–21.
34. Blann, A.D., et al., *Neutrophil elastase, von Willebrand factor, soluble thrombomodulin and percutaneous oxygen in peripheral atherosclerosis*. Eur J Vasc Endovasc Surg, 1996. **12**(2): p. 218–22.
35. Salvesen G, T.J., *Properties of natural occuring leastase inhibitors.*, in *Elastin and elastases*. 1989, CRC Press Inc.: Boca Raton.
36. Sallenave, J.M. and A. Silva, *Characterization and gene sequence of the precursor of elafin, an elastase-specific inhibitor in bronchial secretions*. Am J Respir Cell Mol Biol, 1993. **8**(4): p. 439–45.

37. Robert, L., A.M. Robert, and B. Jacotot, *Elastin-elastase-atherosclerosis revisited.* Atherosclerosis, 1998. **140**(2): p. 281–95.

38. Rao, S.K., et al., *Reduced capacity to inhibit elastase in abdominal aortic aneurysm.* J Surg Res, 1999. **82**(1): p. 24–7.

39. Oho, S., et al., *Increased elastin-degrading activity and neointimal formation in porcine aortic organ culture. Reduction of both features with a serine proteinase inhibitor.* Arterioscler Thromb Vasc Biol, 1995. **15**(12): p. 2200–6.

40. Oho, S. and M. Rabinovitch, *Post-cardiac transplant arteriopathy in piglets is associated with fragmentation of elastin and increased activity of a serine elastase.* Am J Pathol, 1994. **145**(1): p. 202–10.

41. Zaidi, S.H., et al., *Targeted overexpression of elafin protects mice against cardiac dysfunction and mortality following viral myocarditis.* J Clin Invest, 1999. **103**(8): p. 1211–9.

42. Zaidi, S.H., et al., *Suppressed smooth muscle proliferation and inflammatory cell invasion after arterial injury in elafin-overexpressing mice.* J Clin Invest, 2000. **105**(12): p. 1687–95.

43. O'Blenes, S.B., et al., *Gene transfer of the serine elastase inhibitor elafin protects against vein graft degeneration.* Circulation, 2000. **102**(19 Suppl 3): p. III289–95.

44. Thompson, K., et al., *Endothelial and serum factors which include apolipoprotein A1 tether elastin to smooth muscle cells inducing serine elastase activity via a tyrosine kinase-mediated transcription and translation.* J Cell Physiol, 1998. **174**(1): p. 78–89.

45. Nuchprayoon, I., et al., *PEBP2/CBF, the murine homolog of the human myeloid AML1 and PEBP2 beta/CBF beta proto-oncoproteins, regulates the murine myeloperoxidase and neutrophil elastase genes in immature myeloid cells.* Mol Cell Biol, 1994. **14**(8): p. 5558–68.

46. Wigle, D.A., et al., *AML1-like transcription factor induces serine elastase activity in ovine pulmonary artery smooth muscle cells.* Circ Res, 1998. **83**(3): p. 252–63.

47. Kuzuya, M. and A. Iguchi, *Role of matrix metalloproteinases in vascular remodeling.* J Atheroscler Thromb, 2003. **10**(5): p. 275–82.

48. Aimes, R.T. and J.P. Quigley, *Matrix metalloproteinase-2 is an interstitial collagenase. Inhibitor-free enzyme catalyzes the cleavage of collagen fibrils and soluble native type I collagen generating the specific 3/4- and 1/4-length fragments.* J Biol Chem, 1995. **270**(11): p. 5872–6.

49. Okada, Y., et al., *Localization of matrix metalloproteinase 9 (92-kilodalton gelatinase/type IV collagenase = gelatinase B) in osteoclasts: implications for bone resorption.* Lab Invest, 1995. **72**(3): p. 311–22.

50. Kahari, V.M. and U. Saarialho-Kere, *Matrix metalloproteinases in skin.* Exp Dermatol, 1997. **6**(5): p. 199–213.

51. Libby, P., *Molecular bases of the acute coronary syndromes.* Circulation, 1995. **91**(11): p. 2844–50.

52. Ross, R., *The pathogenesis of atherosclerosis: a perspective for the 1990s.* Nature, 1993. **362**(6423): p. 801–9.

53. Dollery, C.M., J.R. McEwan, and A.M. Henney, *Matrix metalloproteinases and cardiovascular disease.* Circ Res, 1995. **77**(5): p. 863–8.

54. Celentano, D.C. and W.H. Frishman, *Matrix metalloproteinases and coronary artery disease: a novel therapeutic target.* J Clin Pharmacol, 1997. **37**(11): p. 991–1000.

55. Galis, Z.S., et al., *Increased expression of matrix metalloproteinases and matrix degrading activity in vulnerable regions of human atherosclerotic plaques.* J Clin Invest, 1994. **94**(6): p. 2493–503.

56. Knox, J.B., et al., *Evidence for altered balance between matrix metalloproteinases and their inhibitors in human aortic diseases.* Circulation, 1997. **95**(1): p. 205–12.

57. Carmeliet, P., et al., *Urokinase-generated plasmin activates matrix metalloproteinases during aneurysm formation.* Nat Genet, 1997. **17**(4): p. 439–44.

58. Newman, K.M., et al., *Cellular localization of matrix metalloproteinases in the abdominal aortic aneurysm wall.* J Vasc Surg, 1994. **20**(5): p. 814–20.

59. Patel, M.I., et al., *Increased synthesis of matrix metalloproteinases by aortic smooth muscle cells is implicated in the etiopathogenesis of abdominal aortic aneurysms.* J Vasc Surg, 1996. **24**(1): p. 82–92.

60. Strauss, B.H., et al., *Extracellular matrix remodeling after balloon angioplasty injury in a rabbit model of restenosis.* Circ Res, 1994. **75**(4): p. 650–8.

61. Strauss, B.H., et al., *In vivo collagen turnover following experimental balloon angioplasty injury and the role of matrix metalloproteinases.* Circ Res, 1996. **79**(3): p. 541–50.

62. Barolet, A.W., et al., *Arterial elastase activity after balloon angioplasty and effects of elafin, an elastase inhibitor.* Arterioscler Thromb Vasc Biol, 2001. **21**(8): p. 1269–74.

63. Bendeck, M.P., et al., *Smooth muscle cell migration and matrix metalloproteinase expression after arterial injury in the rat.* Circ Res, 1994. **75**(3): p. 539–45.

64. Zempo, N., et al., *Matrix metalloproteinases of vascular wall cells are increased in balloon-injured rat carotid artery.* J Vasc Surg, 1994. **20**(2): p. 209–17.

65. Tyagi, S.C., et al., *Proteinases and restenosis in the human coronary artery: extracellular matrix production exceeds the expression of proteolytic activity.* Atherosclerosis, 1995. **116**(1): p. 43–57.

66. Bendeck, M.P., C. Irvin, and M.A. Reidy, *Inhibition of matrix metalloproteinase activity inhibits smooth muscle cell migration but not neointimal thickening after arterial injury.* Circ Res, 1996. **78**(1): p. 38–43.

67. Zempo, N., et al., *Regulation of vascular smooth muscle cell migration and proliferation in vitro and in injured rat arteries by a synthetic matrix metalloproteinase inhibitor.* Arterioscler Thromb Vasc Biol, 1996. **16**(1): p. 28–33.

68. Thompson, K. and M. Rabinovitch, *Exogenous leukocyte and endogenous elastases can mediate mitogenic activity in pulmonary artery smooth muscle cells by release of extracellular-matrix bound basic fibroblast growth factor.* J Cell Physiol, 1996. **166**(3): p. 495–505.

69. Jones, P.L., K.N. Cowan, and M. Rabinovitch, *Tenascin-C, proliferation and subendothelial fibronectin in progressive pulmonary vascular disease.* Am J Pathol, 1997. **150**(4): p. 1349–60.

70. Jones, P.L. and M. Rabinovitch, *Tenascin-C is induced with progressive pulmonary vascular disease in rats and is functionally related to increased smooth muscle cell proliferation.* Circ Res, 1996. **79**(6): p. 1131–42.

71. Jones, P.L., J. Crack, and M. Rabinovitch, *Regulation of tenascin-C, a vascular smooth muscle cell survival factor that interacts with the alpha v beta 3 integrin to promote epidermal growth factor receptor phosphorylation and growth.* J Cell Biol, 1997. **139**(1): p. 279–93.

72. Feng, Y., et al., *Transcriptional profile of mechanically induced genes in human vascular smooth muscle cells.* Circ Res, 1999. **85**(12): p. 1118–23.

73. Chung, C.Y., J.E. Murphy-Ullrich, and H.P. Erickson, *Mitogenesis, cell migration, and loss of focal adhesions induced by tenascin-C interacting with its cell surface receptor, annexin II.* Mol Biol Cell, 1996. **7**(6): p. 883–92.

74. Chung, C.Y. and H.P. Erickson, *Cell surface annexin II is a high affinity receptor for the alternatively spliced segment of tenascin-C.* J Cell Biol, 1994. **126**(2): p. 539–48.

75. End, P., et al., *Tenascin: a modulator of cell growth.* Eur J Biochem, 1992. **209**(3): p. 1041–51.

76. Rabinovitch, M., *Elastase and the pathobiology of unexplained pulmonary hypertension.* Chest, 1998. **114**(3 Suppl): p. 213S–224S.

77. Zhu, L., et al., *A developmentally regulated program restricting insolubilization of elastin and formation of laminae in the fetal lamb ductus arteriosus*. Lab Invest, 1993. **68**(3): p. 321–31.

78. Hinek, A., S. Molossi, and M. Rabinovitch, *Functional interplay between interleukin-1 receptor and elastin binding protein regulates fibronectin production in coronary artery smooth muscle cells*. Exp Cell Res, 1996. **225**(1): p. 122–31.

79. Cowan, B., et al., *Elafin, a serine elastase inhibitor, attenuates post-cardiac transplant coronary arteriopathy and reduces myocardial necrosis in rabbits after heterotopic cardiac transplantation*. J Clin Invest, 1996. **97**(11): p. 2452–68.

80. Yanagisawa, H., et al., *Fibulin-5 is an elastin-binding protein essential for elastic fibre development in vivo*. Nature, 2002. **415**(6868): p. 168–71.

81. Nakamura, T., et al., *Fibulin-5/DANCE is essential for elastogenesis in vivo*. Nature, 2002. **415**(6868): p. 171–5.

82. Nakamura, T., et al., *DANCE, a novel secreted RGD protein expressed in developing, atherosclerotic, and balloon-injured arteries*. J Biol Chem, 1999. **274**(32): p. 22476–83.

83. Kowal, R.C., et al., *EVEC, a novel epidermal growth factor-like repeat-containing protein upregulated in embryonic and diseased adult vasculature*. Circ Res, 1999. **84**(10): p. 1166–76.

84. Evan, G. and T. Littlewood, *A matter of life and cell death*. Science, 1998. **281**(5381): p. 1317–22.

85. Michel, J.B., *Anoikis in the cardiovascular system: known and unknown extracellular mediators*. Arterioscler Thromb Vasc Biol, 2003. **23**(12): p. 2146–54.

86. Ingber, D.E., *Mechanical signaling and the cellular response to extracellular matrix in angiogenesis and cardiovascular physiology*. Circ Res, 2002. **91**(10): p. 877–87.

87. Gartner, S. and H.S. Kaplan, *Long-term culture of human bone marrow cells*. Proc Natl Acad Sci U S A, 1980. **77**(8): p. 4756–9.

88. Tzima, E., et al., *Activation of integrins in endothelial cells by fluid shear stress mediates Rho-dependent cytoskeletal alignment*. Embo J, 2001. **20**(17): p. 4639–47.

89. Howe, A.K., A.E. Aplin, and R.L. Juliano, *Anchorage-dependent ERK signaling–mechanisms and consequences*. Curr Opin Genet Dev, 2002. **12**(1): p. 30–5.

90. Han, D.K., et al., *Evidence for apoptosis in human atherogenesis and in a rat vascular injury model*. Am J Pathol, 1995. **147**(2): p. 267–77.

91. Isner, J.M., et al., *Apoptosis in human atherosclerosis and restenosis*. Circulation, 1995. **91**(11): p. 2703–11.

92. Kockx, M.M., et al., *Foam cell replication and smooth muscle cell apoptosis in human saphenous vein grafts*. Histopathology, 1994. **25**(4): p. 365–71.

93. Clowes, A.W., M.A. Reidy, and M.M. Clowes, *Kinetics of cellular proliferation after arterial injury. I. Smooth muscle growth in the absence of endothelium*. Lab Invest, 1983. **49**(3): p. 327–33.

94. Perlman, H., et al., *Evidence for the rapid onset of apoptosis in medial smooth muscle cells after balloon injury*. Circulation, 1997. **95**(4): p. 981–7.

95. Kocher, O., et al., *Cytoskeleton of rat aortic smooth muscle cells. Normal conditions and experimental intimal thickening*. Lab Invest, 1984. **50**(6): p. 645–52.

96. Bochaton-Piallat, M.L., et al., *Apoptosis participates in cellularity regulation during rat aortic intimal thickening*. Am J Pathol, 1995. **146**(5): p. 1059–64.

97. Flynn, P.D., et al., *Thrombin generation by apoptotic vascular smooth muscle cells*. Blood, 1997. **89**(12): p. 4378–84.

98. Bombeli, T., et al., *Apoptotic vascular endothelial cells become procoagulant*. Blood, 1997. **89**(7): p. 2429–42.

99. Bennett, M.R. and J.J. Boyle, *Apoptosis of vascular smooth muscle cells in atherosclerosis*. Atherosclerosis, 1998. **138**(1): p. 3–9.

100. Cowan, K.N., P.L. Jones, and M. Rabinovitch, *Regression of hypertrophied rat pulmonary arteries in organ culture is associated with suppression of proteolytic activity, inhibition of tenascin-C, and smooth muscle cell apoptosis*. Circ Res, 1999. **84**(10): p. 1223–33.

101. O'Blenes, S.B., et al., *Hemodynamic unloading leads to regression of pulmonary vascular disease in rats*. J Thorac Cardiovasc Surg, 2001. **121**(2): p. 279–89.

102. Cowan, K.N., et al., *Complete reversal of fatal pulmonary hypertension in rats by a serine elastase inhibitor*. Nat Med, 2000. **6**(6): p. 698–702.

103. Merklinger, S.L., et al., *Epidermal growth factor receptor blockade mediates smooth muscle cell apoptosis and improves survival in rats with pulmonary hypertension*. Circulation, 2005. **112**(3): p. 423–31.

104. Campbell, A.I., et al., *Cell-based gene transfer of vascular endothelial growth factor attenuates monocrotaline-induced pulmonary hypertension*. Circulation, 2001. **104**(18): p. 2242–8.

105. Indolfi, C., et al., *Effects of hydroxymethylglutaryl coenzyme A reductase inhibitor simvastatin on smooth muscle cell proliferation in vitro and neointimal formation in vivo after vascular injury*. J Am Coll Cardiol, 2000. **35**(1): p. 214–21.

106. Nishimura, T., et al., *Simvastatin rescues rats from fatal pulmonary hypertension by inducing apoptosis of neointimal smooth muscle cells*. Circulation, 2003. **108**(13): p. 1640–5.

107. Laufs, U., V.L. Fata, and J.K. Liao, *Inhibition of 3-hydroxy-3-methylglutaryl (HMG)-CoA reductase blocks hypoxia-mediated down-regulation of endothelial nitric oxide synthase*. J Biol Chem, 1997. **272**(50): p. 31725–9.

108. Dimmeler, S., et al., *HMG-CoA reductase inhibitors (statins) increase endothelial progenitor cells via the PI 3-kinase/Akt pathway*. J Clin Invest, 2001. **108**(3): p. 391–7.

Pulmonary Arterial Hypertension: Genetics and Gene Therapy

6

Paul E. Szmitko and Duncan J. Stewart

6.1 Introduction

The pulmonary circulation differs considerably from its systemic counterpart. The delicate pulmonary microvasculature consists mainly of an endothelial monolayer, with scant support from the matrix, and incomplete muscularization. Under normal circumstances, the pulmonary vascular bed functions as a high-flow, low-impedance system that must accommodate the entire cardiac output with low arterial pressures [1]. In patients with pulmonary arterial hypertension, in contrast, this unique hemodynamic system is compromised due to vasoconstriction, the narrowing of arterioles, and the obliteration and remodeling of the pulmonary microvessels leading to a progressive and persistent elevation in pulmonary arterial pressure [2]. Clinically, pulmonary arterial hypertension is defined as a sustained elevation of pulmonary arterial pressure to more than 25 mmHg at rest, or to more than 30 mmHg with exercise [3]. Despite improvements in symptomatic treatments, no current therapy can improve the underlying pathological abnormalities of this devastating condition. As our insight into the pathogenesis of its *primary* or idiopathic form evolves, it is hoped that a better understanding of the complex molecular pathways that interact to maintain the homeostatic balance of the pulmonary vascular bed will lead to the development of innovative new strategies that may provide clinicians with the ability not only to stabilize, but also to reverse, the progression of the disease.

6.2 The Precapillary Arterioles: The "Achilles' Heel" of the Lung Vasculature?

The pathobiology behind the development of pulmonary arterial hypertension remains elusive. It is widely held to be instigated by perturbations in the normal relationships between vasodilators and vasoconstrictors, and inhibitors of growth and mitogenic factors, which affect endothelial homeostasis [3]. The primary feature is a striking reduction in the pulmonary microcirculation, particularly at the level of the distal arteriolar bed [2]. The precapillary arterioles, which consist primarily of endothelial cells with and scant support from the matrix, are little more than endothelial tubes. Coupled with the paucity in surrounding smooth muscle cells, the rather fragile, distal pulmonary arteriole structure makes it susceptible to regression upon exposure to endothelial stress [4]. Damage to the endothelium at the level of the precapillary arterioles could then result in vascular discontinuity, progressively leading to the exclusion of alveolar–capillary units from the pulmonary circulation [5]. In the monocrotaline-induced model of pulmonary hypertension model, the loss of precapillary arteriolar continuity, in part by apoptosis of the endothelial cells, precedes the development of hypertension [5]. As more alveolar–capillary units are excluded from the pulmonary circulation, the cross-sectional microvascular area is reduced, and ultimately the pulmonary pressure rises, with the onset of pulmonary arterial hypertension.

In addition to this loss of pulmonary microvessels, the pathological features include hypertrophy of the layers of medial smooth muscle, hypertrophy and fibrosis of the intima, and occasionally the appearance of plexiform lesions, which often occur distal to regions of arteriolar occlusion [1]. Postmortem investigations revealed that children with pulmonary arterial hypertension had more pulmonary vascular medial hypertrophy, and less intimal fibrosis and fewer plexiform lesions, than their adult counterparts [6]. These observations suggest that pulmonary arterial remodeling may predominate in earlier stages of

P.E. Szmitko (✉)
Department of Internal Medicine, St Michael's Hospital, University of Toronto, Toronto, ON, Canada

disease, with increased intimal fibrosis and hyperproliferative plexiform lesions dominating in advanced stages of disease. An important component of these plexiform lesions appears to be hyperproliferative endothelial cells, sometimes monoclonal, that may emerge secondary to selection pressures created by early loss of endothelial cells and arteriolar occlusion [7, 8]. Efforts to prevent proliferation of the endothelial cells in experimental models of hypoxia-induced pulmonary hypertension by blocking vascular endothelial growth factor receptor-2 resulted in a paradoxical worsening in pulmonary arterial remodeling [9]. These detrimental changes were abrogated with the co-administration of an inhibitor of lung cell apoptosis, the broad-spectrum caspase inhibitor Z-Asp-2,6-dichlorobenzoyloxymethylketone, suggesting an important role for vascular endothelial growth factor in the maintenance of the surviving endothelial cells [9]. These observations raise the possibility that the abnormalities of the pulmonary vasculature may be secondary to inheritable or acquired mutations of genes involved in regulating the survival, proliferation, and differentiation of vascular cells. Unlocking the molecular processes behind these complex vascular changes will likely lead to potential therapeutic targets.

6.3 Genetic Abnormalities in Idiopathic Pulmonary Arterial Hypertension

New insights into the pathogenesis of pulmonary hypertension have emerged from an examination of the genes involved in familial pulmonary arterial hypertension. The familial form accounts for at least 6% of all cases [3]. Germline mutations in the familial form have been mapped to a single locus on chromosome 2q31–32 [10]. In approximately two-fifths of familial cases, mutations were found in the open reading frame of the bone morphogenetic protein receptor-2 gene [11–13]. More than 45 different mutations in the gene have been identified, with some point mutations resulting in a loss of receptor function, which may have different effects depending on the cell type involved [14, 15]. It is likely that the mutations alone are not sufficient for the clinical expression of pulmonary arterial hypertension, but likely make the individual more susceptible to developing the condition [16].

The gene belongs to the transforming growth factor superfamily of transmembrane serine/threonine kinase receptors that are expressed ubiquitously by a wide variety of different cell types, including both pulmonary arterial smooth muscle and endothelial cells. Signal transduction by bone morphogenetic proteins involves heterodimerization of BMPR2 with the type 1 BMP receptor. Activation

of BMPR1 results in the phosphorylation of downstream regulatory proteins, Smad (mothers against decapentaplegic) proteins (R-Smad: 1, 5, and 8), which then dimerize with Smad-4 (coSmad). The resulting complex is then translocated to the nucleus, where it regulates the transcription of target genes containing the Smad-binding sequences (5′-CAGAC-3′ and 5′-GTCTG-3′) in their promoter, among which are genes that control survival and proliferation of cells [8, 17].

In pulmonary arterial smooth muscle cells isolated from normal subjects, bone morphogenetic proteins inhibited the cellular proliferation and induced apoptosis. These observed effects were reduced in smooth muscle cells derived from patients with idiopathic pulmonary arterial hypertension [18, 19]. The antiproliferative and proapoptotic effects of bone morphogenetic proteins in normal pulmonary arterial smooth muscle cells could result in the maintenance of a normal, thin pulmonary vascular wall by preserving a balance in the ratio of proliferation as compared to apoptosis. In patients with idiopathic pulmonary arterial hypertension, however, impairment in signaling could lead to excessive pulmonary arterial muscularization by reducing apoptosis and promoting growth. In contrast, bone morphogenetic proteins protect against apoptosis in both human pulmonary arterial endothelial cells and their progenitor cells [20], circulating stem cells derived from the bone marrow which possess the ability to differentiate into functional and mature endothelial cells [21]. Furthermore, reducing expression of BMPR2 using a small interfering RNA significantly increased apoptosis in human pulmonary arterial endothelial cells, supporting the hypothesis that loss-of-function mutations in BMPR2 could lead to increased death of pulmonary endothelial cells [20]. Thus, taken together, the opposite consequences of mutations of BMPR2 in the two primary vascular cell types may jointly contribute to the development of pulmonary arterial hypertension. Increased apoptosis of endothelial cells leading to the loss of distal arteriolar integrity may serve as an initiating trigger. Subsequently, enhanced pulmonary arteriolar remodeling may be driven mainly by overly exaggerated growth of smooth muscle cells, contributing to the full spectrum of pathology [8].

Heterozygous mice deficient in BMPR2, however, show only a very mild phenotype, with only a slight increase in pulmonary arterial pressures [22]. Furthermore, transgenic mice expressing a dominant-negative BMPR2 gene in smooth muscle cells have more substantial elevations in pulmonary arterial pressures, but do not develop significant increases in the extent of arteriolar muscularization [23]. Thus, these findings reinforce the concept that additional genetic or environmental factors in addition to BMPR2 mutations are likely required to develop pulmonary arterial hypertension.

In addition to the identified mutations in BMPR2, overexpression of the serotonin transporter 5-HTT has been found in specimens obtained from patients with idiopathic pulmonary arterial hypertension [24]. The L-allelic variant of the 5HTT gene appears to be more prevalent, and is associated with increased expression of the transporter, leading to increased serotonin-dependent proliferation of vascular smooth muscle cells [24]. Mutations in another member of the TGF-β receptor family, Alk-1, which has previously been implicated in hereditary hemorrhagic telangectasia, have also been recently linked to pulmonary arterial hypertension [25]. As expression of Alk-1 is largely restricted to the endothelium, this finding provides additional genetic evidence that abnormalities in endothelial cellular biology serve as the primary mechanism in the pathogenesis of this disease. As with mutations in BMPR2, mutations in Alk-1 are believed to result in growth-promoting Smad dependent signalling [3]. Since Alk-1 also signals via Smad 1/5/8, it is likely that genetic mutations in Alk-1 will also predispose individuals to microvascular loss of pulmonary endothelial cells.

6.4 Endothelial Cellular Apoptosis: The Initiating Event in Pulmonary Arterial Hypertension?

The sequence of cellular events behind the complex vascular changes associated with pulmonary hypertension is not entirely clear. It appears to be initiated by injury to the endothelial cells (See Fig. 6.1). In the normal lung, the vascular endothelium is believed to be quiescent. The lung microvasculature, nonetheless, is exposed directly to the environment with every breath, by virtue of its proximity to the distal airways. Thus, it is likely that periodically there are waves of damage to endothelial cells induced by exposure to toxins or other dangerous stimuli. Damage to the pulmonary endothelium subsequently stimulates proliferation, and/or recruitment of endothelial proliferative cells to mediate vascular repair, restoring the normal architecture to the pulmonary vasculature. Thus, in healthy individuals, endothelial function and microvascular structure is maintained by a continuous cycle of damage and repair to the endothelial cells.

If there is disruption to this delicate balance, the pulmonary vasculature may sustain permanent damage. Individuals with genetic mutations in BMPR2 are likely more susceptible to endothelial injury. In the context of severe environmental triggers, such as toxins, anorexigens, hypoxia, shear stress, and infection with the human immunodeficient virus, the level of endothelial injury sustained may overwhelm endogenous repairing mechanisms, which themselves may be impaired, and microvascular loss occurs. Specific factors for survival, such as bone morphogenetic proteins and possibly angiopoietin-1, may be essential for the maintenance of endothelial integrity and survival. Ang-1, a ligand of the endothelial-specific tyrosine kinase receptor Tie-2, has been shown to play an essential role in embryonic vascular development, like vascular endothelial growth factor, though at a later stage [26]. Ang-1 induces the activation of Tie-2, stimulating the Akt/phosphatidylinositol-3 kinase pathway, inhibiting apoptosis and functioning to recruit and sustain periendothelial support cells, allowing the endothelial cells to stabilize the structure of the vessels, modulate their function, and maintain microvascular homeostasis [27].

Apoptosis localized to the precapillary arterioles may lead not only to microvascular obliteration and dropout, but may also promote endothelial dysfunction, thus providing another mechanism that could contribute to abnormal vascular tone and remodeling. Endothelial dysfunction is a broad term that implies diminished production or availability of vasodilator mediators, such as nitric oxide and prostacyclin, and/or an imbalance in the relative contribution of endothelium-derived relaxing and contracting factors such as endothelin-1 and thromboxane [28]. An imbalance of vasodilatory and vasoconstrictive factors, including an altered ratio of thromboxane and prostacyclin [29], decreased expression of endothelial nitric oxide synthase [30], and increased endothelin-1 [31], have been reported in experimental and human pulmonary hypertension.

Nitric oxide and prostacyclin are both vasodilators with antiproliferative effects. Nitric oxide is a potent, endogenous, endothelium-derived vasodilator that directly relaxes vascular smooth muscle. It is produced by the sequential oxidation of the guanidino group at the N-terminus of L-arginine, mediated by nitric oxide synthases, of which eNOS appears to be the dominant form expressed in the lung [32, 33]. In addition to its vasodilatory properties, it is also a potent angiogenic agent, playing a critical role in postnatal angiogenesis [34]. It stimulates endothelial proliferation and migration, and eNOS has been implicated as a downstream mediator of Vegf in the angiogenic cascade [35]. Nitric oxide also appears to play a critical role in fetal lung vascular development, with mice deficient in eNOS having a phenotype characterized by a marked paucity of precapillary arterioles that closely resemble alveolar capillary dysplasia in humans [33, 36]. Nitric oxide has been shown both to inhibit the growth, and to promote apoptosis, of vascular smooth muscle cells [37, 38]. Likewise, prostacyclin or prostaglandin I₂, the main product of arachidonic acid in the vascular endothelium, induces

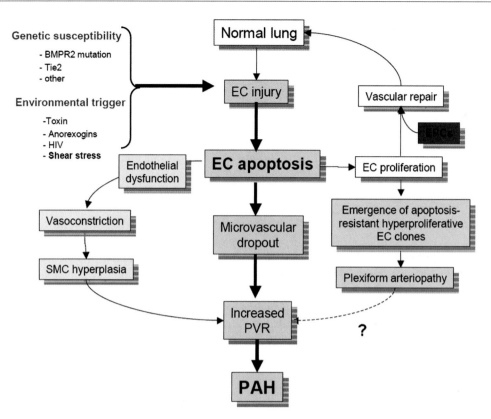

Fig. 6.1 The hypothesis relating idiopathic pulmonary arterial hypertension to apoptosis of endothelial cells. The normal pulmonary vascular endothelium is believed to be quiescent. The lung microvasculature, nonetheless, is constantly exposed to environmental insults that may lead to injury and death of endothelial cells (EC). In healthy individuals, the endothelium is repaired by proliferation of these cells, and likely recruitment of endothelial progenitor cells (EPC) to maintain the microvascular structure. In individuals with genetic mutations in BMPR2, however, who are more susceptible to injury of the endothelial cells, the level of endothelial damage sustained from environment triggers may overwhelm the endogenous repairing mechanisms, leading to endothelial dysfunction, excessive vasoconstriction, smooth muscle cell (SMC) hyperplasia, and microvascular dropout, which lead to increased pulmonary vascular resistance (PVR) and pulmonary artery hypertension (PAH). Once microvascular changes occur, plexiform lesions may develop, characterized by hyperproliferative endothelial cells that appear to be resistant to apoptosis

relaxation of vascular smooth muscle cells by stimulating the production of cyclic AMP, which inhibits both growth of the muscle cells and platelet activation [32, 39]. In pulmonary arterial hypertension, the production of prostacyclin synthase appears to be decreased in the small- and medium-sized pulmonary arteries [40]. Decreases in both nitric oxide and prostacyclin, combined with elevations in endothelin-1, a potent vasoconstrictor which stimulates the proliferation of pulmonary arterial smooth muscle cells [41], promote vasoconstriction and hyperplasia of the muscular cells. Coupled with microvascular dropout secondary to endothelial apoptosis, these molecular changes result in increased pulmonary vascular resistance, remodeling of the pulmonary microvasculature, and the eventual development and progression of pulmonary arterial hypertension.

Understanding the molecular pathways contributing to the vascular changes observed in idiopathic pulmonary arterial hypertension forms the basis for several of its current treatments. For example, prostacyclin therapy, endothelin-receptor antagonists, and phosphodiesterae type 5 inhibitors, which enhance pulmonary vasodilation dependent on nitric oxide, have been applied clinically [32]. Despite these advances, the prognosis remains poor. Novel therapeutic approaches capable of reversing vascular structural changes and regenerating pulmonary microvasculature are needed to restore healthy pulmonary hemodynamics in patients with advanced idiopathic pulmonary arterial hypertension.

6.5 Gene Therapy Approaches for Pulmonary Arterial Hypertension

Ideally, a treatment for any disease should result in a cure, or at the very least halt further progression. Understanding the cellular mechanisms behind development and identifying the genes involved presents targets for intervention. Genetic therapeutic strategies attempt to deliver functional copies of genes to tissues that may have nonfunctional genes or abnormal levels of a particular gene product. In pulmonary arterial hypertension, such strategies have primarily focused on improving the vasodilatory function of the endothelium, maintaining survival of the endothelial cells, or promoting an environment that is more conducive to restoring the normal pulmonary vasculature.

In order to transfer genes efficiently to the lung vasculature, different vector systems have been employed. One system entails the use of viral vectors, usually an adenovirus, adeno-associated virus, or negative strand RNA virus, to deliver the therapeutic gene to the target organ. An immune response develops which may limit subsequent treatments, and the cells transfected may not be the intended targets. Nevertheless, using a hemagglutinating virus of Japan-liposome method to transfer the gene for human prostacyclin synthase ameliorated pulmonary hypertension induced experimentally in rats [42]. The use of nonviral vectors for lung gene transfer includes delivery of naked plasmid DNA or liposomal gene transfer agents. Our group has successfully employed a cell-based gene transfer method in animal models of pulmonary arterial hypertension, whereby autologous cells transfected with the gene of interest are injected back into the subject. Various cell types have been employed, including smooth muscle cells, fibroblasts, and most recently, endothelial proliferative cells. The cells overexpressing the therapeutic gene are injected into the venous circulation and make their way to the distal pulmonary circulation, being trapped at the site of disease by the natural filtering properties of the pulmonary microvasculature. This approach may offer significant advantages over other strategies to achieve selective pulmonary vascular cell gene transfer as endotracheal gene delivery using either viral or nonviral vectors results predominantly in epithelial overexpression.

Since pulmonary arterial hypertension is characterized by increased pulmonary vascular resistance secondary to a decrease in the caliber and number of pulmonary vascular channels, the targeted overexpression of an angiogenic factor within the lung could potentially prevent the loss of existing vessels or induce the development of new vessels. Using a monocrotaline-induced rat model, syngeneic smooth muscle cells overexpressing Vegf were injected into rats simultaneously at the time of endothelial injury [43]. Four weeks after gene transfer, the plasmid VEGF transcript was still detectable in the pulmonary tissue of animals receiving the treatment, suggesting the survival of the delivered cells and persistent transgene expression. Also, transfer reduced caspase-3 activation,

a marker of apoptosis, in pulmonary arteriolar endothelium, suggesting it may prevent apoptotic cell loss induced by endothelial injury. The treated animals had significantly decreased right ventricular hypertension and hypertrophy, compared to controls, suggesting the treatment was effective in inhibiting the development of pulmonary arterial hypertension. Likewise, delayed transfer after the development of pulmonary hypertension also resulted in a significant decrease in the progression of right ventricular hypertension and hypertrophy [43].

Limiting apoptosis after endothelial injury is the basis for strategies involving the use of Ang-1 gene transfer. Smooth muscle cells from rat pulmonary arteries transfected with Ang-1 cDNA were injected into rats treated with monocrotaline at the time of endothelial injury [5]. Treatment resulted in increased apoptosis, mainly in the pulmonary microvasculature, reduced eNOS mRNA expression, and downregulated Tie-2 receptor expression. The cell-based gene transfer of Ang-1 significantly reduced right ventricular systolic pressure, as well as the measurement of right to left ventricular plus septal weight. These beneficial effects with Ang-1 gene transfer were accompanied by a significant reduction in apoptosis, and the restoration of Tie-2 and eNOS mRNA expression [5]. Similar findings with Ang-1 gene transfer were also observed in rats with hypoxia-induced pulmonary arterial hypertension [4].

Endothelial dysfunction, marked by the reduction in release of nitric oxide from the vascular endothelium, appears to assume a prominent role in facilitating the changes observed in idiopathic pulmonary arterial hypertension. Transfer of the cell-based eNOS gene to the pulmonary microvasculature attenuated the chronic increase in pulmonary arterial pressures in a monocrotaline model of pulmonary vascular remodeling [44]. Using a reversal model, in which gene therapy was delayed until 3 weeks after administration of monocrotaline, at which point pulmonary arterial hypertension and the associated vascular remodeling were well developed, delivery of syngeneic fibroblasts transfected with eNOS resulted in a reversal of established hypertension [45]. Cell-based transfer of the eNOS gene was found to be more effective than transfer of the Vegf gene. Transfer of eNOS significantly reduced right ventricular hypertrophy and systolic pressure at the 35th compared with the 21st day. Using fluorescent microangiography, widespread occlusion of the precapillary arterioles was observed at the 21st day after treatment. In the animals receiving the eNOS gene, however, a normal pattern of pulmonary microvasculature and alveolar capillary perfusion were seen on the 35th day, supporting the concept that the reestablishment of continuity between the pulmonary arterioles and the capillaries is an important mechanism for improving the hemodynamic abnormalities in experimental pulmonary arterial hypertension. Thus, promoting angiogenesis may serve as a potential therapeutic mechanism for pulmonary arterial hypertension.

To further promote therapeutic angiogenesis, endothelial progenitor cells have been utilized as the cell type for

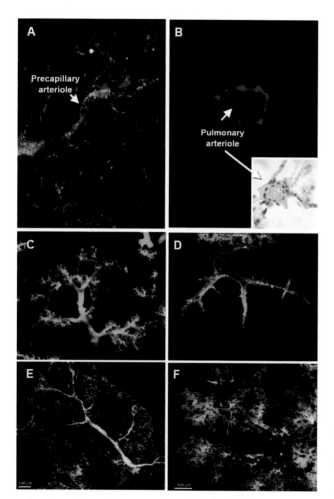

Fig. 6.2 Engraftment of endothelial progenitor cells into the lung microcirculation leads to re-endothelialization of distal arterioles and improves the appearance of the microvasculature. Progenitor cells (EPC) transfected with eNOS were injected into rats treated with monocrotaline. (**A**) Injected cells (*red*) were seen to engraft into the endothelial layer of distal precapillary arterioles as confirmed by fluorescent microangiography, where lung sections are perfused with fluorescent microspheres (*green*) suspended in agarose (*green*). (**B**) In some areas, complete luminal incorporation was observed. (**C–F**) Confocal projection images of lung sections perfused with fluorescent microspheres (*green*) and counterstained for α-smooth muscle actin (*red*). (**C**) Normal filling of the microvasculature is seen in control rats, whereas rats treated with monocrotaline showed a marked loss of microvascular perfusion and widespread precapillary occlusion 35 days after injection, (**D**) In the reversal model, eNOS-transfected cells dramatically improved the appearance of the pulmonary microvasculature (**F**) whereas infusion of cells alone resulted in more modest increases in perfusion and little noticeable reduction in arteriolar muscularization. (**E**) Scale bar 100 μm. Modified from reference #47

cell-based transfer of genes. Transplantation of such cells has been shown to inhibit the progression of pulmonary arterial hypertension induced by monocrotaline in the models depending on both prevention and reversal [46, 47]. The administration of the cells 3 days after treatment with monocrotaline nearly completely prevented the increase in right ventricular systolic pressure seen at 3 weeks with monocrotaline alone, while the injection of skin fibroblasts had no protective effect [47]. The delayed administration of progenitor cells 3 weeks after treatment with monocrotaline prevented further progression of pulmonary hypertension, albeit that only animals receiving progenitor cells transduced with human eNOS exhibited significant reversal of established disease at the 35th day compared with the 21st day. The mechanism of benefit appears to involve repair of the damaged lung mediated by the endothelial progenitor cells, and restoration of microvasculature structure and function (See Fig. 6.2) [47]. Thus, gene transfer based on endothelial progenitor cells provides both the cells required to repair endothelial damage as well as the overexpression of a therapeutic gene, such as eNOS, which provides the molecular environment to further promote angiogenesis, endothelial function, inhibition of smooth muscle cells, and survival of endothelial cells. Even though these novel therapeutic strategies have shown promising results in experimental animals, the key will be applying these techniques in patients, and assessing their utility.

6.6 From Bench to Bedside

The Pulmonary Hypertension and Cell Therapy (PHACeT) trial, currently underway at St. Michael's Hospital, Toronto, Canada, will assess the tolerability of cell-based gene therapy in patients with pulmonary arterial hypertension refractory to all standard therapies. Autologous-circulating endothelial progenitor cells are isolated from patients, cultured, and transfected with human eNOS via electroporation. The transfected autologous cells are then delivered via a Swan-Ganz catheter directly into the right ventricle. Up to 150×10^6 cells are delivered over a period of 3 days in divided doses, while the patient undergoes continuous hemodynamic monitoring. Early safety end-points, assessed prior to discharge from hospital, include testing for the presence of the transfected plasmid in the arterial circulation, and noting any hemodynamic changes or adverse reactions during administration of cells. Late safety end-points include overall survival, time to clinical worsening, and changes to pulmonary function tests, or echocardiography. Though not the primary goal of this study, efficacy is also assessed with all patients undergoing a repeated hemodynamic assessment 3 months after transfer of cells, an assessment of expired NO as a marker of activity of eNOS, a 6-min walk test, and a score for quality of life.

6.7 Conclusion

The ideal therapy for pulmonary arterial hypertension will reverse pathologic remodeling and restore a normal pulmonary vasculature. Understanding the molecular mechanisms that mediate the initiation and progression of the disease will provide directed therapeutic targets. Limiting the apoptosis of endothelial cells, and the resulting microvascular degeneration at the critical precapillary level, and promoting angiogenesis to reverse the exclusion of large portions of the pulmonary microvasculature from the pulmonary circulation will likely guide future therapies. Using endothelial progenitor cells to deliver the eNOS gene appears to be capable of addressing both these issues, with this approach being successful in animal models. The results of the ongoing PHACeT trial will determine if this therapeutic strategy is safe in the clinical situation, and hopefully, it will serve as the first step toward developing a treatment that can halt the progression and reverse the vascular changes in pulmonary arterial hypertension.

References

1. Gaine SP, Rubin LJ. Primary pulmonary hypertension. Lancet. 1998;352:719–25.
2. Widlitz A, Barst RJ. Pulmonary arterial hypertension in children. Eur Respir J. 2003;21:155–76.
3. Farber HW, Loscalzo J. Pulmonary arterial hypertension. N Engl J Med. 1004;351:1655–65.
4. Kugathasan L, Dutly AE, Zhao YD, et al. Role of angiopoietin-1 in experimental and human arterial hypertension. Chest. 2005;128:633S–642S.
5. Zhao YD, Campbell AI, Robb M, Ng D, Stewart DJ. Protective role of angiopoietin-1 in experimental pulmonary hypertension. Circ Res. 2003;92:984–91.
6. Wagenvoort CA, Wagenvoort N. Primary pulmonary hypertension. A pathological study of the lung vessels in 156 clinically diagnosed cases. Circulation. 1970;42:1163–84.
7. Lee SD, Shroyer KR, Markham NE, et al. Monoclonal endothelial cell proliferation is present in primary but not secondary pulmonary hypertension. J Clin Invest. 1998;101: 927–34.
8. Stewart DJ. Bone morphogenic protein receptor-2 and pulmonary arterial hypertension. Unraveling a riddle inside an enigma? Cir Res. 2005;96:1033–35.
9. Taraseviciene-Stewart L, Kasahara Y, Alger L, et al. Inhibition of the VEGF receptor 2 combined with chronic hypoxia causes cell death-dependent pulmonary endothelial cell proliferation and severe pulmonary hypertension. FASEB J. 2001;15: 427–38.
10. Nichols WC, Koller DL, Slovis B, et al. Localization of the gene for familial primary pulmonary hypertension to chromosome 2q31-32. Nat Genet. 1997;15:277–80.
11. Lane KB, Machado RD, Pauciulo MW, et al. Heterozygous germline mutations in BMPR2, encoding a TGF-beta receptor, cause familial primary pulmonary hypertension. The International PPH Consortium. Nat Genet. 2000; 26:81–4.
12. Machado RD, Pauciulo MW, Thomson JR, et al. BMPR2 haploinsufficiency as the inherited molecular mechanism for primary pulmonary hypertension. Am J Hum Genet. 2001;68:92–102.
13. Deng Z, Morse JH, Slager SL, et al. Familial primary pulmonary hypertension (gene PPH1) is caused by mutations in the bone morphogenetic protein receptor-II gene. Am J Hum Genet. 2000;67:737–44.
14. Newman JH, Wheeler L, Lane KB, et al. Mutation in the gene for bone morphogenetic protein receptor II as a cause of primary pulmonary hypertension in a large kindred. N Engl J Med. 2001;345:319–24. [Errata, N Engl J Med. 2001;345: 1506, 2002;346:1258.]
15. Newman JH, Trembath RC, Morse JA, et al. Genetic basis of pulmonary arterial hypertension: current understanding and future directions. J Am Coll Cardiol. 2004;43:Suppl S:33S–39S.
16. Yuan JX, Rubin LJ. Pathogenesis of pulmonary arterial hypertension. The need for multiple hits. Circulation. 2005;111: 534–38.
17. Shi Y, Massague J. Mechanisms of TGF-beta signaling from cell membrane to the nucleus. Cell. 2003;113:685–700.
18. Zhang S, Fantozzi I, Tigno DD, et al. Bone morphogenetic proteins induce apoptosis in human pulmonary vascular smooth muscle cells. Am J Physiol Lung Cell Mol Physiol. 2003;285:L740–54.
19. Morrell NW, Yang X, Upton PD, et al. Altered growth responses of pulmonary artery smooth muscle cells from patients with primary pulmonary hypertension to transforming growth factor-beta(1) and bone morphogenetic proteins. Circulation. 2001;104:790–5.
20. Teichert-Kuliszewska K, Kutryk MJ, Kuliszewski MA, et al. Bone morphogenetic protein receptor-2 signaling promotes pulmonary arterial endothelial cell survival. Implications for loss-of-function mutations in the pathogenesis of pulmonary hypertension. Circ Res. 2006;98:209–217.
21. Szmitko PE, Fedak PWM, Weisel RD, et al. Endothelial Progenitor Cells: New hope for a broken heart. Circulation. 2003;107:3093–100.
22. Beppu H, Ishinose F, Kawai N, et al. BMPR-II heterozygous mice have mild pulmonary hypertension and an impaired pulmonary vascular remodeling response to prolonged hypoxia. Am J Physiol Lung Cell Mol Physiol. 2004;287: L1241–47.
23. West J, Fagan K, Steudel W, et al. Pulmonary hypertension in transgenic mice expressing a dominant-negative BMPRII gene in smooth muscle. Circ Res. 2004;94:1109–114.
24. Eddahibi S, Humbert M, Fadel E, et al. Serotonin transporter overexpression is responsible for pulmonary artery smooth muscle hyperplasia in primary pulmonary hypertension. J Clin Invest. 2001;108:1141–50.
25. Harrison RE, Flanagan JA, Sankelo M, et al. Molecular and functional analysis identifies ALK-1 as the predominant cause of pulmonary hypertension related to hereditary haemorrhagic telangiectasia. J Med Genet. 2003;40:865–71.
26. Gale NW, Yancopoulos GD. Growth factors acting via endothelial cell-specific receptor tyrosine kinases: VEGFs, angiopoietins, and ephrins in vascular development. Genes Dev. 1999;13:1055–66.
27. Kim I, Kim HG, So JN, et al. Angiopoietin-1 regulates endothelial cell survival through the phosphatidylinositol 3'-kinase/Akt signal transduction pathway. Circ Res. 2000;86:24–9.

28. Verma S, Anderson TJ. Fundamentals of endothelial function for the clinical cardiologist. Circulation. 2002;105:546–9.

29. Christman BW, McPherson CD, Newman JH, et al. An imbalance between the excretion of thromboxane and prostacyclin metabolites in pulmonary hypertension. N Engl J Med. 1992;327:70–5.

30. Giadi A, Saleh D. Reduced expression of endothelial nitric oxide synthase in the lungs of patients with pulmonary hypertension. N Engl J Med. 1995;333:214–21.

31. Giaid A, Yanagisawa M, Langleben D, et al. Expression of endothelin-1 in the lungs of patients with pulmonary hypertension. N Engl J Med. 1993;328:1732–39.

32. Humbert M, Sitbon O, Simonneau G. Treatment of pulmonary arterial hypertension. N Engl J Med. 2004:351:1425–36.

33. Han RN, Stewart DJ. Defective lung vascular development in endothelial nitric oxide synthase-deficient mice. Trends Cardiovasc Med. 2006;16:29–34.

34. Aicher A, Heeschen C, Mildner-Rihm C, et al. Essential role of endothelial nitric oxide synthase for mobilzation of stem and progenitor cells. Nat Med. 2003;9:1370–76.

35. Ziche M, Morbidelli L, Choudhuri R, et al. Nitric oxide synthase lies downstream from vascular endothelial growth factor-induced but not basic fibroblast growth factor-induced angiogenesis. J Clin Invest. 1997;99:2625–34.

36. Han RN, Babaei S, Robb M, et al. Defective lung vascular development and fatal respiratory distress in endothelial NO synthase-deficient mice: A model of alveolar capillary dysplasia? Circ Res. 2004;94:1115–23.

37. Sato J, Nair K, Hiddinga J, et al. eNOS gene transfer to vascular smooth muscle cells inhibits cell proliferation via upregulation of p27 and p21 and not apoptosis. Cardiovasc Res. 2000;47:697–706.

38. Ambalavanan N, Mariani G, Bulger A, Philips JB III. Role of nitric oxide in regulating neonatal procine pulmonary artery smooth muscle cell proliferation. Biol Neonate. 1999;76:291–300.

39. Clapp LH, Finney P, Turcato S, et al. Differential effects of stable prostacyclin analogues on smooth muscle proliferation and cyclic AMP generation in human pulmonary artery. Am J Respir Cell Mol Biol. 2002;26:194–201.

40. Tuder RM, Coo CD, Geraci MW, et al. Prostacyclin synthase expression is decreased in lungs from patients with severe pulmonary hypertension. Am J Respir Crit Care Med. 1999;159: 1925–32.

41. Hassoun PM, Thappa V, Landman MJ, Fanburg BL. Endothelin 1 mitogenic activity on pulmonary artery smooth muscle cells and release from hypoxic endothelial cells. Proc Soc Exp Biol Med. 1992;199:165–70.

42. Nagaya N, Yokoyama C, Kyotani S, et al. Gene transfer of human prostacyclin synthase ameliorates monocrotaline-induced pulmonary hypertension in rats. Circulation. 2000; 102:2005–2010.

43. Campbell AI, Zhao Y, Sandu R, Stewart DJ. Cell-based gene transfer of vascular endothelial growth factor attenuates monocrotaline-induced pulmonary hypertension. Circulation. 2001;104:2242–48.

44. Campbell AI, Kuliszewski MA, Stewart DJ. Cell-based gene transfer to the pulmonary vasculature: endothelial nitric oxide synthase overexpression inhibits monocrotaline-induced pulmonary hypertension. Am J Respir Cell Mol Biol. 1999;21: 567–75.

45. Zhao YD, Courtman DW, Ng DS, et al. Microvascular regeneration in established pulmonary hypertension by angiogenic gene transfer. Am J Respir Cell Mol Biol. 2006;35:182–89.

46. Nagaya N, Kangawa K, Kanda M, et al. Hybrid cell-gene therapy for pulmonary hypertension based on phagocytosing action of endothelial progenitor cells. Circulation. 2003; 108:889–95.

47. Zhao YD, Courtman DW, Deng Y, et al. Rescue of monocrotaline-induced pulmonary arterial hypertension using bone marrow-derived endothelial-like progenitor cells. Efficacy of combined cell and eNOS gene therapy in established disease. Circ Res. 2005;96:442–50.

Christopher K. Macgowan and Andrea Kassner

7.1 Introduction

A common consequence of cardiopulmonary disease is the disruption and redistribution of blood flow within the lungs. Chronic increases in pulmonary blood pressure and flow cause abnormal growth and function of the pulmonary vascular wall [1–3], and increased pulmonary vascular resistance [4, 5]. Eventually, irreversible dysfunction of the lungs and right ventricle can occur, so it is important to evaluate the function of the pulmonary vasculature in the early stages of pathological change [6, 7]. Because changes in flow likely precede gross remodeling, flow measurement may provide early information about disease progression and response to therapy [8]. Such hemodynamic information is relevant to the study of many pathologies ranging from pulmonary hypertension (PH) to chronic thromboembolism [9–11]. Furthermore, most of the hypoxemia and carbon dioxide retention observed in patients with various pulmonary diseases are caused by mismatching of ventilation and perfusion in the lung [12]. Therefore, the accurate estimation of pulmonary perfusion is important to understand physiology and pathophysiology of the lung.

At the Hospital for Sick Children, we have recently investigated how normal flow volumes and patterns are distributed through the main and branch pulmonary arteries in both normal subjects and those with congenital heart disease [13, 14]. This chapter introduces the related topic of *perfusion* – blood flow in the parenchymal microcirculation of the lungs. Because the definition of perfusion varies in the literature, we begin the chapter with a description of qualitative, semi-quantitative, and quantitative methods to assess pulmonary perfusion. The utility of different imaging modalities for the measurement of perfusion is then discussed. The chapter concludes with an overview of several recent publications pertaining to perfusion measurement in PH.

7.2 Definitions of Perfusion

The perfusion data obtained using different modalities can be qualitative (descriptive), semi-quantitative, or quantitative, depending on how the images are acquired and analyzed.

A. Qualitative methods include the subjective evaluation of diagnostic scans, relating the appearance of an image to a disease. An example of this is the mottled scintigraphy pattern obtained from scans of subjects with PH, indicative of an abnormal flow distribution [15].

B. Semi-quantitative methods do not attempt to measure absolute perfusion, but instead characterize the pathology based on other numerical properties of the images (which are often easier to measure). For example, the time-to-peak (TTP) concentration of contrast agent may indicate perfusion delays related to embolism. Although they do not provide values for absolute perfusion, such methods are often more clinically practical and may be useful for studying relative changes during therapy.

A common approach is to inject a short bolus of contrast agent into the venous system and then acquire time-resolved images of its passage through the pulmonary tree. To characterize perfusion, the enhancement curve in a parenchymal volume-of-interest, C_{VOI}, is fitted using the following expression for a gamma-variate function:

$$C_{VOI}(t) = A \cdot t^{\alpha} \cdot e^{-t/\beta}, \tag{7.1}$$

where A is a constant scaling factor, and α and β define the shape of the curve [16]. From the fit, the TTP and

C.K. Macgowan (✉)
Department of Medical Biophysics & Medical Imaging, Hospital for Sick Children, Toronto, ON, Canada

A.N. Redington et al. (eds.), *Congenital Diseases in the Right Heart*, DOI 10.1007/978-1-84800-378-1_7,
© Springer-Verlag London Limited 2009

mean transit time (MTT) can be derived using the following two expressions:

$$TTP = \alpha \cdot \beta, \qquad (7.2)$$

$$MTT = \beta \cdot (\alpha + 1) \qquad (7.3)$$

An example of fitted pulmonary data is presented in Fig. 7.1. Note that the start and end points of the fitted data must be specified to define the first-pass of the contrast agent and to exclude data affected by recirculation. Provided the signal-to-noise ratio (SNR) is sufficient, this analysis can also be performed on a pixel-by-pixel basis rather than on VOIs, allowing spatial maps of TTP and MTT to be calculated.

In practice, more simplistic approaches for a semi-quantitative analysis of contrast-enhanced perfusion MR imaging data are used. They consist of the calculation of signal intensity time curves, SNR, and contrast-to-noise ratios (CNR) using region-of-interest (ROI) analysis of the signal of the lung tissue.

C. Quantitative methods attempt to measure absolute blood perfusion in mL/min per gram of tissue and blood volume in mL. An adult cardiac output of 5 L/min passing through lungs with a typical 2–3 L volume would create an average local perfusion of about 1.7–2.5 mL/min mL^{-1} of tissue.

An important hemodynamic parameter that can be obtained from contrast-enhanced perfusion is pulmonary blood volume (PBV). This parameter can be determined from the ratio of the areas under the parenchymal and arterial concentration time curves:

$$PBV = \int C_{VOI}(t)dt / \int C_a(t)dt, \qquad (7.4)$$

where C_a is the arterial contrast-agent concentration.

Once PBV and MTT are known, parenchymal pulmonary blood flow (PBF) can be estimated using the central volume theorem [17, 18]. This is defined as follows:

$$PBF = PBV/MTT \qquad (7.5)$$

Alternatively, a more complex model for perfusion quantification can be used based on tracer kinetic principles for nondiffusible (i.e., intravascular) tracers [19, 20]. Using this model, PBF can be determined if the arterial input function (i.e., the concentration vs. time of the feeding artery) of the contrast agent entering the VOI is known. For an injection which gives rise to an arterial input function $C_a(t)$, the concentration of the contrast agent in the parenchymal VOI is:

$$C_{VOI}(t) = PBF \cdot C_a(t) \otimes R(t) \qquad (7.6)$$

where $\otimes$ denotes a mathematical operation known as "convolution" between the two functions $C_a(t)$ and $R(t)$. Convolution represents blurring of the arterial input function as contrast moves into smaller vessels. $R(t)$ is the residue function, which is the relative amount of contrast agent in the VOI in an idealized perfusion experiment, and determines how blurred $C_a(t)$ becomes.

In order to derive PBF from this equation, the impulse response has to be determined by a process called *deconvolution*. A more detailed description on deconvolution methods is available by Calamante et al. [21].

7.3 Modalities

Perfusion can be measured indirectly using a variety of noninvasive imaging modalities, including scintigraphy [22], computed tomography (CT) [23, 24], positron emission tomography (PET) [25], and magnetic resonance (MR) imaging [16]. These methods may be based on projections, single two-dimensional (2D) slices, or fully resolved two-dimensional (3D) volumes of the lungs. The strengths and weaknesses of each of these modalities, specifically in the context of pediatric pulmonary disease, are discussed below.

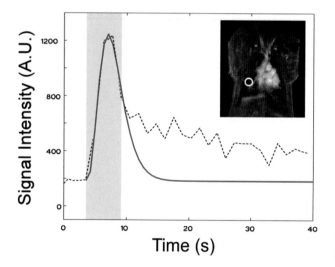

Fig. 7.1 Gamma-variate fit (*red line*) to contrast-enhancement curve (*dashed black line*). The gray area indicates the bounds of the data used for fitting. Data were measured in a region of interest in a time-resolved MR angiogram (*white circle* in inset image)

7.3.1 Scintigraphy

For prediction of functional loss, quantitative radionuclide pulmonary perfusion scintigraphy is the current most widely applied clinical tool. A radiolabeled tracer such as a ^{99m}Tc-labeled macroaggregate of albumin is injected via a peripheral vein. As this agent passes through the lungs, it becomes lodged in a fraction of the capillary bed in proportion to tissue perfusion. Anterior and posterior coronal projections of the chest, and possibly other oblique views, are then acquired using a gamma camera to record nuclear emissions from this tracer (Fig. 7.2). Multiple views are acquired to compensate for the greater attenuation of emissions from deeper tissues.

Scintigraphic images display perfusion irregularities associated with diffuse small-vessel diseases such as primary PH [15]. It is also possible to quantify relative differences in volumetric flow, for example, between left lung and right, based on the integrated activity over each lung. However, the relatively low-spatial resolution of the method (approximately 1–2 cm) results in poor depiction of focal defects and contributes to the low specificity of chest scintigraphy [26]. It is also limited by artifacts from the diaphragm and breast tissue, and overlap due to projection. As a result, contrast-enhanced CT or MR pulmonary angiography is often indicated after an inconclusive scintigraphy study. Pulmonary scintigraphy results in relatively low radiation doses of approximately 1 mSv (50 chest X-rays), but this may limit longitudinal studies in young patients.

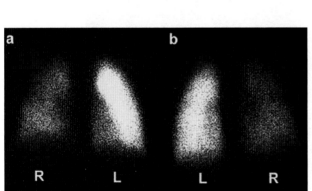

Fig. 7.2 Lung perfusion scintigraphy images of a patient with a Fontan circulation. (a) Lung fields in anterior plane and (b) lung fields in posterior plane. L: left side; R: right side. True differential pulmonary blood flow cannot be depicted by lung perfusion scintigraphy, as it is influenced by the site of injection. Preferential flow of radio isotope to the left lung was caused by the geometric orientation of the Fontan and cavopulmonary pathways
Reproduced with kind permission of Springer Science and Business Media (Fig. 4, Roman et al. [53])

7.3.2 Computed Tomography

Early applications of contrast-enhanced CT to the study of pulmonary perfusion were hindered by slow gantry rotation speeds and the viscosity of available nondiffusible ionic contrast agents [27]. With the introduction of multidetector CT (MDCT), 64 axial slices spanning approximately 4 cm can now be acquired on modern systems in only 0.3 s. This permits whole lung volumes to be scanned within a 5 s breath-hold, but temporal resolution remains too low to quantify perfusion throughout the lungs using these systems. MDCT-based perfusion measurement is therefore restricted to a segment of the lung pending inevitable increases in detector number or rotation speed.

A more advanced but less common form of CT, known as electron-beam CT (EBCT), achieves higher temporal resolution by electrically sweeping an electron beam to generate X-rays from each angle. This removes the hindrance of a mechanical gantry and provides single axial images at a temporal resolution of approximately 0.1 s. However, only one slice is acquired at a time making this approach impractical for volumetric studies.

An average chest CT scan deposits between 8 and 12 mSv of dose to a patient. This number could be considerably higher when time-resolved CT angiography is performed, depending on the duration of data acquisition.

7.3.3 Positron Emission Tomography

This modality involves the injection of a radiopharmaceutical that emits subatomic particles known as positrons. These particles quickly interact with electrons, and the two annihilate to produce two high-energy photons traveling in opposite directions. The photons are detected by the PET scanner, which can determine their point of origin to reconstruct 3D maps of tracer distribution.

For pulmonary perfusion studies, a radioactive gas of low solubility (e.g., $^{13}N_2$) is dissolved in saline and injected intravenously over 3–5 s [25]. Volumetric PET data are then acquired repeatedly for approximately 30 s while the subject holds their breath. The low solubility of the gas in blood ensures that most of gas leaves the blood as it passes through the capillaries of aerated alveoli, and so the distribution of the gas in these areas is indicative of regional perfusion.

Signal characteristics are dramatically different in nonaerated regions of the lung, which will not take up gas. Signal intensity in these areas will rise and fall as the first-pass of the agent washes through the pulmonary system. Perfusion in these regions can then be calculated using tracer-kinetic theory, described earlier.

Once the subject begins to breath, PET data continue to be collected and clearance of the gas via the airways can be imaged to assess ventilation. Aerated but unventilated portions of the lung will retain gas during breathing, thus allowing gas trapping to be visualized.

The spatial resolution of PET is determined by several factors, including the size of the detector and the range positrons travel before annihilation. The resolution of modern PET systems is approximately 3 mm, which is much greater than that of SPECT. The recent production of combined PET/CT scanners marries the physiologic information of PET with the high-resolution anatomical information of CT.

The primary physical limitation of PET imaging is the creation and delivery of appropriate radiopharmaceuticals. Because the half-life of many PET tracers is relatively short (e.g., the half-life of $^{13}N_2$ is 9.96 min), a cyclotron and associated personnel must be part of the imaging facility. Tracers with long half-lives, such as fluorodeoxyglucose (FDG) at 109.8 min, can be produced at off-site facilities and shared between nearby institutions, but this restricts PET use to specific physiologic studies. Furthermore, tracers with short half-lives may be administered several times in one examination, which may be useful for monitoring intervention.

7.3.4 Magnetic Resonance Imaging

The use of MR imaging to measure microvascular characteristics has several advantages. MR imaging is widely available, does not use ionizing radiation, provides high spatial and temporal resolution and can make use of well-tolerated exogenous as well as endogenous contrast agents. In addition, MR perfusion can be combined with other techniques such as diffusion, spectroscopy, and tissue relaxometry. This allows the combined longitudinal assessment of tissue perfusion, morphologic features, metabolism, and function, thus providing a comprehensive understanding of the developing pathophysiologic mechanism.

Perfusion imaging using MR has been accomplished using two techniques: dynamic contrast-enhanced MR imaging, which rapidly monitors the lung parenchyma following an IV injection of a paramagnetic contrast agent; and arterial spin labeling (ASL), which uses magnetically labeled blood water as a contrast agent. Both methods are described in detail below.

A. Dynamic contrast-enhanced (DCE) MR imaging: Contrast-enhanced perfusion MR imaging uses dynamic imaging of the first-pass of a paramagnetic contrast agent bolus (typically Gadolinium) through the pulmonary circulation. Using tracer kinetic principles, hemodynamic parameters such as transit times, blood volume, and blood flow can be derived from these data (see Fig. 7.3).

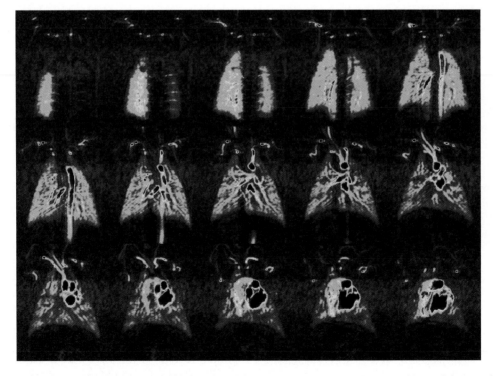

Fig. 7.3 Coronal lung-perfusion maps obtained using time-resolved contrast-enhanced MR imaging (Anterior: top left; Posterior: bottom right)

Since the lung is characterized by a very short transit time (approximately 3–5 s), rapid imaging techniques are required to capture the peak enhancement of the lung parenchyma [28]. Therefore, contrast-enhanced perfusion MR imaging uses ultra-short T1-weighted gradient-echo-pulse sequences [29]. Both 2D and 3D acquisition techniques have been used to track the contrast agent which should be injected as a bolus at a rate 3 ml/s or faster [29, 30]. The advantage of 2D perfusion MR imaging is the excellent temporal resolution of less than 1 s per image. This is beneficial with regard to artifact reduction resulting from patient movement, cardiac, and respiratory motion, as well as quantitative assessment of lung perfusion using deconvolution methods [21, 31].

Although 2D perfusion MR imaging often has sufficient in-plane resolution, its limited anatomic coverage and insufficient spatial resolution in the z-axis are major disadvantages which restrict its clinical value, for example, for the assessment of pulmonary embolism. Hence, 3D MR imaging, which offers improved anatomical coverage, has recently been proposed for the assessment of regional lung perfusion [30, 32–34].

With the implementation of high-performance gradient systems and alternative k-space sampling strategies, such as elliptical k-space sampling, 3D imaging of the entire pulmonary vascular tree in less than 4 s per volume is possible [35]. When combining this with parallel imaging strategies, such as simultaneous acquisitions of spatial harmonics (SMASH) or sensitivity encoding (SENSE) [36, 37] the temporal resolution can be improved several fold as recently published by Fink et al. [34] However, a major drawback of parallel MR imaging is that the time saving achieved is accompanied by an increase of image noise, which is crucial with regards to the low signal-to-noise ratio (SNR) of the lungs. Since the ultimate achievable SNR for parallel MR imaging is closely coupled to the geometry and sensitivity patterns of the coil arrays, dedicated design of coil arrays with regard to parallel imaging might overcome this limitation in the future [38, 39].

B. Other contrast agents: Other contrast agents used for studying lung perfusion include blood pool agents, hyperpolarized helium, and oxygen. The advantage of blood pool agents is the higher relaxivity and longer retention within the intravascular compartment allowing higher spatial resolution of pulmonary angiography with equal or even higher vascular contrast [40, 41]. The single injection of a blood pool contrast agent yielded sufficient SNR and negligible artifact, thus demonstrating its potential for the acquisition of pulmonary perfusion and angiographic imaging [42]. Although the routine clinical application of blood pool contrast agents is still limited, they may soon play an important role in perfusion MR imaging in general and in particular of the lung. Recently, blood-dissolved hyperpolarized ^{3}helium gas was found to be effective as an intravascular contrast agent in animal models [43, 44]. Similarly, ventilation of 100% oxygen has been used to enhance the signal from pulmonary blood at the site absorption.

C. Arterial Spin Labeling (ASL): Arterial spin labeling (ASL) is a general term for techniques which use blood water as an endogenous, freely diffusible contrast agent to detect signal changes due to perfusion. By applying an appropriate series of radiofrequency (RF) pulses, water protons in arterial blood can be magnetically labeled before entering the lung parenchyma. In general, a flow-insensitive and a flow-sensitive image are acquired, which are then subtracted from one another. The key difference of the two images is that for one of them the magnetization of the arterial blood is fully relaxed, while for the other it is inverted. The difference image is thus proportional to the amount of arterial inflow, and thus proportional to perfusion.

The major problem in applying this extremely promising technique to human studies is that the observed signal difference is very small, no more than 1–2%, even at high fields. At 1.5 T, signal-to-noise ratio must be very large, image quantitation must be extremely precise, and instrumental hardware must be very stable to measure perfusion. Furthermore, blood labeling may partially vanish during the imaging process. This technique has only been used in animal experiments or normal subjects, not in experiments using human subjects with lung disease. Therefore, the significance of this technique in the clinical setting must still be determined.

Nevertheless, several techniques have been developed for this purpose, all belonging to one of two distinct categories: continuous (CASL) or pulsed (PASL) arterial spin labeling. However, application of these techniques to the lung is difficult, as the data must be acquired within a breath-hold.

7.3.5 Continuous Arterial Spin Labeling(CASL)

This method was the first ASL method for MR perfusion imaging. It is based on the steady-state magnetic labeling of arterial flow to an organ [45]. The measurable changes in the steady-state magnetization can be used to calculate tissue-specific perfusion. For every voxel in the image PBF can be expressed as:

$$PBF = \lambda/T1_{app} \cdot (M_{cont} - M_{inv})/2 \cdot M_{count} \quad (7.7)$$

where λ is the blood–lung partition coefficient (a ratio quantifying the distribution of tissue water between extra- and intravascular compartments), $T1_{app}$ is the apparent longitudinal relaxation rate (the T1 value as altered by the labeled blood water), M_{cont} is the longitudinal magnetization per gram of lung tissue (i.e., signal intensity) for a control image obtained without spin inversion, and M_{inv} is the magnetization for an image obtained with inversion. Thus the CASL technique allows PBF to be calculated from a set of three separately acquired images: (1) a spin inverted or tagged image, (2) a control image acquired without spin labeling, and (3) a T1 image. To overcome the need for breath-holding, the respiratory-triggered 3D implementation of this technique has been used to depict regional pulmonary perfusion in healthy subjects [46]. The perfusion deficit in pulmonary arterial occlusion in a pig model has also been demonstrated using this technique [47]. Although steady-state ASL techniques theoretically produce larger signal changes compared to PASL, magnetization-transfer and transit-time delays cause signal loss. Furthermore, the specific absorption rate is a concern, especially when imaging at higher field strength (3T and above).

7.3.6 Pulsed Arterial Spin Labeling (PASL)

PASL is a more diverse set of techniques than CASL, with several different variations in use such as, for example, EPISTAR or FAIR. Like CASL, PASL techniques involve the subtraction of two images: one a spin-labeled or tagged image acquired after putting arterial blood water and lung tissue into different magnetization states (flow-sensitive), the other a control image acquired with blood and tissue water in identical states (flow-insensitive).

The major difference between PASL and CASL, as well as between the various PASL techniques, is in the method by which arterial blood water and lung tissue are put into differing magnetization states prior to acquiring the tagged image. For example, in the EPISTAR (echo-planar imaging and signal targeting with alternating RF) technique, a slice-selective RF pulse pre-saturates the imaging slice just prior to labeling, and a single RF inversion pulse labels the arterial spins in a proximal slab [48]. In the FAIR (flow-sensitive alternating inversion recovery) technique, the roles of inverted and noninverted spins are reversed, that is, to acquire the tagged image, the imaging slice is subjected to a slice-selective inversion pulse and relaxed arterial spins are allowed to flow into the slice, whereas the control image is acquired after a global inversion pulse inverts the spins of both blood and tissue water [49, 50].

Instead of EPISTAR, Hatabu et al. used a fast gradient-echo [51] or single-shot half-Fourier turbo spin-echo (HASTE) pulse sequence [52] to acquire perfusion images of lung tissue. Two sets of images are acquired during each breath-holding period. In order to invert the magnetization of blood within those structures in only one set of images, an RF pulse is applied to the right ventricle and main pulmonary artery. The subtraction of the two images results in the perfusion image. However, both methods suffer from magnetic susceptibility artifacts. Recently, FAIR with extra radiofrequency pulse (FAIRER), another pulsed ASL technique, was introduced by Mai and Berr (1999). This technique is a modification of the FAIR technique and provides high-resolution perfusion images of the pulmonary parenchyma with negligible artifacts.

The equations for calculating PBF vary with the technique, but they typically assume a signal intensity difference between tagged and control images, which is a function of many variables, some measured during the scan and some assumed from empirical data. These variables include M0 (the longitudinal magnetization at equilibrium), TI (the inversion time), $T1_{app}$ (the apparent T1 of lung tissue in the presence of labeled blood water), $T1_{blood}$ (the T1 of arterial blood), λ (lung-blood partition coefficient), α (the degree of spin inversion), and τ (the arterial transit time). As in CASL, the equation relating the difference signal to PBF is solved for every voxel to generate a quantitative PBF map.

7.4 Quantitative Perfusion Measurement in PH – Recent Literature

Qualitative imaging of gross perfusion defects has been possible for decades, and remains important today for the detection of pulmonary thromboembolism and other pathologies. However, improvements to 3D time-resolved imaging now permit quantitative perfusion measurement throughout the lungs at high-spatial resolution. This has broadened the applications of pulmonary perfusion measurement to pathologies associated with more subtle perfusion changes, including PH [8, 53–56].

Only a handful of recent publications have explored the capabilities of time-resolved CT angiography and MR angiography to study PH.

Jones et al. showed that large-scale gravity-dependent changes in perfusion could be detected using EBCT [56]. However, they also showed that perfusion differences between adjacent parenchyma were too large to be attributed to gravity alone. This supported previous animal work using high-spatial-resolution microspheres that suggested pulmonary branching is a major determinant of perfusion heterogeneity [57]. The group then showed that supine subjects with PH had no significant gravity dependence in perfusion. These findings are in agreement with perfusion scintigraphy studies by Horn et al. which, after correcting for lung volume based on xenon-133 equilibrium ventilation scans, found reduced gravity dependence in subjects with PH [58].

Ohno et al. instead used rapid MR imaging to quantify the spatial distribution of perfusion in both normal subjects and those with PH related to chronic pulmonary thromboembolism (CPTE), chronic obstructive pulmonary disease (COPD), and primary pulmonary hypertension (PPH) [55]. Regions of pathology in the CPTE subjects were visible in the MR images and possessed a significant decrease in PBF and PBV compared with normal subjects. The MTT in these segments was significantly larger. Similarly, PBF and PVB were significantly reduced in subjects with COPD, but the MTT was also shorter. In PPH, a decrease in PBF was measured, but no significant difference in PBV was detected relative to the normal population.

7.5 Conclusion

This chapter described several exciting new methods for the noninvasive measurement of pulmonary perfusion. The recent improvements in both the temporal and spatial resolutions of these methods will allow 3D imaging of perfusion in a variety of pediatric pathologies. At the same time, more robust mathematical algorithms are being developed to calculate perfusion. The combination of imaging technology, new contrast-agents, and improved analysis tools sets the stage for direct application of perfusion measurement to pediatric pulmonary disease. The methods hold promise for detecting early therapeutic changes and may one day help to guide therapy.

References

1. Patel DJ, Schilder DP, Mallos AJ. Mechanical properties and dimensions of the major pulmonary arteries. J Appl Physiol. 1960;15:92–6.
2. Rabinovitch M. Pulmonary hypertension: updating a mysterious disease. Cardiovasc Res. 1997;34:268–72.
3. Hoffman JI, Rudolph AM, Heymann MA. Pulmonary vascular disease with congenital heart lesions: pathologic features and causes. Circulation. 1981;64:873–7.
4. Palevsky HI, Gurughagavatula I. Pulmonary hypertension in collagen vascular disease. Compr Ther. 1999;25:133–43.
5. Weitzenblum E, Loiseau A, Hirth C, et al. Course of pulmonary hemodynamics in patients with chronic obstructive pulmonary disease. Chest. 1979;75:656–62.
6. Bogren HG, Klipstein RH, Mohiaddin RH, et al. Pulmonary artery distensibility and blood flow patterns: a magnetic resonance study of normal subjects and of patients with pulmonary arterial hypertension. Am Heart J. 1989;118: 990–9.
7. Wagenvoort CA. Open lung biopsies in congenital heart disease for evaluation of pulmonary vascular disease. Predictive value with regard to corrective operability. Histopathology. 1985;9:417–36.
8. Fukuchi K, Hayashida K, Nakanishi N, et al. Quantitative analysis of lung perfusion in patients with primary pulmonary hypertension. J Nucl Med. 2002;43:757–61.
9. Roman KS, Kellenberger CJ, Farooq S, et al. Differential pulmonary blood flow in patients with congenital heart disease: Magnetic resonance imaging versus lung perfusion scintigraphy. Pediatr Radiol. In Press.
10. Rubin LJ. Primary pulmonary hypertension. N Engl J Med. 1997;336:111–7.
11. Agata Y, Hiraishi S, Oguchi K, et al. Changes in pulmonary venous flow pattern during early neonatal life. Br Heart J. 1994;71:182–6.
12. West J, Wagner, PD. Ventilation-perfusion relationships. Philadelphia: Lippincott-Raven; 1997.
13. Kang IS, Redington AN, Benson LN, et al. Differential regurgitation in branch pulmonary arteries after repair of tetralogy of Fallot: a phase-contrast cine magnetic resonance study. Circulation. 2003;107:2938–43.
14. Kellenberger CJ, Macgowan CK, Roman KS, et al. Hemodynamic evaluation of the peripheral pulmonary circulation by cine phase-contrast magnetic resonance imaging. J Magn Reson Imaging. 2005;22:780–7.
15. Fishman AJ, Moser KM, Fedullo PF. Perfusion lung scans vs pulmonary angiography in evaluation of suspected primary pulmonary hypertension. Chest. 1983;84:679–83.
16. Hatabu H, Tadamura E, Levin DL, et al. Quantitative assessment of pulmonary perfusion with dynamic contrast-enhanced MRI. Magn Reson Med. 1999;42:1033–8.
17. Stewart GN. Researches on the circulation time in organs and on the influences which affect it. Parts I-III. J. Physiol. 1894;15:1–89.
18. Meir P ZK. On the theory of the indicatir-dilution method for measurement of blood flow and volume. J Appl Physiol. 1954;6:731–44.
19. Zierler K. Theoretical basis of indicator-dilution methods for measuring flow and volume. Circ Res. 1962;137:677–84.
20. Axel L. Cerebral blood flow determination by rapid-sequence computed tomography: theoretical analysis. Radiology. 1980;137:679–86.
21. Calamante F, Thomas DL, Pell GS, et al. Measuring cerebral blood flow using magnetic resonance imaging techniques. J Cereb Blood Flow Metab. 1999;19:701–35.
22. Johnson K. Ventilation and perfusion scanning in children. Paediatr Respir Rev. 2000;1:347–53.
23. Hoffman EA, Chon D. Computed tomography studies of lung ventilation and perfusion. Proc Am Thorac Soc. 2005;2: 492–8, 506.
24. Boll DT, Lewin JS, Young P, et al. Perfusion abnormalities in congenital and neoplastic pulmonary disease: comparison of MR perfusion and multislice CT imaging. Eur Radiol. 2005;15:1978–86.
25. Musch G, Venegas JG. Positron emission tomography imaging of regional pulmonary perfusion and ventilation. Proc Am Thorac Soc. 2005;2:522–7, 508–9.

26. Investigators TP. Value of the ventilation/perfusion scan in acute pulmonary embolism. Results of the prospective investigation of pulmonary embolism diagnosis (PIOPED). JAMA. 1990;263:2753–59.

27. Tonge KA, Wright CH, Mathew J, et al. Flow rate determination using computed tomography. Br J Radiol. 1980;53:946–9.

28. Macgowan CK, Al-Kwifi O, Varodayan F, et al. Optimization of 3D contrast-enhanced pulmonary magnetic resonance angiography in pediatric patients with congenital heart disease. Magn Reson Med. 2005;54:207–12.

29. Hatabu H GJ, Kim D et al. Pulmonary perfusion: qualitative assessment with dynamic contrast-enhanced MRI using ultrashort TE and inversion recovery turbo FLASH. Magn Reson Med. 1996a;36:503–508.

30. Matsuoka S UK, Chima H et al. Effect of the rate of gadolinium injection on magnetic resonance pulmonary perfusion imaging. J Magn Reson Imaging. 2002;15:108–113.

31. Ostergaard L WR, Chesler DA et al. High resolution measurement of cerebral blood flow using intravascular tracer bolus passages, Part I. Mathematical approach and statistical analysis. Magn Reson Med. 1996;36:715–25.

32. Iwasawa T SK, Ogawa N et al. Prediction of postoperative pulmonary function using perfusion magnetic resonance imaging of the lung. J Magn Reson Imaging. 2002;15:685–92.

33. Nikolaou K SS, Nittka M et al. Magnetic resonance imaging in the diagnosis of pulmonary arterial hypertension: High resolution angiography and fast perfusion imaging using intelligent parallel acquistion techniques (IPAT) (abstract). Radiology. 2002;225:473.

34. Fink C BM, Puderbach M et al. partially parallel three-dimensional magnetic resonance imaging for the assessment of lund perfusion - initial results. Invest Radiol. 2003;38:482–88.

35. Goyen M, Laub G, Ladd ME, et al. Dynamic 3D MR angiography of the pulmonary arteries in under four seconds. J Magn Reson Imaging. 2001;13:372–7.

36. Sodickson DK, Manning WJ. Simultaneous acquisition of spatial harmonics (SMASH): fast imaging with radiofrequency coil arrays. Magn Reson Med. 1997;38:591–603.

37. Pruessmann KP, Weiger M, Scheidegger MB, et al. SENSE: sensitivity encoding for fast MRI. Magn Reson Med. 1999;42:952–62.

38. Sodickson DK, McKenzie CA, Ohliger MA, et al. Recent advances in image reconstruction, coil sensitivity calibration, and coil array design for SMASH and generalized parallel MRI. Magma. 2002;13:158–63.

39. Madore B, Pelc NJ. SMASH and SENSE: experimental and numerical comparisons. Magn Reson Med. 2001;45:1103–11.

40. Ahlstrom KH, Johansson LO, Rodenburg JB, et al. Pulmonary MR angiography with ultrasmall superparamagnetic iron oxide particles as a blood pool agent and a navigator echo for respiratory gating: pilot study. Radiology. 1999;211:865–9.

41. Nolte-Ernsting CC, Krombach G, Staatz G, et al. [Virtual endoscopy of the upper urinary tract based on contrast-enhanced MR urography data sets]. Rofo. 1999;170:550–6.

42. Zheng J, Carr J, Harris K, et al. Three-dimensional MR pulmonary perfusion imaging and angiography with an injection of a new blood pool contrast agent B-22956/1. J Magn Reson Imaging. 2001;14:425–32.

43. Viallon M, Berthezene Y, Decorps M, et al. Laser-polarized (3)He as a probe for dynamic regional measurements of lung perfusion and ventilation using magnetic resonance imaging. Magn Reson Med. 2000;44:1–4.

44. Callot V, Canet E, Brochot J, et al. MR perfusion imaging using encapsulated laser-polarized 3He. Magn Reson Med. 2001;46:535–40.

45. Detre JA, Leigh JS, Williams DS, et al. Perfusion imaging. Magn Reson Med. 1992;23:37–45.

46. Roberts DA, Gefter WB, Hirsch JA, et al. Pulmonary perfusion: respiratory-triggered three-dimensional MR imaging with arterial spin tagging–preliminary results in healthy volunteers. Radiology. 1999;212:890–5.

47. Roberts DA, Rizi RR, Lipson DA, et al. Dynamic observation of pulmonary perfusion using continuous arterial spin-labeling in a pig model. J Magn Reson Imaging. 2001;14:175–80.

48. Edelman RR, Siewert B, Darby DG, et al. Qualitative mapping of cerebral blood flow and functional localization with echo-planar MR imaging and signal targeting with alternating radio frequency. Radiology. 1994;192:513–20.

49. Kwong KK, Belliveau JW, Chesler DA, et al. Dynamic magnetic resonance imaging of human brain activity during primary sensory stimulation. Proc Natl Acad Sci U S A. 1992;89:5675–9.

50. Kim SG. Quantification of relative cerebral blood flow change by flow-sensitive alternating inversion recovery (FAIR) technique: application to functional mapping. Magn Reson Med. 1995;34:293–301.

51. Hatabu H, Wielopolski PA, Tadamura E. An attempt of pulmonary perfusion imaging utilizing ultrashort echo time turbo FLASH sequence with signal targeting and alternating radio-frequency (STAR). Eur J Radiol. 1999e;29:160–3.

52. Hatabu H, Tadamura E, Prasad PV, et al. Noninvasive pulmonary perfusion imaging by STAR-HASTE sequence. Magn Reson Med. 2000;44:808–12.

53. Roman KS, Kellenberger CJ, Farooq S, et al. Comparative imaging of differential pulmonary blood flow in patients with congenital heart disease: magnetic resonance imaging versus lung perfusion scintigraphy. Pediatr Radiol. 2005;35:295–301.

54. Nikolaou K, Schoenberg SO, Attenberger U, et al. Pulmonary arterial hypertension: diagnosis with fast perfusion MR imaging and high-spatial-resolution MR angiography–preliminary experience. Radiology. 2005;236:694–703.

55. Ohno Y, Hatabu H, Murase K, et al. Quantitative assessment of regional pulmonary perfusion in the entire lung using three-dimensional ultrafast dynamic contrast-enhanced magnetic resonance imaging: Preliminary experience in 40 subjects. J Magn Reson Imaging. 2004;20:353–65.

56. Jones AT, Hansell DM, Evans TW. Quantifying pulmonary perfusion in primary pulmonary hypertension using electron-beam computed tomography. Eur Respir J. 2004;23:202–7.

57. Glenny RW, Robertson HT. Fractal modeling of pulmonary blood flow heterogeneity. J Appl Physiol. 1991;70:1024–30.

58. Horn M, Hooper W, Brach B, et al. Postural changes in pulmonary blood flow in pulmonary hypertension: a noninvasive technique using ventilation-perfusion scans. Circulation. 1982;66:621–6.

Functional Evaluation of Pulmonary Circulation: With Special Emphasis on Magnetic Resonance Imaging

Shi-Joon Yoo and Lars Grosse-Wortmann

Complete assessment of the pulmonary circulation should include not only the anatomy of the pulmonary arteries and veins but also the functional and hemodynamic consequences of the pathology. The available tools for the pulmonary vascular assessment include: catheterization with x-ray angiography, echocardiography, magnetic resonance (MR), computed tomography (CT), and radioisotope scintigraphy. As each has its own advantages and disadvantages, proper selection of a diagnostic tool or tools should be tailored to the specific purpose of the study in a given patient. Utilization of the imaging resources for anatomical depiction of the pulmonary arteries and veins has well been described in the literature. This chapter discusses the functional and hemodynamic assessment of the pulmonary circulation with particular emphasis on utilization of MR and how we perform functional and hemodynamic evaluation of the pulmonary circulation in a few selected clinical situations.

8.1 Overview

The functional and hemodynamic aspects of pulmonary circulation include: (1) flow velocities, volumes, and patterns, (2) blood pressures and vascular resistance, (3) oxygen saturation, (4) pulmonary perfusion, and (5) secondary changes in right and left ventricular anatomy and function.

8.1.1 Flow Velocities, Volumes, and Patterns

The blood flow velocities of the pulmonary arteries and veins can be evaluated by using either ultrasound Doppler

technique or phase-contrast MR imaging [1–4]. The former technique utilizes the shift of the sound frequency, while the latter utilizes the shift of the magnetic axis of the nuclei on exposure to a magnetic gradient for calculation of the blood-flow velocity. For accurate estimation of blood-flow velocities, the imaging plane should be aligned as parallel as possible with the flow direction in ultrasound Doppler technique, while the plane should be as perpendicular as possible to the flow direction in MR phase-contrast imaging. Therefore, ultrasound Doppler provides the velocity data for only a part of the flow stream where the sample volume is placed in the vessel, while MR phase-contrast imaging provides the velocity data for the whole cross-section of the vessel. As a consequence, ultrasound Doppler technique has significant limitation in depicting the whole spectrum of velocity profile across the vessel and accurate flow-volume calculation is limited. On the contrary, MR phase-contrast imaging provides both the velocity profile across the vessel and the cross-sectional area simultaneously at each time point of data sample, allowing accurate calculation of the flow volume through the target vessel. The other major disadvantage of ultrasound is the need for a proper sonic window to the target vessel, which not only limits parallel alignment of the sonic beam with the flow direction but also disallows approach to the pulmonary vessels behind the bones or within the lungs. However, MR imaging is not significantly influenced by the vessel location and alignment. The major disadvantage of the MR phase-contrast imaging is its relatively low spatial and temporal resolutions as compared to ultrasound Doppler technique. Although high-spatial resolution MR imaging is possible, it not only increases the scan time but also reduces the signal-to-noise ratio. In most currently available scanners, accurate flow data are obtainable for the vessels > 3 mm in diameter. Although maximum achievable temporal resolution with the current MR technology can be as low as 10 ms, it takes several minutes to achieve

S.–J. Yoo (✉)
Department of Diagnostic Imaging, Hospital for Sick Children, University of Toronto, Canada
e-mail: shi-joon.yoo@sickkids.ca

A.N. Redington et al. (eds.), *Congenital Diseases in the Right Heart*, DOI 10.1007/978-1-84800-378-1_8,
© Springer-Verlag London Limited 2009

high temporal and spatial resolutions, even with a new fast data-acquisition method called parallel imaging technique [5]. Therefore, a compromise between the temporal resolution and scanning time is inevitable when multiple vessels are to be investigated. When the data are acquired with lower temporal resolution, the peak-flow velocity is underestimated and high-frequency peaks are not clearly shown, while the accuracy of the flow volumes is less significantly affected. Although cardiac catheterization is regarded as the gold standard tool for hemodynamic evaluation, calculation of the pulmonary blood flow volumes using Fick principle at catheterization is associated with a number of potential errors [6]. Catheterization is only needed when the pulmonary vascular pressures are to be measured and the vascular resistance calculated or when catheter intervention is indicated.

8.1.2 Blood Pressure and Resistance

Currently, measurement of the pulmonary vascular pressure and resistance requires catheterization. The pulmonary arterial pressure can be estimated with Doppler echocardiography or MR phase-contrast imaging only when there is tricuspid and pulmonary regurgitation by using Bernoulli's equation. Therefore, great reliance has been placed on catheterization data in deciding treatment plan, especially when the patient has or is at risk of pulmonary hypertension. Calculation of pulmonary vascular resistance requires accurate measurement of pulmonary arterial pressure and flow volume. Although the pressure is directly measured by using a manometer, the flow volume is calculated by using the Fick principle [6]. As the Fick principle requires measurement of multiple parameters and introduces assumptions, a certain degree of inaccuracy is inevitable in measuring the pulmonary blood flow, and, consequently, in calculating the vascular resistance. Recent introduction of the combined MR and catheterization unit allows simultaneous measurement of the blood pressure through a catheter and the blood flow volume by MR phase-contrast imaging [7]. As MR phase-contrast imaging measures flow directly without relying on assumptions, the combined MR and catheterization method is considered to be the most accurate for invasive measurement of the vascular resistance.

8.1.3 Oxygen Saturation

The blood-oxygen saturation is routinely measured by blood sampling during catheterization. MRI oximetry,

which is now available, is based on the mathematical relationship between the T2 relaxation time of blood and the %HbO2 [8]. This relationship can be expressed by the equation: $1/T_2 = 1/T_2O + K\{(1 - \%O_2)/100\}^2$, where T_2O is the T2 signal decay of fully oxygenated blood and K is a constant. Thus, the %HbO2 can be estimated by a T2 weighted imaging sequence after a calibration to determine the T_2O and K in the subject. Recent studies found that both T_2O and the constant K can be estimated if the patient's hematocrit and fibrinogen concentrations are known [9]. Nield et al. showed that the oxygen saturation measurements using MR strongly correlated with the measurements at cardiac catheterization ($r = 0.825$, $p < 0.001$) [9]. MRI oximetry can be applied to detect intra- or extracardiac shunts, such as pulmonary arteriovenous fistulous communications. Although this method is presently limited to dedicated centers, it is expected to become more prevalent with a general trend for avoiding cardiac catheterization.

8.1.4 Pulmonary Perfusion

Scintigraphy with intravenous administration of radiolabeled macro-aggregated serum albumin or red blood cells is the most widely used technique for the assessment of pulmonary thromboembolism and blood flow distribution in the lungs [10]. The spatial resolution of scintigraphy, however, is inferior to that of CT and MR imaging. MR imaging offers a noninvasive assessment of pulmonary perfusion without radiation. Two general types of MR techniques have been introduced for this purpose, one with and the other without using contrast medium [11]. The most commonly adopted noncontrast technique is the arterial spin labeling sequence in which the nuclei in the pulmonary arteries are tagged and their movements to the lung parenchyma are traced [12]. Although this technique is very useful in the evaluation of the cerebral blood flow, its use in the evaluation of pulmonary perfusion is limited because of poor signal-to-noise ratio and strong artifacts from air in the lungs. Also used is a subtraction technique in which the lung perfusion is correlated with the signal difference between the systolic and diastolic images obtained by fast spin-echo technique [13]. Contrast-enhanced technique traces the bolus of gadolinium-based contrast agent in the pulmonary vasculature and the lung parenchyma [14]. It provides the highest temporal and spatial resolutions among all perfusion imaging techniques. Recent introduction of fast-imaging techniques such as parallel imaging and under-sampling algorithm allows time-resolved image acquisition in an interval of <150 ms for 2D images or 1–3 s for 3D images. Both noncontrast and contrast techniques may be used for quantitative assessment of the regional blood flow and mean transit time, although the accuracies should further be improved. Electron-beam or multidetector CT with a rapid bolus injection of contrast medium is also a promising technique for evaluation of the regional lung perfusion, albeit its use is limited in children by the use of ionizing radiation [15]. Positron emission tomography (PET) with bolus infusion of $^{13}N_2$-saline has also been used to study pulmonary perfusion and ventilation [16] but its use in children has not yet been reported.

8.1.5 Secondary Changes in Right and Left Ventricular Function

Pulmonary vascular abnormalities result in altered hemodynamics and anatomy of the right heart and systemic veins and, ultimately, in left ventricular functional impairment. Although ventricular function can be assessed by echocardiography, radioisotope scintigraphy, and catheterization with angiography, MR is regarded as the gold standard method. It does not make any geometric assumption for the calculation of ventricular volumes and ejection fraction and it images the complete right ventricle in every patient without the using ionizing radiation.

8.2 Clinical Applications

8.2.1 Pulmonary Arterial or Venous Stenosis

Echocardiography is able to visualize only the pulmonary arteries and veins within the mediastinum. Contrast-enhanced CT or MR angiography is best suited for anatomical assessment of the obstructive lesions of the pulmonary arteries and veins. As the scanning time for multidetector CT angiography takes only a few seconds, sedation or general anesthesia can be avoided in most cases, unlike in MR where it is needed for younger and uncooperative children. Whenever the hemodynamic significance of an obstructive lesion is in question, MR is preferable over CT [17, 18]. The hemodynamic importance of the pulmonary arterial or venous stenosis can be evaluated by measuring the velocity across the stenosis with MR-velocity mapping or Doppler echocardiography. The pressure gradient is estimated using Bernoulli's equation. However, the pressure gradient does not necessarily represent the severity of stenosis, because the blood

flow is redistributed to the unaffected lung region and the stenotic artery or vein carries a reduced amount of blood flow. MR is able to detect redistribution of blood flow between the right and the left lung as well as within the same lung. When there is significant pulmonary vein stenosis, the pulmonary arteries supplying the affected lung show reduced systolic forward flow and reversed diastolic flow, while the pulmonary artery supplying the unaffected lung show increased systolic forward flow and continuous diastolic forward flow (Fig. 8.1) [19, 20]. The ratio of the blood-flow volumes between the right and left lungs is a simple but valuable parameter of the pathologic status when the disease is unilateral or the pathology of one lung is worse than that of the other. In addition, pulmonary arterial blood flow pattern may show the typical signs of pulmonary hypertension when pulmonary vein stenosis is severe. The lung region that is drained by the stenotic pulmonary vein may show a perfusion defect in time-resolved MR angiography [21] Rarely, the lung affected by severe pulmonary vein stenosis may recruit the systemic arterial collaterals. As the collateral systemic arterial blood to the pulmonary artery cannot be drained through the pulmonary vein, the collateral blood flow refluxes into the central pulmonary artery to eventually flow into the unaffected lung. Catheterization with angiography is performed only when a catheter intervention is indicated.

8.2.2 Congenital Heart Diseases with Left-to-Right Shunt

When there is congenital heart disease, the amount and direction of shunting, the ratio between the pulmonary and systemic blood flow volumes (Q_p/Q_s), pulmonary arterial blood pressure, and pulmonary vascular resistance are important hemodynamic parameters for determination of the surgical approach as well as patient's prognosis. Catheterization is the only tool for direct measurement of pulmonary arterial pressure and calculation of vascular resistance. Q_p/Q_s can be measured by first-pass radionuclide angiography or MR phase-contrast velocity mapping as well as catheterization. As compared to radionuclide technique, MR velocity mapping provides more accurate Q_p/Q_s data with low interobserver variability and is not limited by other factors such as valvular regurgitation and slow circulation [22, 23]. Q_p is generally measured by sampling the branch pulmonary arteries or the main pulmonary artery. Q_p also can be measured by sampling the pulmonary venous return, especially when there is extracardiac shunt. Q_s is the

(a)   (b)

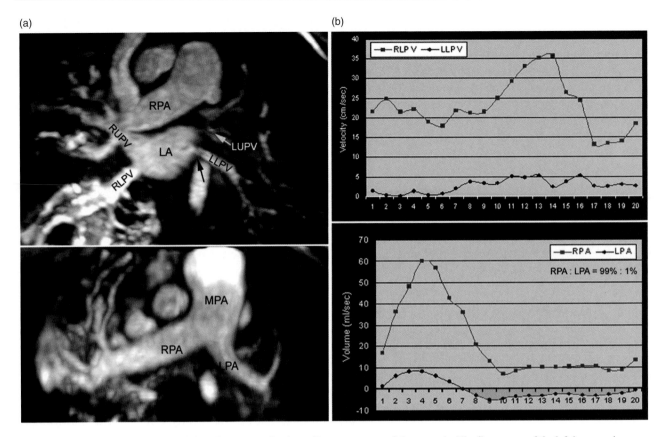

Fig. 8.1 Recurrent stenosis of the left pulmonary veins in a 18-month-old girl who underwent surgery for congenital stenosis at 10 months of age. **A**. Contrast-enhanced MR angiograms show tight stenosis of the left upper pulmonary vein (LUPV) and less severe narrowing of the left lower pulmonary vein (LLPV). The left pulmonary artery (LPA) is much smaller than the right pulmonary artery (RPA) due to redistribution of blood flow. **B**. Time–volume curves of the pulmonary veins (upper panel) and pulmonary arteries (lower panel) obtained from phase-contrast MR imaging. The flow data of the left lower pulmonary vein was obtained from the upstream of the stenosis. The flow curve of the left lower pulmonary vein shows markedly reduced flow velocity and loss of phasic changes. There is severe redistribution of the blood flow to the right pulmonary artery. The left pulmonary arterial flow curve shows reduced systolic forward flow and reversed flow in diastole. Note the continuous forward flow in the right pulmonary artery. LA = left atrium, MPA = main pulmonary artery, RLPV = right lower pulmonary vein, RUPV = right upper pulmonary vein. (*Reprinted from Reference with permission[20].*)

blood flow through the ascending aorta when there is no extracardiac shunt. When there is extracardiac shunt, Q_s can be measured by sampling the superior and inferior venae cavae. MR velocity mapping of the pulmonary arteries provides additional information about pulmonary hypertension, which is characterized by distinct changes in flow curve pattern that will be discussed later in this chapter. MR velocity mapping can be repeated after administration of pulmonary vasodilator such as oxygen, nitrogen or sildenafil to assess the pulmonary vascular reactivity. Catheterization is performed only when the pulmonary hypertension is considered severe or when the defect can be closed by catheter intervention. Simultaneous measurement of pulmonary arterial pressure and blood flow volume at a combined MR and catheterization unit will likely advance as the most accurate method for the hemodynamic study of the left-to-right shunt [7].

8.2.3 Aortopulmonary Collateral Circulation

The anatomy of the major aortopulmonary collateral arteries in patients with pulmonary atresia and ventricular septal defect can be assessed with either CT or MR angiography. In MR, the pulmonary blood flow volumes supplied by the major aortopulmonary collateral arteries can be estimated by measuring the pulmonary venous return. Total pulmonary blood flow can also be calculated by subtracting the amount of systemic venous return from the blood flow through the ascending aorta.

Systemic-to-pulmonary arterial collaterals often develop after bidirectional cavopulmonary anastomosis or Fontan or modified Fontan operation. As the systemic-to-pulmonary collaterals are inefficient recirculation pathways, compete with the systemic venous return to the pulmonary circulation and increase the ventricular volume load, larger collaterals are occluded with coil embolization. However, this procedure has been performed without any quantitative criteria. Theoretically, the amount of systemic-to-pulmonary arterial collateral circulation is the difference between the pulmonary venous and arterial blood flow volumes, although normal bronchial circulation may contribute a small amount to the difference. MR velocity mapping can then be used to quantify the systemic-to-pulmonary arterial collateral blood flow volume by measuring the blood flow volumes of the branch pulmonary arteries and individual pulmonary veins [24].

8.2.4 Pulmonary Hypertension

Catheterization is the ultimate diagnostic tool for pulmonary hypertension. Yet, the patients with pulmonary hypertension are usually critically ill and have a limited reserve capacity to tolerate any physiologic or hemodynamic changes that can be induced in the catheterization laboratory. Therefore, noninvasive diagnostic approaches are advised. CT angiography has become the standard imaging method for the evaluation of pulmonary embolism

[25]. Both echocardiography and MR can be used for the evaluation of pulmonary hypertension of nonembolic origin. MR approaches to the evaluation of pulmonary hypertension include: first, measurement of the pulmonary arterial size; second, quantitative and qualitative evaluation of the pulmonary arterial flow; and third, measurement of the right ventricular volume, ejection fraction, and myocardial mass. A simple measurement of the pulmonary arterial size is a good screening tool for patients with significant chronic pulmonary hypertension. Murray et al. showed strong correlation between the mean pulmonary arterial pressure (PAP) and the ratio of the diameters of the main pulmonary artery (MPA) and descending aorta (AO): mean $PAP = 24 \times MPA/AO + 3.7$ ($r = 0.7$, $p < 0.01$) [26]. MR phase-contrast imaging provides direct information regarding blood flow in the pulmonary circulation. The findings in patients with pulmonary hypertension include: inhomogeneous flow profile, early systolic peak with diminished peak systolic velocity, diminished acceleration time and acceleration volume, a second peak in mid-systole, early decline of systolic velocity, and greater retrograde flow after middle or late systole (Fig. 8.2) [27–29]. The pathophysiology of these findings is not altogether understood, but they are

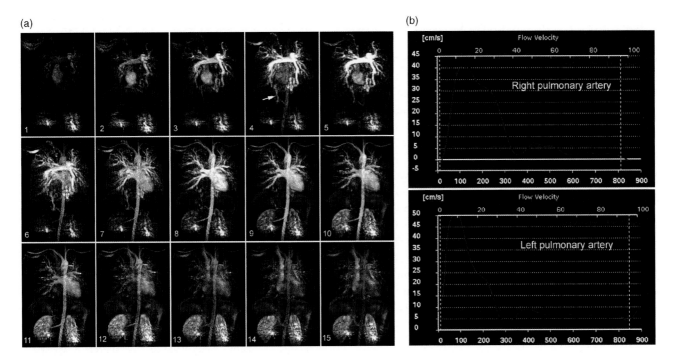

Fig. 8.2 Pulmonary hypertension and desaturation in the lower limbs in a 10-year-old boy. **A**. Time-resolved contrast enhanced MR angiograms show that the abdominal aorta opacifies earlier than the thoracic aorta (refer to the frames 4 and 6). The early opacification of the abdominal aorta is through the aberrant channel (arrow in frame 4) connecting the pulmonary and systemic arterial circulation. It is speculated that the aberrant channel is an

acquired decompressing channel of the hypertensive pulmonary circulation. **B**. Time–velocity curves obtained from phase-contrast imaging of the right and left pulmonary arteries. The left pulmonary arterial flow curve shows an earlier systolic peak and earlier cessation of the systolic forward flow as compared to the right pulmonary arterial flow curve. The difference suggests that the pulmonary resistance is higher than the systemic resistance the results of not only changes in resistance, impedance, and compliance of the peripheral vascular bed but also an abnormal capacitance and shape of the pulmonary arteries in pulmonary hypertension. It is possible to trace simultaneously the changes in flow velocity/volume and cross-sectional area of the pulmonary artery, enhancing our understanding of the interplay between blood flow and arterial wall properties [30]. Laffon et al. [30] suggested that mean pulmonary arterial pressure can be estimated by calculating the pressure-wave velocity from MR data. MR findings of right heart changes secondary to pulmonary hypertension include: right ventricular enlargement with hypertrophy, enlargement of the right atrium and inferior vena cava, abnormal ventricular septal motion with leftward bowing in early diastole, diminished right ventricular ejection fraction, and tricuspid regurgitation [31, 32].

8.2.5 Pulmonary Regurgitation

Pulmonary regurgitation is an unavoidable consequence of surgery for tetralogy of Fallot. As it causes right ventricular dysfunction with exercise intolerance, arrhythmia, and sudden death, quantification of pulmonary regurgitation and timely surgical intervention is very important. Pulmonary regurgitation can best be quantified by using MR phase-contrast imaging of the main pulmonary artery [33]. Kang et al. [34] showed that the degree of flow reversal is greater in the left than in the right pulmonary artery in the majority of cases after repair of tetralogy of Fallot. They also showed that decreased net blood flow to the left lung in these patients was due mostly to increased regurgitation rather than to decreased systolic forward flow. Subsequently, we have seen a similar phenomenon after the repair of truncus arteriosus and pulmonary atresia with intact ventricular septum, and after arterial switch operation for complete transposition of the great arteries. Roest et al. [35] utilized an MR-compatible bicycle ergometer to assess the responses of pulmonary regurgitation and biventricular function in patients who underwent tetralogy repair. Their study showed decreased pulmonary regurgitation during exercise as well as abnormal response of right ventricular function to exercise. They correlated this phenomenon with an increase in right ventricular end-diastolic pressure secondary to the right ventricular diastolic dysfunction. They suggested that exercise MR may allow detection of early right ventricular dysfunction in patients with normal right ventricular function at rest.

References

1. Lee VS, Spritzer CE, Carroll BA, et al. Flow quantification using fast cine phase-contrast MR imaging, conventional cine phase-contrast MR imaging, and Doppler sonography: *in vitro* and *in vivo* validation. Am J Roentgenol. 1997;169:1125–31.
2. Lotz J, Meier C, Leppert A, Galanski M. Cardiovascular flow measurement with phase-contrast MR imaging: basic facts and implementation. Radiographics. 2002;22:651–71.
3. Powell AJ, Maier SE, Chung T, Geva T. Phase-velocity cine magnetic resonance imaging measurement of pulsatile blood flow in children and young adults: *in vitro* and *in vivo* validation. Pediatr Cardiol. 2000;21:104–10.
4. Greil G, Geva T, Maier SE, Powell AJ. Effect of acquisition parameters on the accuracy of velocity encoded cine magnetic resonance imaging blood flow measurements. J Magn Reson Imaging. 2002;15:47–54.
5. Beerbaum P, Korperich H, Gieseke J, Barth P, Peuster M, Meyer H. Blood flow quantification in adults by phase-contrast MRI combined with SENSE–a validation study. J Cardiovasc Magn Reson. 2005;7:361–9.
6. Rudolph AM. Functional assessment. In: Congenital diseases of the heart: clinical-physiological considerations, 2nd ed, p. 45–84. Futura, Armonk, New York.
7. Muthurangu V, Taylor A, Andriantsimiavona R, et al. Novel method of quantifying pulmonary vascular resistance by use of simultaneous invasive pressure monitoring and phase-contrast magnetic resonance flow. Circulation 2004;110:826–34.
8. Wright GA, Hu BS, Macovski A. Estimating oxygen saturation of blood *in vivo* with MR imaging at 1.5T. J Mag Rson Imaging. 1991;1:275–83.
9. Nield LE, Qi X, Valsangiacomo ER, et al. *In vivo* MRI measurement of blood oxygen saturation in children with congenital heart disease. Pediatr Radiol. 2005;193:1253–1259.
10. Kim JH, Lee DS, Chung JK, Lee MC, Kim YW, Yun YS, et al. Quantitative lung perfusion scintigraphy in postoperative evaluation of congenital right ventricular outflow tract obstructive lesions. Clin Nucl Med. 1996;21:471–6.
11. Pedersen MR, Fisher MT, van Beek EJ. MR imaging of the pulmonary vasculature–an update. Eur Radiol. 2006;16:1374–86.
12. Mai VM, Berr SS. MR perfusion imaging of pulmonary parenchyma using pulsed arterial spin labeling techniques: FAIRER and FAIR. J Magn Reson Imaging. 1999;9:483–7.
13. Ogasawara N, Suga K, Zaki M, Okada M, Kawakami Y, Matsunaga N. Assessment of lung perfusion impairment in patients with pulmonary artery-occlusive and chronic obstructive pulmonary diseases with noncontrast electrocardiogram-gated fast-spin-echo perfusion MR imaging. J Mag Reson Imaging. 2004; 20:601–611.
14. Ohno Y, Hatabu H, Murase K, Higashino T, Kawamitsu H, Watanabe H, et al. Quantitative assessment of regional pulmonary perfusion in the entire lung using three-dimensional ultrafast dynamic contrast-enhanced magnetic resonance imaging: Preliminary experience in 40 subjects. J Magn Reson Imaging. 2004;20:353–65.
15. Won C, Chon D, Tajik J, et al. CT-based assessment of regional pulmonary microvascular blood flow parameters. J Appl Physiol 2003;94:2483–93.
16. Musch G, Venegas G. Positron emission tomography imaging of regional pulmonary perfusion and ventilation. Proc Am Thorac Soc. 2005;2:522–7.
17. Videlefsky N, Parks WJ, Oshinski J, et al. Magnetic resonance phase-shift velocity mapping in pediatric patients with pulmonary venous obstruction. J Am Coll Cardiol. 2001;38:262–7.

18. Valsangiacomo ER, Barrea C, Macgowan CK, Smallhorn JF, Coles JG, Yoo SJ. Phase-contrast MR assessment of pulmonary venous blood flow in children with surgically repaired pulmonary veins. Pediatr Radiol. 2003;33:607–13.

19. Roman K, Kellenberger C, Macgowan CK, et al. How is pulmonary arterial blood flow affected by pulmonary venous obstruction in children? A phase-contrast magnetic resonance study. Pediatr Radiol. Jan 19 2005; [Epub ahead of print].

20. Grosse-Wortmann L, Al-Otay A, Goo HW, et al. Anatomical and functional evaluation of pulmonary veins in children by magnetic resonance imaging. J Am Coll Cardiol. 2007; 49(9): 993–1002.

21. Kluge A, Dill T, Ekinci O, et al. Decreased pulmonary perfusion in pulmonary vein stenosis after radiofrequency ablation. Chest 2004;126:428–37.

22. Arheden H, Holmqvist C, Thilen U, Hanseus K, Bjorkhem G, Pahlm O, et al. Left-to-right cardiac shunts: comparison of measurements obtained with MR velocity mapping and with radionuclide angiography. Radiology 1999;211:453–8.

23. Powell AJ, Tsai-Goodman B, Prakash A, Greil GF, Geva T. Comparison between phase-velocity cine magnetic resonance imaging and invasive oximetry for quantification of atrial shunts. Am J Cardiol. 2003;91:1523–5.

24. Grosse-Wortmann L, Hamilton RM, Yoo SJ. Massive systemic-to-pulmonary collateral arteries in the setting of a cavopulmonary shunt and pulmonary venous stenosis. Cardiol. Young. 2007; 17(5):548–50.

25. Stein PD, Beemath A, Olson RE. Trends in the incidence of pulmonary embolism and deep venous thrombosis in hospitalized patients. Am J Cardiol. 2005;95:1525–6.

26. Murray TI, Boxt L, Katz J, Reagan K, Barst RJ. Estimation of pulmonary artery pressure in patients with primary pulmonary hypertension by quantitative analysis of magnetic resonance images. J Thorac Imaging. 1994;9:198–204.

27. Kondo C, Caputo GR, Masui T, et al. Pulmonary hypertension: pulmonary flow quantification and flow profile analysis with velocity-encoded cine MR imaging. Radiology. 1992;183:751–8.

28. Tardivon AA, Mousseaux E, Brenot F, et al. Quantification of hemodynamics in primary pulmonary hypertension with magnetic resonance imaging. Am J Respir Crit Care Med. 1994;150:1075–80.

29. Mousseaux E, Tasu JP, Jolivet O, Simonneau G, Bittoun J, Gaux JC. Pulmonary arterial resistance: noninvasive measurement with indexes of pulmonary flow estimated at velocity-encoded MR imaging—preliminary experience. Radiology. 1999;212:896–902.

30. Laffon E, Laurent F, Bernard V, De Boucaud L, Duccassou D, Marthan R. Noninvasive assessment of pulmonary arterial hypertension by MR phase-mapping method. J Appl Physiol. 2001;90:2197–202.

31. Saba TS, Foster J, Cockburn M, Cowan M, Peacock AJ. Ventricular mass index using magnetic resonance imaging accurately estimates pulmonary artery pressure. Eur Respir J. 2002;20:1519–24.

32. Hoeper MM, Tongers J, Leppert A, Baus S, Maier R, Lotz J. Evaluation of right ventricular performance with a right ventricular ejection fraction thermodilution catheter and MRI in patients with pulmonary hypertension. Chest. 2001;120:502–7.

33. Helbing WA, de Roos A. Clinical applications of cardiac magnetic resonance imaging after repair of tetralogy of Fallot. Pediatr Cardiol. 2000;21:70–9.

34. Kang IS, Redington AN, Benson LN, et al. Differential regurgitation in branch pulmonary arteries after repair of tetralogy of Fallot. A phase-contrast cine magnetic resonance study. Circulation. 2003;107:2928–43.

35. Roest AAW, Helbing WA, Kunz P, et al. Exercise MR imaging in the assessment of pulmonary regurgitation and biventricular function in patients after tetralogy of Fallot repair. Radiology. 2002;223:204–11.

Transcatheter Intervention on the Central Pulmonary Arteries—Current Techniques and Outcomes

Kyong-Jin Lee

9.1 Introduction

The spectrum of obstruction of the pulmonary arterial vascular bed ranges from discrete isolated stenosis of the central branch pulmonary artery to multiple lesions affecting peripheral intralobar branches. It may be congenital or acquired (Table 9.1). Difficulties with surgical management of pulmonary artery stenosis have shifted responsibility to a balloon-catheter-based approach [1–4]. This chapter (1) provides an overview of the current catheter-based techniques of increasing pulmonary vessel size, (2) describes application of these techniques in specific settings of congenital heart disease, and (3) discusses the impact of pulmonary artery intervention on right heart hemodynamics.

9.1.1 Technical Aspects and Results of Catheter-Based Intervention of Pulmonary Arteries

The histology of congenital pulmonary artery stenosis ranges from normal to significant hyperplasia of the intima and/or media with altered proportions of smooth muscle, elastin, and collagen [5]. Stenosis in the post-operative setting may include mural and perivascular fibrosis [5]. Effective balloon angioplasty involves a longitudinal or oblique tearing of all of the vascular intima and ideally a portion of the media [5–7]. This gap is eventually filled with organization of the intramural hemorrhage and ultimately scar formation (collagen and elastin fibers) enabling the vessel to *heal* at a larger diameter. Re-endothelialization is usually complete by 2 months after angioplasty [6]. Areas of mural thinning may predispose for aneurysm formation [8].

General consensus regarding indications for pulmonary artery intervention are outlined in Table 9.2 [9–11].

Successful dilation is defined as an increase in vessel diameter greater than or equal to 150%, increase in lung perfusion of greater than 20% to the affected lung, decrease in ratio of the right ventricular to aortic pressures greater than 20%, and a decrease in the pressure gradient across the obstructive segment [3, 10, 12–18]. Current markers of successful pulmonary artery intervention are insufficiently comprehensive. Two-dimensional (2D) diameters fail to represent three-dimensional (3D) vessel volumes, the majority of perfusion studies fail to quantitate segmental

Table 9.1 Causes of pulmonary artery obstruction

Congenital	Acquired
Ductal constriction	Postoperative for:
	Arterial switch operation for transposition of great arteries
	Central or Blalock–Taussig shunt
	Pulmonary artery banding
	Reimplantation of pulmonary artery (e.g., truncus arteriosus, aortopulmonary collaterals)
	Pulmonary arterioplasty
Tetralogy of Fallot	Fibrosing mediastinitis
Pulmonary atresia/ VSD/MAPCAs	Mediastinal tumors
Alagille syndrome	
Williams–Beuren syndrome	
Noonan syndrome	
Congenital rubella syndrome	
Cutix laxa	
Ehlers–Danlos syndrome	
Silver syndrome	
Takayasu's arteritis	

K.-J. Lee (✉)
Department of Paediatrics, Hospital for Sick Children, Toronto, ON, Canada

A.N. Redington et al. (eds.), *Congenital Diseases in the Right Heart*, DOI 10.1007/978-1-84800-378-1_9,
© Springer-Verlag London Limited 2009

Table 9.2 Indication for pulmonary artery intervention

RV pressure > 50–75% systemic

Hypertension in unaffected segments secondary to increased flow

Marked decrease in flow in affected segments (as assessed by radionuclide scan)

RV dysfunction or cyanosis aggravated by pulmonary artery stenosis

Symptoms

RV; right ventricle

flows, and ultimately, analyses of quantitative changes in diffusing lung capacity and reduction of right ventricular pressure load effect are lacking. However, such criteria do allow for consistency of reporting.

9.1.2 Pulmonary Balloon Aangioplasty— Standard and High Pressure

Balloon dilation of pulmonary arteries was first reported in the early 1980s [6]. The optimal balloon has a low-profile, high-burst pressure, short length and tip. Balloon catheters are made of transparent polyethylene with diameters ranging from 2.5 to 25 mm with lengths from 2 to 10 cm. Standard or conventional balloon catheters have a burst pressure between 1.5 and 10 atmospheres (ATM). High-pressure balloons have burst pressures greater than 10 and up to 20 ATM. These catheters in general have higher profiles, stiffer shafts, longer balloon lengths, and are more difficult to manipulate within the heart and pulmonary arteries. Coronary balloons have diameters between 2.5 and 5 mm, and are 20 mm length. They offer the advantageous features of high-burst pressures up to 18 ATM with a low profile. Recommended balloon diameters are 3–4 times the narrowed segment [10, 11, 17, 19] but generally not greater than 2 times the diameter of the adjacent normal vessel. The waist should be >50% of the inflated balloon diameter as very tight waists predispose to vessel rupture. Inflation pressures are increased incrementally until the balloon waist disappears or to the maximum burst pressure. Inflation times vary between 5 and 30 s and generally multiple inflations are performed. Unnecessarily large or long balloons may predispose to rupture of the thin-walled poststenotic vessel segments or outflow tract as they straighten during inflation [20].

The success rate of standard balloon angioplasty is approximately 30–60% in the larger case series [11, 13–15, 17]. High-pressure balloons have a 63% success rate in vessels resistant to standard balloon with an 81%

success rate with primary application [9]. Stenoses at surgical anastomoses sites respond better to dilatation compared with congenital subtypes (87% vs. 48%, respectively) [9]. Pulmonary artery stenosis located peripherally is more refractory to dilation compared to proximal lesions (34–71% vs. 56–72%, respectively) [21].

9.1.3 Stent Implantation of Pulmonary Arteries

Endovascular stents were first described in 1989 [22] and have subsequently been widely implanted into pulmonary arteries [23–29]. Intravascular stents achieve high success rates (>90%) in increasing vessel diameter [3, 24, 29–31]. The ideal stent has a low profile, high trackability, flexibility, predictable expansion with minimal foreshortening, sufficient radial strength, resistance to thrombosis and corrosion, side-branch accessibility, biodegradability, good redilation capabilities, and good visibility [8]. Stents may be either closed or open cell design, made of stainless steel, platinum, or polymer balloon expandable or self-expanding [8, 23, 27, 32–34]. More widespread clinical application of drug eluting and biodegradable stents is in the horizon [35–37]. Open cell stents have advantages of less foreshortening, allowing for side-branch access and favorable bending performance but disadvantages of less radial strength, more recoil, and protrusion of stent struts into side branches and vessel wall [33, 34]. Standard stents have recommended expansion ranges from 4 to 20 mm. Coronary stents have diameters between 3.5 and 5 mm with lengths between 13 and 28 mm. A smaller balloon to stenosis ratio is required during stent implantation than with standard angioplasty alone.

Stents provide a framework which address vessel recoil and maintains dilatation of the vessel wall. It is particularly effective when the mechanism of pulmonary artery obstruction is kinking, twisting, or tension as can be seen after the LeCompte maneuver for transposition of the great vessels [28, 38] from extrinsic compression as in left pulmonary artery compression from a Damus–Kaye–Stanzel anastomosis, intimal flap complications of balloon dilation [15, 38–40], and pulmonary artery obstruction in patients with cavopulmonary connections [22, 25, 29, 41].

Within days to weeks of implantation, the initial reactive thrombotic layer covering the stent struts is progressively replaced by neointima [8, 23]. The medial layer is compressed by the stent wires display varying degrees of fibrosis, some loss of smooth muscle fibers, and fragmentation of the elastic lamellae within the inner half of media. The adventitia may be normal or demonstrate fibrosis [23, 27].

Disadvantages include possibly higher restenosis rates than with angioplasty alone (2–3% in some series and up to 15–35% in other series) particularly with smaller stents (< 5 mm diameter) and when there is significant mismatch between the stented and nonstented vessels [24, 28, 31, 40–43], risk of straddling or *jailing* of side branches and limited expansion abilities [23, 40]. Implanted stents are amenable to future re-dilation, thus initial selection should factor reexpansion potential [24, 40, 43–45]. Drug-eluting stents may decrease restenosis rates and self-dissolving stents may address the issues of future expansion limitations [35–37].

9.1.4 Cutting or Bladed Balloon Angioplasty

The bladed balloon was first introduced to successfully treat coronary artery stenoses resistant to dilation with high-pressure balloons [46, 47]. Its use has been extrapolated to pulmonary artery stenosis [12, 48–52]. The design of the Cutting Balloon^{TM} (Boston Scientific, San Diego, California) consists of 3 or 4 microsurgical stainless steel blades bound longitudinally onto balloons at 90° or 120° angles. The blades have a working height of 0.127 mm. Balloon diameters range from 2 to 8 mm introduced through 4–7 French systems. Balloon burst pressure is 10 ATM. The dilatation concept consists of controlled scoring of the vessel wall into the medial layer which creates sites for tears to propagate during subsequent balloon dilation [46]. Recommendations for the diameter of the bladed balloon include at least twice the diameter of the stenotic vessel [52], equal to or 1 mm greater than the size of the persistent waist of the high-pressure balloon [51] and no larger than the adjacent vessel diameter. A long guiding sheath allows for better trackability over the required small 0.014 or 0.018 inch wires. Cutting balloon angioplasty is generally followed by high-pressure balloon dilatation.

Effectiveness of cutting balloon technology has been demonstrated by successful dilatations in vessel stenoses resistant to high-pressure balloons [12, 48, 51, 52] (Fig. 9.1). Cutting balloon angioplasty yielded an 81–92% [12, 48, 50, 52] increase in lesion diameter at intermediate term follow-up. Cutting balloons have been utilized successfully for the full spectrum of pulmonary artery stenoses, including aortopulmonary collaterals (APCs), unifocalized APCs, postsurgical lesions, intrastent stenosis, multiple pulmonary peripheral stenoses including those of Williams and Alagille syndromes [12, 52–54]. Complication rates are not higher, possibly lower, compared with conventional balloon angioplasty in reported series [48, 51, 52]. In Bergersen et al., of the 79 dilated vessels, aneurysm was acutely observed in three but no new aneurysms were noted at a median follow-up of 6 months (range 3–24 months) [51]. There was an 11% incidence of stent placement for acute dissection complications.

Although most commonly indicated for vessels which demonstrate resistance to high-pressure balloon angioplasty, its utilization as the initial choice may evolve with further use and availability.

9.1.5 Restenosis

Restenosis (≥50% loss in initial diameter gain) rates are 10–16% in the early stage [9, 13, 17, 51] and 5–43% on longer-term follow-up [9, 13, 15, 17, 55, 56]. Mechanisms of restenosis include elastic recoil of a transiently stretched vessel and intimal hyperplasia. There is some evidence to suggest that there is less restenosis with cutting balloon angioplasty by reduction in traumatic triggers of inflammation and neointimal proliferation compared with standard angioplasty [12, 46, 57]. Ongoing

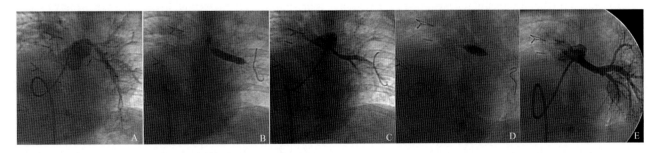

Fig. 9.1 Cutting-balloon angioplasty of unifocalized aortopulmonary collateral. **A**. Severe stenosis of unifocalized aortopulmonary collateral supplying left lower pulmonary artery lobe (indicated by arrow). **B**. Standard balloon angioplasty with high-pressure coronary balloon. **C**. Follow-up angiogram post-balloon angioplasty. **D**. Cutting-balloon angioplasty **E**. Post-cutting balloon angiogram demonstrating significantly improved vessel diameter and flow

monitoring and repeated procedures of initially successful dilations should be anticipated.

9.1.6 Complications

Pulmonary artery interventions are technically demanding, time consuming, and regarded as relatively higher risk cardiac catheterizations. The Valvuloplasty and Angioplasty for Congenital Anomalies Registry reported an overall complication rate of 13% on 182 pulmonary artery dilations performed on 156 patients [19]. Mortality rates are 0.8–3% overall and as high as 7.7% in the early experience with Williams Syndrome patients [15, 17, 19, 20, 51, 58, 59].

Pulmonary artery rupture is the most frequent serious morbidity occurring in as high as 2.3–4.9% [19, 20]. Baker et al. report on 1286 pulmonary artery balloon dilation catheterizations of 782 patients. Pulmonary artery trauma occurred in 29 (2.2%) procedures and 26 (3.3%) patients [20]. Unconfined transmural tears result in free extravasation of contrast or blood and communication with the pleural space, airway, or progressive lobar opacification. Tears generally occur distal to the site of obstruction [20]. Resuscitative measures include selective mainstem intubation for management of unilateral pulmonary hemorrhage, blood transfusions, and catheter-delivered therapy, including balloon tamponade proximal to the site of rupture, stent (covered and uncovered) placement, and extracorporeal membrane oxygenation support for low cardiac output [20]. Coil occlusion of the damaged pulmonary artery may prevent fatal hemorrhage [20]. Late (5 days and 2 weeks postdilation) hemorrhage has been reported [20, 60]. Risk factors for unconfined tears include recent pulmonary artery surgery, peripheral pulmonary artery stenoses, and in the setting of elevated pulmonary artery pressures [17, 58].

Successful dilatation may result in markedly increased local pulmonary blood flow and pressure in previously underperfused segments causing the so-called reperfusion injury in which an acute increase in capillary perfusion pressure results in pulmonary edema and hemoptysis [17, 61]. The angiographic appearance and hemodynamic status differentiate reperfusion injury from unconfined pulmonary artery tear. In these patients with no evidence of extravasation and stable hemodynamics, monitoring in the intensive care setting and medical management including diuretics and ventilatory support result in resolution within 24–72 hours.

Aneurysm is defined as saccular deformation of a vessel which tapers abruptly and measures at least twice the diameter of the adjacent pulmonary artery. It occurs in 3–18% of arteries, the highest being in the peripheral pulmonary arteries of Williams syndrome [15, 17, 59]. Rothman et al. demonstrated no correlation between aneurysm formation and balloon to stenosis ratio or maximal inflation pressures [17]. Aneurysms occurred most frequently in small branches distal to the targeted stenosis. The natural history of aneurysms is widely variable ranging from spontaneous resolution, no change, and to both decrease and increase in vessel diameter [17].

9.2 Pulmonary Angioplasty in Congenital Heart Disease

The overall impact of catheter-based interventions of pulmonary artery stenosis on the clinical course of patients appears to be favorable [15, 18]. The heterogeneity of scenarios invites selected discussion.

9.2.1 Preoperative Tetralogy of Fallot

Early primary repair of congenital heart defects can be accomplished with low mortality [62–64]. In tetralogy of Fallot, the complications associated with the Blalock–Taussig shunt can be avoided and early increased pulmonary blood flow may ultimately promote better lung growth [65–68]. The enthusiasm for neonatal repair has been to a degree tempered by emerging recognition of comorbidities including prolonged intensive care unit stay and impaired neurodevelopmental outcomes associated with early circulatory arrest and cardiopulmonary bypass [69–71].

Palliation of pulmonary arteries and the pulmonary valve by balloon dilation may postpone surgery in the neonatal period and allow for interim vessel growth [72–74]. Kreutzer et al. report such intervention on 10 patients with severe tetralogy of Fallot with diminutive pulmonary arteries deemed unsuitable for primary repair [75]. Nine patients underwent complete single-stage correction at an average of 8.5 ± 7.6 months (range 1–23 months) following initial catheterization. At a mean follow-up of 2.6 ± 2 years, the right ventricular pressure was < 70% in all patients and < 50% in seven patients. The incidence of the procedure-induced hypercyanotic spells is reportedly low [72–74]. Furthermore, in patients with tetralogy of Fallot with diminuitive pulmonary arteries, partial repair including a preemptive fenestration patch closure of the ventricular septal defect (VSD) may allow for catheter-based recruitment of the pulmonary vasculature prior to VSD closure [76].

In the unusual setting of tetralogy of Fallot with an isolated pulmonary artery with blood flow being maintained through a patent ductus arteriosus (PDA), stenting of the PDA may obviate the need for prolonged prostaglandin therapy and defer neonatal surgery allowing for growth of the hilar pulmonary artery [77].

9.2.2 Immediate Postoperative Period

Stenotic pulmonary arteries may create critical pulmonary blood flow states in the immediate postoperative period manifesting as elevated right ventricular to aortic pressure ratios, profound desaturation, and low cardiac output. Pulmonary blood flow is further compromised by cardiopulmonary bypass-induced lung injury and increased right ventricular dysfunction [78, 79]. Balloon angioplasty of new surgical anastomotic sites of branch pulmonary arteries in the early postoperative period (less than 7 weeks) is associated with increased risk of rupture and mortality up to 20% [17, 20, 58]. More favorably, Zahn et al. reported no deaths, vessel rupture, or transmural tear in 19 pulmonary artery interventions at a median time of 9 days (range 0–42 days) after surgery [80]. Transcatheter pulmonary artery intervention before 6 weeks in the postoperative setting must be approached conservatively and cautiously but is not absolutely prohibitive during critical hemodynamic states. Recommended balloon to stenosis ratios are less than 2.5:1. For this reason, stent implantation may be preferable to balloon angioplasty. A multidisciplinary team approach including the cardiovascular surgeon and the cardiac intensivist is advocated and in exceptionally high-risk patients, a cardiopulmonary support unit on standby should be considered.

9.2.3 Pulmonary Atresia/Ventriculo-Septal Defect/Multiple Aortopulmonary Collaterals

The spectrum of congenital heart disease challenges the adaptive mechanisms of the pulmonary vascular bed. This is nowhere as apparent as in pulmonary atresia/ventriculo-septal defect/multiple aortopulmonary collaterals (PA/VSD/MAPCAs). In this complex lesion, great morphologic variability exists regarding sources of pulmonary blood flow. A given segment of lung may be supplied solely from the true central pulmonary artery, solely from an APC, or from both with connections which are single or multiple, central or peripheral [67, 81]. Rabinovitch et al. [67] demonstrate the histology of APCs to be muscular systemic arteries replaced by an elastic pulmonary artery, the junction being marked by eccentric mounds of intimal hyperplasia. There is speculation that APCs react to the abnormal hemodynamics of a systemic-pulmonary artery connection by developing myointimal hyperplasia and the natural history of some APCs is progressive stenosis and occlusion. This may deem vessels inaccessible for future surgical unifocalization, which may result in iatrogenic stenosis or occlusion. Diminished pulmonary blood flow appears to result in distal arterial hypoplasia and underdevelopment of preacinar and acinar vessels and alveoli. In contrast, pulmonary vascular occlusive disease may be a consequence of APCs without obstruction and after placement surgical aortopulmonary shunts [67]. High postoperative right ventricular pressures are predictive of unfavorable outcomes [82]. Right ventricular pressure relies not only on the number of communicating lung segments but also on the integrity of the pulmonary microvasculature of those segments.

While debate continues regarding the virtues of early one-stage complete unifocalization versus initial palliation with aortopulmonary shunt [68, 82–86], there is general consensus that any successful strategy requires a combination of surgical and interventional catheterization techniques. Catheter-based pulmonary artery interventions, both balloon dilation and stent implantation of central and aortopulmonary collateral vessels, have been performed successfully in preoperative patients with subsequent increase in saturation, improved pulmonary blood flow and growth of peripheral vessels [53, 87–89]. Maneuvers to increase antegrade flow to central pulmonary arteries such as radiofrequency of atretic pulmonary valves and balloon dilation of central pulmonary arteries may ultimately result in a healthier pulmonary vascular bed [82, 90, 91]. Early catheterization after surgical recruitment identifies stenotic vessels, generally at anastomotic sites, at risk for complete occlusion [42, 54]. Lengthy and repeated procedures are to be expected. Outcomes of this disease remain suboptimal almost entirely related to the state of the pulmonary vascular bed [92].

9.2.4 Single Ventricle Physiology

In the Fontan circulation, the primary determinants of pulmonary blood flow are pulmonary vascular resistance, pulmonary vascular compliance, and the function of the ventricle as a flow generator [93]. In such a series circuit, optimizing factors of blood oxygenation are critical and as such aggressive pulmonary artery interventions should be the rule for maintaining single-ventricle circulation integrity [22, 29, 41, 94].

9.2.5 Diffuse Peripheral Pulmonary Artery Stenoses

Genetic syndromes may be associated with pulmonary artery stenosis. It may be discrete and isolated but often there may be severe diffuse peripheral pulmonary artery stenoses often involving the intralobar arteries, the extent of which may cause systemic to suprasystemic right ventricular pressures [95]. The incidence of peripheral pulmonary artery stenosis is 83% in Williams syndrome [96] and 85% in Alagille syndrome [97]. Williams syndrome in particular may be associated with other cardiovascular anomalies, including supravalvar aortic stenosis, coronary ostial obstruction, coarctation of the aorta, and supravalvar pulmonary stenosis [95, 97–99]. High mortality, particularly sudden death, appears to be associated with these conditions [97, 98, 100]. The incidence of sudden death was 1 death per 1,000 patient-years [98] and 3% in 104 patients with Williams syndrome followed for 30 years [100]. In Alagille syndrome, 7.5% of deaths were attributed to a cardiac cause [97]. In the total 19 deaths reported among six pediatric cardiology centers in the United States, 11 (58%) were associated with anesthesia administered for cardiac catheterization [99].

The reported literature regarding not only the cardiovascular outcomes but also, in particular, the experience with these multiple peripheral pulmonary artery stenoses is limited [98, 99, 101]. Histology of pulmonary artery stenoses of Williams syndrome shows diffuse wall thickening consisting of intimal proliferation, medial dysplasia with hypertrophy, fibrosis, and nonparallel mosaic arrangement of smooth muscle cells, the latter being hypothesized as the basis of less-successful outcomes of angioplasty in this patient population, and adventitial fibroelastosis [102, 103]. Often, *successful* pulmonary artery dilatation does not manifest as a decrease in right ventricular pressures [59]. As an exception to the general principle that proximal lesions are more amenable to dilation, balloon angioplasty is more successful in the distal vessels of these *syndromic* pulmonary arteries [59]. Cutting balloons have been applied and are shown to be effective [52]. Often the distensible proximal portions are best addressed with surgical patching or stent implantation [22, 104, 105]. Geggel et al. [59] report a mortality rate of 7.7% and an aneurysm rate of 18% during balloon angioplasties of pulmonary arteries

in Williams syndrome. The high rate of procedural complication and the natural history for spontaneous improvement in many patients (not only well documented in Williams syndrome but also reported in Alagille syndrome) [95–97, 101, 106, 107] may advocate for noninvasive monitoring and intervention to be reserved for symptomatic patients, those with at least systemic right ventricular pressures and severe left ventricular outflow obstruction. It may be considered in order to reduce risks of other interventions such as liver transplantation (Alagille syndrome) and supravalvar aortic surgery [108–111]. In Alagille syndrome patients who underwent liver transplantation, two (33%) deaths were attributed to heart failure induced by pulmonary hypertension and cardiac defects [111].

9.3 Hemodynamic Consequences of Pulmonary Arterial Obstruction

The consequence of pulmonary artery stenosis is far reaching in the spectrum of congenital heart disease. Pulmonary artery obstruction cannot be regarded in isolation but within the context of the entire cardiopulmonary unit (Fig. 9.2). Lung maturity relies on adequate pulmonary blood flow and its compromise may be profound during critical growth periods. Pulmonary artery obstruction independently creates a pressure load on the right ventricle but in conjunction with pulmonary regurgitation adds a simultaneous volume load. The consequences of chronic pressure and volume loading of the right ventricle are discussed extensively in other chapters. Increased afterload of the right ventricle increases myocardial oxygen consumption which alters coronary flow patterns predisposing to coronary ischemia and risk of sudden death [112, 113]. The intimate spatial relationship of the right to the left ventricle translates to

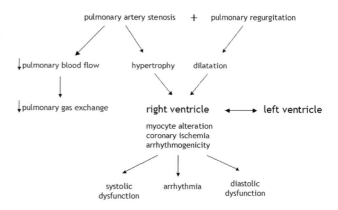

Fig. 9.2 Consequences of pulmonary artery stenosis

physiological interdependence. Ultimately, obstruction of the pulmonary vascular bed results in ventilation to perfusion mismatch, decreased exercise endurance, low cardiac output, and susceptibility to life-threatening arrhythmias.

9.3.1 Pulmonary Artery Stenosis and Right Ventricular Hypertension

Chronic right ventricular pressure load can be guardedly tolerated in the settings of postoperative Mustard or Senning operations, Williams and Alagille syndromes, and single-ventricle hemodynamics such as hypoplastic left heart syndrome [114].

Pulmonary artery dilation and stenting has been documented to reduce right ventricular pressure, particularly with improvements in the central segments [9, 15, 17, 18]. As such, hypertension in the unaffected portions of the vascular bed presumably secondary to increased flow may also be ameliorated. The degree of right ventricular hypertension to cause detrimental hypertrophy, impairment of systolic and diastolic function, and predisposition to coronary ischemia is not known [112]. As a corollary, the degree of reduction to be of clinical significance remains undefined.

9.3.2 Pulmonary Artery Stenosis and Pulmonary Regurgitation

The morbidity of chronic pulmonary regurgitation has become apparent [115–117]. Its adverse effects are best documented in the model of the postoperative tetralogy of Fallot patient with decreased exercise endurance and increased risk of sudden death. Right ventricular pressure-volume loops and magnetic resonance imaging (MRI) have been utilized to demonstrate an increase in pulmonary regurgitant volume when there is concurrent branch pulmonary artery stenosis [118].

The left pulmonary artery appears to be predisposed to regurgitation possibly related to higher impedance of the smaller left lung in a levocardic heart position [119]. Kang et al. [119] demonstrated by MRI that despite higher forward flow in the left pulmonary artery, the larger regurgitant fraction resulted in a lower net flow compared with the right side. The combination of stenosis and regurgitation of the left pulmonary artery synergistically may create particularly unfavorable right ventricular hemodynamics.

9.3.3 Pulmonary Artery Stenosis and Gas Exchange

The functional unit of the cardiorespiratory system lies at the capillary–alveolar interface. In the laws of lung development as stated by Reid et al., in the pre-acinar region of the lung, the branching pattern of arteries and airways is complete by the 16th week of intrauterine life, alveoli develop after birth, increasing in number until the age of 8 years (most rapidly within in the first 10 months to 3 years) and in size until growth of the chest wall is finished, and blood vessels are remodeled and increase concurrently with growth of the alveoli [120, 121].

The spectacular adaptive compensatory mechanisms of the cardiorespiratory unit is highlighted by two models—unilateral pneumonectomy and ligation of unilateral pulmonary artery. Unilateral pneumonectomy in the dog provides an insightful model for characterizing sources, mechanisms, and limits of adaptation to the loss of a known number of lung units [122]. To compensate, there is recruitment of the tremendous preexisting alveolar-capillary reserves. Furthermore, regenerative growth is manifested by acinar tissue, alveolar capillaries, alveolar septae, and bronchioles. In contrast, blood vessels incapable of regeneration adapt by elongation and dilatation of existing branches manifesting compensatory growth [123]. In immature dogs, unilateral lung resection simulated vigorous alveolar regeneration that returned lung volume, diffusing capacity, and extravascular septal tissue volume to completely normal and maintained up to somatic maturity [124]. Compensatory mechanisms were significantly more robust in puppies than in adult dogs [124, 125].

There appears to be a critical environment of pulmonary artery blood supply that is required to ensure normal development of the intra-acinar arteries [67]. Tetralogy of Fallot is associated with a decrease in size and number of alveoli and small intra-acinar arteries despite the larger than normal preacinar arteries [67, 68]. Pulmonary atresia is associated with reduced pre- and intra-acinar arterial size and number in the neonatal period [126, 127]. Lung hypoplasia and impaired diffusing capacity is reported in adults with congenital pulmonary valve stenosis [128].

Ligation of the left pulmonary artery in the pig provides a model of the most extreme pulmonary artery stenosis [129]. Ipsilateral lung volume is decreased associated with reduction in size and number of alveoli. Total lung volume was within normal limits because of compensation by the right lung. Unique to the lung are the two sources of pulmonary blood flow with the bronchial circulation, with its prolific capacity for angiogenesis, maintaining normal or near normal intra-acinar arteries [126, 127, 130, 131]. This is in contrast to the hypoplasia or obliteration of the underperfused pre-acinar arteries. There is a risk of pulmonary hypertension in the contralateral lung [131–133]. Insights from a review of 81 cases of congenital unilateral absence of a pulmonary artery highlighted the importance of pressure and flow in the genesis of pulmonary hypertension, particularly when regression of the fetal pulmonary vascular pattern has not been allowed to occur. Furthermore, the incidence of pulmonary hypertension was 19% in isolated cases versus 88% when combined with a cardiovascular shunt [132].

Such models provide evidence that normal pulmonary blood flow hemodynamics should be restored as soon as possible. It should occur before reduction in luminal diameter and changes in elastic wall structure increase the technical difficulty and subsequent outcomes of surgical anastomosis. Improving pulmonary blood flow before the critical growth period of the lung is over presumably encourages normal alveolar development [68, 134]. As demonstrated in the animal model, lung-diffusing capacity measured physiologically at peak exercise provides a noninvasive sensitive indicator of the integrity of the pulmonary vascular bed during lung growth, subclinical cardiopulmonary disease, and a response to therapeutic interventions [125, 135, 136].

9.3.4 Pulmonary Artery Stenosis and Exercise Capacity

Exercise is associated with a large increase in pulmonary blood flow. In order to accommodate, recruitment of blood vessels ensues with a corresponding decrease in pulmonary vascular resistance. Pulmonary vascular obstruction compromises these adaptive responses, thus resulting in excessive right ventricular pressure and volume loading and ultimately decreases ventricular output [137]. In adults with peripheral pulmonary artery stenoses manifesting as progressive dyspnea and fatigue, pulmonary balloon angioplasty targeted at normalizing ventilation to perfusion mismatch abnormalities improved symptoms (NYHA class I–II) in 82% and this was sustained in 64% at a mean follow-up period of 52 ± 32 months [16].

Decreased exercise capacity in postoperative patients with tetralogy of Fallot is well described. [137–141]. Severe pulmonary regurgitation is one of the most frequent and important of the multifactorial causes [116, 117, 138, 141]. Its magnitude and effect on exercise capacity appears to be heightened when pulmonary artery stenosis is also present [118, 137, 140, 142]. During exercise, patients with pulmonary artery stenosis exhibit higher VE/VCO2 slopes (the slope of relation between minute ventilation and carbon dioxide production, an index of the degree of excessive ventilation as a result of pulmonary blood flow maldistribution, ventilation–perfusion mismatch, and inefficient gas exchange) during exercise compared with their counterparts without stenosis [137].

There exists no report specifically comparing exercise parameters before and after pulmonary artery intervention, particularly in the absence of significant pulmonary regurgitation.

9.4 Summary

Evidence supports that catheter-based angioplasty and stenting of pulmonary arteries can effectively increase vessel diameter and flow resulting in decrease in right ventricular pressure and degree of pulmonary regurgitation. The lung-gas exchange unit displays remarkable adaptive mechanisms but time appears to be of the essence in order to obtain maximal benefit for ultimate lung development. It has become apparent that current catheter-based therapies have limitations and are inadequate for significant future advancements. Pulmonary angiogenesis agents appear to be in foreseeable future and are eagerly anticipated. Much remains unknown about the magnitude of impact of pulmonary artery interventions at clinical, functional, and microscopic levels. As such, more sophisticated methods of analyzing and quantifying changes in the pulmonary microvascular bed are needed. Rehabilitation and manipulation of the pulmonary vascular bed remains one of the most important challenges in the management of congenital heart disease.

References

1. Cohn LH, Sanders JH Jr, Collins JJ, Jr. Surgical treatment of congenital unilateral pulmonary arterial stenosis with contralateral pulmonary hypertension. Am J Cardiol. Aug 1976;38(2): 257–60.
2. Fuster V, McGoon DC, Kennedy MA, Ritter DG, Kirklin JW. Long-term evaluation (12–22 years) of open heart surgery for tetralogy of Fallot. Am J Cardiol. Oct 1980;469(4):635–42.
3. Trant CA Jr, O'Laughlin MP, Ungerleider RM, Garson A Jr. Cost-effectiveness analysis of stents, balloon angioplasty, and surgery for the treatment of branch pulmonary artery stenosis. Pediatr Cardiol. Sep–Oct 1997;18(5):339–44.
4. Stamm C, Friehs I, Zurakowski D, Scheule AM, Moran AM, Lock JE, et al. Outcome after reconstruction of discontinuous pulmonary arteries. J Thorac Cardiovasc Surg. Feb 2002;123(2): 46–57.

5. Edwards BS, Lucas RV Jr, Lock JE, Edwards JE. Morphologic changes in the pulmonary arteries after percutaneous balloon angioplasty for pulmonary arterial stenosis. Circulation. Feb 1985;71(2):195–201.

6. Lock JE, Niemi T, Einzig S, Amplatz K, Burke B, Bass JL. Transvenous angioplasty of experimental branch pulmonary artery stenosis in newborn lambs. Circulation. Nov 1981;64(5):886–93.

7. Ino T, Kishiro M, Okubo M, Akimoto K, Nishimoto K, Yabuta K, et al. Dilatation mechanism of balloon angioplasty in children: assessment by angiography and intravascular ultrasound. Cardiovasc Intervent Radiol. Mar–Apr 1998;21(2): 102–8.

8. Palmaz JC. Intravascular stents: tissue-stent interactions and design considerations. Am J Roentgenol. Mar 1993; 160(3):613–8.

9. Gentles TL, Lock JE, Perry SB. High pressure balloon angioplasty for branch pulmonary artery stenosis: early experience. J Am Coll Cardiol. Sep 1993;22(3):867–72.

10. Lock JE, Castaneda-Zuniga WR, Fuhrman BP, Bass JL. Balloon dilation angioplasty of hypoplastic and stenotic pulmonary arteries. Circulation. May 1983;67(5):962–7.

11. Ring JC, Bass JL, Marvin W, Fuhrman BP, Kulik TJ, Foker JE, et al. Management of congenital stenosis of a branch pulmonary artery with balloon dilation angioplasty. Report of 52 procedures. J Thorac Cardiovasc Surg. Jul 1985;90(1):35–44.

12. Butera G, Antonio LT, Massimo C, Mario C. Expanding indications for the treatment of pulmonary artery stenosis in children by using cutting balloon angioplasty. Catheter Cardiovasc Interv. Mar 2006;67(3):460–5.

13. Bartolomaeus G, Radtke WA. Patterns of late diameter change after balloon angioplasty of branch pulmonary artery stenosis: evidence for vascular remodeling. Catheter Cardiovasc Interv. Aug 2002;56(4):533–40.

14. Bush DM, Hoffman TM, Del Rosario J, Eiriksson H, Rome JJ. Frequency of restenosis after balloon pulmonary arterioplasty and its causes. Am J Cardiol. Dec 1 2000;86(11):1205–9.

15. Hosking MC, Thomaidis C, Hamilton R, Burrows PE, Freedom RM, Benson LN. Clinical impact of balloon angioplasty for branch pulmonary arterial stenosis. Am J Cardiol. Jun 1 1992;69(17):1467–70.

16. Kreutzer J, Landzberg MJ, Preminger TJ, Mandell VS, Treves ST, Reid LM, et al. Isolated peripheral pulmonary artery stenoses in the adult. Circulation. Apr 1 1996;93(7):1417–23.

17. Rothman A, Perry SB, Keane JF, Lock JE. Early results and follow-up of balloon angioplasty for branch pulmonary artery stenoses. J Am Coll Cardiol. Apr 1990;15(5):1109–17.

18. Zeevi B, Berant M, Blieden LC. Midterm clinical impact versus procedural success of balloon angioplasty for pulmonary artery stenosis. Pediatr Cardiol. Mar–Apr 1997;18(2):101–6.

19. Kan JS, Marvin WJ, Jr., Bass JL, Muster AJ, Murphy J. Balloon angioplasty—branch pulmonary artery stenosis: results from the Valvuloplasty and Angioplasty of Congenital Anomalies Registry. Am J Cardiol. Mar 15 1990;65(11):798–801.

20. Baker CM, McGowan FX, Jr, Keane JF, Lock JE. Pulmonary artery trauma due to balloon dilation: recognition, avoidance and management. J Am Coll Cardiol. Nov 1 2000;36(5):1684–90.

21. Bergersen L, Gauvreau K, Lock JE, Jenkins KJ. Recent results of pulmonary arterial angioplasty: the differences between proximal and distal lesions. Cardiol Young. Dec 2005;15(6): 597–604.

22. O'Laughlin MP, Perry SB, Lock JE, Mullins CE. Use of endovascular stents in congenital heart disease. Circulation. Jun 1991;83(6):1923–39.

23. Benson LN, Hamilton F, Dasmahapatra H, Rabinowitch M, Coles JC, Freedom RM. Percutaneous implantation of a balloon-expandable endoprosthesis for pulmonary artery stenosis: an experimental study. J Am Coll Cardiol. Nov 1 1991;18(5):1303–8.

24. Fogelman R, Nykanen D, Smallhorn JF, McCrindle BW, Freedom RM, Benson LN. Endovascular stents in the pulmonary circulation. Circulation. Aug 15 1995;92(4):881–5.

25. McMahon CJ, El Said HG, Vincent JA, Grifka RG, Nihill MR, Ing FF, Fraley JK, Mullins CE. Refinements in the implantation of pulmonary arterial stents: impact on morbidity and mortality of the procedure over the last two decades. Cardiol Young. Oct 2002;12(5):445–52.

26. Mendelsohn AM, Bove EL, Lupinetti FM, Crowley DC, Lloyd TR, Fedderly RT, Beekman RH 3rd. Intraoperative and percutaneous stenting of congenital pulmonary artery and vein stenosis. Circulation. Nov 1993;88(5 Pt 2):II210–7.

27. Mullins CE, O'Laughlin MP, Vick GW III, Mayer DC, Myers TJ, Kearney DL, et al. Implantation of balloon-expandable intravascular grafts by catheterization in pulmonary arteries and systemic veins. Circulation. Jan 1988;77(1):188–99.

28. Shaffer KM, Mullins CE, Grifka RG, O'Laughlin MP, McMahon W, Ing FF, et al. Intravascular stents in congenital heart disease: short- and long-term results from a large single-center experience. J Am Coll Cardiol. 1998;31:661–7.

29. O'Laughlin MP, Slack MC, Grifka RG, Perry SB, Lock JE, Mullins CE. Implantation and intermediate-term follow-up stents in congenital heart disease. Circulation. Aug 1993;88(2):605–14.

30. Hijazi ZM, al-Fadley F, Geggel RL, Marx GR, Galal O, al-Halees Z, et al. Stent implantation for relief of pulmonary artery stenosis: immediate and short-term results. Cathet Cardiovasc Diagn. May 1996;38(1):16–23.

31. Spadoni I, Giusti S, Bertolaccini P, Maneschi A, Kraft G, Carminati M. Long-term follow-up of stents implanted to relieve peripheral pulmonary arterial stenosis: hemodynamic findings and results of lung perfusion scanning. Cardiol Young. Nov 1999;9(6):585–91.

32. Forbes TJ, Rodriguez-Cruz E, Amin Z, Benson LN, Fagan TE, Hellenbrand WE, et al. The Genesis stent: a new low-profile stent for use in infants, children, and adults with congenital heart disease. Cathet Cardiovasc Intervent. Jul 2003;59(3):406–14.

33. Rutledge JM, Mullins CE, Nihill MR, Grifka RG, Vincent JA. Initial experience with IntraTherapeutics IntraStent Double Strut LD stents in patients with congenital heart defects. Cathet Cardiovasc Intervent. 2002;56:541–8.

34. Kreutzer J, Rome JJ. Open-cell design stents in congenital heart disease: a comparison of IntraStent vs. Palmaz stents. Cathet Cardiovasc Intervent. 2002;56:400–409.

35. Peuster M, Hesse C, Schloo T, Fink C, Beerbaum P, von Schnakenburg C. Long-term biocompatibility of a corrodible peripheral iron stent in the porcine descending aorta. Biomaterials. Oct 2006;27(28):4955–62.

36. Peuster M, Wohlsein P, Brugmann M, Ehlerding M, Seidler K, Fink C, et al. A novel approach to temporary stenting: degradable cardiovascular stents produced from corrodible metal-results 6–18 months after implantation into New Zealand white rabbits. Heart. Nov 2001;86(5):563–9.

37. Stone GW, Ellis SG, Cox DA, Hermiller J, O'Shaughnessy C, Mann JT, et al. A polymer-based, paclitaxel-eluting stent in patients with coronary artery disease. N Engl J Med. Jan 15 2004;350(3):221–3.

38. Formigari R, Santoro G, Guccione P, Giamberti A, Pasquini L, et al. Treatment of pulmonary artery stenosis after arterial switch operation: stent implantation vs. balloon angioplasty. Catheter Cardiovasc Interv. Jun 2000;50(2):207–11.

39. Hashmi A, Benson LN, Nykanen D. Endovascular stent implantation to relieve extrinsic right pulmonary artery

compression due to an enlarged neoaorta. Catheter Cardiovasc Interv. Apr 1999;46(4):430–3.

40. Schneider MB, Zartner P, Duveneck K, Lange PE. Various reasons for repeat dilatation of stented pulmonary arteries in paediatric patients. Heart. Nov 2002;88(5):505–9.

41. Moore JW, Spicer RL, Perry JC, Mathewson JW, Kirkpatrick SE, George L, et al. Percutaneous use of stents to correct pulmonary artery stenosis in young children after cavopulmonary anastomosis. Am Heart J. Dec 1995;130(6):1245–9.

42. Vranicar M, Teitel DF, Moore P. Use of small stents for rehabilitation of hypoplastic pulmonary arteries in pulmonary atresia with ventricular septal defect. Catheter Cardiovasc Interv. Jan 2002;55(1):78–82.

43. Ing FF, Grifka RG, Nihill MR, Mullins CE. Repeat dilation of intravascular stents in congenital heart defects. Circulation. Aug 15 1995;92(4):893–7.

44. Morrow WR, Palmaz JC, Tio FO, Ehler WJ, VanDellen AF, Mullins CE. Re-expansion of balloon-expandable stents after growth. J Am Coll Cardiol. Dec 1993;22(7):2007–13.

45. Trerotola SO, Lund GB, Newman J, Olson JL, Widlus DM, Anderson JH, et al. Repeat dilation of Palmaz stents in pulmonary arteries: study of safety and effectiveness in a growing animal model. J Vasc Interv Radiol. May–Jun 1994;5(3):425–32.

46. Barath P, Fishbein MC, Vari S, Forrester JS. Cutting balloon: a novel approach to percutaneous angioplasty. Am J Cardiol. Nov 1 1991;68(11):1249–52.

47. Unterberg C, Buchwald AB, Barath P, Schmidt T, Kreuzer H, et al. Cutting balloon coronary angioplasty: initial clinical experience. Clin Cardiol. 1993;16:660–4.

48. Rhodes JF, Lane GK, Mesia CI, Moore JD, Nasman CM, Cowan DA, et al. Cutting balloon angioplasty for children with small-vessel pulmonary artery stenoses. Catheter Cardiovasc Interv. Jan 2002;55(1):73–7.

49. Magee AG, Wax D, Saiki Y, Rebekya I, Benson LN. Experimental branch pulmonary artery stenosis angioplasty using a novel cutting balloon. Can J Cardiol. Aug 1998;14(8):1037–41.

50. Bergersen LJ, Perry SB, Lock JE. Effect of cutting balloon angioplasty on resistant pulmonary artery stenosis. Am J Cardiol. Jan 15 2003;91(2):185–9.

51. Bergersen L, Jenkins KJ, Gauvreau K, Lock JE. Follow-up results of Cutting Balloon angioplasty used to relieve stenoses in small pulmonary arteries. Cardiol Young. Dec 2005;15(6):605–10.

52. Sugiyama H, Veldtman GR, Norgard G, Lee KJ, Chaturvedi R, Benson LN. Bladed balloon angioplasty for peripheral pulmonary artery stenosis. Catheter Cardiovasc Interv. May 2004;62(1):71–7.

53. Mertens L, Dens J, Gewillig M. Use of a cutting balloon catheter to dilate resistant stenoses in major aortic-to-pulmonary collateral arteries. Cardiol Young. Sep 2001;119(5):574–7.

54. De Giovanni JV. Timing, frequency, and results of catheter intervention following recruitment of major aortopulmonary collaterals in patients with pulmonary atresia and ventricular septal defect. J Interv Cardiol. Feb 2004;17(1):47–52.

55. Bush A, Busst CM, Haworth SG, Hislop AA, Knight WB, Corrin B, et al. Correlations of lung morphology, pulmonary vascular resistance, and outcome in children with congenital heart disease. Br Heart J. Apr 1988;59(4):480–5.

56. Mori Y, Nakanishi T, Niki T, Kondo C, Nakazawa M, Imai Y, et al. Growth of stenotic lesions after balloon angioplasty for pulmonary artery stenosis after arterial switch operation. Am J Cardiol. Mar 15 2003;91(6):693–8.

57. Inoue T, Sakai Y, Hoshi K, Yaguchi I, Fujito T, Morooka S. Lower expression of neutrophil adhesion molecule indicates less vessel wall injury and might explain lower restenosis rate after

cutting balloon angioplasty. Circulation. Jun 30 1998;97(25):2511–8.

58. Rosales AM, Lock JE, Perry SB, Geggel RL. Interventional catheterization management of perioperative peripheral pulmonary stenosis: balloon angioplasty or endovascular stenting. Catheter Cardiovasc Interv. Jun 2002;56(2):272–7.

59. Geggel RL, Gauvreau K, Lock JE. Balloon dilation angioplasty of peripheral pulmonary stenosis associated with Williams syndrome. Circulation. May 1 2001;103(17):2165–70.

60. Zeevi B, Berant M, Blieden LC. Late death from aneurysm rupture following balloon angioplasty for branch pulmonary artery stenosis. Cathet Cardiovasc Diagn. Nov 1996;39(3):284–6.

61. Arnold LW, Keane JF, Kan JS, Fellows KE, Lock JE. Transient unilateral pulmonary edema after successful balloon dilation of peripheral pulmonary artery stenosis. Am J Cardiol. Aug 1 1988;62(4):327–30.

62. Reddy VM, Liddicoat Jr, McElhinney DB, Brook MM, Stanger P, Hanley FL. Routine primary repair of tetralogy of Fallot in neonates and infants less than three months of age. Ann Thorac Surg. Dec 1995;60(Suppl 6):S592–6.

63. Pigula FA, Khalil PN, Mayer JE, del Nido PJ, Jonas RA. Repair of tetralogy of Fallot in neonates and young infants. Circulation. Nov 9 1999;100(Suppl 19):II157–61.

64. Hirsch JC, Mosca RS, Bove EL. Complete repair of tetralogy of Fallot in the neonate: results in the modern era. Ann Surg. Oct 2000;232(4):508–14.

65. Gladman G, McCrindle BW, Williams WG, Freedom RM, Benson LN. The modified Blalock–Taussig shunt: clinical impact and morbidity in Fallot's tetralogy in the current era. J Thorac Cardiovasc Surg. Jul 1997;114(1):25–30.

66. Sachweh J, Dabritz S. Didilis V, Vazquez-Jiminez JF, Bernuth G, Messmer BJ. Pulmonary artery stenosis after systemic-to-pulmonary shunt operations. Eur J Cardiothorac Surg. Sep 1998;14(3):229–34.

67. Rabinovitch M, Herrera-deLeon V, Castaneda AR, Reid L. Growth and development of the pulmonary vascular bed in patients with tetralogy of Fallot with or without pulmonary atresia. Circulation. Dec 1981;64(6):1234–49.

68. Johnson RJ, Haworth SG. Pulmonary vascular and alveolar development in tetralogy of Fallot: a recommendation for early correction. Thorax. Dec 1982;37(12):893–901.

69. Hovels-Gurich HH, Konrad K, Skorzenski D, Nacken C, Minkenberg R, et al. Long-term neurodevelopmental outcome and exercise capacity after corrective surgery for tetralogy of Fallot or ventricular septal defect in infancy. Ann Thorac Surg. Mar 2006;81(3):958–66.

70. Shillingford AJ, Wernovsky G. Academic performance and behavioral difficulties after neonatal and infant heart surgery. Pediatr Clin North Am. Dec 2004;51(6):1625–39.

71. Bellinger DC, Wypij D, duDuplessis AJ, Rappaport LA, Jonas RA, et al. Neurodevelopmental status at eight years in children with dextro-transposition of the great arteries: the Boston Circulatory Arrest Trial. J Thorac Cardiovasc Surg. Nov 2003;126(5):1385–96.

72. Sluysmans T, Neven B, Rubay J, Lintermans J, Ovaert C, Mucumbitsi J, et al. Early balloon dilatation of the pulmonary valve in infants with tetralogy of Fallot. Risks and benefits. Circulation. Mar 1 1995;91(5):1506–11.

73. Sreeram N, Saleem M, Jackson M, Peart I, McKay R, Arnold R, Walsh K. Results of balloon pulmonary valvuloplasty as a palliative procedure in tetralogy of Fallot. J Am Coll Cardiol. Jul 1991;18(1):159–65.

74. Hwang B, Lu JH, Lee BC, Hsieng JH, Meng CC. Palliative treatment for tetralogy of Fallot with percutaneous balloon

dilatation of right ventricular outflow tract. Jpn Heart J. Nov 1995;36(6):751–61.

75. Kreutzer J, Perry SB, Jonas RA, Mayer JE, Castaneda AR, Lock JE. Tetralogy of Fallot with diminutive pulmonary arteries: preoperative pulmonary valve dilation and transcatheter rehabilitation of pulmonary arteries. J Am Coll Cardiol. Jun 1996;27(7):1741–7.

76. Marshall AC, Love BA, Lang P, Jonas RA, del Nido PJ, et al. Staged repair of tetralogy of Fallot and diminuitive pulmonary arteries with a fenestrated ventricular septal defect patch. J Thorac Cardiovasc Surg. Nov 2003;126(5):1427–1433.

77. Peirone A, Lee KJ, Yoo SJ, Musewe N, Smallhorn J, Benson l. Staged rehabilitation of ductal origin of left pulmonary artery in an infant Fallot's tetralogy. Cath Cardiovasc Interv. Jul 2003;59(3):392–5.

78. Clark SC. Lung injury after cardiopulmonary bypass. Perfusion. Jul 2006;21(4):225–8.

79. Schultz JM, Karamlou T, Swanson J, Shen I, Ungerleider RM. Hypothermic low-flow cardiopulmonary bypass impairs pulmonary and right ventricular function more than circulatory arrest. Ann Thorac Surg. Feb 2006;81(2):474–80.

80. Zahn EM, Dobrolet NC, Nykanen DG, Ojito J, Hannan RL, Burke RP. Interventional catheterization performed in the early postoperative period after congenital heart surgery in children. J Am Coll Cardiol. Apr 7 2004;43(7):1264–9.

81. Haworth SG, Rees PG, Taylor JF, Macartney FJ, de Leval M, Stark J. Pulmonary atresia with ventricular septal defect and major aortopulmonary collateral arteries. Effect of systemic pulmonary anastomosis. Br Heart J. Feb 1981;45(2):133–41.

82. Reddy VM, Petrossian E, McElhinney DB, Moore P, Teitel DF, Hanley FL. One-stage complete unifocalization in infants: when should the ventricular septal defect be closed? J Thorac Cardiovasc Surg. May 1997;113(5):858–66; discussion 66–8.

83. Reddy VM, McElhinney DB, Amin Z, Moore P, Parry AJ, Teitel DF, et al. Early and intermediate outcomes after repair of pulmonary atresia with ventricular septal defect and major aortopulmonary collateral arteries: experience with 85 patients. Circulation. Apr 18 2000;101(15):1826–32.

84. d'Udekem Y, Alphonso N, Norgaard MA, Cochrane AD, Grigg LE, et al. Pulmonary atresia with ventricular septal defects and major aortopulmonary collateral arteries: unifocalization brings no long-term benefits. J Thorac Cardiovasc Surg. Dec 2005;130(6):1496–502.

85. Yagihara T, Yamamoto F, Nishigaki K, Matsuki O, Uemura H. Isizaka T, et al. Unifocalization for pulmonary atresia with ventricular septal defect and major aortopulmonary collaterals. J Thorac Cardiovasc Surg. 1996;109:832–44.

86. Gupta A, Odim J, Levi D, Chang RK, Laks H. Staged repair of pulmonary atresia with ventricular septal defect and major aortopulmonary collateral arteries: experience with 104 patients. J Thorac Cardiovasc Surg. 2003;126:174652.

87. Brown SC, Eyskens B, Mertens L, Dumoulin M, Gewillig M. Percutaneous treatment of stenosed major aortopulmonary collaterals with balloon dilatation and stenting: what can be achieved? Heart. Jan 1998;79(1):24–8.

88. Vance MS. Use of Palmaz stents to palliate pulmonary atresia with ventricular septal defect and stenotic aortopulmonary collaterals. Cathet Cardiovasc Diagn. Apr 1997;40(4):387–9.

89. El-Said HG, Clapp S, Fagan TE, Conwell J, Nihill MR. Stenting of stenosed aortopulmonary collaterals and shunts for palliation of pulmonary atresia/ventricular septal defect. Catheter Cardiovasc Interv. Apr 2000;49(4):430–6.

90. Veldtman GR, Hartley A, Visram N, Benson LN. Radiofrequency applications in congenital heart disease. Expert Rev Cardiovasc Ther. Jan 2004;2(1):117–26.

91. Hausdorf G, Schulze-Neick I, Lange PE. Radiofrequency-assisted "reconstruction" of the right ventricular outflow tract in muscular pulmonary atresia with ventricular septal defect. Br Heart J. Apr 1993;69(4):343–6.

92. Bull K, Somerville J, Ty E, Spiegelhalter D. Presentation and attrition in complex pulmonary atresia. J Am Coll Cardiol. Feb 1995;25(2):491–9.

93. Senzaki H, Isoda T, Ishizawa A, Hishi T. Reconsideration of criteria for the Fontan operation. Circulation. 1994;89:266–71.

94. Petit CJ, Gillespie MJ, Kreutzer J, Rome JJ. Endovascular stents for relief of cyanosis in single-ventricle patients with shunt or conduit-dependent pulmonary blood flow. Catheter Cardiovasc Interv. Aug 2006;68(2):280–6.

95. Zalzstein E, Moes CA, Musewe NN, Freedom Rm. Spectrum of cardiovascular anomalies in Williams-Beuren syndrome. Pediatr Cardiol. Oct 1991;12(4):219–23.

96. Wessel A, Pankau R, Kececioglu D. Ruschewski W. Bursch JH. Three decades of follow-up of aortic and pulmonary vascular lesions in the Williams-Beuren syndrome. Am J Med Genet. Sep 1 1994;52(3):297–301.

97. Alagille D Estrada A, Hadchouel M, Gautier M, Odievre M, Dommergues JP. Syndromic paucity of interlobular bile ducts (Alagille syndrome or ariohepatic dysplasia): Review of 80 cases. J Pediatr. 1987;110:195–200.

98. Wessel A, Gravenhorst V, Buchhorn R, Gosch A, Partsch CJ, Pankau R. Risk of sudden death in the Williams-Beuren syndrome. Am J Med Genet A. Jun 15 2004;127(3):234–7.

99. Bird LM, Billman GF, Lacro RV, Spicer RL, Jariwala LK, Hoyme HE, et al. Sudden death in Williams syndrome: report of ten cases. J Pediatr. Dec 1996;129(6):926–31.

100. Kececioglu D. Kotthoff S, Vogt J. Williams-Beuren syndrome: a 30-year follow-up of natural and postoperative course. Eur Heart J. Nov 1993;14(11):1458–64.

101. Miyamura H, Watanabe H, Tatebe S, Eguchi S. Spontaneous regression of peripheral pulmonary artery stenosis in Williams syndrome. Jpn Circ J. May 1996;60(5):311–4.

102. van Son JA, Edwards WD, Danielson GK. Pathology of coronary arteries, myocardium, and great arteries in supravalvular aortic stenosis. Report of five cases with implications for surgical treatment. J Thorac Cardiovasc Surg. Jul 1994;108(1):21–8.

103. Geggel < !AU: Ref. 103 Geggel RL et al. not cited in the text. Please cite it or delete from the list.– > RL, Gauvreau K, Lock JE. Balloon dilation angioplasty of peripheral pulmonary stenosis associated with Williams syndrome. Circulation. May 1 2001;103(17):2165–70.

104. Fraser CD, Jr., Latson LA, Mee RB. Surgical repair of severe bilateral branch pulmonary artery stenosis. Ann Thorac Surg. Mar 1995;59(3):738–40.

105. Saidi AS, Kovalchin JP, Fisher DJ, Ferry GD, Grifka RG. Balloon pulmonary valvuloplasty and stent implantation. For peripheral pulmonary artery stenosis in Alagille syndrome. Tex Heart Inst J. 1998;25(1):79–82.

106. Wren C, Oslizlok P, Bull C. Natural history of supravalvular aortic stenosis and pulmonary artery stenosis. J Am Coll Cardiol. Jun 1990;15(7):1625–30.

107. Giddins NG, Finley JP, Nanton MA, Roy DL. The natural course of supravalvar aortic stenosis and peripheral pulmonary artery stenosis in Williams syndrome. Br Heart J. Oct 1989;62(4):315–9.

108. Stamm C, Friehs I, Moran A, Zurakowski D, Bacha E, Mayer JE, Jonas RA, del Nido PF. Surgery for bilateral outflow tract obstruction in elastin arteriopathy. J Thorac Cardiovasc Surg. 2000;120:75563.

109. Razavi RS, Baker A, Qureshi SA, Rosenthal E, Marsh MJ, Leech SC, Rela M, Mieli-Vergani G. Hemodynamic response

to continuous dobutamine in Alagille's syndrome. Transplantation. Sep 15 2001;72(5):823–8.

110. EmerickKM, Rand EB, Goldmuntz E, Krantz ID, Spinner NB, Picooli DA. Features of Alagille syndrome in 92 patients; frequency and relation to prognosis. Hepatology. 1999; 29(3):822–9.

111. Marino IR, ChapChap P, Esquivel CO, Zetti G, Carone E, Borland L, Tzakis AG, Todo S. Rowe MI, Starzl TE. Liver transplantation for arteriohepatic dysplasia (Alagille's syndrome). Transpl Int. May 1992;5(2):61–4.

112. Gomez A, Bialostozky D, Zajarias A, Santos E, Palomar A, Martinez ML, et al. Right ventricular ischemia in patients with primary pulmonary hypertension. J Am Coll Cardiol. Oct 2001;38(4):1137–42.

113. Mebazaa A, Karpati P, Renaud E, Algotsson L. Acute right ventricular failure—from pathophysiology to new treatments. Intensive Care Med. Feb 2004;30(2):185–96.

114. Cheung MM, Smallhorn JF, McCrindle BW, Van Arsdell GS, Redington AN. Non-invasive assessment of ventricular force-frequency relations in the univentricular circulation by tissue Doppler echocardiography: a novel method of assessing myocardial performance in congenital heart disease. Heart. Oct 2005;91(10):1338–42.

115. Redington AN. Physiopathology of right ventricular failure. Semin Thorac Cardiovasc Surg Pediatr Card Surg Annu. 2006;3–10.

116. Carvalho JS, Shinebourne EA, Busst C, Rigby ML, Redington AN. Exercise capacity after complete repair of tetralogy of Fallot: deleterious effects of residual pulmonary regurgitation. Br Heart J. Jun 1992;67(6):470–3.

117. Rowe SA, Zahka KG, Manolio TA, Horneffer PJ, Kidd L. Lung function and pulmonary regurgitation limit exercise capacity in postoperative tetralogy of Fallot. J Am Coll Cardiol. Feb 1991;17(2):461–6.

118. Chaturvedi RR, Kilner PJ, White PA, Bishop A, Szwarc R, Redington AN. Increased airway pressure and simulated branch pulmonary artery stenosis increase pulmonary regurgitation after repair of tetralogy of Fallot. Real-time analysis with a conductance catheter technique. Circulation. Feb 4 1997;95(3):643–9.

119. Kang I-S, Redington AN, Benson LN, MacGowan C, Valsangiacomo ER, Roman K, et al. Differential regurgitation in branch pulmonary arteries after repair of tetralogy of Fallot. Circulation. Jun 17 2003;107(23):2938–2943.

120. Davies G, Reid L. Growth of the alveoli and pulmonary arteries in childhood. Thorax. Nov 1970;25(6):669–81.

121. Hislop A, Reid L. Pulmonary arterial development during childhood: branching pattern and structure. Thorax. Mar 1973;28(2):129–35.

122. Hsia CC, Herazo LF, Ramanathan M, Johnson RL Jr. Cardiopulmonary adaptations to pneumonectomy in dogs. IV. Membrane diffusing capacity and capillary blood volume. J Appl Physiol. Aug 1994;77(2):998–1005.

123. Hsia CC. Signals and mechanisms of compensatory lung growth. J Appl Physiol. Nov 2004;97(5):1992–8.

124. Takeda SI, Ramanathan M, Estrera AS, Hsia CC. Postpneumonectomy alveolar growth does not normalize hemodynamic and mechanical function. J Appl Physiol. Aug 1999;87(2):491–7.

125. Hsia CC, Herazo LF, Johnson RL, Jr. Cardiopulmonary adaptations to pneumonectomy in dogs. I. Maximal exercise performance. J Appl Physiol. Jul 1992;73(1):362–7.

126. Haworth SG, Reid L. Quantitative structural study of pulmonary circulation in the newborn with pulmonary atresia. Thorax. Apr 1977;32(2):129–33.

127. Haworth SG, Macartney FJ. Growth and development of pulmonary circulation in pulmonary atresia with ventricular septal defect and major aortopulmonary collateral arteries. Br Heart J. Jul 1980;44(1):14–24.

128. De Troyer A, Yernault JC, Englert M. Lung hypoplasia in congenital pulmonary valve stenosis. Circulation. Oct 1977;56(4 Pt 1):647–51.

129. Haworth SG, McKenzie SA, Fitzpatrick ML. Alveolar development after ligation of left pulmonary artery in newborn pig: clinical relevance to unilateral pulmonary artery. Thorax. Dec 1981;36(12):938–43.

130. Mitzner W, Wagner EM. Vascular remodeling in the circulations of the lung. J Appl Physiol. Nov 2004;97(5): 1999–2004.

131. Haworth SG, de Leval M, Macartney FJ. Hypoperfusion and hyperperfusion in the immature lung. Pulmonary arterial development following ligation of the left pulmonary artery in the newborn pig. J Thorac Cardiovasc Surg. Aug 1981;82(2):281–92.

132. Pool PE, Vogel JH, Blount SG, Jr. Congenital unilateral absence of a pulmonary artery. The importance of flow in pulmonary hypertension. Am J Cardiol. Nov 1962;10: 706–32.

133. Vogel JH, Averill KH, Pool PE, Bount SG Jr. Experimental pulmonary arterial hypertension in the newborn calf. Circ Res. Dec 1963;13:55771.

134. Haworth SG, Rees PG, Taylor JF, Macartney FJ, de Leval M, Stark J. Pulmonary atresia with ventricular septal defect and major aortopulmonary collateral arteries. Effect of systemic pulmonary anastomosis. Br Heart J. Feb 1981;45(2): 133–41.

135. Hsia CC. Recruitment of lung diffusing capacity: update of concept and application. Chest. Nov 2002;122(5):1774–83.

136. Hsia CC, Herazo LF, Ramanathan M, Claassen H, Fryder-Doffey F, Hoppeler H, et al. Cardiopulmonary adaptations to pneumonectomy in dogs. III. Ventilatory power requirements and muscle structure. J Appl Physiol. May 1994;76(5): 2191–8.

137. Rhodes J, Dave A, Pulling MC, Geggel RL, Marx GR, Fulton DR, et al. Effect of pulmonary artery stenoses on the cardiopulmonary response to exercise following repair of tetralogy of Fallot. Am J Cardiol. May 15 1998;81(10):1217–9.

138. Wessel HU, Cunningham WJ, Paul MH, Bastanier CK, Muster AJ, Idriss FS. Exercise performance in tetralogy of Fallot after intracardiac repair. J Thorac Cardiovasc Surg. Oct 1980;80(4):582–93.

139. Yetman AT, Lee KJ, Hamilton R, Morrow WR, McCrindle BW. Exercise capacity after repair of Tetralogy of Fallot in infancy. Am J Cardiol. Apr 15 2001;87(8):1021–3; A5.

140. Marx GR, Hicks RW, Allen HD, Goldberg SJ. Noninvasive assessment of hemodynamic responses to exercise in pulmonary regurgitation after operations to correct pulmonary outflow obstruction. Am J Cardiol. Mar 1 1988;61(8): 595–601.

141. Eyskens B, Reybrouck T, Bogaert J, Dymarkowsky S, Daenen W, Dumoulin M, et al. Homograft insertion for pulmonary regurgitation after repair of tetralogy of fallot improves cardiorespiratory exercise performance. Am J Cardiol. Jan 15 2000;85(2):221–5.

142. Ruzyllo W, Nihill MR, Mullins CE, McNamara DG. Hemodynamic evaluation of 221 patients after intracardiac repair of tetralogy of Fallot. Am J Cardiol. Oct 3 1974;34(5): 565–76.

Surgical Repair of Pulmonary Arterial Stenosis 10

Michael E. Mitchell and James S. Tweddell

10.1 Introduction

The surgical repair of pulmonary arterial stenosis, be the obstruction congenital or acquired, remains a challenge to cardiac surgeons dealing with congenital malformations, pediatric cardiologists, and most importantly, the patients and families whose lives are affected. Obstructive lesions of the right ventricular outflow tract and pulmonary arteries are found in one-quarter to one-third of children with congenitally malformed hearts. The spectrum of diagnoses includes tetralogy of Fallot with pulmonary stenosis or atresia, heterotaxy syndromes, transposition, double-outlet right ventricle, atrioventricular septal defect with common atrioventricular junction, common arterial trunk, elastin arteriopathy, and Noonan's syndrome, in addition to others. The indications for surgery are often the presence of ductal-dependent flow of blood to the lungs with hypoxia, and careful technical management of stenotic and hypoplastic pulmonary arteries is critical to success. In this review, we discuss surgical techniques to manage congenital and acquired pulmonary stenosis. In most cases, a combination of approaches is required. Our review will concentrate on three standard surgical strategies, including (1) the promotion of growth and relief of cyanosis through the use of systemic-to-pulmonary arterial shunts, (2) reconstruction and/or unifocalization of discontinuous pulmonary arteries or major aortopulmonary collateral arteries, and (3) the selection of conduits from the right ventricle to the pulmonary arteries as part of reparative procedures. To finish, we discuss the current state of advanced strategies, including the application of hybrid procedures and the use of tissue-engineered grafts for reconstruction.

J.S. Tweddell (✉)
Children's Hospital of Wisconsin, MS 715, 9000 W. Wisconsin Ave., Milwaukee, WI, 53226
e-mail: jtweddell@chw.org

10.2 Preoperative Planning and Diagnostic Imaging

Careful preoperative imaging for evaluation and surgical planning is essential to consistent operative success. Angiography is the gold standard for delineating anatomic and physiologic details relevant to the repair of the stenotic pulmonary arterial bed. Although angiography is invasive, and exposes the patient to radiation and iodinated contrast, it provides the only means of obtaining data concerning pressures and saturations of oxygen. As the number and complexity of the patients increase, less invasive methods, including computerized tomographic scanning, magnetic resonance imaging, and quantitative lung perfusion scintigraphy, can contribute to preoperative and preinterventional evaluation, as well as providing for less-invasive postoperative follow-up. These techniques may permit more targeted angiography, limiting exposure to radiation and dyes. Both computerized tomographic and magnetic resonance imaging have shown excellent correlation with angiography in identifying localized stenosis, as well as the diameter of the pulmonary arteries. [1, 2]

For evaluating the flow of blood through the pulmonary arteries subsequent to reconstruction, quantitative lung perfusion scintigraphy is a useful technology. In this respect, Kim et al. [3] compared the use of imaging of the lungs with technetium perfusion, resonance imaging, and cine-angiography in patients with congenital obstruction of the right ventricular outflow tract. They found reasonable correlation between the different techniques, and concluded that quantitative perfusion scanning is an excellent technique for ongoing follow-up of the patterns of pulmonary arterial flow.

10.3 Systemic-to-Pulmonary Arterial Shunts

Shunts are used to increase the flow of blood to the lungs, and thereby relieve cyanosis prior to anticipated biventricular repair, or as part of a staged functionally univentricular

A.N. Redington et al. (eds.), *Congenital Diseases in the Right Heart*, DOI 10.1007/978-1-84800-378-1_10,
© Springer-Verlag London Limited 2009

strategy. In lesions requiring shunting, the goals of surgery are, first, to provide a stable source of pulmonary arterial flow, and second, to induce growth of the native pulmonary arteries. Successful accomplishment of both goals depends on technical and anatomic factors. Following shunting procedures, it is common to find hypoplasia of the pulmonary artery on the opposite side to the insertion of the shunt. In a retrospective review of 101 patients with modified Blalock–Taussig shunts undergoing subsequent catheterization, Barta and colleagues [4] found that, when there was no antegrade flow through the pulmonary trunk, the pulmonary artery on the opposite side to the shunt was significantly smaller than the one to which the distal anastomosis had been constructed. They concluded that, in the absence of antegrade flow of blood, a shunt to the pulmonary trunk or the bifurcation of the pulmonary arteries may promote more uniform growth [4].

In a study designed to analyze the relationship of shunting to the subsequent development of pulmonary arterial stenosis, Sachweh and associates [5] looked at the angiograms taken before and after construction of shunts in 59 patients. They concluded that stenosis is not a rare event after the operative procedure, and that stenoses were found on the same side and the opposite side to the shunt in essentially equal numbers. Patency of the arterial duct, with or without administration of prostaglandin E1, correlated with the development of stenosis on the side of the duct. Stenosis on the side of the shunt was attributed to inappropriate surgical technique, increased intimal proliferation, or to kinking of the pulmonary arteries.

The size of the bifurcation of the pulmonary trunk, and the proximal right and left pulmonary arteries, is important in patients with functionally univentricular anatomy, and is a risk factor for staged palliation when creating the Fontan circulation [6]. Recently, modification of the Norwood procedure by placing a conduit from the right ventricle to the pulmonary arteries has been introduced as an alternative to creating a shunt from the brachiocephalic arteries. Rumball and colleagues [7] found better growth of the central pulmonary arteries when a conduit was placed from the right ventricle. Despite the increase in size of the central arteries, the ratio of pulmonary-to-systemic flows was, in some cases, less. Patients with a conduit also need the second stage of palliation more rapidly than patients undergoing construction of a modified Blalock–Taussig shunt, presumably due to increased cyanosis [8]. Patients receiving the conduit frequently had stenoses in the distal branches of the pulmonary arteries, and although the size of the arteries proximal to their first branches was satisfactory, the proximal narrowing may account for the increased cyanosis and lower ratio of pulmonary-to-systemic flows [7]. Although such proximal stenosis would seem to be amenable to surgical rehabilitation at the second stage of

Norwood palliation, in at least one study these patients did remain at risk for late mortality following the superior cavopulmonary anastomosis [8]. Ultimately, the ongoing multicentered trial may answer some of these questions.

10.4 Reconstruction and Unifocalization

10.4.1 Discontinuous Pulmonary Arteries

Discontinuity of the right and left pulmonary arteries may be the result of anomalous origin of one of the arteries from the aorta or arterial duct, or the discontinuity may result from ductal involution in the setting of hypoplastic pulmonary arteries. The use of prosthetic material, or bilateral construction of shunts and a staged approach, is sometimes necessary, particularly if there is limited intrapericardial pulmonary arterial tissue. When possible, primary repair by means of direct primary anastomosis of the discontinuous arteries offers the best potential for growth [9, 10]. Luhmer and associates [11] observed that it is necessary to remove the ductal tissue in the artery completely at the time of reconstruction in order to prevent recurrent stenosis. Stamm and colleagues [10] reported on 200 patients undergoing reconstruction of congenital or acquired discontinuity, and found that a direct anastomosis was associated with significantly better survival, and that the presence of aortopulmonary collateral arteries was a risk factor for late occlusion of the pulmonary arteries. Reconstruction of discontinuous pulmonary arteries can result in a durable outcome, with potential for growth. Murphy et al. [12] reported late outcome in a small group of patients followed for less than 5 years, with lung scans demonstrated flow of less than half through the affected lung, albeit with growth in the diameter of the recruited native arteries in all patients.

10.4.2 Unifocalization

Despite encouraging results with reconstruction of discontinuous pulmonary arteries, the outcomes of unifocalization of patients with tetralogy of Fallot with pulmonary atresia and major aortopulmonary collateral arteries remain a challenge. It was Haworth and colleagues at Great Ormond Street Hospital who first suggested that unifocalization of such collateral arteries could increase the flow of blood to the lungs, and hence permit anatomic reconstruction in this group of patients. The same group subsequently reported disappointing results with a strategy of staged unifocalization, with half of the patients deemed unsuitable for complete repair, and only one-eighth achieving correction [13]. In 1995, Reddy et al. [14] described primary midline unifocalization, reporting that nine of their 10 survivors of the operation were doing well at median follow-up of 8 months (Fig. 10.1). They concluded that this single-stage approach establishes normal cardiovascular physiology early in life, minimizing the potential for development of pulmonary vascular obstructive disease, eliminates the need for multiple shunts and the use of prosthetic material, and minimizes the number of operations required.

Late results of the unifocalization suggest, nonetheless, that there are problems with growth and development of the collateral arteries. D'Udekem and colleagues [15] from the Royal Children's Hospital in Melbourne reviewed serial angiographies of 82 consecutive patients with who had undergone repair of tetralogy of Fallot with pulmonary atresia and systemic-to-pulmonary collateral arteries, and demonstrated that late survival depended primarily on the rowth of the native pulmonary circulation. More discouragingly, the unifocalized collateral arteries had a high rate of thrombosis, with little evidence of growth (Fig. 10.2). The available evidence suggests that a direct anastomosis between diminutive pulmonary arteries and the ascending aorta in order to promote growth of the native pulmonary arteries appears to be a reasonable first step with reproducible results [16, 17]. The proportion of patients with the diagnosis of tetralogy of Fallot and

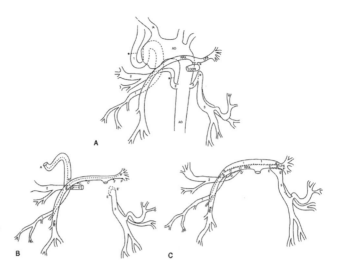

Fig. 10.1 Schematic diagram of a patient with tetralogy of Fallot with pulmonary atresia and major aortopulmonary collateral arteries undergoing one-stage unifocalization via a median sternotomy. The collateral arteries are anastomosed to the native pulmonary arteries. The goal is to supply as many lung segments as possible, and reconstruction is performed early in life to avoid development of pulmonary vascular obstructive disease
Reprinted from Circulation 2000;101:1826–1832.; Reddy MV, McElhinney DB, Amin Z, et al., Early and intermediate outcomes after repair of pulmonary atresia with ventricular septal defect and major aortopulmonary collateral arteries. Copyright 2000 with permission from Elsevier.

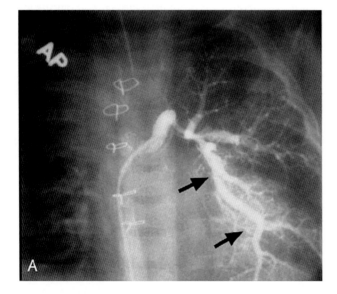

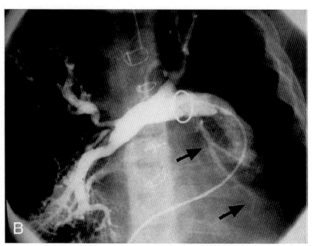

Fig. 10.2 Failure of growth of unifocalized major aortopulmonary collaterals. A large aortopulmonary collateral supplying the left lower lobe is shown prior to unifocalization and 4 years after unifocalization. The angiograms demonstrate growth of the native intrapericardial pulmonary arteries, but no growth in the unifocalized collateral vessel.

Reprinted from J Thorac Cardiovasc Surg. 2005;130:1496–502;. d'Udekem Y, Alphonso N, Norgaard MA, et al. Pulmonary atresia with ventricular septal defects and major aortopulmonary collateral arteries: unifocalization brings no long-term benefits. Copyright 2005, with permission from Elsevier

Table 10.1 Published reports for treatment of tetralogy of Fallot with pulmonary atresia and major aortopulmonary collateral arteries

Institution	n	Complete repair (%)	Hosp survival (%)	Intraop RV/LV pressure	Long-term survival (%)	Latest RV/LV pressure	Length of follow-up (months)
Mayo Clinic 1989 [18]	38	61	96	0.63	91	N/R	32
Royal Children's Hosp, Melbourne, 1991 [19]	58	52	97	0.51	90	N/R	43
Children's Hospital Boston, 1993 [20]	48	29	73	N/R	56	0.71	120
University of California, Los Angeles, 1997 [21]	26	38	100	0.45	100	N/R	9
University of Michigan, 1995 [22]	14	57	79	0.57	64	N/R	9
Children's Hospital, Los Angeles, 1997 [23]	10	80	100	NR	100	0.44	17
Montreal Children's Hospital, 1997 [24]	12	92	92	0.47	83	N/R	19
Children's Mercy Hospital, Kansas City, 2000 [25]	11	N/A	91	<0.5	91	N/R	N/R
University of California, San Francisco, 2000 [26]	85	80	89	0.44	81	N/R	22
Children's Hospital La Timone, Marseille, 2001 [27]	10	70	90	0.5	80	0.6	45
Bambino Gesu, Rome 2003 [28]	37	78	85	0.5	81	0.48	43
Cleveland Clinic Children's Hospital, 2003 [16]	46	61	100	0.36	98	0.50	44

RV/LV = right ventricular/left ventricular pressure ratio; N/A = not available; N/R = not recorded (adapted from Duncan et al. 2003 [16])

pulmonary atresia with systemic-to-pulmonary collateral arteries in whom complete repair can be accomplished with an acceptable right ventricular pressure of less than half systemic is not precisely known, since not all series include all patients with the diagnosis, and variable follow-up is available. Taken at a rough estimate, it appears to be between one-half and four-fifths (Table 10.1).

10.5 Conduits from the Right Ventricle to the Pulmonary Arteries

Valved conduits are commonly used in cardiac reconstruction for lesions in which there is hypoplasia of the right ventricular outflow tract or pulmonary arteries, and/or in which the postoperative right-sided pressures may be elevated, such as common arterial trunk, and pulmonary atresia with ventricular septal defect. The ideal valved conduit, one which is readily available, durable, and accommodates growth, remains to be found. In neonates and infants, homografts are generally preferable, because of their ease of use and durability. Among such conduits, smaller relative size at implantation, use of aortic versus pulmonary homografts, and placement in extra-anatomic

positions were associated with earlier need for reintervention [29–31]. In older children and adults, it is difficult to identify a difference in durability between homografts and xenografts [32, 33].

Availability of homograft conduits remains a problem necessitating the development of alternatives. Among the available alternatives, bovine jugular vein conduits are increasingly used. Shebani et al. [34] examined the early outcomes using such conduits in a group of 64 patients. After a mean follow-up of 14 months, four conduits had been explantated, one for endocarditis and three because of dilatation, but that catheter intervention was needed in one-quarter. Risk factors for failure seemed to be related less to the use of the bovine conduit than to factors related to the underlying congenital cardiac disease, specifically, the small size of the conduit and the higher ratio of right-to-left ventricular pressures. Others have identified factors specific to the use of bovine conduits [35]. Gober et al. [36] studied a series of 38 patients, and found that five conduits needed to be replaced because of severe stenosis at the distal anastomosis, while moderate to severe dilation occurred in two proximal to the valve. They noted excessive formation of intimal peel, and severe perigraft scarring reaction in all cases, after a mean follow-up of around 18 months. Proximal dilatation of the conduits may result in the early development of regurgitation [37]. In younger patients, nevertheless, these being the group in whom an alternative to homografts is most desperately needed, the bovine veins performed well when compared to homografts. A recent multicentered study from the Congenital Heart Surgeons' Society [38] showed that bovine venous conduits had a similar freedom from reintervention to homografts when used in children under the age of 2 years.

As conduits fail, reoperation becomes necessary. Options at this time include complete replacement as opposed to removal of peel. In this respect, Bermudez et al. [39] reported on the late results from follow-up of a cohort for 102 patients aged from 5 to 58 years who underwent placement of a prosthetic roof over the fibrous bed of the explanted conduit. In nine patients, reoperation related to the peel operation, with regurgitation in the nonvalved conduit in seven, moderate stenosis of the pulmonary bioprosthesis in one, and endocarditis in the other. Overall survival free from reoperation for failure of peel reconstruction at 10 and 15 years was 90.7 and 82%, respectively [39].

The optimal material for reconstruction of the right ventricular outflow tract, including its valve, has not been discovered. Decisions are based on the age and diagnosis of the patient, pulmonary arterial pressure, and availability of materials. At present, most institutions employ all of the above techniques in combination. Reoperations are predictable.

10.6 Hybrid Procedures

Catheter-based interventions, with dilations of both native and acquired pulmonary arterial stenosis, are a cornerstone of management for this difficult group of patients, and sometimes provide the definitive solution. Although serial surgical and interventional efforts performed at intervals have been routine, simultaneous hybrid procedures are becoming more common.

Early postoperative intervention for stenoses in the pulmonary arteries might salvage patients who would otherwise require complex and hazardous reoperation. Zahn and colleagues [40] have suggested that transcatheter interventions, including angioplasty of stenotic suture lines and implantation of stents, can safely be performed even in the early postoperative period. Difficult stenoses of the right or left pulmonary arteries can successfully be managed with a combined transcatheter and surgical approach. Mendelsohn and colleagues [41] demonstrated that a hybrid approach with intraoperative angioplasty extends the implantation of

stents to smaller children, who may have limited percutaneous access. Certain lesions, such as supravalvar pulmonary stenosis or stenosis at the bifurcation of the pulmonary trunk, are better dealt with at surgery [42]. After reviewing 134 dilations for stenosis in the setting of Williams' syndrome, Geggel et al. [43] concluded that a serial approach of distal dilations followed by surgical repair of proximal obstruction may be rational and successful. Ungerleider et al. [44] reported on their experience using stents placed intraoperatively to rehabilitate severely stenotic pulmonary vessels in the context of the need for a concomitant cardiac surgical procedure in 16 cases, because of limited vascular access for placement of the stents in the catheterization laboratory in 11 instances, or to *rescue* of patients with complications after attempted placement of stents in four cases. They concluded that intraoperative stenting is an attractive option, commenting that insertion during cardiopulmonary bypass using direct vision is quick and immediately effective. Once stented, they found that the vessels remained open, and were amenable to future surgical intervention as necessary.

10.7 Tissue Engineering

The ideal reconstructive material for the stenotic pulmonary artery would be both easy to work with, allowing reconstruction of even the most delicate vessels, and would have the capacity to grow and develop with the native arteries. Shin'oka et al. [45] reported implanting tissue-engineered grafts seeded with autologous bone marrow cells in 42 patients requiring reconstructions of the pulmonary arteries. After a mean follow-up of up to 2 years, they reported patency in all arteries, as well as a growth of the grafts to over 100% of the implanted size. Their report represents one of the first successful reports of tissue-engineered vascular autografts for use in reconstructing the pulmonary vascular bed (Fig. 10.3).

10.8 Conclusion

The management of congenital and acquired pulmonary arterial stenosis remains a challenge. Surgical strategies include relief of cyanosis, and induction of growth, through the use of shunting procedures; reconstructive and recruitment procedures on the pulmonary arteries; as well as reconstruction of the right ventricular outflow tract using valved conduits. The best results

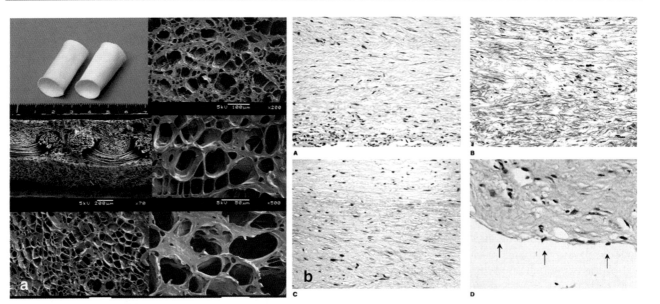

Fig. 10.3 Tissue-engineered conduit. **a** shows how biodegradable scaffolds are created using L-lactide and epsilon caprolactone. Scanning electromicroscopic findings of polymer scaffolds demonstrate the interstices that host cells will occupy following implantation. **b** shows histopathologic findings of explanted graft in a patient requiring reoperation. *Arrows* indicate endothelium-like cells.

Reprinted from J Thorac Cardiovasc Surg. 2005;129:1330–8, Shin'oka T, Matsumura G, Hibino N, et al. Midterm clinical result of tissue-engineered vascular autografts seeded with autologous bone marrow cells Copyright 2005, with permission from Elsevier

with the most complex and difficult patients clearly reflect successful combination of preoperative evaluation, meticulous surgical technique, informed surgical decision making, and close collaboration with interventional cardiologists. New advances in operative materials and interventional technologies are short-term goals to improve outcomes.

References

1. Ley S, Zaporozhan J, Arnold R, et al. Preoperative assessment and follow-up of congenital abnormalities of the pulmonary arteries using CT and MRI. Eur Radiol. 2006 Jun 24; [Epub ahead of print]
2. Kondo C, Takada K, Yokoyama U, et al. Comparison of three-dimensional contrast-enhanced magnetic resonance angiography and axial radiographic angiography for diagnosing congenital stenoses in small pulmonary arteries. Am J Cardiol. 2001;87:420–4.
3. Kim JH, Lee DS, Chung JK, et al. Quantitative lung perfusion scintigraphy in postoperative evaluation of congenital right ventricular outflow tract obstructive lesions. Clin Nucl Med. 1996;21:471–6.
4. Batra AS, Starnes VA, Wells WJ. Does the site of insertion of a systemic–pulmonary shunt influence growth of the pulmonary arteries? Ann Thorac Surg. 2005;79:636–40.
5. Sachweh J, Dabritz S, Didilis V, et al. Pulmonary artery stenosis after systemic-to-pulmonary shunt operations. Eur J Cardiothorac Surg. 1998;14:229–34.
6. Gentles TL, Mayer JE Jr, Gauvreau K, et al. Fontan operation in five hundred consecutive patients: factors influencing early and late outcome. J Thorac Cardiovasc Surg. 1997;114:376–91.
7. Rumball EM, McGuirk SP, Stumper O, et al. The RV-PA conduit stimulates better growth of the pulmonary arteries in hypoplastic left heart syndrome. Eur J Cardiothorac Surg. 2005;27:801–6.
8. Tabbutt S, Dominguez TE, Ravishankar C, et al. Outcomes after the stage I reconstruction comparing the right ventricular to pulmonary artery conduit with the modified Blalock Taussig shunt. Ann Thorac Surg. 2005;80:1582–90
9. Shanley CJ, Lupinetti FM, Shah NL, et al. Primary unifocalization for the absence of intrapericardial pulmonary arteries in the neonate. J Thorac Cardiovasc Surg. 1993;106:237–47.
10. Stamm C, Friehs I, Zurakowski D, et al. Outcome after reconstruction of discontinuous pulmonary arteries. J Thorac Cardiovasc Surg. 2002;123:246–57.,
11. Luhmer I, Ziemer G. Coarctation of the pulmonary artery in neonates. Prevalence, diagnosis, and surgical treatment. J Thorac Cardiovasc Surg. 1993;106:889–94.
12. Murphy DN, Winlaw DS, Cooper SG, et al. Successful early surgical recruitment of the congenitally disconnected pulmonary artery. Ann Thorac Surg. 2004;77:29–35.
13. Haworth SG, Rees PG, Taylor JF, et al. Pulmonary atresia with ventricular septal defect and major aortopulmonary collateral arteries. Effect of systemic pulmonary anastomosis. Br Heart J. 1981;45:133–41.
14. Reddy VM, Liddicoat JR, Hanley FL, et al. Midline one-stage complete unifocalization and repair of pulmonary atresia with ventricular septal defect and major aortopulmonary collaterals. J Thorac Cardiovasc Surg. 1995;109:832–44
15. d'Udekem Y, Alphonso N, Norgaard MA, et al. Pulmonary atresia with ventricular septal defects and major

aortopulmonary collateral arteries: unifocalization brings no long-term benefits. J Thorac Cardiovasc Surg. 2005;130: 1496–502.

16. Duncan BW, Mee RB, Prieto LR, et al. Staged repair of tetralogy of Fallot with pulmonary atresia and major aortopulmonary collateral arteries. J Thorac Cardiovasc Surg. 2003;126:694–702.

17. Rodefeld MD, Reddy VM, Thompson LD, et al. Surgical creation of aortopulmonary window in selected patients with pulmonary atresia with poorly developed aortopulmonary collaterals and hypoplastic pulmonary arteries. J Thorac Cardiovasc Surg. 2002;123:1147–54.

18. Puga FJ, Leoni FE, Julsrud PR et al. Complete repair of pulmonary atresia, ventricular septal defect, and severe peripheral arborization abnormalities of the central pulmonary arteries. Experience with preliminary unifocalization procedures in 38 patients. J Thorac Cardiovasc Surg. 1989;98:1018–28.

19. Iyer KS, Mee RB. Staged repair of pulmonary atresia with ventricular septal defect and major systemic to pulmonary artery collaterals. Ann Thorac Surg. 1991;51:65–72.

20. Rome JJ, Mayer JE, Castaneda AR, et al. Tetralogy of Fallot with pulmonary atresia. Rehabilitation of diminutive pulmonary arteries. Circulation. 1993;88:1691–8.

21. Marelli AJ, Perloff JK, Child JS. et al. Pulmonary atresia with ventricular septal defect in adults. Circulation. 1994;89:243–51.

22. Pagani FD, Cheatham JP, Beekman RH, et al. The management of tetralogy of Fallot with pulmonary atresia and di minutive pulmonary arteries. J Thorac Cardiovasc Surg. 1995;110:1521–32.

23. Luciani GB, Wells WJ, Khong A, et al. The clamshell incision for bilateral pulmonary artery reconstruction in tetralogy of Fallot with pulmonary atresia. J Thorac Cardiovasc Surg. 1997;113:443–52.

24. Tchervenkov CI, Salasidis G, Cecere R, et al., One-stage midline unifocalization and complete repair in infancy versus multiple-stage unifocalization followed by repair for complex heart disease with major aortopulmonary collaterals. J Thorac Cardiovasc Surg. 1997;114:727–35.

25. Lofland GK, The management of pulmonary atresia, ventricular septal defect, and multiple aorta pulmonary collateral arteries by definitive single stage repair in early infancy. Eur J Cardiothorac Surg. 2000;18:480–6.

26. Reddy MV, McElhinney DB, Amin Z, et al. Early and intermediate outcomes after repair of pulmonary atresia with ventricular septal defect and major aortopulmonary collateral arteries. Circulation. 2000;101:1826–32.

27. Metras D, Chetaille P, Kreitmann B, et al. Pulmonary atresia with ventricular septal defect, extremely hypoplastic pulmonary arteries, major aorto-pulmonary collaterals. Eur J Cardiothorac Surg. 2001;20:590–7.

28. Carotti A, Albanese SB, Minniti G, et al. Increasing experience with integrated approach to pulmonary atresia with ventricular septal defect and major aortopulmonary collateral arteries. Eur J Cardiothorac Surg. 2003;23:719–26.

29. Tweddell JS, Pelech AN, Frommelt PC, et al. Factors affecting longevity of homograft valves used in right ventricular outflow

tract reconstruction for congenital heart disease. Circulation. 2000;102(19 Suppl 3):III130–5.

30. Meyns B, Jashari R, Gewillig M, et al. Factors influencing the survival of cryopreserved homografts. The second homograft performs as well as the first. Eur J Cardiothorac Surg. 2005;28(2):211–6.

31. Bando K, Danielson GK, Schaff HV, et al. Outcome of pulmonary and aortic homografts for right ventricular outflow tract reconstruction. J Thorac Cardiovasc Surg. 1995;109:509–17.

32. Homann M, Haehnel JC, Mendler N, et al. Reconstruction of the RVOT with valved biological conduits: 25 years experience with allografts and xenografts. Eur J Cardiothorac Surg. 2000;17:624–30.

33. Dearani JA, Danielson GK, Puga FJ, et al. Late follow–up of 1095 patients undergoing operation for complex congenital heart disease utilizing pulmonary ventricle to pulmonary artery conduits. Ann Thorac Surg. 2003;75:399–410

34. Shebani SO, McGuirk S, Baghai M, et al. Right ventricular outflow tract reconstruction using Contegra valved conduit: natural history and conduit performance under pressure. Eur J Cardiothorac Surg. 2006;29:397–405.

35. Meyns B, Van Garsse L, Boshoff D, et al. The Contegra conduit in the right ventricular outflow tract induces supravalvular stenosis. J Thorac Cardiovasc Surg. 2004;128:834–40.

36. Gober V, Berdat P, Pavlovic M, et al. Adverse mid-term outcome following RVOT reconstruction using the Contegra valved bovine jugular vein. Ann Thorac Surg. 2005;79:625–31.

37. Bove T, Demanet H, Wauthy P, et al. Early results of valved bovine jugular vein conduit versus bicuspid homograft for right ventricular outflow tract reconstruction. Ann Thorac Surg. 2002;74:536–41.

38. Karamlou T, Blackstone EH, Hawkins JA, et al. Can Pulmonary Conduit Dysfunction and Failure Be Reduced in Infants Less Than Age Two Years at Implantation? J Thorac Cardiovasc Surg. 2006;132(4):829–38.

39. Bermudez CA, Dearani JA, Puga FJ, et al. Late results of the peel operation for replacement of failing extracardiac conduits. Ann Thorac Surg. 2004;77:881–7.

40. Zahn EM, Dobrolet NC, Nykanen DG, et al. Interventional catheterization performed in the early postoperative period after congenital heart surgery in children. J Am Coll Cardiol. 2004;43:1264–9.

41. Mendelsohn AM, Bove EL, Lupinetti FM, et al. Intraoperative and percutaneous stenting of congenital pulmonary artery and vein stenosis. Circulation. 1993;88(suppl 2):II 210–7.

42. Bacha EA, Kreutzer J. Comprehensive management of branch pulmonary artery stenosis. J Interv Cardiol. 2001;14:367–75.

43. Geggel RL, Gauvreau K, Lock JE. Balloon dilation angioplasty of peripheral pulmonary stenosis associated with Williams syndrome. Circulation. 2001;103:2165–70.

44. Ungerleider RM, Johnston TA, O'Laughlin MP, et al. Intraoperative stents to rehabilitate severely stenotic pulmonary vessels. Ann Thorac Surg. 2001;71:476–81.

45. Shin'oka T, Matsumura G, Hibino N, et al. Midterm clinical result of tissue-engineered vascular autografts seeded with autologous bone marrow cells. J Thorac Cardiovasc Surg. 2005;129:1330–8.

Mechanisms of Late Systemic Right Ventricular Failure

Andrew S. Mackie and Judith Therrien

A morphologic right ventricle (RV) supports the systemic circulation in patients who have undergone an atrial baffle palliation of transposition of the great arteries (TGA), in patients with congenitally corrected transposition of the great arteries (CCTGA), and in patients with hypoplastic left syndrome (HLHS) or other functional single ventricle lesions of right ventricular morphology. The RV has important morphologic differences relative to the normal left ventricle (LV), which is believed to account for abnormalities of right ventricular function, both at rest and in response to exercise, that have been described in patients with a RV supporting the systemic circulation. The increased risk of premature death related to right ventricular dysfunction after atrial baffle procedures for TGA highlights the importance of this problem [1–3]. Novel noninvasive imaging modalities have recently contributed to our understanding of the mechanisms by which the systemic RV fails. However, the etiology of systemic right ventricular dysfunction remains incompletely understood. This chapter summarizes the current body of knowledge in this field.

11.1 Natural History of the Systemic Right Ventricle

Numerous authors have described the long-term sequelae of the Mustard and Senning procedures for TGA [1–9]. Roos-Hesselink and colleagues, in the longest prospective study to date of patients who have undergone a Mustard procedure, found that moderate or severe right ventricular dysfunction, as assessed by echocardiography, was present in none of 47 patients after a median follow-up of 14 years, but developed in 61% of the same patients when reassessed 11 years later.[4] Independent predictors of moderate or severe right ventricular dysfunction were atrial flutter and the combination of Mustard surgery with ventricular septal defect or pulmonary stenosis repair. The prevalence of severe tricuspid regurgitation (TR) increased from 2% at the initial evaluation to 20% at a median follow-up of 25 years. A corresponding decline in exercise capacity was also observed, with a median maximal exercise capacity of 84% predicted at 14 years, declining to 72% at 25 years.

The natural history of CCTGA shares some parallels with TGA following atrial switch procedures. However, there are important factors that distinguish these lesions. CCTGA is more commonly associated with a ventricular septal defect, pulmonary stenosis or atresia, variable degrees of atrioventricular block, and Ebstein's anomaly of the tricuspid valve [10]. The majority of patients with associated lesions and CCTGA have undergone cardiac surgery [10], which may impact long-term outcome. Although some patients remain asymptomatic [11, 12], many develop significant clinical manifestations. Graham et al., in a large multicenter study of adults with CCTGA and two functional ventricles, found that clinical congestive heart failure (CHF) was more common in patients with *significant* associated lesions (defined as a large VSD, moderate-severe pulmonary stenosis, pulmonary atresia, moderate-severe TR, or Ebstein's anomaly) than in those with insignificant or no associated abnormalities. CHF also increased in prevalence with increasing age [10]. By age 45 years, 67% of patients with significant lesions had CHF, compared to 25% of those without associated lesions. Moderate-severe right ventricular dysfunction was present in approximately one-third of patients, both with and without associated lesions, and also increased in prevalence with increasing age. In the largest single-center cohort published to date, Rutledge and colleagues found that complete atrioventricular block was an independent risk factor for progressive right ventricular dysfunction [13]. Additional risk factors were prior *conventional*

A.S. Mackie (✉)
MAUDE Unit, McGill University Health Center, Montreal, Canada

A.N. Redington et al. (eds.), *Congenital Diseases in the Right Heart*, DOI 10.1007/978-1-84800-378-1_11,
© Springer-Verlag London Limited 2009

biventricular repair (repair of ventricular septal defect and/or pulmonary stenosis) and moderate-severe TR.

Relative to TGA and CCTGA, the long-term prognosis of the single systemic RV is less well documented. Although the atrial switch procedures were introduced in the late 1950s and early 1960s, Norwood surgery for HLHS was first described in the early 1980s and in most centers has been associated with higher mortality than the atrial switch procedures. For these reasons, a shorter duration of follow-up and a smaller population of single RV patients exist relative to TGA and CCTGA. The presence of HLHS was a risk factor for perioperative mortality early in the Fontan era [14], but in a more recent cohort the morphology of the systemic ventricle was not a risk factor [15]. In an echocardiographic analysis of systemic right ventricular function following the Fontan procedure in school-age children (mean age 7.8 years), systolic function was diminished when compared to healthy controls, with a lower fractional area change (42.7% vs. 54.6%, $p = 0.001$). In addition, the Fontan group had a greater reliance on atrial contraction for ventricular filling, consistent with reduced diastolic function [16]. The subjects in this study were asymptomatic, implying that the results may underestimate the true degree of right ventricular dysfunction in this patient population.

11.2 Right Versus Left Ventricles: Morphologic Differences

Several fundamental distinctions exist between the morphologic right and left ventricles. These include differences in atrioventricular valve morphology, myocardial architecture, ventricular shape, coronary perfusion, and the presence of a hypokinetic segment in the normal RV (the infundibulum).

1. Morphology of the atrioventricular valves. Unlike the mitral valve, the tricuspid valve has a papillary muscle that inserts into the ventricular septum. The papillary muscles of the tricuspid valve are small relative to those of the mitral valve. These factors reduce the geometric integrity of the tricuspid valve, relative to the mitral valve, when guarding a systemic circular orifice. In the setting of a systemic RV, the altered position of the ventricular septum results in an abnormal shape of the tricuspid valve annulus and reduced coaptation of the tricuspid leaflets in systole, with tricuspid regurgitation. In addition, among patients with CCTGA there is a high prevalence of morphologic abnormalities of the tricuspid valve (> 90%), the most common being Ebstein's anomaly [17].

2. Myocardial architecture. The ventricular myocardium is arranged in three layers in the LV, but only two layers in the RV. A superficial (subepicardial) and deep (subendocardial) layer are present in both ventricles, whereas a middle layer is unique to the left ventricle [18, 19]. The middle layer is circumferentially oriented and is responsible for the greater myocardial mass of the LV relative to the RV in the normal heart. The majority of RV myocardial fibers are longitudinally oriented, originating at the cardiac apex and inserted into the right atrioventricular junction [20].

3. Ventricular shape. From the three-dimensional perspective, the normal LV approximates a truncated ellipsoid. Relative to a spherical or conical chamber, this shape minimizes the sum of energy expenditures in systole and diastole [21]. In comparison, the RV is a tripartite chamber with a complex three-dimensional shape which is suited to adapting to changes in preload that normally occur with changes in intrathoracic pressure, but not suited to significant increases in afterload [22].

4. Coronary perfusion. Although the origin of the coronary arteries in TGA varies widely [23], the RV is consistently supplied by the right coronary artery. Likewise, the usual arrangement of the coronary arteries in patients with CCTGA is that the RV is supplied by a single right coronary artery [24]. The LV is supplied by two epicardial arteries, the left anterior descending and the circumflex coronary arteries. Therefore, the systemic RV, with its single coronary artery, is at a potential disadvantage with regard to myocardial perfusion, resulting in ischemia. particularly in the setting of myocardial hypertrophy which develops when the RV functions at systemic pressure over long periods of time (mismatch phenomenon).

5. The infundibulum. The infundibulum (conus) of the RV does not contribute significantly to right ventricular ejection. The normal LV does not have an equivalent noncontractile segment [25].

11.3 Mechanisms of Systemic Right Ventricular Dysfunction

1. *Tricuspid regurgitation.* Moderate or severe tricuspid regurgitation is common in patients with a systemic RV. Moderate-severe TR and a prior history of tricuspid valve surgery are both strong risk factors for clinical CHF and RV dysfunction in adults with CCTGA [10]. However, whether patients have TR secondary to ventricular dysfunction, or the presence of TR promotes the development of ventricular dysfunction, has

been the subject of much speculation. Among patients with intrinsic abnormalities of the tricuspid valve, as in patients with Ebstein's anomaly and CCTGA, it seems likely that TR is independent of the development of right ventricular dysfunction. Indeed, Prieto et al. showed that moderate-severe TR preceded right ventricular dysfunction in a cohort of 40 patients with CCTGA [26]. Forty patients were followed for a median of 19 years; 17 (43%) had moderate-severe TR during their clinical course. The presence of a morphologically abnormal tricuspid valve predicted the development of moderate-severe TR, whereas right ventricular dysfunction, open-heart surgery, complete heart block, and pulmonary overcirculation did not. Of 36 patients who had documentation of right ventricular function before the onset of moderate-severe TR, only 2 had impaired function. Among patients in whom the tricuspid valve remained competent, all had normal RV function at last follow-up. These data support a temporal course of TR preceding RV dysfunction in the majority of patients. Furthermore, moderate-severe TR was an independent risk factor for mortality in this cohort, highlighting the importance of this complication (Fig. 11.1). Presumably, the inability of the RV to cope with TR results in a vicious cycle of right ventricular dilation, increasing wall stress, annular dilation, and increasing TR.

2. *Impaired myocardial perfusion.* Radionuclide techniques have demonstrated that perfusion defects, both at rest and during stress, are common in patients who have undergone a Mustard palliation of TGA as well as in patients with CCTGA. Millane and colleagues studied 22 patients (age range 10–25 years, median

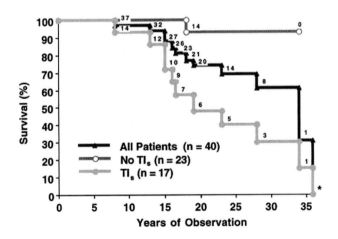

Fig. 11.1 Kaplan–Meier estimate of survival for patients with CCTGA ($n = 40$). Patients with moderate-severe tricuspid regurgitation/insufficiency (TI$_s$) had lower survival than those with mild or no TI$_s$ ($p = 0.01$).
Prieto et al. Circulation 1998;98:997–1005 (page 1000)

15.5 years) status postatrial baffle procedure [9]. Perfusion defects were present in all patients in at least one segment. Twelve patients (55%) had fixed defects only, nine (41%) had fixed and reversible defects, and one (4.5%) had reversible defects only. Fixed perfusion defects, representing areas of infarction or fibrosis, correlated strongly with abnormalities of wall thickening and reduced wall motion. In turn, wall-thickening abnormalities correlated with right ventricular ejection fraction, and there was a trend toward a greater number of perfusion defects in patients with an ejection fraction less than 40%. The same group did a similar study in a small group of children and adults with CCTGA (without associated lesions) and found similar results [27]. None of the patients in this latter study were operated, implying that perfusion defects seen in patients who have had atrial baffle procedures are due at least in part to right ventricular ischemia or infarction, rather than solely to the effects of cardiopulmonary bypass.

Positron emission tomography (PET) has also been used to evaluate myocardial blood flow in patients with CCTGA. Hauser and colleagues showed that myocardial blood flow did not differ at rest between unoperated patients with CCTGA and controls. However, adenosine-induced vasodilation resulted in significantly less hyperemic blood flow in the CCTGA group [28]. Coronary flow reserve correlated positively with maximum oxygen consumption on bicycle ergometry, indicating the clinical significance of these findings. PET has also demonstrated reduced coronary flow reserve as compared to controls in a small study of adolescents and young adults after Mustard palliation of TGA [29].

The pathogenesis of right ventricular ischemia and infarction is likely multifactorial. Right ventricular hypertrophy increases myocardial oxygen requirements, and the right coronary system with a single coronary artery may provide insufficient flow. Animal experiments have shown reduced right-coronary artery flow in the setting of elevated right ventricular pressure [30]. Other investigators have shown that the hypertrophied heart is prone to subendocardial hypoperfusion, even in the absence of macroscopic coronary abnormalities [31]. Myocardial ischemia results from an imbalance between oxygen supply and demand. Reduced oxygen supply relates to decreased effective coronary perfusion caused by impaired diastolic function. In the systemic RV, reduced oxygen supply [28] coexists with an increased oxygen demand (increased wall stress). This mismatch of supply and demand predisposes to subendocardial ischemia and right ventricular dysfunction. Hornung and colleagues showed that following the Mustard procedure, RV mass index correlated inversely with right ventricular ejection fraction determined by MRI [32], supporting this notion that demand ischemia, related to myocardial hypertrophy, results in impaired RV systolic function. Left ventricular ejection fraction was lower in patients with higher RV mass index (> 95 g/m^2), implying that RV hypertrophy impacts LV perfusion and systolic function as well. The inverse correlations between RV mass index and both RV and LV ejection fraction have subsequently been reproduced in a similar population [33].

3. *Myocardial fibrosis.* Magnetic resonance imaging with late gadolinium enhancement (LGE) can detect the presence of myocardial fibrosis of the LV in ischemic and nonischemic cardiomyopathies [34]. In an analysis of 36 adults with TGA who had undergone an atrial baffle procedure, 22 (61%) had evidence of fibrosis of the RV using this technique (Fig. 11.2) [33]. The

presence of fibrosis correlated with increasing age, increased RV end-systolic volume, decreased RV ejection fraction, increased QT dispersion, and increased QRS duration. Although the cross-sectional nature of this study did not allow conclusions about the mechanisms of fibrosis, this data suggests that RV fibrosis contributes to RV dysfunction.

Other mechanisms. This is not an exhaustive list of mechanisms contributing to systemic right ventricular dysfunction; it is likely that other mechanisms remain to be described. Specific patient-related factors probably play a contributing role. These include the influence of cardiopulmonary bypass and myocardial protection, particularly in patients who had cardiac surgery in the more remote past, and the impact of discordant ventricular contraction in patients who have ventricular pacing related to complete heart block. The concept of interventricular dependence as well should not be overlooked.

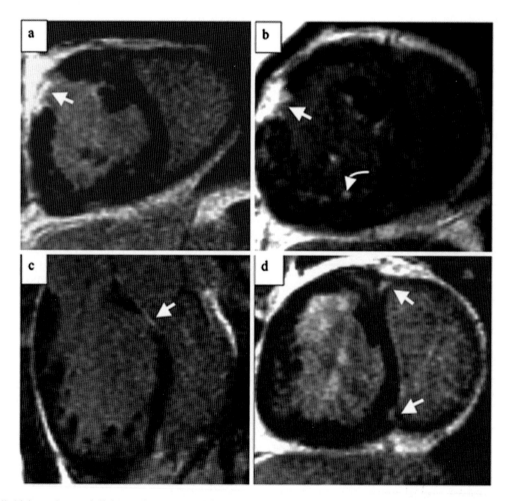

Fig. 11.2 Full-thickness late-gadolinium enhancement of the anterior right ventricular wall (*arrow*) in a patient with previous atrial baffle palliation of transposition of the great arteries.

Babu-Narayan SV et al. Circulation 2005;111:2091–98, Fig. 3a, page 2096

11.4 Conclusion

The majority of patients with a RV in the systemic position develop right ventricular dysfunction over time. The prevalence of this complication increases with age, is frequently accompanied by symptoms and/or impaired exercise capacity, and carries a poor prognosis. Multiple factors contribute to the development of right ventricular dysfunction, tricuspid regurgitation from abnormal tricuspid valve morphology or septal leaflet displacement being probably the most important. Right ventricular ischemia resulting from an imbalance between myocardial oxygen supply and demand also plays a significant role. However, much of the work in this field has been cross-sectional in nature. The challenge now is to follow these cohorts over the long term, in order to improve our understanding of the timing and relative contribution of these and other potential risk factors as they relate to the onset of right ventricular dysfunction. Potential drug therapies such as beta-blockade [44] and angiotensin inhibition [45–47] have recently been reported, but require further evaluation. Surgical interventions, including tricuspid valve replacement in CCTGA [48] and two-stage arterial switch [49, 50], will probably play an increasingly important role, but optimal timing and indications remain to be elucidated. The influence of coronary artery disease on right ventricular performance may become relevant as this population ages.

The number of adolescents and adults with a Fontan circulation and functional single RV will rise significantly in the next 10 years. This group will require further study, using techniques that have been applied to patients with CCTGA and an atrial baffle repair of TGA, and employing new methods of functional and anatomic assessment as they are developed. The evolution of novel therapies for this population will depend on advancing our knowledge of the mechanisms of RV failure.

References

1. Gewillig M, et al. Risk factors for arrhythmia and death after Mustard operation for simple transposition of the great arteries. Circulation. 1991;84(5 Suppl):III187–92.
2. Myridakis DJ, Ehlers KH, Engle MA. Late follow-up after venous switch operation (Mustard procedure) for simple and complex transposition of the great arteries. Am J Cardiol. 1994;74(10):1030–6.
3. Piran S, et al. Heart failure and ventricular dysfunction in patients with single or systemic right ventricles. Circulation. 2002;105(10):1189–94.
4. Roos-Hesselink JW, et al. Decline in ventricular function and clinical condition after Mustard repair for transposition of the great arteries (a prospective study of 22–29 years). Eur Heart J. 2004;25(14):1264–70.
5. Wilson NJ, et al. Long-term outcome after the mustard repair for simple transposition of the great arteries. 28-year follow-up. J Am Coll Cardiol. 1998;32(3):758–65.
6. Gelatt M, et al. Arrhythmia and mortality after the Mustard procedure: a 30-year single-center experience. J Am Coll Cardiol. 1997;29(1):194–201.
7. Warnes CA, Somerville J. Transposition of the great arteries: late results in adolescents and adults after the Mustard procedure. Br Heart J. 1987;58(2):148–55.
8. Puley G, et al. Arrhythmia and survival in patients >18 years of age after the mustard procedure for complete transposition of the great arteries. Am J Cardiol. 1999;83(7):1080–4.
9. Millane T, et al. Role of ischemia and infarction in late right ventricular dysfunction after atrial repair of transposition of the great arteries. J Am Coll Cardiol. 2000;35(6):1661–8.
10. Graham TP Jr, et al. Long-term outcome in congenitally corrected transposition of the great arteries: a multi-institutional study. J Am Coll Cardiol. 2000;36(1):255–61.
11. Ikeda U, et al. Long-term survival in aged patients with corrected transposition of the great arteries. Chest. 1992;101(5):1382–5.
12. Presbitero P, et al. Corrected transposition of the great arteries without associated defects in adult patients: clinical profile and follow up. Br Heart J. 1995;74(1):57–9.
13. Rutledge JM, et al. Outcome of 121 patients with congenitally corrected transposition of the great arteries. Pediatr Cardiol. 2002;23(2):137–45.
14. Gentles TL, et al. Fontan operation in five hundred consecutive patients: factors influencing early and late outcome. J Thorac Cardiovasc Surg. 1997;114(3):376–91.
15. Gaynor JW, et al. Predictors of outcome after the Fontan operation: is hypoplastic left heart syndrome still a risk factor? J Thorac Cardiovasc Surg. 2002;123(2):237–45.
16. Mahle WT, et al. Quantitative echocardiographic assessment of the performance of the functionally single right ventricle after the Fontan operation. Cardiol Young. 2001;11(4):399–406.
17. Van Praagh R, et al. Pathologic anatomy of corrected transposition of the great arteries: medical and surgical implications. Am Heart J. 1998;135(5 Pt 1):772–85.
18. Fernandez-Teran MA, JM. Hurle. Myocardial fiber architecture of the human heart ventricles. Anat Rec. 1982;204(2):137–47.
19. Sanchez-Quintana D, et al. Morphological changes in the normal pattern of ventricular myoarchitecture in the developing human heart. Anat Rec. 1995;243(4):483–95.
20. Rushmer RF, Crystal DK, Wagner C. The functional anatomy of ventricular contraction. Circ Res. 1953;1(2):162–70.
21. Hutchins GM, et al. Shape of the human cardiac ventricles. Am J Cardiol. 1978;41(4):646–54.
22. Kvasnicka J, Vokrouhlicky L. Heterogeneity of the myocardium. Function of the left and right ventricle under normal and pathological conditions. Physiol Res. 1991;40(1):31–7.
23. Smith A, et al. An anatomical study of the patterns of the coronary arteries and sinus nodal artery in complete transposition. Int J Cardiol. 1986;12(3):295–307.
24. Allwork SP, et al. Congenitally corrected transposition of the great arteries: morphologic study of 32 cases. Am J Cardiol. 1976;38(7):910–23.
25. van Praagh R, van Praagh S. Morphologic anatomy. In: Hanley and Belfus, editor. Nadas' pediatric cardiology. I. 1992. pp. 17–26.
26. Prieto LR, et al. Progressive tricuspid valve disease in patients with congenitally corrected transposition of the great arteries. Circulation. 1998;98(10):997–1005.
27. Hornung TS, et al. Myocardial perfusion defects and associated systemic ventricular dysfunction in congenitally

corrected transposition of the great arteries. Heart. 1998;80(4):322–6.

28. Hauser M, et al. Impaired myocardial blood flow and coronary flow reserve of the anatomical right systemic ventricle in patients with congenitally corrected transposition of the great arteries. Heart. 2003;89(10):1231–5.

29. Singh TP, et al. Myocardial flow reserve in patients with a systemic right ventricle after atrial switch repair. J Am Coll Cardiol. 2001;37(8):2120–5.

30. Lowensohn HS, et al. Phasic right coronary artery blood flow in conscious dogs with normal and elevated right ventricular pressures. Circ Res. 1976;39(6):760–6.

31. Bache RJ, Vrobel TR. Effects of exercise on blood flow in the hypertrophied heart. Am J Cardiol. 1979;44(5):1029–33.

32. Hornung TS, et al. Excessive right ventricular hypertrophic response in adults with the mustard procedure for transposition of the great arteries. Am J Cardiol. 2002;90(7):800–3.

33. Babu-Narayan SV, et al. Late gadolinium enhancement cardiovascular magnetic resonance of the systemic right ventricle in adults with previous atrial redirection surgery for transposition of the great arteries. Circulation. 2005;111(16):2091–8.

Pharmacologic Approaches to the Failing Systemic Right Ventricle

12

Annie Dore and Paul Khairy

Excellent survival has been reported in patients with a systemic right ventricle (RV) [1, 2]. However, long-term complications, including progressive RV dilatation, systolic and diastolic ventricular dysfunction [2–5], impaired exercise tolerance [6, 7], arrhythmias [1, 2], and sudden death [1] raise concern over the ability of the morphologic RV to sustain an increased afterload over a prolonged period of time.

Over the past 20 years, numerous randomized prospective clinical trials were conducted in patients with acquired left ventricular (LV) systolic heart failure [8]. Collectively, these important studies elucidated underlying pathophysiological mechanisms, provided insights into potential novel pharmacological targets, and established evidence-based indications for therapy. Such pharmacological therapy has resulted in improvements in diverse outcomes, including cardiac index, left ventricular pressures, symptoms, exercise tolerance, quality of life, and survival.

Given the limitations in data that specifically pertain to adults with congenital heart disease, studies performed on the failing LV are often extrapolated to patients with systemic RVs. Not uncommonly, similar pharmacological regimens are empirically initiated. It is unclear, however, whether such practices are justified. The overall objective of this chapter is to provide a contemporary perspective on pharmacological therapy in patients with a systemic RV in light of recent developments and current evidence.

12.1 The Asymptomatic Patient with a Failing LV

Although the heart failure literature has predominantly focused on patients with symptoms, evidence now indicates that asymptomatic LV dysfunction is more common than previously presumed. It is increasingly recognized that a latency period often exists between a reduction in LV ejection fraction and onset of symptoms. Advances in pharmacological therapies aimed at symptomatic patients with LV dysfunction have, therefore, been extended to the asymptomatic patient. The 2006 Canadian consensus conference guidelines on heart failure [8] recommend that angiotensin-converting enzyme (ACE) inhibitors be given to all asymptomatic patients with an LV ejection as fraction less than 35% (class I, level A). It is further recommended that all patients with an LV ejection fraction equal to or less than 40% receive a beta-blocker proven to be beneficial in large-scale clinical trials (class I, level A).

Favorable effects of ACE inhibitors in asymptomatic patients with a decreased LV ejection fraction were reported in the studies of left ventricular dysfunction (SOLVD) prevention trial [9]. This trial is the largest clinical study to assess the impact of an ACE inhibitor on mortality in New York Heart Association (NYHA) class I patients with LV dysfunction. Over 4000 asymptomatic patients with an ejection fraction less than 35% and no other pharmacological therapy for heart failure were randomized to treatment with enalapril or placebo for a 3-year period. Despite the lack of a demonstrated survival advantage of enalapril over placebo, enalapril significantly reduced the incidence of symptomatic heart failure and need for hospitalization. ACE inhibitors have since been recommended to all asymptomatic patients with a reduced LV ejection fraction to prevent or delay the onset of heart failure symptoms.

Large-scale clinical studies have not focused of beta-blockers in NYHA class I patients with a decreased LV ejection fraction. Nevertheless, all consensus guidelines recommend their use in asymptomatic patients on the basis of consistent benefits noted across a range of subgroups with LV dysfunction, including patients without overt heart failure following an acute myocardial infarction [8, 10–11]. The CAPRICORN study examined the

A. Dore (✉)
From the Adult Congenital Heart Disease Center, Montreal Heart Institute, Montreal, Canada

A.N. Redington et al. (eds.), *Congenital Diseases in the Right Heart*, DOI 10.1007/978-1-84800-378-1_12,
© Springer-Verlag London Limited 2009

effects of carvedilol in asymptomatic patients with a reduced LV ejection fraction postinfarction and found a lower incidence of the combined end-point of mortality and recurrent myocardial infarction [11]. No trial has specifically investigated the effect of beta-blockers on mortality in asymptomatic patients with a decreased LV ejection fraction but without a recent myocardial infarction.

12.2 The Asymptomatic Patient with a Failing RV

Data on the use of ACE inhibitors or angiotensin receptor blockers in patients with a systemic RV was initially limited to nonrandomized studies involving few patients. In seven patients over 13 years of age with a Mustard repair for transposition of the great arteries (TGA), Lester et al. [12] found a small but statistically significant increase in exercise duration following 8 weeks of losartan therapy. The Toronto group reported their results with cardiopulmonary testing and magnetic resonance imaging in 14 adults late after a Mustard operation treated with ACE inhibitors for a minimum of 6 months [13]. No change in exercise time, VO2 max, ejection fraction, or RV volume was noted. In a subsequent nonrandomized and unblinded study of eight young patients who underwent a Mustard operation for TGA, Robinson et al. [14] reported a baseline reduction in VO_2 max and exercise duration that did not improve after 12 months of enalapril therapy.

More recently, a multicenter prospective randomized double-blind, placebo-controlled clinical trial assessed the effects of an angiotensin receptor blocker in patients with a systemic RV [15]. In this study, 29 adults (mean age 30 years; 21 with D-TGA after a Mustard or Senning repair and 8 with congenitally corrected TGA and no other hemodynamic lesion) were randomly assigned to 15 weeks of treatment with losartan or placebo, with crossover for an additional 15 weeks. At baseline, the RV was dilated in 97% of patients (mildly in 45%, moderately to severely in 52%). The mean RV ejection fraction was 41% with a mean VO_2 max of 29 mL/kg/min (73.5 ± 12.9% predicted value). Serological studies revealed a mean NT-proBNP level of 257 pg/mL (normal <125 pg/mL) and angiotensin II level of 5.7 pg/mL (normal <5.0 pg/mL). Comparing losartan to placebo, no differences were observed in VO_2 max, exercise duration, and NT-proBNP levels despite a trend toward increased angiotensin II levels.

Reasons underlying the lack of an observed benefit remain speculative. Interestingly, minimal activation of the renin angiotensin system (RAS) was noted at baseline, thus raising the possibility that, unlike patients with LV dysfunction, activation of the RAS is not a dominant pathophysiologic contributor to impaired exercise tolerance in patients with a systemic RV [15]. Bolger AP et al. [16] measured neurohormonal levels in a heterogeneous group of 53 adults with chronic heart failure secondary to complex congenital heart disease, most of them with underlying univentricular physiology, tetralogy of Fallot, or systemic RV. In this diverse patient population, levels of ANP, BNP, epinephrine, norepinephrine, renin, and aldosterone were higher than in healthy controls. However, renin and aldosterone levels were not significantly different between congenital patients in NYHA functional class I and healthy controls, providing further evidence that the renin angiotensin axis is not significantly activated in asymptomatic patients with congenital heart disease.

Pathophysiological insights from animal models suggest that when the RV is submitted to a pressure overload, activation of the RAS is not a necessary component of the RV hypertrophic response [17]. In a feline model subjected to pulmonary artery banding, Koide et al. found a level of angiotensin II similar to nonbanded controls despite a substantial RV hypertrophic response. The authors concluded that hypertrophy resulting from RV pressure overload could occur without RAS activation.

From a clinical perspective, despite the vast majority of patients with a systemic RV reporting symptoms consistent with a NYHA class I designation, impaired exercise capacity has been well demonstrated [7, 8, 15, 16]. Discrepancies between the NYHA functional class category and cardiopulmonary exercise testing are not uncommon, with reports suggesting less than 50% concordance [18]. In NYHA class I patients with systemic LV dysfunction, the observed reduction in exercise tolerance has been attributed to a combination of various cardiovascular and peripheral factors. Potential cardiovascular factors include chronotropic incompetence and the inability to sufficiently increase stroke volume as a result of preload anomalies, impaired contractility, and/or increased afterload. Peripheral factors include endothelial dysfunction, abnormal skeletal muscle metabolism, suboptimal distribution of the cardiac output, reflex sympathetic activation, and hyperventilation.

While the predominant factor underlying a reduction in exercise capacity in the asymptomatic patient with a systemic RV remains unknown, afterload reduction by inhibiting the RAS system does not appear to appreciably improve exercise capacity. Results from a study by Derrick et al. [19] in patients with a prior Mustard or Senning operation, the largest subgroup of patients with a systemic RV, are consistent with these findings. The authors suggest that exercise intolerance primarily results from preload anomalies with failure to augment RV filling rates during tachycardia, presumably due to abnormal intra-atrial pathways with impaired atrioventricular transport.

If the main factor limiting an appropriate increase in stroke volume relates to preload in the setting of exercise-induced tachycardia, beta-blocker therapy may prove beneficial by blunting the chronotropic response and increasing diastolic filling time. In this population of patients, case reports have described favorable effects of beta-blocker therapy [20–22]. In an observational study, Giardini et al. [21] assessed the effects of carvedilol on RV remodeling and exercise tolerance in eight adults with systemic RV dysfunction. All patients were in NYHA functional class I–III and treated with ACE inhibitors. Cardiovascular magnetic resonance and cardiopulmonary exercise testing were performed prior to and 12 months after receiving the maximum tolerated dose of carvedilol. Results were encouraging, in that improvements in RV end-diastolic volume, RV end-systolic volume, and RV and LV ejection fractions were noted. However, no improvement in VO2 max was observed. This pilot study concluded that carvedilol administration is safe and associated with positive RV remodeling. It remains to be determined whether such favorable effects will translate into clinically meaningful outcomes.

12.3 The Symptomatic Patient with a Failing LV

In patients with symptomatic LV dysfunction, the primary objectives of therapy include improving symptoms and quality of life, halting progressive heart failure, and reducing mortality. Beta-blockers, ACE inhibitors, or angiotensin receptor blockers, and diuretics have become the cornerstone of pharmacological therapy [8, 10]. A diuretic is recommended to relieve congestive symptoms and prevent the recurrence of fluid retention. ACE inhibitors and beta-blockers have been the subject of numerous large-scale clinical investigations and both have been demonstrated to alleviate symptoms, ameliorate clinical status, improve survival, and reduce the combined risk of death and hospitalization.

In addition to these agents, digoxin can improve symptoms, quality of life, and exercise tolerance in patients with mild-to-moderate heart failure [8, 10]. These benefits have been observed independent of the underlying rhythm, the etiology of LV systolic dysfunction, and concomitant heart failure therapy. In patients with NYHA class IV symptoms or NYHA class III symptoms and a recent hospitalization, low-dose spironolactone can be added to the medical regimen. This aldosterone antagonist has been associated with a 30% relative risk reduction in mortality, 35% reduction in hospitalizations for heart failure, and an improvement in functional class [23].

12.4 The Symptomatic Patient with a Failing RV

Designing a prospective randomized clinical study to assess the impact of medical therapy on patients with a systemic RV and NYHA class III or IV symptoms is greatly hampered by the limited number of such patients and heterogeneity of underlying congenital heart defects. To date, there exists no evidence-based data on pharmacological therapies in the setting of symptomatic systemic RV failure. In the absence of data, clinicians have traditionally prescribed diuretics (especially loop diuretics) to relieve signs and symptoms of congestion and digoxin for its positive inotropic effects. Over the past 10 years, ACE inhibitors and beta-blockers were empirically added.

As patients with systemic RVs thrive into their adult years, clinicians should be cognizant of the fact that all cardiovascular risk factors need to be aggressively managed, with appropriate lifestyle modifications and drug therapies. Manifestations of coronary artery disease are beginning to surface in adults with congenital heart disease [24].

12.5 Conclusion

In patients with a systemic RV, heart failure is a feared long-term complication. Although a minority report NYHA class III or IV symptoms, exercise intolerance is prevalent even among those who consider themselves asymptomatic. There is, therefore, much interest in developing and defining pharmacological strategies that support the systemic RV. Initial enthusiasm for RAS antagonists has not been borne out by prospective randomized assessment. It has become increasingly apparent that caution is warranted in extrapolating results from trials assessing pharmacological therapy for the failing LV without independent validation in the systemic RV. Despite discouraging initial results, insights gained into potentially different pathophysiological mechanisms that underlie the failing systemic LV versus RV may ultimately lead to more appropriate tailored therapy. Currently, data do not support using RAS antagonists in the asymptomatic patient with a failing systemic RV. Initial observational data with beta-blocker therapy appear encouraging and merit further prospective study. Results of large-scale clinical trials in LV dysfunction should spark enthusiasm within the adult congenital medical community to pursue collaborative research in an effort to provide our patients with evidence-based guidelines for care-limiting questions.

References

1. Myridakis DJ, Ehlers KH, Engle MA. Late follow-up after venous switch operation (Mustard Procedure) for simple and complex transposition of the great arteries. Am J Cardiol. 1994;74(1030):–36.
2. Graham TP Jr, Bernard YD, Mellen BG, Celermajer D, Baumgartner H, Cetta F, et al. Long-term outcome in congenitally corrected transposition of the great arteries : a multi-institutional study. J Am Coll Cardiol. 2000;36(1):255–61.
3. Hurwitz RA, Caldwell RL, Girod DA, Brown J. Right ventricular systolic function in adolescents and young adults after Mustard operation for transposition of the great arteries. Am J Cardiol. 1996;77(294):–7.
4. Piran S, Veldtman G, Siu S, Webb GD, Liu PP. Heart failure and ventricular dysfunction in patients with single or systemic right ventricles. Circulation. 2002;105(1189):–94.
5. Reich O, Voriskova M, Ruth C, Krejcir M, Marek J, Skovranek J, Hucin B, Samanek M. Long term ventricular performance after intra-atrial correction of transposition: left ventricular filling is the major limitation. Heart. 1997;78(376):–81.
6. Musewe NN, Reisman J, Benson LN, Wilkes D, Levison H, Freedom RM, et al. Cardiopulmonary adaptation at rest and during exercise 10 years after Mustard atrial repair for transposition of the great arteries. Circulation. 1988;77(1055):–61.
7. Fredriksen PM, Veldtman G, Hechter S, Therrien J, Chen A, Warsi MA, et al. Aerobic capacity in adults with various congenital heart diseases. Am J Cardiol. 2001;87(310):–4.
8. Arnold JM, Liu P, Demers C, Dorian P, Gianetti N, Haddad H, et al. Canadian Cardiovascular Society consensus conference recommendations on heart failure 2006: diagnosis and management. Can J Cardiol. 2006;22(1):23–45.
9. The SOLVD Investigators. Effect of enalapril on mortality and the development of heart failure in asymptomatic patients with reduced left ventricular ejection fractions. N Engl J Med. 1992;327;685–91.
10. Hunt SA, Abraham WT, Chin MH, Feldman AM, Francis GS, Ganiats TG, et al. ACC/AHA 2005 Guideline Update for the diagnosis and management of chronic heart failure in the adult: a report of the American College of Cardiology/American Heart Association task Force on Practice Guidelines (Writing Committee to Update the 2001 Guidelines for the Evaluation and Management of Heart Failure). American College of Cardiology Web Site. Available at: http://www.acc.org/clinical/guidelines/failure//index.pdf.
11. Dargie HJ. Effect of carvedilol on outcome after myocardial infarction in patients with left ventricular dysfunction: the CAPRICORN randomised trial. Lancet. 2001; 357(9266):1385–90.
12. Lester SJ, McElhinney DB, Viloria E, Reddy GP, Ryan E, Tworetzky W, et al. Effects of losartan in patients with a systemically functioning morphologic right ventricle after atrial repair of transposition of the great arteries. Am J Cardiol. 2001;88(1314):–16.
13. Hechter SJ, Fredriksen PM, Liu P, Veldtman G, Merchant N, Freeman M, et al. Angiotensin-Converting Enzyme Inhibitors in Adults After the Mustard Procedure. Am J Cardiol. 2001;87(310):–14.
14. Robinson B, Heise CT, Moore JW, Anella J, Sokoloski M, Eshaghpour E. Afterload reduction therapy in patients following intraatrial baffle operation for transposition of the great arteries. Pediatr Cardiol. 2002;23(618):–23.
15. Dore A, Houde C, Chan KL, Ducharme A, Khairy P, Juneau M, et al. Angiotensin receptor blockade and exercise capacity in adults with systemic right ventricles: a multicenter, randomized, placebo-controlled clinical trial. Circulation. 2005;112(2411):–16.
16. Bolger AP, Sharma R, Wei L, Leenarts M, Kalra PR, Kemp M, et al. Neurohormonal activation and the chronic heart failure syndrome in adults with congenital heart disease. Circulation. 2002;106(92):–9.
17. Koide M, Carabello BA, Conrad CC, Buckley JM, DeFreyte G, Barnes M, et al. Hypertrophic response to hemodynamic overload: role of load vs renin–angiotensin system activation. Am J Physiol. 1999;276:H350–8.
18. Rostagno C, Galanti G, Comeglio M, Boddi V, Olivo G, Gastone Neri Serneri G. Comparison of different methods of functional evaluation in patients with chronic heart failure. Eur J Fail. 2000;2(273):–80.
19. Derrick GP, Narang I, White PA, Kelleher A, Bush A, Penny DJ, et al. Failure of stroke volume augmentation during exercise and dobutamine stress is unrelated to load-independaent indexes of right ventricular performance after the Mustard operation. Circulation. 2000;102:III-154–9.
20. Lindenfeld J, Keller K, Campbell DN, Wolfe RR, Quaife RA. Improved systemic ventricular function after cardvedilol administration in a patient with congenittaly corrected transposition of the great arteries. J Heart L Transplant. 2003;22(2):198–201.
21. Giardini A, Lovato L, Donti A, Formigari R, Gargiulo G, Picchio FM, et al. A pilot study on the effects of carvedilol on right ventricular remodelling and exercise tolerance in patients with systemic right ventricle. Int J Cardiol. 2006 Jun 10; (Epub ahead of print).
22. Josephson CB, Howlett JG, Jackson SD, Finley J, Kells CM. A case series of systemic right ventricular dysfunction post atrial switch for simple D-transposition of the great arteries: The impact of beta-blockade. Can J Cardiol. 2006;22(9):769–72.
23. Pitt B, Zannad F, Remme WJ, Cody R, Castaigne A, Perez A, et al. The effect of spironolactone on morbidity and mortality in patients with severe heart failure. Randomized Aldactone Evaluation Study Investigators. N Engl J Med. 1999;341(10):709–17.
24. Coutu M, Poirier NC, Dore A, Carrier M, Perrault LP. Late myocardial revascularisation in patients with tetralogy of Fallot. Ann Thorac Surg. 2004;77(4):1454–5.

Congenitally Corrected Transposition: Replacement of the Tricuspid Valve or Double Switch?

Jennifer C. Hirsch and Edward L. Bove

13.1 Anatomy

Congenitally corrected transposition is produced by the combination of discordant atrioventricular and ventriculoarterial connections. In this condition, the morphologically right atrium receives the systemic venous return, which then enters the morphologically left ventricle via the mitral valve. In the setting of usual atrial arrangement, this morphologically left ventricle is usually right sided. The morphologically left atrium then receives the pulmonary venous return, which enters the morphologically right ventricle, usually left sided, via the tricuspid valve. The morphologically left ventricle supports the pulmonary trunk, while the morphologically right ventricle is connected to the aorta. In consequence of the double discordance, there is a physiologically *normal* pattern of circulation, with the deoxygenated systemic venous return entering the pulmonary circulation, and oxygenated pulmonary venous return entering the systemic circulation. It is possible, of course, to find discordant atrioventricular connections with other ventriculoarterial connections, such as double-outlet ventricle, usually the right, or single outlet with pulmonary atresia. These variants are close cousins, but do not produce congenitally corrected transposition.

The pattern described above is the commonest form of the lesion, with usual atrial arrangement, but congenitally corrected transposition can also be found in the mirror-imaged variant, when the atrial chambers are mirror imaged, but the ventricular mass show the usual pattern of right-hand ventricular topology. There can then be a multitude of other conditions, found in nine-tenths of more of cases. These include ventricular septal defects, seen in three-quarters of patients, pulmonary stenosis or

atresia, present in half, disturbances of atrioventricular conduction, tricuspid regurgitation, atrial septal defect, and right-sided heart. Anomalies of the morphologically tricuspid valve, including Ebstein's malformation, are particularly common, seen in perhaps more than half of patients, and achieve clinical significance because the morphologically tricuspid valve is the systemic atrioventricular valve in the setting of discordant atrioventricular connections.

The atrioventricular conduction system is abnormally positioned due to malalignment between the atrial and ventricular septal structures. The result is a superiorly displaced atrioventricular node, which is positioned anteriorly on the atrial septum at the junction of the superior rim of the oval fossa and the vestibule of the morphologically mitral valve. The node attaches to the bundle of His, which travels anterior to the pulmonary outflow tract, coursing in the subendocardial layer of the morphologically left ventricle, usually found, as already discussed, on the right side [1]. It has been theorized that the long course traveled by the bundle of His predisposes it to damage from ischemia or stretch, which can result in variable degrees of heart block [1].

13.2 Physiology

Patients without associated anomalies have normal physiology. Most patients, however, will present as a consequence of an associated condition. Patients with significant pulmonary stenosis or atresia generally present early in life due to cyanosis. Those with significant regurgitation across the morphologically tricuspid valve, or those with a large ventricular septal defect with minimal obstruction to the outlet from the left ventricle, may develop congestive heart failure symptoms early in life. Additional conditions include bradycardia from heart block, congestive heart failure from systemic ventricular failure and/or tricuspid

E.L. Bove (✉)
F7830, Mott Children's Hospital, 1500 East Medical Center Drive, Ann Arbor, MI 48109
e-mail: elbove@umich.edu

A.N. Redington et al. (eds.), *Congenital Diseases in the Right Heart*, DOI 10.1007/978-1-84800-378-1_13,
© Springer-Verlag London Limited 2009

regurgitation, and cyanosis from progressive pulmonary stenosis. Death from congestive heart failure occurs with increasing frequency in the third to fifth decade of life [2].

Regurgitation across the morphologically tricuspid valve is an important determinant of long-term outcome. In a study from Prieto and colleagues [3], who analyzed 40 patients, tricuspid valvar regurgitation was found to be an independent risk factor for death. At 20 years, over nine-tenths of those without significant regurgitation survived, in comparison to just under half of those with tricuspid valvar regurgitation [3]. Regurgitation may result from a multitude of causes, including Ebstein's malformation of the valve, and annular dilation from progressive right ventricular dysfunction. More recently, it has been recognized that the shift of the ventricular septum to the right, into the morphologically left ventricle, can also result in tricuspid valvar regurgitation. The etiology of the regurgitation is likely due to the *septophilic* nature of the valve, which is altered when the pressure in the morphologically right ventricle exceeds that of the left ventricle, resulting in shift of the septum to the right. The regurgitation has also been shown to improve after banding of the pulmonary trunk, which increases left ventricular pressure and produces a shift of the ventricular septum to the left, that is, toward the morphologically right ventricle.

13.3 Surgical Management

13.3.1 Nonanatomic Repair

Traditional methods of surgical repair had been aimed at the treatment of the associated lesions. Early and late results of such an approach have not been optimal. In series published recently, operative mortality for repair of associated conditions ranges from 4% to 15%, with a 15% to 30% incidence of postoperative complete heart block [4–6]. Furthermore, there is a high rate of reoperation for replacement of the tricuspid valve and insertion of pacemakers. In another series, the late survival was less than 70% at 10 years [7].

Right ventricular dysfunction and tricuspid valvar regurgitation are common late sequels. Survival after the development of significant tricuspid valvar regurgitation is poor. In the study of Prieto and colleagues [3], survival was no more than 70% at 1 year after the diagnosis of tricuspid valvar regurgitation. This had decreased to 38% by 10 years, regardless of treatment. Even in patients undergoing replacement of the tricuspid valve, survival at 10 years was a dismal 14% [3]. The potential benefit of replacement of the valve for tricuspid regurgitation is impacted significantly by the presence of right ventricular

dysfunction. In a study from the Mayo Clinic [5], patients with an ejection fraction less than 44% undergoing valvar replacement had survivals at 5 and 10 years of 49% and 20%, respectively. For patients with an ejection fraction above 44%, comparable survival was 100% at both 5 and 10 years, this being highly statistically significant. In another study evaluating outcomes following traditional repairs, progressive right ventricular dysfunction occurred in over two-fifths of patients in whom the morphologically right ventricle remained as the systemic ventricle. In that study [8] significant predictors of right ventricular dysfunction included Ebstein's malformation of the tricuspid valve, tricuspid valvar replacement, and postoperative complete heart block.

13.3.2 Anatomic Repair

In the 1990s, the focus of surgical treatment shifted toward anatomic repair, allowing the morphologically left ventricle to support the systemic circulation. To achieve this, it is necessary to retrain the morphologically left ventricle, so that it can function at systemic pressures. This can be achieved by banding the pulmonary trunk. It is essential to gradually increase pressure so as to avoid dysfunction of the ventricle. When the band is first placed, a reasonable goal is to achieve a left ventricular pressure half the systemic pressure, which should achieve a shift of the ventricular septum to the left. Tricuspid valvar regurgitation often improves as the septum moves into the cavity of the morphologically right ventricle. In many instances, it is not possible to achieve adequate pressures in the left ventricle subsequent to initial banding due to the potential of left ventricular dysfunction. Repetitive banding will be required to achieve sufficient ventricular retraining. Anatomic repair can be carried out when the ratio of right to left ventricular pressures is around 80%, and left ventricular function is normal. The pressure in the morphologically left ventricle may have remained at or near systemic levels in presence of a nonrestrictive ventricular septal defect, or if there had been sufficient preexisting obstruction in the left ventricular outflow tract. In these circumstances, retraining of the left ventricle is not necessary.

To achieve anatomical repair in the presence of a normal pulmonary valve, a Senning procedure is combined with an arterial switch operation. The Senning technique mobilizes a flap of atrial septum to begin the redirection of venous return (Fig. 13.1). The right atrial free wall is then used to create a systemic venous pathway, which carries the blood towards the tricuspid valve. (Fig. 13.2A) The pulmonary venous pathway passes

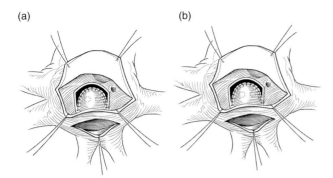

Fig. 13.1 To achieve the Senning procedure, the atrial septum is first mobilized, closing any atrial septal defect (a) If the atrial septal defect is large, it is often easier to resect the septum and use a patch. The mobilized atrial septum (b) is then sutured above the left pulmonary veins to create the floor of the systemic venous atrium
Reprinted with permission

around the systemic venous chamber to communicate with the mitral valve (Fig. 13.2B). The pulmonary venous atrium may require augmentation to prevent obstruction of pulmonary venous return.

The arterial switch operation is performed using traditional techniques as employed for patients with regular transposition. This involves transecting both the pulmonary trunk and the aorta at the level of the bifurcation of the trunk. The coronary arteries are mobilized with generous buttons of arterial wall. The distal part of the pulmonary trunk is translocated anterior to the aorta, following which the ascending aorta is anastomosed to the proximal part of the pulmonary trunk, and the coronary arterial buttons placed into the appropriate sinuses of Valsalva. The resected sinuses of the proximal aorta, soon to become the pulmonary trunk, are reconstructed with autologous pericardium, and the proximal channel is

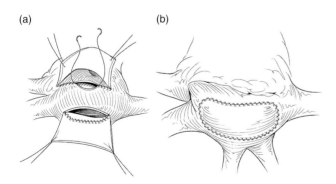

Fig. 13.2 The systemic venous atrium is completed by suturing the posterior aspect of the right atriotomy over the caval venous orifices and along the prior attachment of the atrial septum (a). The roof the left atrium is then opened posterior to the interatrial groove. The pulmonary venous atrium is completed (b) by augmenting the left atriotomy with a patch to the anterior aspect of the right atriotomy
Reprinted with permission

anastomosed to the right and left pulmonary arteries. This connection needs to be shifted leftward onto the proximal part of the left pulmonary artery to prevent distortion.

Patients with significant obstruction in the left ventricular outflow tract that cannot be resected, or those with pulmonary atresia, are unsuitable for an arterial switch. In this situation, the Senning procedure can be combined with the Rastelli operation. The Senning procedure is performed as previously described. An intraventricular baffle is then placed to channel the interventricular communication from the left ventricle to the aorta, and a conduit is inserted from the right ventricle to the pulmonary arteries. The sutures securing the baffle are kept on the morphologically right ventricular side of the septum to avoid damage to the conduction tissue. The defect itself may need to be enlarged to allow unobstructed flow from the morphologically left ventricle. The anterior and superior position of the conduction system must be kept in mind to avoid complete heart block.

13.4 Results

We have reported previously the results obtained at the University of Michigan for the Senning procedure combined with an arterial switch operation [5]. Our series now includes a total of 55 patients, in 30 of whom we combined the Senning and arterial switch procedures, and in the other 25 using the Senning procedure combined with a Rastelli operation. Our overall hospital survival is 95%, with one patient dying following the Senning and arterial switch procedures, and two following the combined Senning and Rastelli operations. There were no new cases of complete heart block, albeit those four patients had preoperative block. In a 7-year-old patient, who had undergone retraining of the left ventricle, left ventricular failure developed subsequently due to diastolic dysfunction. This patient ultimately required heart transplantation, following initial Senning and arterial switch operations. Late reoperations included replacement of a conduit in one, relief of pulmonary venous obstruction in another, and relief of superior caval venous obstruction in still another patient. Other potential complications, not seen in our cohort of patients, include neoaortic valvar regurgitation and coronary arterial obstruction following the combined Senning and arterial switch procedures, and late conduit failure and obstruction of the left ventricular outflow tract by the intraventricular baffle in the patients having combined Senning and Rastelli procedures. When present, tricuspid valvar regurgitation improved significantly following anatomic repair [5].

13.5 Discussion

Traditional approaches to repair underlying anomalies associated with congenitally corrected transposition are now accepted to result in unsatisfactory long-term outcomes, with high late rates of mortality, progressive right ventricular dysfunction, and progressive tricuspid valvar regurgitation. Following traditional repairs, such as closure of an interventricular communication, or relief of obstruction within the left ventricular outflow tract, left ventricular pressure is reduced, resulting in a shift of the ventricular septum to the right. This impairs tricuspid valvar function, and may lead to tricuspid valvar regurgitation. The resultant volume overload on the morphologically right ventricle leads to a relatively rapid decline in ventricular function, perhaps due to impaired coronary arterial flow as mural tension increases. Tricuspid valvar replacement in the face of existing right ventricular dysfunction results in high operative risk and poor long-term survival.

When feasible, therefore, complete anatomic repair has become the preferred approach. Following this procedure, the morphologically left ventricle and mitral valve, better suited for long-term performance under high pressure, are placed in the systemic circulation. The combined Senning and arterial switch operations can be performed with low morbidity and mortality. Among the group of patients repaired at the University of Michigan, early and intermediate survival has been excellent, with a low incidence of significant residual lesions.

Elective retraining of the morphologically left ventricle by banding the pulmonary trunk can be accomplished in younger patients who have developed right ventricular dysfunction, and/or tricuspid valvar regurgitation. Left ventricular retraining may not be appropriate in older patients, who may be prone to the development of late left ventricular failure following a double-switch operation. This group may better be managed with heart transplantation. Longer follow-up will be necessary to assess survival, ventricular function, arrhythmias, and surgical complications.

At the University of Michigan, the use of combined Senning and arterial switch procedures for patients with an isolated ventricular septal defect is preferred. The presence of the interventricular communication maintains left ventricular pressures at elevated levels if it is nonrestrictive, and retraining of the left ventricle is not necessary. For those patients also having pulmonary stenosis, surgery is reserved for those who are symptomatic. In this group, the combined Senning and Rastelli approach is typically adopted. Closure of the ventricular septal defect, with partial relief of pulmonary stenosis, may also be considered for patients who are not candidates for anatomic repair. In those patients, it is preferable to leave some pulmonary stenosis to minimize septal shift. Lastly, there are some patients with subpulmonary stenosis and a normal pulmonary valve who may be suitable for the combined Senning and arterial switch operations if it is possible to resect the obstructive lesions in the left ventricular outflow tract. Older patients with tricuspid regurgitation should be considered for early valvar replacement, before the onset of right ventricular dysfunction. Alternatively, even in older patients, it is possible to band the pulmonary trunk. Even if left ventricular training is ultimately unsuccessful, some reduction in tricuspid regurgitation may result in an improved clinical condition.

References

1. Anderson RH, Arnold R, Wilkinson JL. The conducting system in congenitally corrected transposition. Lancet. 1973;1:1286.
2. Kirklin JW, Barratt-Boyes BG. Congenitally corrected transposition of the great arteries. In: Cardiac surgery. New York, Churchill Livingstone. 1993.
3. Prieto LR, Hordof AJ, Secic M, et al. Progressive tricuspid valve disease in patients with congenitally corrected transposition of the great arteries. Circulation 1998;98:997–1005.
4. Termignon JL, Leca F, Couhe, PR, et al. "Classic" repair of congenitally corrected transposition and ventricular septal defect. Ann Thorac Surg. 1996;62:199–206.
5. Devaney EJ, Charpie JR, Ohye RG, Bove EL. Combined arterial switch and Senning operation for congenitally corrected transposition of the great arteries: patient selection and intermediate results. J Thorac Cardiovasc Surg. 2003; 125:500–7.

Section 4
Disease in The Absence of Structural Malformations

Right Ventricular Tachycardia

Shubhayan Sanatani and Gil J. Gross

Right ventricular ectopy preempts normal activation of the ventricular myocardium through pacemaking and conduction pathways comprising the sinoatrial node, atriums, atrioventricular node, and His–Purkinje system. Ectopic activity ranging from isolated ventricular premature beats to sustained ventricular tachycardia (VT) frequently arises in right ventricular myocardium affected by native and especially by surgically palliated structural congenital heart disease, as well as by various cardiomyopathic processes. However, the right ventricle also serves as the most common source of ventricular ectopy in hearts with no other detectable structural or functional abnormality.

14.1 Ventricular Extrasystoles

A ventricular extrasystole has been defined as an impulse which arises in an ectopic ventricular focus and which is premature in relation to the prevailing rhythm [1]. There are several terms used to describe this electrical event, the most common being *premature ventricular contraction* (PVC). This term has the disadvantage of linking an assumed hemodynamic event with the electrical event. Other terms such as *ventricular premature beat*, *premature ventricular depolarization*, or *ventricular ectopic beat* are also used. For simplicity, we will use the term PVC. This is manifest on the electrocardiogram as an atypical, usually wide QRS complex that is not preceded by a conducted P wave. Ventriculo-atrial conduction of the ectopic beat can activate the atria and produce a retrograde P wave, resetting the timing of the next normal beat if the sinus node is captured along with the bulk of the atrial tissue. More commonly, however, the sinus node is not captured or reset by a PVC, yielding the so-called *compensatory pause* whereby the normally timed sinus beat coincident with or immediately following the PVC cannot be conducted due to ventricular refractoriness, and the latency of the next normally conducted QRS complex thus precisely offsets the degree of prematurity of the PVC. The repolarization that follows a PVC is also abnormal, reflecting the abnormal ventricular depolarization sequence. PVC's frequently occur in patterns alternating with one or more normal sinus beats; this incompletely understood phenomenon is known as bigeminy, trigeminy, and so forth, and forms the subject of sophisticated modeling work [2].

PVC's are observed in up to 2.8% of electrocardiograms recorded in presumably healthy children [3, 4]. Using ambulatory continuous electrocardiographic recording, Nagashima and colleagues found an incidence of 18% in newborns on the first day of life and 27% in school children aged 13–15 years. However, the great majority of these patients had fewer than four PVC's in a 24 h period [5].

The evaluation of patients with isolated PVC's has not been standardized. A history of exercise-induced symptoms, particularly syncope, might suggest catecholamine-sensitive ion channelopathies such as polymorphic ventricular tachycardia. The family history can be informative in these typically hereditary conditions. Clues about underlying structural heart disease should be sought, such as failure to thrive, respiratory difficulties, and exercise intolerance. The physical exam and ancillary investigations should focus on the following key questions:

a. Is there evidence of structural heart disease?

The role of testing beyond basic surface electrocardiography (ECG) has not been clarified. Echocardiography might reveal evidence of cardiomyopathy or mitral valve prolapse in the setting of ventricular ectopy [6]. The balance of currently available evidence supports the widely held view that low-grade ventricular ectopy occurring in the absence of structural heart disease generally carries a benign prognosis [7].

S. Sanatani (✉)
British Columbia Children's Hospital, , Vancouver, BC, Canada

A.N. Redington et al. (eds.), *Congenital Diseases in the Right Heart*, DOI 10.1007/978-1-84800-378-1_14,
© Springer-Verlag London Limited 2009

There is a paucity of literature examining ectopy in the young in the presence of structural heart disease. While one study found that ventricular couplets in the presence of structural heart disease did carry a worse prognosis than those occurring in the absence of structural heart disease, and that patients with couplets and structural heart disease were more likely to have inducible ventricular tachycardia at electrophysiology study [8], the same question has not been addressed with respect to isolated PVC's. In the absence of structural heart disease, repolarization abnormalities including QT interval prolongation were found in a higher percentage of patients with PVC's than in a matched group without PVC's [9]. QT dispersion, another marker of susceptibility to arrhythmias, was found to be increased in a similar pediatric population [10].

(b) Is the ectopy monomorphic or polymorphic?

An attempt should be made to record the ectopic beats in 12 ECG leads to help define their origin. In patients with infrequent ectopy, running all 12 leads simultaneously might provide this information, and reducing the gain will render the tracing more easily interpretable. The literature has not emphasized the site of origin of the ectopic beats to date. PVC's originate from the right ventricle more commonly than the left. This represents one end of the continuum of ectopy typically originating in the right ventricular outflow tract. Zweytick et al. prospectively evaluated 56 patients with ectopy arising in the right ventricle. Only 16% were asymptomatic. More than half of the patients had echocardiographic abnormalities including focal dilatation and wall motion abnormalities. Left ventricular function was depressed in two patients. From an electrophysiologic perspective, isolated ectopy from the right ventricular outflow tract carried a benign prognosis and there were no cases of sustained ventricular tachycardia or sudden death over the mean follow-up period of 7 years [11]. However, in view of the frequency of associated symptoms and echocardiographic abnormalities, it is not surprising that many such patients are offered catheter ablation in the current era (see below).

(c) How frequent is the ectopy?

Ambulatory electrocardiography (Holter monitoring) can be useful to quantify the ectopy, although the correlation between the burden of ectopy and prognosis has not been established in children. Percentage of total beats and PVC's per hour are two common ways to quantify low-grade ectopy. Somewhat arbitrary definitions of terms such as *frequent* and *occasional* limit their usefulness. The variability of ectopy frequency between sampling intervals in individuals is substantial [12–14]. The distribution of ectopy may or may not follow a distinct circadian pattern.

The impact of low-grade ventricular ectopy on contractile function, particularly in relation to the prevalence of ectopic beats, has not been systematically studied in a pediatric population. One study involving 40 patients found that function was reduced in the 13 patients with frequent PVC's (>10/min) as compared with those having less frequent ectopy [15]. In an adult population, no difference was found in arrhythmia burden among those patients with and without reduced ventricular function in one study [16], while another report indicated that left ventricular dysfunction did, in fact, correlate with the frequency of ventricular ectopy [17].

(d) What is the degree of complexity of the ectopy?

The complexity of ventricular ectopy has been classified by the Lown criteria (Table 14.1). These are based on Holter data [18]. The utility of such a classification is primarily as a means of comparison of ectopy between two states or time points. However, as mentioned above, Holter monitoring does have limitations in this role. The apparent normalization of the Holter recording can be transient and might not accurately predict eventual outcome [8].

The significance of PVC's provoked by exercise testing in the adult population has been the subject of some debate. PVC's that occur during exercise are differentiated from those occurring in the recovery period. An increased sympathetic drive in the recovery phase may indicate an increase risk of cardiac death [19]. However, cardiac events and all-cause mortality are not consistently found to be increased in patients with exercise-induced PVC's [20–22].

PVC's do not require any specific treatment once the evaluation has excluded an arrhythmogenic substrate or underlying structural heart disease. In fact, the cardiac arrhythmia suppression trial (CAST) trial firmly ended the practice of ectopy suppression as a means of improving

Table 14.1 Modified Lown criteria for Holter classification of ventricular ectopy [18]

Grade	Description
0	No ventricular ectopic beats
1	Occasional, isolated PVC
2	Frequent VPC (>1/min or 30/hr)
3	Multiform VPC
4	Repetitive VPC:
	a) Couplets
	b) Salvos
5	Ventricular tachycardia

Reprinted from Circulation 1971;44:130–142. Lown B, Wolf M. Approaches to sudden death from coronary heart disease. Copyright 1971, with permission from Elsevier survival following myocardial infarction [23, 24]. Despite their acknowledged benign nature, symptomatic PVC's have been treated by catheter ablation [25, 26], with salutary effects on ventricular function claimed by at least two groups of investigators [16, 17]. There are limitations in measuring cardiac function in the presence of frequent ectopic beats. The role of catheter ablation in low-grade ventricular ectopy thus remains controversial [27, 28].

14.2 Primary or Idiopathic Right Ventricular Tachycardia

Ventricular tachycardia is conventionally defined as the occurrence of at least three consecutive PVC's at a rate beyond the upper limit of normal for sinus rhythm in the affected individual's age group and physiologic state. Ventricular tachycardia is generally considered to be sustained if spontaneous termination fails to occur within 30 sec of onset. QRS morphology reminiscent of left bundle branch block is the electrocardiographic hallmark of VT arising in the right ventricle (Fig. 14.1).

14.2.1 Right ventricular outflow tract (RVOT) tachycardia

RVOT tachycardia is widely recognized as being the most commonly observed form of ventricular tachycardia in otherwise healthy young individuals. The reasons for predominance of this anatomic focus as a source of presumably benign ectopy are unknown. We recently summarized the pediatric RVOT tachycardia literature in the context of a more extensive review of pediatric VT occurring in the absence of structural congenital heart disease [29]. Since completion of that review, further evidence of the generally benign nature of this condition among young patients has come from a multicenter retrospective study undertaken by the Canadian Pediatric Electrophysiology Working Group [30]. The records of 48 RVOT tachycardia patients at 5 participating pediatric tertiary care institutions were examined with the aim of characterizing the clinical spectrum and management of this condition. The median age at presentation was 8.2 years, and 15% of patients were referred for evaluation of syncope or near-syncope whose temporal and etiologic relationship to the rhythm disturbance was not specifically addressed. Our experience, however, has been that syncope, when present in these patients, is typically an incidental event that brings RVOT tachycardia to medical attention but is etiologically unrelated to it. Central findings of the multicenter study included lack of mortality and a tendency toward resolution of RVOT ectopy during a median follow-up duration of 22 months, irrespective of medical therapy. Interestingly, symptoms thought to be related to ectopy were more likely to resolve with antiarrhythmic therapy, raising the possibility of a placebo effect [30].

Notwithstanding the broadly reassuring nature of the pediatric RVOT tachycardia experience published to date, adult cardiologists have recently raised concerns

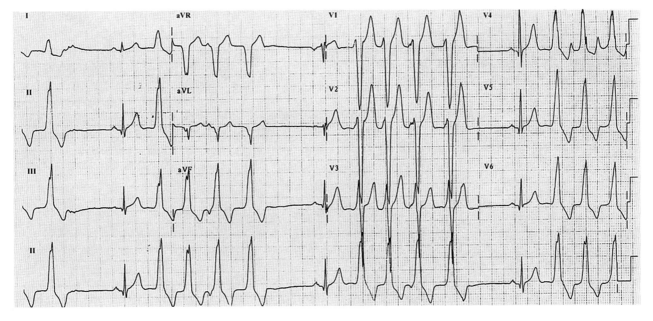

Fig. 14.1 Typical ECG in RVOT tachycardia. Note inferior QRS axis and left bundle branch block QRS morphology

about unexpected adverse outcomes in patients presumed to have benign ventricular ectopy, and have begun to identify prognostically distinct subgroups of RVOT ectopy associated with more serious conditions including idiopathic ventricular fibrillation [31]. These distinctions have important management implications that are discussed below. As often seems to be the case with cardiac rhythm disturbances, it will likely be just a matter of time before some of the less favorable observations in adults begin to *trickle down* to the pediatric age group. Thus, this section is meant to raise a cautionary note against the backdrop of what, by all accounts, has thus far been recognized as an essentially benign dysrhythmia in young patients.

Viskin and colleagues observed three cases of adults who developed malignant polymorphic ventricular tachycardia during follow-up for what had been considered typical, essentially benign RVOT ectopy. In one of their patients, syncope associated with polymorphic ventricular tachycardia began at age 47, some 12 years after initial diagnosis. Noting that each of these three patients had episodically *short-coupled* PVC's falling on the preceding T wave, they proceeded to demonstrate more systematically, albeit retrospectively, that the incidence of *R on T* PVC's bears a direct relationship to the risk of malignant ectopy [32]. Subsequently, Noda and associates reported on the elimination of life-threatening dysrhythmias and symptomatic events among 16 patients who underwent successful transcatheter ablation of otherwise typically benign RVOT ectopy [33].

In an editorial comment accompanying Noda et al.'s report, Viskin and Antzelevitch proposed a set of criteria according to which patients with RVOT ectopy should be advised to undergo transcatheter ablation (Table 14.2) [34]. It must be emphasized that these criteria are based on their authors' perception of *high-risk characteristics* which have not been rigorously proven. Moreover, their applicability to the pediatric population is probably mitigated by the marked rarity of adverse outcomes among children with typical RVOT ectopy, and by the nontrivial technical challenges and potential long-term risks [35] associated with ventricular ablation in this young age group. Based on the 15% incidence of syncope and the median initial ectopy frequency of ~15% noted by Harris et al. [30], a very

substantial minority, if not an outright majority, of pediatric patients with *benign* RVOT ectopy would be referred for ablation if the Viskin and Antzelevitch criteria were to be applied without modification. Nevertheless, these criteria will likely prove conceptually valuable in focusing attention on identifiable features of RVOT ectopy that could be quantified and tested as risk factors for adverse outcomes across all age groups, including the very young.

14.3 Right Ventricular Ectopy in Congenital Heart Disease

There is limited information about the occurrence of ventricular arrhythmias in the unmodified state of most structural congenital heart lesions [36–38]. Sullivan and colleagues described a cohort of patients with tetralogy of Fallot evaluated for preoperative arrhythmias. They documented a 45% incidence of frequent or complex ventricular ectopy in older patients [37]. The practical relevance of these data in the current era, with its emphasis on primary tetralogy repair during infancy, is unclear. A study in the early days of the arterial switch operation identified preoperative arrhythmias in 5 of 41 infants with transposed great arteries, consisting mainly of isolated PVC's, with one patient having nonsustained ventricular tachycardia. In the same study, postoperative arrhythmias were seen in 8 of 40 patients, with the majority once again experiencing isolated PVC's [39].

Rhythm disturbances have been more commonly observed and documented in palliated as opposed to unmodified congenital heart disease [38, 40]. In the early postoperative period, junctional ectopic tachycardia with bundle branch block can be difficult to differentiate from ventricular tachycardia. Ventricular ectopy is occasionally encountered in the acute postoperative recovery period in the absence of recognized systemic triggers such as electrolyte imbalances; this is most often a form of accelerated ventricular rhythm similar to that seen in postmyocardial infarction patients. Although its pathophysiology is not clearly established, inflammation and edema causing enhanced automaticity likely play a role.

There is limited information about ventricular arrhythmias in the chronic setting following repair or palliation of most congenital heart defects. The creation of myocardial conduction barriers including fibrous scar tissue undoubtedly contributes to the increased incidence of ventricular arrhythmias noted in relation to follow-up duration as well as older age at repair [41]. The Second Natural History study examined the incidence of ventricular arrhythmias in patients with pulmonary stenosis.

Table 14.2 Suggested criteria for ablation of RVOT ectopy (Viskin and Antzelevitch) [34]

History of syncope
Fast ventricular tachycardia (>230/min)
Frequent ectopy (>20,000 PVC's/day)
Short-coupled ventricular ectopy

Most of the patients had undergone surgical valvotomy; the incidence of arrhythmic complications was 3.6% in this group and was associated with increased age at admission [40]. Houyel et al. studied patients who underwent closure of ventricular septal defects through a ventriculotomy and those repaired via atriotomy. The hospital records of 262 patients were reviewed, of whom 185 had been repaired via a ventriculotomy and 77 via an atriotomy. Fifty were randomly chosen from each group for evaluation comprising ECG, Holter monitoring, and exercise testing. No patients had sustained ventricular tachycardia. PVC's were common in both groups. In a theme common to a variety of lesions, older age at surgery and duration of follow-up were risk factors for arrhythmias [42]. The incidence of ventricular ectopy on Holter monitoring was 65% in a large cohort of transposition patients following arterial switch [43]. A more recent study found occasional ventricular ectopy in 20%, with only 1 patient out of 60 having > 30 PVC's/hour some 10 years after arterial switch. No patient had ventricular tachycardia on ambulatory monitoring [44].

There are two lesions in particular in which long-term postoperative follow-up is associated with the late appearance of ventricular arrhythmias that can be associated with sudden death: tetralogy of Fallot, and transposition of the great arteries palliated with an atrial switch (Mustard or Senning) procedure. Chronically abnormal right ventricular loading conditions are thought to play a role in the pathogenesis of ectopy in both of these settings. Interestingly, ventricular arrhythmias are much less common in the atrial switch population, and the absence of a ventriculotomy scar in these patients might be significant in this regard. Importantly, the surgical management of these conditions has evolved significantly over the past 4–5 decades, such that many of the recognized or presumed risk factors for late postoperative ventricular ectopy have been reduced or eliminated. The arterial switch has supplanted the atrial switch as the standard procedure for transposition, eliminating the systemic right ventricle. Tetralogy of Fallot repair is routinely done at a younger age and includes measures to minimize pulmonary insufficiency [45]. The anticipated long-term benefits of these altered approaches remain to be confirmed.

In tetralogy of Fallot, several risk factors for sudden death have been identified [46–49]. The arrhythmic substrate in tetralogy includes the ventriculotomy scar and outflow tract patches, creating a substrate for reentrant tachycardia [50, 51]. In the case of the atrial switch, sinus node dysfunction and atrial arrhythmias are prevalent and likely account for many cases of sudden death [52]. There is very little information about ventricular arrhythmias in the Mustard population, although right ventricular pressure load might contribute to their development [53].

There is no uniform approach to the electrophysiologic evaluation or management of congenital heart disease patients. This relates to the lack of data on the incidence and significance of ventricular arrhythmias in congenital heart disease. The investigation of newly detected ventricular ectopy should include assessment of acute illness, medication effects, and hemodynamically significant residual such as outflow tract obstruction and valvar insufficiency. There is a general consensus that symptomatic patients should undergo further evaluation that typically includes an intracardiac electrophysiology study. However, the detection of asymptomatic nonsustained ventricular tachycardia on routine follow-up surveillance studies such as ambulatory Holter monitoring does not always prompt an electrophysiology study. This is due in part to the lack of specificity of this testing in congenital heart disease patients. Alexander et al. reported a single-center experience with programmed electrical stimulation in a variety of congenital heart defects. Failure to induce VT was a favorable prognostic sign, but the frequency of false-negative studies was high [54]. Khairy and associates reported a multicenter study of programmed electrical stimulation in postoperative tetralogy of Fallot. Over 60% had symptoms prompting electrophysiologic testing. Induction of sustained ventricular tachycardia was a powerful predictor of subsequent events. In patients being evaluated as part of routine testing, a negative test was associated with a high probability of event-free survival [47].

Among patients found to be at risk for sustained or otherwise concerning ventricular arrhythmias in the setting of congenital heart disease, the therapeutic options fall under four broad categories: (1) medical management; (2) catheter-based therapies [50, 55]; (3) surgical revision aimed at mitigating hemodynamically significant residual lesions that predispose to arrhythmias [49, 56, 57]; and (4) implantable devices.

There are no studies evaluating the efficacy of medications in the current era. Sotalol and amiodarone appear to be the most commonly used antiarrhythmic agents for ventricular arrhythmias in congenital heart disease [55]. There are no prospective data evaluating these medications for ventricular arrhythmias in the specific setting of palliated congenital heart disease.

Catheter ablation has been used for ventricular arrhythmias in congenital heart disease patients; the experience with this is limited [50, 55, 58].

Finally, in patients who are likely to have life-threatening ventricular arrhythmias, implantable defibrillators have gained acceptance in the treatment of this group of patients, using novel lead configurations when necessary [59].

14.4 Summary

Ventricular arrhythmias are an increasingly recognized feature of late follow-up in patients with palliated structural congenital heart disease. Because of the potentially serious nature of ventricular arrhythmias in this growing population, a cooperative effort is required to develop an effective, evidence-based approach to diagnosis and management.

Reference

1. Schamroth L. Ventriculare extrasystoles. The disorders of cardiac rhythm. Philadelphia: Blackwell Scientific Publications, 1971: pp. 85–94.
2. Ikeda N, Takeuchi A, Hamada A, Goto H, Mamorita N, Takayanagi K. Model of bidirectional modulated parasystole as a mechanism for cyclic bursts of ventricular premature contractions. Biol Cybern. 2004;91:37–47.
3. Jacobsen JR, Garson A Jr, Gillette PC, McNamara DG. Premature ventricular contractions in normal children. J Pediatr. 1978;92(1):36–38.
4. Jones RW, Sharp C, Rabb LR, Lambert BR, Chamberlain DA. 1028 neonatal electrocardiograms. Arch Dis Child. 1979;54:427–31.
5. Nagashima M, Matsushima M, Ogawa A, Ohsuga A, Kaneko T, Yazaki T, et al. Cardiac arrhythmias in healthy children revealed by 24-hour ambulatory ECG monitoring. Pediatr Cardiol. 1987;8(2):103–108.
6. Alexander ME, Berul CI. Ventricular arrhythmias: when to worry. Pediatr Cardiol. 2000;21(6):532–41.
7. Kennedy HL. Ventricular ectopy in athletes: don't worry..more good news! J Am Coll Cardiol. 2002;40:453–56.
8. Paul T, Marchal C, Garson A Jr. Ventricular couplets in the young: prognosis related to underlying substrate. Am Heart J. 1990;119:577–82.
9. Miga DE, Case CL, Gillette PC. High prevalence of repolarization abnormalities in children with simple ventricular ectopy. Clin Cardiol. 1996;19:726–8.
10. Das BB, Sharma J. Repolarization abnormalities in children with a structurally normal heart and ventricular ectopy. Pediatr Cardiol. 2004;25:354–6.
11. Zweytick B, Pignoni-Mory P, Zweytick G, Steinbach K. Prognostic significance of right ventricular extrasystoles. Europace. 2004;6:123–9.
12. Raeder EA, Hohnloser SH, Graboys TB, Podrid PJ, Lampert S, Lown B. Spontaneous variability and circadian distribution of ectopic activity in patients with malignant ventricular arrhythmia. J Am Coll Cardiol. 1988;12:656–61.
13. Massin MM, Maeyns K, Withofs N, Gerard P. Dependency of premature ventricular contractions on heart rate and circadian rhythms during childhood. Cardiology. 2000;93 (1–2):70–3.
14. Anderson JL, Anastasiou-Nana MI, Menlove RL, Moreno FL, Nanas JN, Barker AH. Spontaneous variability in ventricular ectopic activity during chronic antiarrhythmic therapy. Circulation 1990; 82:830–40.
15. Sun Y, Blom NA, Yu Y, Ma P, Wang Y, Han X, et al. The influence of premature ventricular contractions on left ventricular function in asymptomatic children without structural heart disease: an echocardiographic evaluation. Int J Cardiovasc Imaging. 2003;19:295–9.
16. Yarlagadda RK, Iwai S, Stein KM, Markowitz SM, Shah BK, Cheung JW, et al. Reversal of cardiomyopathy in patients with repetitive monomorphic ventricular ectopy originating from the right ventricular outflow tract. Circulation. 2005; 112:1092–97.
17. Takemoto M, Yoshimura H, Ohba Y, Matsumoto Y, Yamamoto U, Mohri M, et al. Radiofrequency catheter ablation of premature ventricular complexes from right ventricular outflow tract improves left ventricular dilation and clinical status in patients without structural heart disease. J Am Coll Cardiol. 2005;45:1259–65.
18. Lown B, Wolf M. Approaches to sudden death from coronary heart disease. Circulation. 1971;44:130–42.
19. Lombardi F. Do we still need to count premature ventricular contractions? Eur Heart J. 1995;16:582–3.
20. Frolkis JP, Pothier CE, Blackstone EH, Lauer MS. Frequent ventricular ectopy after exercise as a predictor of death. N Engl J Med. 2003;348:781–90.
21. Morshedi-Meibodi A, Evans JC, Levy D, Larson MG, Vasan RS. Clinical correlates and prognostic significance of exercise-induced ventricular premature beats in the community: the Framingham Heart Study. Circulation. 2004;109:2417–22.
22. Selzman KA, Gettes LS. Exercise-induced premature ventricular beats: should we do anything differently? Circulation. 2004;109:2374–5.
23. Echt DS, Liebson PR, Michell LB, Peters RW, Obias-Manno D, Barker AH, Areusberg D, Baker A, Friedman L, Greene HL, et al. Preliminary report: effect of encainide and flecainide on mortality in a randomized trial of arrhythmia suppression after myocardial infarction. The Cardiac Arrhythmia Suppression Trial (CAST) Investigators. N Engl J Med. 1989;321:406–12.
24. Akhtar M, Breithardt G, Camm AJ, Coumel P, Janse MJ, Lazzara R, et al. CAST and beyond. Implications of the Cardiac Arrhythmia Suppression Trial. Task Force of the Working Group on Arrhythmias of the European Society of Cardiology. Circulation. 1990;81:1123–27.
25. Zhu DW, Maloney JD, Simmons TW, Nitta J, Fitzgerald DM, Trohman RG, et al. Radiofrequency catheter ablation for management of symptomatic ventricular ectopic activity. J Am Coll Cardiol. 1995;26:843–9.
26. Gumbrielle T, Bourke JP, Furniss SS. Is ventricular ectopy a legitimate target for ablation? Br Heart J. 1994;72:492–4.
27. Wellens HJ. Radiofrequency catheter ablation of benign ventricular ectopic beats: a therapy in search of a disease? J Am Coll Cardiol. 1995;26:850–1.
28. Garratt CJ. Appropriate indications for radiofrequency catheter ablation. Br Heart J. 1994;72:407.
29. Gross GJ, Zhu W, Chiu C, Hamilton RM, Kirsh JA. Ventricular Tachycardia. In: Freedom RM, Yoo S-J, Mikailian H, Williams WG, eds. The natural and modified history of congenital heart disease. New York: Blackwell Publishing, Inc, 2004: pp.587–96.
30. Harris KC, Potts JE, Fournier A, Gross GJ, Kantoch MJ, Cote JM, et al. Right ventricular outflow tract tachycardia in children. J Pediatr. 2006;149:822–6.
31. Haissaguerre M, Shoda M, Jais P, Nogami A, Shah DC, Kautzner J, et al. Mapping and ablation of idiopathic ventricular fibrillation. Circulation. 2002;106:962–7.
32. Viskin S, Rosso R, Rogowski O, Belhassen B. The "short-coupled" variant of right ventricular outflow ventricular tachycardia: a not-so-benign form of benign ventricular tachycardia? J Cardiovasc Electrophysiol. 2005;16:912–6.
33. Noda T, Shimizu W, Taguchi A, Aiba T, Satomi K, Suyama K, et al. Malignant entity of idiopathic ventricular fibrillation and polymorphic ventricular tachycardia initiated by premature extrasystoles originating from the right ventricular outflow tract. J Am Coll Cardiol. 2005;46:1288–94.

34. Viskin S, Antzelevitch C. The cardiologists' worst nightmare sudden death from "benign" ventricular arrhythmias. J Am Coll Cardiol. 2005;46:1295–7.

35. Saul JP, Hulse JE, Papagiannis J, Van Praagh R, Walsh EP. Late enlargement of radiofrequency lesions in infant lambs. Implications for ablation procedures in small children. Circulation. 1994;90(1):492–9.

36. Deanfield JE, McKenna WJ, Presbitero P, England D, Graham GR, Hallidie-Smith K. Ventricular arrhythmia in unrepaired and repaired tetralogy of Fallot. Relation to age, timing of repair, and haemodynamic status. Br Heart J. 1984;52:77–81.

37. Sullivan ID, Presbitero P, Gooch VM, Aruta E, Deanfield JE. Is ventricular arrhythmia in repaired tetralogy of Fallot an effect of operation or a consequence of the course of the disease? A prospective study. Br Heart J. 1987;58:40–44.

38. Balaji S, Silka MJ, McAnulty JH. Arrhythmias in patients with congenital heart disease. Card Electrophysiol Rev. 2002;6:42–44.

39. Martin RP, Radley-Smith R, Yacoub MH. Arrhythmias before and after anatomic correction of transposition of the great arteries. J Am Coll Cardiol. 1987;10:200–204.

40. Wolfe RR, Driscoll DJ, Gersony WM, Hayes CJ, Keane JF, Kidd L, et al. Arrhythmias in patients with valvar aortic stenosis, valvar pulmonary stenosis, and ventricular septal defect. Results of 24-hour ECG monitoring. Circulation. 1993;87:I89–101.

41. Anderson RH, Ho SY. The morphologic substrates for pediatric arrhythmias. Cardiol Young. 1991;1:159–76.

42. Houyel L, Vaksmann G, Fournier A, Davignon A. Ventricular arrhythmias after correction of ventricular septal defects: importance of surgical approach. J Am Coll Cardiol. 1990;16:1224–8.

43. Rhodes LA, Wernovsky G, Keane JF, Mayer JE Jr., Shuren A, Dindy C, et al. Arrhythmias and intracardiac conduction after the arterial switch operation. J Thorac Cardiovasc Surg. 1995;109:303–10.

44. Hovels-Gurich HH, Seghaye MC, Ma Q, Miskova M, Minkenberg R, Messmer BJ, et al. Long-term results of cardiac and general health status in children after neonatal arterial switch operation. Ann Thorac Surg. 2003;75:935–43.

45. Shinebourne EA, Babu-Narayan SV, Carvalho JS. Tetralogy of Fallot: from fetus to adult. Heart. 2006;92:1353–9.

46. Gatzoulis MA, Balaji S, Webber SA, Siu SC, Hokanson JS, Poile C, et al. Risk factors for arrhythmia and sudden cardiac death late after repair of tetralogy of Fallot: a multicentre study. Lancet. 2000;356(9234):975–81.

47. Khairy P, Landzberg MJ, Gatzoulis MA, Lucron H, Lambert J, Marcon F, et al. Value of programmed ventricular stimulation after tetralogy of fallot repair: a multicenter study. Circulation. 2004;109:1994–2000.

48. Nakazawa M, Shinohara T, Sasaki A, Echigo S, Kado H, Niwa K, et al. Arrhythmias late after repair of tetralogy of fallot: a Japanese Multicenter Study. Circ J. 2004;68:126–30.

49. Karamlou T, Silber I, Lao R, McCrindle BW, Harris L, Downar E, et al. Outcomes after late reoperation in patients with repaired tetralogy of Fallot: the impact of arrhythmia and arrhythmia surgery. Ann Thorac Surg. 2006;81:1786–93.

50. Gonska BD, Cao K, Raab J, Eigster G, Kreuzer H. Radiofrequency catheter ablation of right ventricular tachycardia late after repair of congenital heart defects . Circulation. 1996;94:1902–1908.

51. Downar E, Harris L, Kimber S, Mickleborough L, Williams W, Sevaptsidis E, et al. Ventricular tachycardia after surgical repair of tetralogy of Fallot: results of intraoperative mapping studies. J Am Coll Cardiol. 1992;20:648–55.

52. Kammeraad JA, van Deurzen CH, Sreeram N, Bink-Boelkens MT, Ottenkamp J, Helbing WA, et al. Predictors of sudden cardiac death after Mustard or Senning repair for transposition of the great arteries. J Am Coll Cardiol. 2004;44:1095–102.

53. Hornung TS, Kilner PJ, Davlouros PA, Grothues F, Li W, Gatzoulis MA. Excessive right ventricular hypertrophic response in adults with the mustard procedure for transposition of the great arteries. Am J Cardiol. 2002;90:800–803.

54. Alexander ME, Walsh EP, Saul JP, Epstein MR, Triedman JK. Value of programmed ventricular stimulation in patients with congenital heart disease. J Cardiovasc Electrophysiol. 1999;10(8):1033–1044.

55. Furushima H, Chinushi M, Sugiura H, Komura S, Tanabe Y, Watanabe H, et al. Ventricular tachycardia late after repair of congenital heart disease: efficacy of combination therapy with radiofrequency catheter ablation and class III anti-arrhythmic agents and long-term outcome. J Electrocardiol. 2006;39:219–24.

56. Therrien J, Siu SC, Harris L, Dore A, Niwa K, Janousek J, et al. Impact of pulmonary valve replacement on arrhythmia propensity late after repair of tetralogy of Fallot. Circulation. 2001;103(20):2489–94.

57. Stephenson EA, Redington AN. Reduction of QRS duration following pulmonary valve replacement in tetralogy of Fallot: implications for arrhythmia reduction? Eur Heart J. 2005;26:863–4.

58. Morwood JG, Triedman JK, Berul CI, Khairy P, Alexander ME, Cecchin F, et al. Radiofrequency catheter ablation of ventricular tachycardia in children and young adults with congenital heart disease. Heart Rhythm. 2004;1:301–308.

59. Stephenson EA, Batra AS, Knilans TK, Gow RM, Gradaus R, Balaji S, et al. A multicenter experience with novel implantable cardioverter defibrillator configurations in the pediatric and congenital heart disease population. J Cardiovasc Electrophysiol. 2006;17:41–6.

Genetic Origins of Right Ventricular Cardiomyopathies

Deirdre Ward, Srijita Sen-Chowdhry, Maria Teresa Tome Esteban, Giovanni Quarta, and William J. McKenna

Arrhythmogenic right ventricular cardiomyopathy (AVRC), also known as arrhythmogenic right ventricular dysplasia, is a myocardial disease characterized histologically by loss of myocardial cells, with replacement by fibrous and/or fatty tissue, and clinically by ventricular arrhythmia, cardiac failure, and sudden death [1–5]. When first described in 1978 on the basis of four cases [6], and subsequently in the landmark series of Marcus and colleagues [1], the typical patient was a middle-aged male, who presented with arrhythmias arising from the right ventricle, which also exhibited structural abnormalities on imaging. Experience of the last 20 years has broadened our understanding of the condition, but many controversies still exist in clinical diagnosis, etiology, prognosis, and management.

The exact prevalence is unknown, but recent estimates of 1 per 5,000 population are likely to be conservative [7]. In a significant proportion of affected individuals, the first presentation may be with sudden death. The limited information available suggests the disease is a significant cause of unexpected, premature, sudden death. Pathological evidence of the condition was found as a likely cause in over one-tenth of cases in a retrospective review of a French population aged from 1 year to 65 years [8]. A prospective study of an Italian cohort, aged from 12 years to 35 years, found evidence of arrhythmogenic cardiomyopathy in 12% of those who suffered sudden cardiac death [9], while a population-based study from Minnesota reported an underlying diagnosis of the condition in 17% of victims of sudden death under 40 years of age [10]. The aim in clinical management of patients and their relatives is, first, accurately to diagnose those affected and, second, to identify those at risk of complications to enable initiation of preventive treatment.

Clinical diagnosis is notoriously problematic. Many of the described abnormalities on the electrocardiogram and imaging are nonspecific, and there are several conditions which predispose to arrhythmia arising from the right ventricle. To resolve this difficulty, a task force of experts was convened under the auspices of the European Society of Cardiology, known as the Working Group on Myocardial and Pericardial Disease, and the Scientific Council on Cardiomyopathies of the International Society and Federation of Cardiology, resulting in the publication in 1994 of the diagnostic criterions which are still in use today (Table 15.1) [11].

Although early reports suggested that the occurrence of familial disease was rare, with only 1 of the 24 cases in the first series having a family history suggestive of arrhythmogenic cardiomyopathy, with a time pattern of familial disease emerged, suggesting autosomal dominant inheritance in most cases, but with variable expression and incomplete penetrance [12, 13]. With the recognition of familial inheritance, the search for chromosomal loci began, and between 1994 and 2002, eight different loci were identified.

15.1 Genetic Loci

Rampazzo and colleagues [14] were the first to publish their results of linkage analysis in two large families, mapping the locus to chromosome 14q23–q24. The same group from Padova, in Northern Italy, identified a second locus 1 year later at chromosome 1q42–q43. The clinical features associated with this second locus were unusual, as the presentation was with effort-induced polymorphic ventricular tachycardia in the absence of clinically evident morphological abnormalities [15]. The families in the original paper, now denoted as ARVC 1, had a more classical pattern of expression of disease. Additional families with clinical diagnoses of arrhythmogenic right ventricular cardiomyopathy did not map to

D. Ward (✉)
Inherited Cardiovascular Disease Group, University College London, London, UK

Table 15.1 Criteria established by the task force for diagnosis of arrhythmogenic right ventricular cardiomyopathy

Major	Minor
I Global and/or regional structural abnormalities or dysfunction of RV	
Severe dilation of RV with ↓ EF	Mild global RV dilation or ↓ EF
Localised RV aneurysms	Mild segmental dilatation
Severe segmental dilation of RV	Regional hypokinesia of RV
II Tissue characterization of walls	
Fibrofatty replacement of myocardium on biopsy	
III Repolarization abnormalities	
	T-wave inversion V2, V3 (subjects ≥ 12 yrs, in absence RBBB)
IV Depolarization/Conduction abnormalities	
Epsilon waves	Late potentials on SAECG
Localized QRS prolongation (>110 msec) in V1–V3	
V Arrhythmias	
	VT or NSVT of LBBB morphology (on ECG, Holter, exercise test) >1,000 ventricular ectopics in 24 hrs
VI Family History	
Familial disease at autopsy/surgery	Family history premature death <35 (suspected ARVC-related)
	Family history clinical diagnosis

Diagnosis is made in the presence of two or more major criteria, or one major and two minor criteria, or four minor criteria. Only one criterion may be counted from each group. RV = right ventricle; EF = ejection fraction; yrs = years; RBBB = right bundle branch block; SAECG = signal averaged ECG; VT = ventricular tachycardia (sustained >30 sec in duration); NSVT = nonsustained ventricular tachycardia (between 3 beats and 30 sec duration, rate >120/min); LBBB = left bundle branch block; hrs = hours

either of the published loci, confirming further genetic heterogeneity.

Shortly thereafter, two additional loci at 14q12–q22, known as ARVC 3, and 2q32.1–q32.3, giving ARVC 4, were identified [16]. The phenotype for the fourth locus was somewhat distinct from the preceding three, with evidence also of left ventricular involvement, although right ventricular abnormalities and arrhythmias were still the dominant feature [17].

In 1998, a large Newfoundland family was studied. Of over 200 relatives spanning seven generations, 10 living subjects were diagnosed using the criteria established by the Task Force. Previously published loci were excluded, and a new locus mapped to chromosome 3p23. The clinical features of this fifth locus appeared similar to the first and third, although with 17 sudden deaths recorded, the associated prognosis appeared worse [18]. Subsequent survival studies confirmed this impression [19].

One year later, the locus in another North American family mapped to chromosome 10p12–p14 [20]. The pattern of expression of the disease in this instance was very distinctive. All the children with the disease haplotype had clinical or pathological evidence of the disease by the age of 10.

At the same time, a Swedish family with skeletal myopathy and cardiomyopathy were linked to a locus on the long arm of chromosome 10, specifically at 10q22.3 [21]. Although many features of the condition were not typical, showing myopathy, conduction disease, atrial arrhythmia, and perhaps premature atherosclerosis, the presence of T-wave inversion on the electrocardiogram, along with imaging and pathological features, were characteristic, notably the presence of gross dilation, significant systolic impairment, and extensive fibrofatty replacement of the right ventricle.

15.2 Identification of the Gene

The first gene identified was that causing the variant of the cardiomyopathy known as Naxos disease (Table 15.2). This was first described in 1986, when physicians noted the association between cardiac arrhythmia, *woolly hair*, and palmoplantar keratoderma in young inhabitants of the Greek island of Naxos [22]. Analysis of the pedigree indicated a pattern of autosomal recessive inheritance, and linkage analysis subsequently mapped the locus to chromosome 17, specifically to 17q21 [23]. The candidate gene *plakoglobin* was identified. Mice with null mutations of *plakoglobin* have skin and cardiac abnormalities analogous to Naxos disease. A two base-pair deletion was identified in *plakoglobin*, and all 19 clinically affected individuals were homozygous for the mutation. An additional 20 relatives who were clinically unaffected were heterozygous for the mutation [24].

Table 15.2 Genes identified in association with the cardiomyopathy

Year	First author	Gene	Mode of inheritance	Clinical characteristics
2000	McKoy	*Plakoglobin*	Autosomal Recessive	'Naxos disease': nine families, woolly hair, PPK, ARVC features
2000	Norgett	*Desmoplakin*	Autosomal Recessive	'Carvajal syndrome': woolly hair, PPK, LV DCM
2001	Tiso	*Ryanodine2*	Autosomal Dominant	Four families, effort-induced polymorphic VT, RV regional WMA
2002	Rampazzo	*Desmoplakin*	Autosomal Dominant	One family, RV disease (ECG, imaging, arrhythmia), 50% penetrance
2004	Gerull	*Plakophilin-2*	Autosomal Dominant	32 probands, RV disease predominantly, 'incomplete' penetrance
2005	Beffagna	*TGF-β3*	Autosomal Dominant	One family, classical ARVC, RV disease with arrhythmia
2005	Norman	*Desmoplakin*	Autosomal Dominant	One family, LV disease predominantly, penetrance 100% ('LV' criteria)
2005	Bauce	*Desmoplakin*	Autosomal Dominant	Four families, RV and LV disease, 64% penetrance
2006	Syrris	*Plakophilin-2*	Autosomal Dominant	Nine families + two probands, RV disease, 66% penetrance (TF criteria)
2006	Dalal	*Plakophilin-2*	Autosomal Dominant	25 probands (43% of all probands), early presentation
2006	van Tintelen	*Plakophilin-2*	Autosomal Dominant	24 probands (43 % of all probands), 70% of 'familial ARVC'
2006	Pilichou	*Desmoglein-2*	Autosomal Dominant	Eight probands, typical ARVC features but frequent LV disease
2006	Awad	*Desmoglein-2*	Autosomal Dominant	Four probands, three families, 'incomplete' penetrance

PPK = palmoplantar keratoderma; ARVC = arrhythmogenic right ventricular cardiomyopathy; LV = left ventricle; DCM = dilated cardiomyopathy; Ryanodine2 = Ryanodine2 receptor mutation; VT = ventricular tachycardia; RV = right ventricle; WMA = wall morion abnormality; TGF-ß3 = transforming growth factor beta-3 mutation; 'LV' criteria = adaptation of Task Force criteria to left ventricular instead of right ventricular abnormalities; TF criterions = Task Force criterions

Plakoglobin is a member of the armadillo protein family. It is a constituent protein in cell adhesion junctions, found in both adherens and desmosomal junctions, with both adhesive and signaling functions. It is found in many tissues, including epidermis and the heart. The adhesive functions of plakoglobin are mediated through its interaction with other desmosomal proteins, which include desmoplakin, plakophilin-2, and desmoglein-2.

A plausible pathogenic mechanism, therefore, is that, by disrupting the cell adhesion structure, a *plakoglobin* mutation would predispose cardiac myocytes and skin epithelial cells to separate, leading to cell death and repair or replacement by fat and fibrous tissue. The ability of epithelial cells to regenerate, in contrast to the almost complete inability in cardiac myocytes, could explain the different dermal and cardiac manifestations.

The genes coding for other desmosomal proteins became candidate genes for other variants of the cardiomyopathy. An Ecuadorian group described three families where affected members had dermal and hair manifestations similar to Naxos disease, but the cardiac phenotype was more suggestive of dilated cardiomyopathy. The pattern of inheritance again suggested autosomal recessive disease. Subsequent genetic analysis identified a deletion in desmoplakin, another desmosomal protein. The mutation produces a premature stop codon, resulting in a truncated protein which is lacking its C-terminal domain. This region of the protein has been shown to interact with

intermediate filaments to anchor them to the desmosome [25].

This led to the identification in 2002 of a desmoplakin mutation as a cause of the cardiomyopathy in a family with a dominant pattern of inheritance, not corresponding to any of the known loci, and designated as ARVC 8. The clinical features at initial evaluation of 11 affected members were of classical right ventricular disease, although during follow-up three individuals developed left ventricular involvement [26]. Another family has been identified where the morphological changes are predominantly in the left ventricle, with arrhythmias also typically arising from the left ventricle. A single adenine insertion in the *desmoplakin* gene was identified, which introduces a premature stop codon. The term arrhythmogenic left ventricular cardiomyopathy has been used to describe this variation in phenotype [27]. Further information on genotype and phenotype is available from four Italian families with novel mutations of *desmoplakin*, suggesting a high prevalence of arrhythmic death, thus affecting 6 of 26 gene positive individuals. Of the 14 who fulfilled the criteria of the task force for clinical diagnosis, there were ventricular arrhythmias in 79%, right ventricular morphological abnormalities in 86%, and left ventricular involvement in almost half [28].

Desmoplakin is the most abundant of the desmosomal proteins. The carboxy terminus tail region is responsible for binding intermediate filaments of the cytoskeleton, while the amino terminus is hypothesized to associate with desmosomal proteins [25]. The cytoskeleton is said to provide a scaffolding, which is important for transmission of force from the sarcomere to the extracellular matrix, and for protection of the myocyte from the consequences of mechanical stress. Mutations in cytoskeletal genes including actin, desmin, and dystrophin have been shown to result in a dilated cardiomyopathic phenotype as a result of this 'defective force transmission' [29]. Mutations in desmoplakin can therefore be predicted to disrupt the desmosome, resulting in classical arrhythmogenic right ventricular cardiomyopathy with separation and death of myocytes, and replacement with fibrofatty tissue, or to disrupt the myocytic cytoskeleton with subsequent dilated cardiomyopathy. While, in theory, the location of the mutation could dictate the resultant phenotype, in practice variations of a composite phenotype often exist within the same family [27].

Between 2004 and 2006, several mutations have been described in plakophilin 2, another desmosomal protein, in approximately one-quarter of a cohort of probands [30]. Evaluation of kindreds suggests gene penetrance of two-thirds using the criteria of the task force, but with some evidence of expression of disease in all gene positive patients [31]. Dutch and North American groups have recently published an even higher prevalence of *plakophilin-2* mutations in cohorts of patients diagnosed with the cardiomyopathy, with 43% of unrelated probands in both populations found to carry mutations in *PKP2*, and in those with confirmed familial disease 70% were due to such mutations. Interestingly, the Dutch group report that no *PKP2* mutations were found in cases of sporadic disease [32, 33]. In total, 46 different novel *PKP2* mutations have been described, of which 8 are missense mutations. Of the 25 mutations initially described by Gerull, 9 were subsequently identified in the cohorts described by Syrris, Dalal, and van Tintelen, with 6 of these mutations occurring in more than one population [30–33].

Most recently, the *desmoglein-2* gene has been implicated. Of 80 probands with a diagnosis of arrhythmogenic cardiomyopathy, 10% were found to have mutations in this gene. The clinical phenotype was suggestive of a high degree of left ventricular involvement, and half had a family history of arrhythmogenic right ventricular cardiomyopathy [34]. Very limited evaluations of the kindred suggest incomplete penetrance.

Other mutations in nondesmosomal proteins have been linked to the condition, but these are subject to much controversy. The gene for *ARVC 2* was identified as the *Ryanodine 2* receptor gene. As previously mentioned, however, the four families had a remarkably similar phenotype, presenting with syncope, sudden death,

and polymorphic ventricular tachycardia on exercise without major structural abnormality on imaging. Interestingly, the 12-lead electrocardiogram was normal in affected individuals, which is very unusual in the setting of arrhythmogenic right ventricular cardiomyopathy. The phenotype of *ARVC 2* is strikingly similar to adrenergically mediated polymorphic ventricular tachycardia, and families with this rare autosomal dominant are now recognized to have a mutation in the *Ryanodine 2* receptor gene [35]. Interestingly, none of the affected individuals had an abnormal electrocardiogram, and rarely were late potentials identified. The function of the *Ryanodine 2* receptor gene is to regulate the flux of calcium in the myocytes, and the mutation appears to result in a gain of function, therefore causing a massive release of calcium from the sarcoplasmic reticulum, and electrical instability. The high levels of calcium may trigger apoptosis or cell death, resulting in the histological features described, specifically fibrofatty replacement of myocardial cells in the apical segments, and an inflammatory T-cell infiltrate [36]. This differs in many ways from classical cell-adhesion cardiomyopathy, and suggests that this is, in fact, a phenocopy of arrhythmogenic right ventricular cardiomyopathy.

Mutations in transforming growth factor ß3 have been detected in some, but not all, of families with *ARVC1*, which has been linked to chromosome 14q24.3 [14, 37]. One of the functions of this gene is to promote fibrosis. Some controversy exists as to the pathogenic importance of this finding. The exons of this gene had previously been screened in these families as transforming growth factor ß3 had been considered a plausible candidate gene following the linkage studies. No mutations were found. Subsequently the promoter and untranslated regions were screened. There is some evidence that these regions may affect translation of the gene, and experimental studies suggest that the mutations found in two families increase expression of the gene, and therefore can result in increased fibrosis. Several other families with ARVC1 on linkage analysis, however, did not have mutations in any of the screened exons or untranslated regions, leaving questions unanswered.

The prevalence of familial disease has been reported to be approximately 30% [38]. The diagnosis within relatives of affected probands depends on the presence of the requisite number of criterions established by the task force, and indeed excludes those with predominant left ventricular disease. As disease expression is very variable, many relatives may have features consistent with a diagnosis of arrhythmogenic right ventricular cardiomyopathy, but insufficient to satisfy the published criterions. The criterions were developed, however, to facilitate diagnosis in a population where the risk of disease is 1 in 5,000.

In familial disease, the risk of inheritance of a disease-causing gene is 1–2 in 5,000. Thus, any clinical findings consistent with a diagnosis in the setting of a family history of proven disease should be considered indicative of expression of the disease. In retrospect, it may have been more appropriate for the task force to produce two diagnostic standards, that is, one for diagnosis in probands, which the original criterions would address, and a second less stringent set for diagnosing the disease in relatives of affected patients. Hamid and colleagues [29] addressed this problem in their cohort of patients. They identified familial disease in 28% of index cases using the criteria established by the task force. In other families, clinical features such as right precordial T-wave inversion, late potentials on the signal averaged electrocardiogram, or ventricular ectopy, less abundant in relatives than proposed by the task force, but more frequent than found in normal controls, was considered to indicate incomplete disease penetrance. Using these modified criteria, they concluded that the true prevalence of familial disease was at least 48% (Table 15.3).

Thus, there is strong evidence for arrhythmogenic right ventricular cardiomyopathy as a disease of the desmosome, with at least 40% of probands carrying mutation in a desmosomal gene in the Italian experience [34], and even higher percentages for *PKP2* alone in other centers [32, 33]. Correlations between genotype and phenotype are typically not very robust, although some patterns have emerged. Future research will focus on identifying the candidate genes at the previously described loci, and

identifying the genetic cause of the additional 30–70% of affected individuals who do not have desmosomal disease. In the absence of a reliable gold standard for clinical diagnosis, the ability to rely on genetic screening to identify populations at risk would be invaluable.

References

1. Marcus FI, et al. Right ventricular dysplasia: a report of 24 adult cases. Circulation. 1982;65(2):384–98.
2. Fontaine G, et al. Arrhythmogenic right ventricular dysplasia and Uhl's disease. Arch Mal Coeur Vaiss. 1982;75(4):361–71.
3. Thiene G, et al. Right ventricular cardiomyopathy and sudden death in young people. N Engl J Med. 1988;318(3):129–33.
4. Basso C, et al. Arrhythmogenic right ventricular cardiomyopathy. Dysplasia, dystrophy, or myocarditis? Circulation. 1996;94(5):983–91.
5. Corrado D, et al. Spectrum of clinicopathologic manifestations of arrhythmogenic right ventricular cardiomyopathy/dysplasia: a multicenter study. J Am Coll Cardiol. 1997;30(6):1512–20.
6. Frank R, et al. [Electrocardiology of 4 cases of right ventricular dysplasia inducing arrhythmia]. Arch Mal Coeur Vaiss. 1978;71(9):963–72.
7. Norman MW and McKenna WJ. Arrhythmogenic right ventricular cardiomyopathy: perspectives on disease. Z Kardiol. 1999;88(8):550–4.
8. Tabib A, et al. Circumstances of death and gross and microscopic observations in a series of 200 cases of sudden death associated with arrhythmogenic right ventricular cardiomyopathy and/or dysplasia. Circulation. 2003;108(24):3000–5.
9. Corrado D, et al. Does sports activity enhance the risk of sudden death in adolescents and young adults? J Am Coll Cardiol. 2003;42(11):1959–63.
10. Shen WK, et al. Sudden unexpected nontraumatic death in 54 young adults: a 30-year population-based study. Am J Cardiol. 1995;76(3):148–52.
11. McKenna WJ, et al. Diagnosis of arrhythmogenic right ventricular dysplasia/cardiomyopathy. Task Force of the Working Group Myocardial and Pericardial Disease of the European Society of Cardiology and of the Scientific Council on Cardiomyopathies of the International Society and Federation of Cardiology. Br Heart J. 1994;71(3):215–8.
12. Nava A, et al. Familial occurrence of right ventricular dysplasia: a study involving nine families. J Am Coll Cardiol. 1988;12(5):1222–8.
13. Nava A, et al. [Analysis of the mode of transmission of right ventricular dysplasia]. Arch Mal Coeur Vaiss. 1990;83(7):923–8.
14. Rampazzo A, et al. The gene for arrhythmogenic right ventricular cardiomyopathy maps to chromosome 14q23-q24. Hum Mol Genet. 1994;3(6):959–62.
15. Rampazzo A, et al. A new locus for arrhythmogenic right ventricular cardiomyopathy (ARVD2) maps to chromosome 1q42-q43. Hum Mol Genet. 1995;4(11):2151–4.
16. Severini GM, et al. A new locus for arrhythmogenic right ventricular dysplasia on the long arm of chromosome 14. Genomics. 1996;31(2):193–200.
17. Rampazzo A, et al. ARVD4, a new locus for arrhythmogenic right ventricular cardiomyopathy, maps to chromosome 2 long arm. Genomics. 1997;45(2):259–63.
18. Ahmad F, et al. Localization of a gene responsible for arrhythmogenic right ventricular dysplasia to chromosome 3p23. Circulation. 1998;98(25):2791–5.

Table 15.3 Proposed modified criteria for diagnosis of familial disease

Proven disease in a first-degree relative plus one of the following	
1. Electrocardiogram	T-wave inversion in the right precordial leads (V2 and V3)
2. Signal-averaged electrocardiogram	Demonstration of late potentials
3. Arrhythmia	Ventricular tachycardia with left bundle branch block morphology (documented on ECG, Holter monitoring or during exercise testing) >200 ventricular extrasystoles over 24 hours (Holter monitor)
4. Structural or functional abnormality of the right ventricle	Mild global RV dilatation of the RV and/or reduction in ejection fraction with normal LV Mild segmental dilatation of the RV Regional RV hypokinesia

LV = left ventricle; RV = right ventricle
Adapted from Hamid et al. [39]

19. Hodgkinson KA, et al. The impact of implantable cardioverter-defibrillator therapy on survival in autosomal-dominant arrhythmogenic right ventricular cardiomyopathy (ARVD5). J Am Coll Cardiol. 2005;45(3):400–8.

20. Li D, et al. The locus of a novel gene responsible for arrhythmogenic right-ventricular dysplasia characterized by early onset and high penetrance maps to chromosome 10p12–p14. Am J Hum Genet. 2000;66(1):148–56.

21. Melberg A, et al. Autosomal dominant myofibrillar myopathy with arrhythmogenic right ventricular cardiomyopathy linked to chromosome 10q. Ann Neurol. 1999;46(5):684–92.

22. Protonotarios N, et al. Cardiac abnormalities in familial palmoplantar keratosis. Br Heart J. 1986;56(4):321–6.

23. Coonar AS, et al. Gene for arrhythmogenic right ventricular cardiomyopathy with diffuse nonepidermolytic palmoplantar keratoderma and woolly hair (Naxos disease) maps to 17q21. Circulation. 1998;97(20):2049–58.

24. McKoy G, et al. Identification of a deletion in plakoglobin in arrhythmogenic right ventricular cardiomyopathy with palmoplantar keratoderma and woolly hair (Naxos disease). Lancet. 2000;355(9221):2119–24.

25. Norgett EE, et al. Recessive mutation in desmoplakin disrupts desmoplakin-intermediate filament interactions and causes dilated cardiomyopathy, woolly hair and keratoderma. Hum Mol Genet. 2000;9(18):2761–6.

26. Rampazzo A, et al. Mutation in human desmoplakin domain binding to plakoglobin causes a dominant form of arrhythmogenic right ventricular cardiomyopathy. Am J Hum Genet. 2002;71(5):1200–6.

27. Norman M, et al. Novel mutation in desmoplakin causes arrhythmogenic left ventricular cardiomyopathy. Circulation. 2005;112(5):636–42.

28. Bauce B, et al. Clinical profile of four families with arrhythmogenic right ventricular cardiomyopathy caused by dominant desmoplakin mutations. Eur Heart J. 2005;26(16):1666–75.

29. Fatkin D, Graham RM. Molecular mechanisms of inherited cardiomyopathies. Physiol Rev. 2002;82(4):945–80.

30. Gerull B, et al. Mutations in the desmosomal protein plakophilin-2 are common in arrhythmogenic right ventricular cardiomyopathy. Nat Genet. 2004;36(11):1162–4.

31. Syrris P, et al. Clinical expression of plakophilin-2 mutations in familial arrhythmogenic right ventricular cardiomyopathy. Circulation. 2006;113(3):356–64.

32. van Tintelen JP, et al. Plakophilin-2 mutations are the major determinant of familial arrhythmogenic right ventricular dysplasia/cardiomyopathy. Circulation. 2006;113(13):1650–8.

33. Dalal D, et al. Clinical features of arrhythmogenic right ventricular dysplasia/cardiomyopathy associated with mutations in plakophilin-2. Circulation. 2006;113(13):1641–9.

34. Pilichou K, et al. Mutations in desmoglein-2 gene are associated with arrhythmogenic right ventricular cardiomyopathy. Circulation. 2006;113(9):1171–9.

35. Marks AR, et al. Involvement of the cardiac ryanodine receptor/calcium release channel in catecholaminergic polymorphic ventricular tachycardia. J Cell Physiol. 2002;190(1):1–6.

36. Tiso N, et al. Identification of mutations in the cardiac ryanodine receptor gene in families affected with arrhythmogenic right ventricular cardiomyopathy type 2 (ARVD2). Hum Mol Genet. 2001;10(3):189–94.

37. Beffagna G, et al. Regulatory mutations in transforming growth factor-beta3 gene cause arrhythmogenic right ventricular cardiomyopathy type 1. Cardiovasc Res. 2005;65(2):366–73.

38. Dalal D, et al. Arrhythmogenic right ventricular dysplasia: a United States experience. Circulation. 2005;112(25):3823–32.

39. Hamid MS, et al. Prospective evaluation of relatives for familial arrhythmogenic right ventricular cardiomyopathy/dysplasia reveals a need to broaden diagnostic criteria. J Am Coll Cardiol. 2002;40(8):1445–50.

The Pathology of Arrhythmogenic Right Ventricular Cardiomyopathy

16

Glenn P. Taylor

Arrhythmogenic right ventricular cardiomyopathy (ARVC), an entity clinically defined less than 30 years ago, is a heart muscle disorder of an unknown cause characterized morphologically by fibrofatty replacement of the right ventricle myocardium [1, 2]. It clinically presents with ventricular arrhythmias, congestive heart failure, or sudden death. ARVC is included in the primary cardiomyopathy group of the WHO/ISFC 1999 Classification and in the genetic primary cardiomyopathy group of the American Heart Association 2006 Classification [3, 4]. However, despite the attention given over the past three decades to the characterization of the pathologic changes occurring with ARVC, there still remain areas of controversy and dispute in the histologic criteria and interpretation of gross anatomical findings that confound the morphologic diagnosis of ARVC [5]. The longer answer, therefore, requires review of the pathology spectrum, the pathology, diagnostic criteria, and consideration of the etiology and pathogenesis of arrhythmogenic right ventricular cardiomyopathy.

16.1 ARVC and Pediatric Pathology

The estimated prevalence of ARVC is 1 in 5000, but parts of Italy have prevalence of 6 per 10,000 and in some areas as high as 44 per 10,000 [6]. It is said to be the most common cause of sudden, unexpected, natural death in the young adult population. Male predominance, up to 80%, is well recognized. ARVC occurs in all ages, but is primarily a disease of the second to fifth decades [7]. The mean age at diagnosis is early to mid-30s but the reported age range spans toddlers to septuagenarians [8]. Children under 11 years comprise less than 2% of cases. There is

G.P. Taylor, MD, FRCPC (✉)
Division of Pathology, Department of Pediatric Laboratory Medicine, Hospital for Sick Children

one report of an antenatal diagnosis [9]. Thirty percent to 50% of cases are familial with generally an autosomal dominant inheritance pattern having variable penetrance and phenotype. The types of ARVC specimens encountered by the pathologist include hearts at autopsy, generally from sudden unexpected death, endomyocardial biopsy, or explanted hearts. Sudden unexpected death is unfortunately a common presentation of ARVC in adults and also can occur in children [10]. Over a 20-year period at the Hospital for Sick Children, Toronto, ARVC accounted for approximately 15% of cases of sudden unexpected death due to antemortem-undiagnosed cardiomyopathy. In comparison, hypertrophic cardiomyopathy accounted for only 6% of such pediatric sudden unexpected deaths [11].

16.2 Pathology of ARVC

The heart pathology in older children and adolescents with ARVC is similar to that documented in adults [12]. Heart weight is generally normal to moderately increased. The hallmark macroscopic feature is fibrofatty replacement of the right ventricle myocardium (Fig. 16.1) [13, 14]. This can be segmental to diffuse. It typically affects the lateral right ventricle inflow or basal free wall, the apical zone and/or the infundibulum of the right ventricle. These three sites represent the so-called *triangle of dysplasia*. Fat extends from epicardium to the endocardium, sparing the trabecular muscle. The amount of fat varies greatly from case to case and may be a minor component of the fibrofatty infiltrate, with fibrosis predominant. In the majority of cases the right ventricle is thinned, permitting trans-illumination to be used as a macroscopic pathology diagnostic aid. In 50% of cases in adults the right ventricle demonstrates aneurysms. Some cases are characterized by fatty thickening of the right ventricle. Although right ventricle involvement defines ARVC the left ventricle is involved in

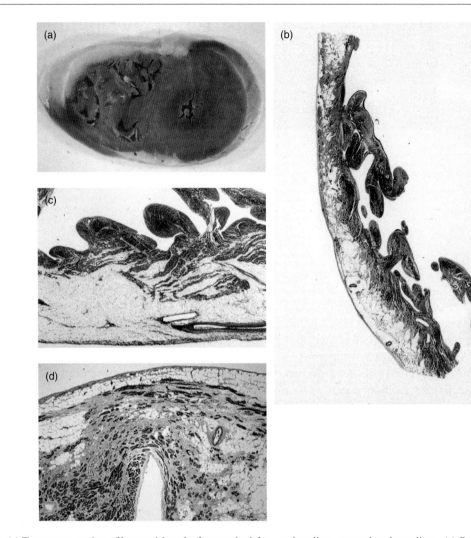

Fig. 16.1 (a) Transverse section of heart with arrhythmogenic right ventricular cardiomyopathy (ARVC) demonstrating fatty replacement of anterior right ventricle wall myocardium, with preservation of posterior free wall myocardium. (b) Longitudinal section of right ventricle outflow tract in ARVC demonstrating marked thinning of myocardium, with fibrous and fatty replacement extending from epicardium toward endocardium. (c) Predominantly fatty infiltration in ARVC, extending from epicardium toward endocardium, sparing trabeculae (hematoxylin and eosin stain, original magnification ×10). (d) Fibrous and fatty replacement of myocardium in ARVC, with atrophy of residual myofibers (Masson trichrome stain, original magnification ×20)

at least 50% of cases, where it is more characterized by fibrosis, generally in a subepicardial distribution, rather than fatty infiltration (Fig. 16.2) [15]. Involvement of the interventricular septum occurs in up to 20% of cases, again primarily fibrous rather than fatty.

Microscopic examination of the affected right ventricle region shows fatty replacement of the myocardium extending from the epicardial surface toward the endocardium. There are variable fibrous replacement, degenerative changes, and atrophy of residual myocytes and often a sparse lymphocytic inflammatory infiltrate. The degenerative changes in the myocardium are progressive. Fibrofatty change is identified initially but appears to become predominantly fatty over time. Involvement of the left ventricle and interventricular septum also tend to occur later in the disease progression. Histologic myocarditis meeting Dallas criteria is seen in 20–80% of cases.

Two patterns for ARVC have been identified [16, 17]. In 20–45% of cases ARVC has a fatty infiltrative pattern characterized by lace-like adipose tissue extending from the epicardium to the endocardium. The residual myocytes may be normal or only mildly atrophic, but do not form a distinct boundary with the epicardium. The right ventricle may be thickened by this infiltration rather than thinned. The more common type is the cardiomyopathic pattern where there is fibrofatty replacement of the right ventricle myocardium, atrophy, and degeneration of residual myocytes and thinning of the right ventricle wall. Aneurysms occur in this form. This type is also biventricular in up to 80% of cases [16].

(a)   (b)

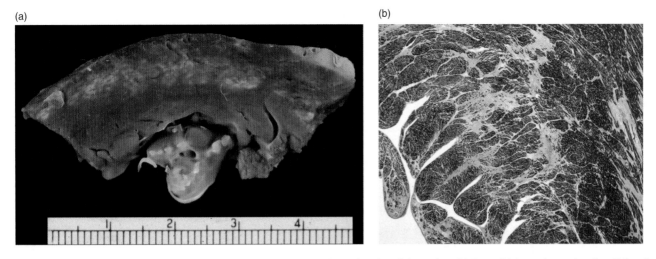

Fig. 16.2 (a) Section of left ventricle free wall in ARVC, demonstrating sub-epicardial scarring. (b) Interstitial scarring, sub-epicardial and intramural, in left ventricle of ARVC (Masson trichrome stain, original magnification ×10)

16.3 Pathology Diagnosis of ARVC

Although fatty infiltration is a hallmark of ARVC it has been said that "fat is the least specific criterion for diagnosis of ARVC" [5]. One differential diagnosis for fatty right ventricle is *core adiposum*. This is abundant epicardial and subepicardial fat associated with obesity. The fat may comprise 50% of the weight of the heart. The myocardial fat increases with age. A second form of fatty right ventricle is *simple* fatty infiltration, which may occur even in the nonobese. This is distinguished from ARVC by the myocardium being displaced by fat, rather than being replaced, with preservation of a distinct boundary between outer epicardium and a resulting *marbled* pattern of fatty infiltration. The intervening myocardium does not show fibrosis or degenerative change. Another consideration is that normal hearts can have varying degrees of myocardial fat, most prominently in the apical and anterolateral right ventricle regions where adipose tissue may constitute up to 15% of the myocardial wall [16].

Combined gross and microscopic findings are required for a reliable pathological diagnosis of ARVC. The three criteria are: (1) fatty and/or fibrofatty replacement of right ventricle myocardium; (2) atrophy, degenerative changes, and/or death of interposed cardiac myocytes; and (3) lymphocytic inflammation (although this is not as important as criteria 1 and 2) [5].

Endomyocardial biopsy has been used in the diagnosis of ARVC but is complicated by false negatives and false positives. Endomyocardial biopsy diagnostic criteria have been presented by Angelini et al. [18]. Their criteria on right ventricle, presumably septal, endomyocardial biopsy is fatty tissue greater than 3.2% of the surface area of the biopsy sample, fibrous tissue greater than

40%, and myocytes less than 45%. As most right ventricle endomyocardial biopsies avoid the free wall, which represents the area of potential greatest diagnostic yield in ARVC, false negatives are a significant concern. However, false positives can also occur if the normal subendocardial fat content of the apical and anterolateral regions of the right ventricle are not considered.

The three ARVC pathologic criteria listed above are not specific to ARVC and can be seen in other types of cardiac myocyte injury. Fibrous and fatty replacement of myocardium occurs with ischemic heart disease and with Chagas' disease. ARVC-like changes have been reported in cardiac allograft failure [19]. ARVC-like changes have also been identified in older children and adolescents that have chronic neurologic and neuromuscular disorders [20]. The suggestion is that fibrofatty replacement is a *common* final pathway for a variety of cardiac myocyte injuries [21]. These include the genetic mutations primarily involved with a cardiac desmosome, as discussed elsewhere in this compendium, myocarditis, immunologic injury, and ischemic injury. Myocyte apoptosis is a well recognized in studies of ARVC and may be the common element for the various potential causes [22].

The identification of desmosome protein mutations in ARVC provides for the molecular genetic diagnostic testing that can now be offered [23]. These protein abnormalities also raise the possibility of more specific diagnostic morphologic studies for ARVC. Immunohistochemical staining for various cardiac desmosome constituents is being explored as is the possibility that *downstream* aberrations of constituents of the intercalated disk such as connexins and other gap junction proteins might represent generic markers for a variety of *upstream* cardiac desmosome protein mutations [24]. Recently, electron microscopic alterations of the intercalated disc have been documented, potentially providing another morphologic diagnostic modality for ARVC [25].

16.4 Summary

In summary, arrhythmogenic right ventricular cardiomyopathy is uncommon in childhood, but can be seen in older children and adolescents, where presentation often is with sudden unexpected death. Pathologic diagnosis can also be made from an explanted heart or on endomyocardial biopsy, although biopsy diagnosis must consider significant false negatives and false positives. In children, the cardiomyopathic fibrofatty form is the most frequent type, but there are other conditions that can mimic the pathology. ARVC most often represents a primary genetic cardiomyopathy for which genetic testing of several variants is available. These genetic abnormalities may also lead to development of morphological tests that are more specific and sensitive for the diagnosis of arrhythmogenic right ventricular cardiomyopathy.

References

1. Frank R, Fontaine G, Vedel J, Mialet G, Sol C, Guiraudon G, et al. [Electrocardiology of 4 cases of right ventricular dysplasia inducing arrhythmia]. Archives des maladies du coeur et des vaisseaux. Sep 1978;71(9):963–72.

2. Marcus FI, Fontaine GH, Guiraudon G, Frank R, Laurenceau JL, Malergue C, et al. Right ventricular dysplasia: a report of 24 adult cases. Circulation. Feb 1982;65(2):384–98.

3. Maron BJ, Towbin JA, Thiene G, Antzelevitch C, Corrado D, Arnett D, et al. Contemporary definitions and classification of the cardiomyopathies: an American Heart Association Scientific Statement from the Council on Clinical Cardiology, Heart Failure and Transplantation Committee; Quality of Care and Outcomes Research and Functional Genomics and Translational Biology Interdisciplinary Working Groups; and Council on Epidemiology and Prevention. Circulation. Apr 11 2006;113(14):1807–16.

4. Richardson P, McKenna W, Bristow M, Maisch B, Mautner B, O'Connell J, et al. Report of the 1995 World Health Organization/International Society and Federation of Cardiology Task Force on the Definition and Classification of cardiomyopathies. Circulation. Mar 1 1996;93(5):841–2.

5. Basso C, Thiene G. Adipositas cordis, fatty infiltration of the right ventricle, and arrhythmogenic right ventricular cardiomyopathy. Just a matter of fat? Cardiovascular Pathology. Jan–Feb 2005;14(1):37–41.

6. Frances RJ. Arrhythmogenic right ventricular dysplasia/cardiomyopathy. A review and update. International Journal of Cardiology. Jun 28 2006;110(3):279–87.

7. Fontaine G, Fontaliran F, Hebert JL, Chemla D, Zenati O, Lecarpentier Y, et al. Arrhythmogenic right ventricular dysplasia. Annu Rev Med. 1999;50:17–35.

8. Tabib A, Loire R, Chalabreysse L, Meyronnet D, Miras A, Malicier D, et al. Circumstances of death and gross and microscopic observations in a series of 200 cases of sudden death associated with arrhythmogenic right ventricular cardiomyopathy and/or dysplasia.[see comment]. Circulation. Dec 16 2003;108(24):3000–5.

9. Rustico MA, Benettoni A, Fontaliran F, Fontaine G. Prenatal echocardiographic appearance of arrhythmogenic right ventricle dysplasia: a case report. Fetal Diagnosis & Therapy. Nov–Dec 2001;16(6):433–6.

10. Pawel BR, de Chadarevian JP, Wolk JH, Donner RM, Vogel RL, Braverman P. Sudden death in childhood due to right ventricular dysplasia: report of two cases. Pediatr Pathol. Nov-Dec 1994;14(6):987–95.

11. Somers G, Perrin D, Taylor GP. Causes of sudden cardiac death in a pediatric population: A review of 105 cases. Pathol Int. 2004;54 Suppl 2:A29.

12. White S, Siebert JR, Kapur RP. Pathologic quiz case: a 10-year-old boy with weakness, lethargy, and edema. Arrhythmogenic right ventricular cardiomyopathy, cardiomyopathic pattern. Archives of Pathology & Laboratory Medicine. Jun 2004;128(6):700–2.

13. Corrado D, Basso C, Thiene G. Arrhythmogenic right ventricular cardiomyopathy: diagnosis, prognosis, and treatment. Heart. May 2000;83(5):588–95.

14. Thiene G, Basso C, Calabrese F, Angelini A, Valente M. Pathology and pathogenesis of arrhythmogenic right ventricular cardiomyopathy. Herz. May 2000;25(3):210–5.

15. Lobo FV, Silver MD, Butany J, Heggtveit HA. Left ventricular involvement in right ventricular dysplasia/cardiomyopathy. Canadian Journal of Cardiology. Nov 1999;15(11):1239–47.

16. Burke AP, Farb A, Tashko G, Virmani R. Arrhythmogenic right ventricular cardiomyopathy and fatty replacement of the right ventricular myocardium: are they different diseases?[see comment]. Circulation. Apr 28 1998;97(16):1571–80.

17. d'Amati G, Leone O, di Gioia CR, Magelli C, Arpesella G, Grillo P, et al. Arrhythmogenic right ventricular cardiomyopathy: clinicopathologic correlation based on a revised definition of pathologic patterns. Human Pathology. Oct 2001;32(10):1078–86.

18. Angelini A, Basso C, Nava A, Thiene G. Endomyocardial biopsy in arrhythmogenic right ventricular cardiomyopathy. American Heart Journal. Jul 1996;132(1 Pt 1):203–6.

19. Shehata BM, Wilson S, Mahle WT, Vincent RN, Kanter KR, Berg AM, et al. Arrhythmogenic right ventricular dysplasia-like changes in cardiac allografts. Mod Pathol. 2004;17(2):273.

20. Martens M, Chiasson DA, Halliday W, Taylor GP. Fatty infiltration of the right ventricular myocardium in children with chronic neurological disorders. Pediatr Develop Pathol. 2008;11(1):75.

21. Vatta M, Marcus F, Towbin JA. Arrhythmogenic right ventricular cardiomyopathy: a 'final common pathway' that defines clinical phenotype. Eur Heart J. Mar 2007;28(5):529–30.

22. Runge MS, Stouffer GA, Sheahan RG, Yamamoto S, Tsyplenkova VG, James TN. Morphological patterns of death by myocytes in arrhythmogenic right ventricular dysplasia. American Journal of the Medical Sciences. Nov 2000;320(5):310–9.

23. Tsatsopoulou AA, Protonotarios NI, McKenna WJ. Arrhythmogenic right ventricular dysplasia, a cell adhesion cardiomyopathy: insights into disease pathogenesis from preliminary genotype–phenotype assessment. Heart. Dec 2006;92(12):1720–3.

24. Kaplan SR, Gard JJ, Protonotarios N, Tsatsopoulou A, Spiliopoulou C, Anastasakis A, et al. Remodeling of myocyte gap junctions in arrhythmogenic right ventricular cardiomyopathy due to a deletion in plakoglobin (Naxos disease).[see comment]. Heart Rhythm. May 2004;1(1):3–11.

25. Yang Z, Bowles NE, Scherer SE, Taylor MD, Kearney DL, Ge S, et al. Desmosomal dysfunction due to mutations in desmoplakin causes arrhythmogenic right ventricular dysplasia/cardiomyopathy. Circulation research. Sep 15 2006; 99(6):646–55.

The Diagnosis of Arrhythmogenic Right Ventricular Cardiomyopathy (ARVC) in Children

17

Robert M. Hamilton

17.1 The Evolution of Diagnosis in Arrhythmogenic Right Ventricular Cardiomyopathy

The diagnosis of arrhythmogenic right ventricular cardiomyopathy (ARVC) has evolved from pathological assessment at postmortem to a recognizable clinical condition during life, and holds promise for definitive genetic diagnosis in the near future. ARVC task force criteria [1], agreed upon by expert consensus, have assisted greatly in identifying symptomatic adults with a high specificity. However, ARVC task force criteria are recognized to be insensitive, in general, and more so in asymptomatic relatives [2, 3] or individuals presenting at an early age [4]. The absence of a definitive gold standard during life makes difficult the evaluation of sensitivity and specificity of individual clinical tests, as well as the estimation of the prevalence of the disease. Using a defined referral population, Peters and colleagues estimate the prevalence of ARVC as 1/1,000 inhabitants [5], although more traditional estimates are from 1/1,667 [6] to 1/5,000 [7].

ARVC diagnosis is now moving into an era of molecular and genetic diagnosis. Although multiple genetic loci have been identified, an evolving common feature is the mutation (usually truncation) of proteins that form desmosomes of the intercalated disks of ventricular myocytes. It is anticipated that a common pathophysiology will underlie the multiple genes and gene loci so far identified, as well as others not yet identified, adding to our understanding and redefinition of this important sudden-death disorder. This chapter evaluates the features that contribute to the diagnosis of ARVC in children based on our current clinical understanding, short of the evolving molecular characterization of this disease.

17.1.1 Symptoms and Assessment

The most common presenting symptoms among a predominantly adult group of ARVC patients were palpitations, syncope, and sudden death in 27%, 26%, and 23%, respectively [8]. Children likely present with similar symptoms, although sudden death is less common. More recently, children are being referred for clinical assessment related only to a positive family history of ARVC or undifferentiated sudden death.

Naxos disease, identified by Protonotarios [9] on the Aegean island of Naxos and subsequently other Hellenic islands, Turkey, Israel, and Saudi Arabia, provided the first paradigm for early and severe presentation in the ARVC spectrum. Children homozygous for Naxos disease can be identified by the associated palmoplantar keratoderma and woolly hair, and present with syncope at puberty. Carvajal syndrome, identified in Ecuador and India, is a similar disease with more pronounced left ventricular involvement and presents even earlier in life [10].

Among patients dying with the more typical autosomal dominant types of ARVC, 10% of deaths occurred before age 19 and 50% occurred before age 35 (Fig. 17.1).

Among children assessed for ARVC in a pediatric arrhythmia clinic, patients rarely met ARVC Task force criteria before the age of 8 years and the rare deaths that occurred were after the age of 12 years. Among children referred with left bundle branch block ventricular tachycardia (LBBB VT) or a positive family history of ARVC, the sensitivity and specificity of each diagnostic test to identify those who met ARVC task force criteria compared to who did not is listed in Table 17.1 [11].

17.1.2 Electrocardiographic Criteria

The electrocardiographic features of ARVC include localized prolonged depolarization, epsilon waves, and T-wave

R.M. Hamilton (✉)
Department of Pediatrics, Hospital for Sick Children, Toronto, ON, Canada

A.N. Redington et al. (eds.), *Congenital Diseases in the Right Heart*, DOI 10.1007/978-1-84800-378-1_17,
© Springer-Verlag London Limited 2009

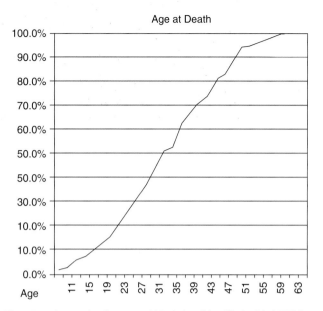

Fig. 17.1 Age at death among 200 victims identified with ARVC at autopsy
(modified from Tabib, 2003)

inversion. Among adults, the incidence in leads V_{1-3} of QRS duration of 110 ms or higher was 75%, that of prolonged right precordial S-wave upstroke of 55 ms or higher was 84%, that of epsilon potentials was 23%, and that of right precordial T-wave inversions was 55%. Neither QRS duration of 110 ms or higher nor epsilon potentials could not be identified in a control group of 52 unaffected individuals. A prolonged S-wave upstroke was present in only two and T-wave inversions were found in three [12].

Among children with LBBB VT or a positive family history of ARVC who were referred for assessment of possible ARVC, total S-wave duration was assessed and compared to a group of 150 normal children [13]. Using a 98th percentile cut-point, S-wave duration in any of leads V_{1-3} was 37% sensitive in identifying children who met ARVC task force criteria, based on an electrocardiography (ECG) at

presentation at an average age of 11.6 years. During follow-up to an average age of 14.2 years, sensitivity increased to 48%. The specificity of this measurement was 94%.

In addition to S-wave duration, T inversion in the right precordial leads is considered a minor criterion for ARVC, but can only be applied to that subset of children of age beyond 12 years. Among children in this age group referred for assessment of ARVC, T inversion was sensitive for meeting ARVC criteria in 66%, but only 64% specific [11]. Finally, a true epsilon wave is found in a minority of adults with ARVC, and even fewer children. However, a sharp spike is not infrequently seen late within the upstroke of the S wave in the right anterior leads in children suspected to have ARVC, and is rarely present in normal ECGs.

17.1.3 Signal-Averaged ECG

Ventricular signal averaging, available as a separated instrument or as an option on many ECG machines, is a method of magnifying and measuring late depolarization occurring within small areas of myocardium. Signal-averaged ECG parameters in adults with ARVC correlate with the extent of myocardial fibrosis on biopsy, reduction in right ventricular ejection fraction, and risk for sustained ventricular arrhythmias. The root-mean-square voltage of the terminal 40 ms at a filter setting of 25 Hz was an independent risk factor for the occurrence of sustained ventricular arrhythmias [14]. Bauce and colleagues, examining two patients with worsening electrical instability, correlated this with rapid progression of abnormal signal-averaged ECG parameters [15]. This same group demonstrated that the filtered QRS duration and duration of high-frequency, low-amplitude signals on a 25–250 Hz signal-averaged ECG identified patients with sustained VT [16]. During follow-up, high-frequency, low-amplitude signals signals increased significantly in the sustained VT group.

Table 17.1 Sensitivity and specificity of clinical test findings to identify patients meeting ARVC task force criteria among patients referred with LBBB VT or a positive family history of ARVC)

Criterion	Sensitivity (%)	Specificity (%)
Major global/regional dysfunction of RV (echo, MRI, or angiography)	30	98
Minor/mild global or segmental dilatation or hypokinesis	58	76
RV wall thinning on MRI	58	79
Tissue characterization on Bx by the pathologist of "fibrofatty replacement"	62	91
Quantitative morphometric analysis on Bx of >18% fibrosis	56	71
T inversion in right precordial ECG	66	64
Epsilon waves or QRS prolongation	39	100
Any SAECG parameter beyond 2 Z-values	66	65
Any SAECG parameter beyond 1.5 Z-values	78	64
Frequent PVCs	48	54

(from MacIntyre et al. [11]

Nasir and colleagues demonstrated that ARVC patients with inducible VT have a longer filtered QRS duration, longer duration of high-frequency, low-amplitude signals, and lower root-mean-square voltage [17, 18]. fQRS duration ≥ 110 ms had a sensitivity of 91%, specificity of 90%, and predictive accuracy of 90% for VT inducibility in these patients.

Signal-averaged ECG parameters in children should be compared to published normals, which are dependent on body surface area [19]. The presence of any signal-averaged ECG parameter beyond two standard deviations identified 66% of children with LBBB VT or a positive family history who met ARVC task force criteria, and this sensitivity increased to 78% if parameters beyond 1.5 standard deviations were included [11].

17.1.4 Exercise Testing

The relationship between exercise and ventricular ectopy in ARVC is unclear. Among 33 exercise tests in 16 children with ARVC, ventricular ectopy was exacerbated in six patients and suppressed in five patients [20]. Nevertheless, there is early evidence in an animal model of ARVC that exercise may speed up the progression of disease [21], and it is recommended that recreational exercise be restricted according American Heart Association guidelines [22].

17.1.5 MRI

Individual MRI criteria have limited sensitivity or specificity for the diagnosis of ARVC. However, similar to the use of task force criteria for the clinical diagnosis of ARVC, an improved MRI score consisting of major and minor criteria has been developed in adults [23]. Major criteria include: fatty infiltration of the RV myocardium, localized RV aneurysm, severe dilatation and reduction in RV ejection fraction with no (or only mild) left ventricular impairment. Minor criteria include regional RV hypokinesia, mild segmental dilatation of RV, mild global RV dilatation, and/or ejection fraction reduction with normal left ventricle and prominent RV trabeculae. The combination of two major criteria, one major and two minor criteria or four minor criteria led to improved diagnostic accuracy with sensitivity of 82.3% and specificity of 88.8%.

Fogel and colleagues evaluated the ability of MRI to detect ARVC in 81 children referred for evaluation due to a broad range of indications [24]. Using the earlier MRI criteria of Midiri and colleagues [25], they found only one patient met the threshold of greater than or equal to three of five criteria to have a high probability of ARVC. An assessment of more recent criteria in a group of children with definitive ARVC would be desirable.

17.1.6 Angiography

Typically, right ventricular biplane angiography is performed with two contrast injections in a total of four views: AP, lateral, 30° RAO, and 60° LAO. Multiple studies assessing the sensitivity and specificity of angiography have been published based on affected adults, and their predictive features are summarized in Table 17.2. Specific assessments of angiography for ARVC in children have not been performed.

Table 17.2 Sensitivity and specificity of angiographic findings in adults with ARVC

Study	Angiographic finding	Sensitivity (%)	Specificity
Daubert (1988)	Slow dye evacuation of RV		low
	Deep fissuring in anterior wall		low
	Localized akinetic or dyskinetic bulges	90	
	Wide, deep fissuring of apex or inferior wall	33	
Chiddo (1989)	Localized Akinesia/dyskinesia	48	
	Small conical outpouchings persisting in systole	40	high
	Apical deep fissuring	8	
Conte (1989)	Aneurysmal formations of the right ventricle		100%
Daliento (1990)	Transversely arranged hypertrophic trabeculae, separated by deep fissures	96	87.50%
	Posterior subtricispid and anterior infuldibular wall bulgings		
Peters (1992)	Segmental Hypokinesia	72	
	Diffuse Hypokinesia	28	
Hebert (2004)	RV ejection fraction <35%	32	100%

Data from Daubert et al. [48], Chido et al. [49], Conte et al. [50], Daliento et al. [51], Peters et al. [52], and Hebert et al. [53]

17.1.7 Electrophysiologic Study

Among adult patients, the electrophysiology study has been used effectively to differentiate ARVC from more benign ventricular tachycardias of RV origin and to assess for concomitant electrophysiologic abnormalities, such as inducible atrial arrhythmias or specialized conduction system disease. Compared to patients with benign idiopathic right ventricular arrhythmias, adults with ARVC have a higher frequency of inducibility with ventricular extrastimuli (93% vs. 0%), multiple VT morphologies (73% vs. 0%) and fragmented diastolic potentials (93% vs. 0%) [26]. Benign RVOT tachycardias have a triggered automatic basis in 97%, whereas ARVC arrhythmias display features of reentry in over 80%. Arrhythmias can be ablated in ARVC, particularly using activation [27, 28] and entrainment mapping [29, 30], with short-term success in 71–82% of ARVC patients, but recur in 47–48%, compared to 95% acute and long-term success in RVOT tachycardias [31, 32]. It is unclear whether inducibility of ventricular arrhythmias is a risk factor for clinical outcome in ARVC (Table 17.3).

Belhassen reported a 19-year-old patient with right ventricular dysplasia and atrial paralysis [33] Proclemer and colleagues reported two brothers with ARVC with early involvement of the right atrium and sustained atrial flutter [34, 35]. Caglar and colleagues reported a right ventricular cardiomyopathy with atrial flutter, [36] as did Nakazato and colleagues [37] and Lui and colleagues [38]. Brembilla-Perrot and colleagues demonstrated that supraventricular arrhythmias could be induced in 65% of ARVC patients compared with 11% of control subjects [39, 40]. Three of 13 patients with inducible atrial arrhythmias went on to have spontaneous atrial fibrillation. Borderline-sustained and sustained-atrial arrhythmias are frequently induced during electrophysiologic (EP) study in children with ARVC, and may be a factor to consider in choosing a defibrillator or interpreting defibrillator events.

17.1.8 Electroanatomic (Voltage) Mapping

Boulos and colleagues first tested the hypothesis that low-amplitude intracardiac electrograms could identify the presence, location, and extent of dysplastic regions in ARVC [41]. Dysplastic areas demonstrated markedly reduced unipolar and bipolar voltages compared to nondysplastic areas or controls. Corrado and colleagues suggested that electroanatomic mapping could be used to guide biopsy for identification of fibrofatty replacement, and demonstrated that patients with normal voltage electrograms typically had inflammatory cardiomyopathy requiring only antiarrhythmic therapy compared to ARVC patients with low-voltage areas who typically required implantable cardioverter-defibrillators (ICD) therapy [42]. Low voltage areas identified by electroanatomical mapping correlate well with areas of dyskinesia identified by echo [42] or MRI [42, 43] and may be useful in characterizing a critical isthmus for catheter ablation [44]. Electroanatomical mapping may provide added diagnostic value in children already scheduled for invasive investigation, but control measurements are not yet available in this population. Ablation is rarely necessary within the pediatric population with ARVC.

17.1.9 Biopsy

The acceptance of endomyocardial biopsy assessment in the diagnosis of ARVC has been hampered by the

Table 17.3 Risk Stratifiers from adult series of ARVC patients

	Pezawas (Vienna)	Piccini (Hopkins)	Roguin (Hopkins)	Lemola (Zurich)	Hulot (Paris)
RV Dysfunction/Dilatation	+		+		+
LV Dysfunction	+				+
Congestive Heart Failure				+	
Left Atrial Dilatation				+	
Antiarrhythmic Therapy	+				
Prolonged PR Interval				+	
Prolonged QRS in Lead V1				+	
Bundle Branch Block				+	
Abnormal SAECG	+				
Spontaneous VT			+		+
Inducible VT at EP Study		−	+		
Meets ARVC Criteria		+			
Male			+		
2° Prevention		+			

Data from Pezawas et al. [54], Piccini et al. [55], Roguin et al. [56], Lemola et al. [57], and Hulot et al. [58]

erroneous anecdote that the ventricular septum is not involved in ARVC, as well as the appropriate concern over the complication rates of endomyocardial biopsy. Compounding this dilemma is the need for multiple samples of endomyocardial septum due to sampling error. Once tissue is obtained, traditional staining may need to be augmented with specific staining for fat or fibrosis [45, 46]. Among 66 children referred for assessment of LBBB VT or a family history of ARVC, quantitative assessment of endomyocardial biopsies from the right ventricular septum demonstrated 23.1 ± 14.8% fibrosis and 6.0 ± 11% fat in patients who met task force criteria for ARVC versus 14.4 ± 9.3% fibrosis and 3.3 ± 7.60% fat in those who did not meet criteria [47]. These differences were significant for fibrosis alone. Recent descriptions on MRI support these findings, in that septal involvement of ARVC can be clearly demonstrated. In addition, MRI techniques such as myocardial delayed enhancement (aimed at identifying fibrotic replacement) are yielding more positive results than previous techniques, which attempted to enhance for fat alone. These MRI findings corroborate the finding of significantly increased fibrosis on endomyocardial biopsy from the right ventricular septum.

As the molecular basis for ARVC becomes more clear, endomyocardial biopsies may play an even more important role in the diagnosis of ARVC, its molecular subtypes, and pathophysiologic mechanisms. Using immunoflorescence, the presence of intercalated disk proteins involved in ARVC, including desmosomal and gap junction proteins, can be characterized.

17.1.10 Risk Stratification

While diagnosis of ARVC in children is often a challenge, a further assessment to risk stratify the patient should also be completed. Thus far, only studies of predominantly adult presentations of ARVD have identified risk stratifiers. These are summarized in Table 17.1 below. Significant risk stratifiers common to two or more studies include right ventricular dysfunction or dilatation, left ventricular dysfunction, and spontaneous ventricular tachycardia (VT). Inducibility of VT at EP study was a significant risk stratifier in a study of Johns Hopkins patients, yet not significant in another study from the same institution. As children become increasingly diagnosed with ARVC, robust risk-stratification strategies for children are needed to identify and treat high-risk patients without exposing all ARVC children to the recognized complications of ICD therapy in the young.

References

1. McKenna WJ, Thiene G, Nava A, Fontaliran F, Blomstrom-Lundqvist C, Fontaine G, et al. Diagnosis of arrhythmogenic right ventricular dysplasia/cardiomyopathy. Task Force of the Working Group Myocardial and Pericardial Disease of the European Society of Cardiology and of the Scientific Council on Cardiomyopathies of the International Society and Federation of Cardiology. Br Heart J. 1994;71:215–8.
2. Nasir K, Bomma C, Tandri H, Roguin A, Dalal D, Prakasa K, et al. Electrocardiographic features of arrhythmogenic right ventricular dysplasia/cardiomyopathy according to disease severity: a need to broaden diagnostic criteria. Circulation. 2004;110:1527–34.
3. Hamid MS, Norman M, Quraishi A, Firoozi S, Thaman R, Gimeno JR, et al. Prospective evaluation of relatives for familial arrhythmogenic right ventricular cardiomyopathy/dysplasia reveals a need to broaden diagnostic criteria. J Am Coll Cardiol. 2002;40:1445–50.
4. Sen-Chowdhry S, Lowe MD, Sporton SC, McKenna WJ. Arrhythmogenic right ventricular cardiomyopathy: clinical presentation, diagnosis, and management. Am J Med. 2004;117:685–95.
5. Peters S, Trummel M, Meyners W. Prevalence of right ventricular dysplasia-cardiomyopathy in a non-referral hospital. Int J Cardiol. 2004;97:499–501.
6. Thiene G, Basso C, Calabrese F, Angelini A, Valente M. Pathology and pathogenesis of arrhythmogenic right ventricular cardiomyopathy. Herz. 2000;25:210–5.
7. Frances RJ. Arrhythmogenic right ventricular dysplasia/cardiomyopathy. A review and update. Int J Cardiol. 2006;110:279–87.
8. Dalal D, Nasir K, Bomma C, Prakasa K, Tandri H, Piccini J, et al. Arrhythmogenic right ventricular dysplasia: a United States experience. Circulation. 2005;112:3823–32.
9. Protonotarios N, Tsatsopoulou A, Patsourakos P, Alexopoulos D, Gezerlis P, Simitsis S, et al. Cardiac abnormalities in familial palmoplantar keratosis. Br Heart J. 1986;56:321–6.
10. Carvajal-Huerta L. Epidermolytic palmoplantar keratoderma with woolly hair and dilated cardiomyopathy. J Am Acad Dermatol. 1998;39:418–21.
11. MacIntyre C, Warren A, Wilson G, Hamilton RM. Sensitivity/Specificity of Clinical Tests/Criteria against ARVC Task Force Criteria in Children Suspected to have ARVC. Canadian Journal of Cardiology. 2006; 22 (Suppl):153D.
12. Peters S, Trummel M, Koehler B, Westermann KU. The value of different electrocardiographic depolarization criteria in the diagnosis of arrhythmogenic right ventricular dysplasia/cardiomyopathy. J Electrocardiol. 2007;40(1):34–7.
13. Buffo-Sequeira I, Gross GJ, Davis AM, Kirsh JA, Hamilton RM. Utility of ECG precordial S-wave duration in diagnosis of arrhythmogenic right ventricular dysplasia/cardiomyopathy (ARVD/C) in pediatric patients. Can J Cardiol. 2003;19A:155A.
14. Turrini P, Angelini A, Thiene G, Buja G, Daliento L, Rizzoli G, et al. Late potentials and ventricular arrhythmias in arrhythmogenic right ventricular cardiomyopathy. Am J Cardiol. 1999;83:1214–9.
15. Bauce B, Basso C, Nava A. Signal-averaged electrocardiographic parameter progression as a marker of increased electrical instability in two cases with an over form of arrhythmogenic right ventricular cardiomyopathy. Pacing Clin Electrophysiol. 2002;25:362–4.
16. Folino AF, Bauce B, Frigo G, Nava A. Long-term follow-up of the signal-averaged ECG in arrhythmogenic right ventricular

cardiomyopathy: correlation with arrhythmic events and echo-cardiographic findings. Europace. 2006;8:423–9.

17. Nasir K, Tandri H, Rutberg J, Tichnell C, Spevak P, Crossan J, et al. Filtered QRS duration on signal-averaged electrocardiography predicts inducibility of ventricular tachycardia in arrhythmogenic right ventricle dysplasia. Pacing Clin Electrophysiol. 2003;26:1955–60.

18. Nasir K, Rutberg J, Tandri H, Berger R, Tomaselli G, Calkins H. Utility of SAECG in arrhythmogenic right ventricle dysplasia. Ann Noninvasive Electrocardiol. 2003;8:112–20.

19. Davis AM, McCrindle BW, Hamilton RM, Moore-Coleman P, Gow RM. Normal values for the childhood signal-averaged ECG. Pacing Clin Electrophysiol. 1996;19:793–801.

20. Buffo-Sequiera I, Hamilton RM, Kirsh JA, Russell JL, Gross GJ. Suppression of ventricular ectopy with exercise may be falsely reassuring in patients with arrhythmogenic right ventricular dysplasia (ARVD). Can J Cardiol. 2003;19A:176A.

21. Kirchhof P, Fabritz L, Zwiener M, Witt H, Schafers M, Zellerhoff S, et al. Age- and training-dependent development of arrhythmogenic right ventricular cardiomyopathy in heterozygous plakoglobin-deficient mice. Circulation. 2006;114:1799–806.

22. Maron BJ, Chaitman BR, Ackerman MJ, Bayes de Luna A, Corrado D, Crosson JE, et al. Recommendations for physical activity and recreational sports participation for young patients with genetic cardiovascular diseases. Circulation. 2004;109:2807–16.

23. Maksimovic R, Ekinci O, Reiner C, Bachmann GF, Seferovic PM, Ristic AD, et al. The value of magnetic resonance imaging for the diagnosis of arrhythmogenic right ventricular cardiomyopathy. Eur Radiol. 2006;16:560–8.

24. Fogel MA, Weinberg PM, Harris M, Rhodes L. Usefulness of magnetic resonance imaging for the diagnosis of right ventricular dysplasia in children. Am J Cardiol. 2006;97:1232–7.

25. Midiri M, Finazzo M, Brancato M, Hoffmann E, Indovina G, Maria MD, et al. Arrhythmogenic right ventricular dysplasia: MR features. Eur Radiol. 1997;7:307–12.

26. Niroomand F, Carbucicchio C, Tondo C, Riva S, Fassini G, Apostolo A, et al. Electrophysiological characteristics and outcome in patients with idiopathic right ventricular arrhythmia compared with arrhythmogenic right ventricular dysplasia. Heart. 2002;87:41–7.

27. Satomi K, Kurita T, Suyama K, Noda T, Okamura H, Otomo K, et al. Catheter ablation of stable and unstable ventricular tachycardias in patients with arrhythmogenic right ventricular dysplasia. J Cardiovasc Electrophysiol. 2006;17:469–76.

28. Zou J, Cao K, Yang B, Chen M, Shan Q, Chen C, et al. Dynamic substrate mapping and ablation of ventricular tachycardias in right ventricular dysplasia. J Interv Card Electrophysiol. 2004;11:37–45.

29. Reithmann C, Hahnefeld A, Remp T, Dorwarth U, Dugas M, Steinbeck G, et al. Electroanatomic mapping of endocardial right ventricular activation as a guide for catheter ablation in patients with arrhythmogenic right ventricular dysplasia. Pacing Clin Electrophysiol. 2003;26:1308–16.

30. Ellison KE, Friedman PL, Ganz LI, Stevenson WG. Entrainment mapping and radiofrequency catheter ablation of ventricular tachycardia in right ventricular dysplasia. J Am Coll Cardiol. 1998;32:724–8.

31. O'Donnell D, Cox D, Bourke J, Mitchell L, Furniss S. Clinical and electrophysiological differences between patients with arrhythmogenic right ventricular dysplasia and right ventricular outflow tract tachycardia. Eur Heart J. 2003;24:801–10.

32. Verma A, Kilicaslan F, Schweikert RA, Tomassoni G, Rossillo A, Marrouche NF, et al. Short- and long-term success of substrate-based mapping and ablation of ventricular tachycardia in arrhythmogenic right ventricular dysplasia. Circulation. 2005;111:3209–16.

33. Belhassen B, Shapira I, Hammerman C. Unusual manifestations of arrhythmogenic right ventricular dysplasia as ventricular fibrillation, atrial paralysis and hypoexcitable right ventricle. Br Heart J. 1988;59:263–5.

34. Proclemer A, Cianci R, Feruglio GA. Atrial involvement in arrhythmogenic right ventricle dysplasia: primary or secondary? Description of a case of occult ventricular dysplasia with right atrial enlargement and exclusively sinoatrial arrhythmia. G Ital Cardiol. 1988;18:671–5.

35. Proclemer A, Cuzzato AL, Morocutti G, Rocco M, Feruglio GA. [Paroxysmal atrial arrhythmias in arrhythmogenic cardiomyopathy of the right ventricle with a familial character: the role of right atrial involvement]. G Ital Cardiol. 1992;22:1315–26.

36. Caglar N, Pamir G, Kural T, Candan I, Kumbasar A, Sonel A. Right ventricular cardiomyopathy similar to Uhl's anomaly with atrial flutter and complete AV block. Int J Cardiol. 1993;38:199–201.

37. Nakazato Y, Nakata Y, Tokano T, Ohno Y, Hisaoka T, Sumiyoshi M, et al. A case of arrhythmogenic right ventricular dysplasia with atrial flutter. Jpn Heart J. 1994;35:689–94.

38. Lui CY, I. MF, Sobonya RE. Arrhythmogenic right ventricular dysplasia masquerading as peripartum cardiomyopathy with atrial flutter, advanced atrioventricular block and embolic stroke. Cardiology. 2002;97:49–50.

39. Brembilla-Perrot B, Terrier de la Chaise A, Buerrier D, Loiuis P, Suty-Selton C, Thiel B. Incidence of inducible supraventricular tachycardia in dysplasia of the right ventricle. Arch Mal Coeur Vaiss. 1993;86:203–7.

40. Brembilla-Perrot B, Jacquemin L, Houplon P, Houriez P, Buerrier D, Berder V, et al. Increased atrial vulnerability in arrhythmogenic right ventricular disease. Am Heart J. 1998;135:748–54.

41. Boulos M, Lashevsky I, Reisner S, Gepstein L. Electroanatomic mapping of arrhythmogenic right ventricular dysplasia. J Am Coll Cardiol. 2001;38:2020–7.

42. Corrado D, Basso C, Leoni L, Tokajuk B, Bauce B, Frigo G, et al. Three-dimensional electroanatomic voltage mapping increases accuracy of diagnosing arrhythmogenic right ventricular cardiomyopathy/dysplasia. Circulation. 2005;111: 3042–50.

43. Roux JF, Dubuc M, Pressacco J, Roy D, Thibault B, Talajic M, et al. Concordance between an electroanatomic mapping system and cardiac MRI in arrhythmogenic right ventricular cardiomyopathy. Pacing Clin Electrophysiol. 2006;29:109–12.

44. Miljoen H, State S, de Chillou C, Magnin-Poull I, Dotto P, Andronache M, et al. Electroanatomic mapping characteristics of ventricular tachycardia in patients with arrhythmogenic right ventricular cardiomyopathy/dysplasia. Europace. 2005;7:516–24.

45. Warren A, MacDonald C, Yoo S-J, Hamilton RM. Diagnostic criteria for arrhythmogenic right ventricular dysplasia in children: separating the fat from the lean. In: Strasbourg: Association of European Pediatric Cardiology; Cardiology in the Young. 2000; 10(Suppl 2):7.

46. Warren A, MacDonald C, Yoo S-J, Hamilton RM. Diagnostic criteria for arrhythmogenic right ventricular dysplasia in children: separating the fat from the lean. Pacing Clin Electrophysiol. 2000;23:598.

47. McIntyre C, Wilson G, Hamilton RM. Quantitative histomorphometric analysis in pediatric patients suspected or confirmed to have arrhythmogenic right ventricular dysplasia (ARVD/C) (manuscript in preparation). 2005.

48. Daubert C, Descaves C, Foulgoc JL, Bourdonnec C, Laurent M, Gouffault J. Critical analysis of cineangiographic criteria for diagnosis of arrhythmogenic right ventricular dysplasia. Am Heart J. 1988;115:448–59.

49. Chiddo A, Locuratolo N, Gaglione A, Bortone A, Troito G, Musci S, et al. Right ventricular dysplasia: angiographic study. Eur Heart J. 1989;10(Suppl. D):42–5.

50. Conte MR, Presbitero P, Gaita F, Tanga M, Massobrio N, Orzan F, et al. Angiographic findings in arrhythmogenic dysplasia of the right ventricle. G Ital Cardiol. 1989;19:580–4.

51. Daliento L, Rizzoli G, Thiene G, Nava A, Rinuncini M, Chioin R, et al. Diagnostic accuracy of right ventriculography in arrhythmogenic right ventricular cardiomyopathy. Am J Cardiol. 1990;66:741–5.

52. Peters S, Hartwig CA, Reil GH. Risk assessment in nonischemic ventricular arrhythmia by left and right ventriculography. Am Heart J. 1992;124:116–22.

53. Hebert JL, Chemla D, Gerard O, Zamani K, Quillard J, Azarine A, et al. Angiographic right and left ventricular function in arrhythmogenic right ventricular dysplasia. Am J Cardiol. 2004;93:728–33.

54. Pezawas T, Stix G, Kastner J, Schneider B, Wolzt M, Schmidinger H. Ventricular tachycardia in arrhythmogenic right ventricular dysplasia/cardiomyopathy: clinical presentation, risk stratification and results of long-term follow-up. Int J Cardiol. 2006;107:360–8.

55. Piccini JP, Dalal D, Roguin A, Bomma C, Cheng A, Prakasa K, et al. Predictors of appropriate implantable defibrillator therapies in patients with arrhythmogenic right ventricular dysplasia. Heart Rhythm. 2005;2:1188–94.

56. Roguin A, Bomma CS, Nasir K, Tandri H, Tichnell C, James C, et al. Implantable cardioverter-defibrillators in patients with arrhythmogenic right ventricular dysplasia/cardiomyopathy. J Am Coll Cardiol. 2004;43:1843–52.

57. Lemola K, Brunckhorst C, Helfenstein U, Oechslin E, Jenni R, Duru F. Predictors of adverse outcome in patients with arrhythmogenic right ventricular dysplasia/cardiomyopathy: long term experience of a tertiary care centre. Heart. 2005;91:1167–72.

58. Hulot JS, Jouven X, Empana JP, Frank R, Fontaine G. Natural history and risk stratification of arrhythmogenic right ventricular dysplasia/cardiomyopathy. Circulation. 2004;110:1879–84.

Clinical Outcomes and Current Therapies in Arrhythmogenic Right Ventricular Cardiomyopathy

18

Deirdre Ward, Srijita Sen-Chowdhry, Giovanni Quarta, and William J. McKenna

18.1 Introduction

Information on the natural history of arrhythmogenic right ventricular cardiomyopathy is somewhat limited by under-recognition of the condition. The prevalence is estimated to be 1 in 5,000, although this may be much higher in reality, and may be subject to regional variation [1]. Autopsy studies from the Veneto region of Italy have identified the condition in over one-fifth of athletes, and one-tenth of nonathletes under the age of 35 [2]. Whether this reflects a *founder effect*, or simply a higher degree of awareness among clinicians and pathologists in this region is unclear.

18.2 Natural History

It has been suggested that the natural history of arrhythmogenic right ventricular cardiomyopathy could be considered to have four distinct phases [3]. In the early *concealed* phase, the patient is usually asymptomatic, albeit still be at risk of sudden death, which typically occurs in young people during competitive sport or intense physical activity. Structural changes, when present are subtle, and may be confined to a region of the *triangle of dysplasia*, which comprises the inflow, apical, and outflow portions of the right ventricle.

Symptoms of ventricular arrhythmia herald the second phase of *overt electrical disorder*. The symptoms may include awareness of palpitation or frequent ectopy, syncope, and in some cases sudden death may occur. Structural and functional changes are usually obvious during this phase, although these are again often regional rather than global, and often only affect the right ventricle.

The third phase of *right ventricular failure* is characterized by diffuse right ventricular disease, with relative preservation of left ventricular function. Progression to *biventricular pump failure* denotes the final *advanced* phase of the disease, which may be confused with dilated cardiomyopathy. In addition to heart failure or sudden arrhythmic death, this phase may be associated with the development of atrial fibrillation and the occurrence of thromboembolic events. A multicentric study [4] involving 42 patients with the condition, 34 of whom died suddenly, 16 during effort, 2 due to heart failure, 2 from other causes, and 6 who had undergone transplantation, showed evidence of left ventricular involvement in three-quarters of the hearts. The occurrence of left ventricular involvement correlated well with increasing age, the occurrence of clinical arrhythmia, more severe cardiomegaly, inflammatory infiltrates, and heart failure.

18.3 Symptoms and Arrhythmia

Patients usually present with symptoms between the second and fifth decades of life. The symptoms usually relate to arrhythmia, with palpitations in up to two-thirds of individuals, and syncope or near-syncope in over one-third [5, 6]. Atypical chest pain may occur in up to one-quarter of affected individuals. The spectrum of ventricular arrhythmias ranges from isolated ventricular ectopy through sustained monomorphic ventricular tachycardia to ventricular fibrillation. The classical morphology of ventricular tachycardia in this setting is left bundle branch block, although patients with predominant left ventricular disease may present with right bundle branch block [7]. Patients with advanced disease may have several different

D. Ward (✉)
Inherited Cardiovascular Disease Group, University College London, London, UK

A.N. Redington et al. (eds.), *Congenital Diseases in the Right Heart*, DOI 10.1007/978-1-84800-378-1_18,
© Springer-Verlag London Limited 2009

morphologies, indicating multiple arrhythmic focuses. The occurrence of this form of tachycardia is not specific for arrhythmogenic right ventricular cardiomyopathy, and the differential diagnosis includes congenital heart disease, primary or secondary pulmonary hypertension, right ventricular infarction, bundle branch reentry, or idiopathic right ventricular outflow tract tachycardia [8].

18.3.1 Sudden Death

In the US, the condition accounts for approximately 5% of sudden cardiac deaths in those aged 1–65 years, and is associated with 3–4% of deaths occurring in relation to physical activity in young athletes [9]. In the Veneto region of Italy, where a comprehensive register has been compiled, and where all competitive athletes are subject by law to preparticipation screening, it is the most common cause of sudden death in those under 35 years, and the most common cause of sudden death in competitive athletes. This may reflect the fact that *concealed* disease may pass even the most rigorous screening tests, whereas those affected with conditions such as hypertrophic cardiomyopathy are more easily identified, and by law excluded from participation.

Annual mortality rates for populations with a diagnosis of arrhythmogenic right ventricular cardiomyopathy have been estimated to be 1% with and 3% without pharmacological treatment in the era prior to the insertion of cardioverter defibrillators [10]. Data from a Parisian tertiary referral hospital showed an annual mortality rate of 2.3%, which may to some extent reflect referral bias [5]. A review of the familial of the disease in Italy showed a favorable prognosis, with only one death over a mean of 8.5 years of follow-up, giving an annual mortality rate in these families of 0.08% [11].

The commonly held theory that death predominantly occurs in relation to exertion is not borne out by all the available information. In studies of athletes in Italy it is suggested that competitive sport doubles the risk of sudden death, but this still only occurs in 2 per 100,000 athletes. Most sudden deaths, however, do not occur in athletes, and in the nonathletic population only 9% of deaths were related to exertion [2]. Furthermore, in a review of autopsies of sudden-death victims in France, death occurred during normal daily activities in 150 of 200 cases of arrhythmogenic right ventricular cardiomyopathy, and during sporting activity in only 3.5% [12]. Review of the circumstances of death in 29 patients from the US who experienced a cardiac arrest also confirms that less than one-third were engaged in active exercise at the time [6].

18.4 Heart Failure

Patients may develop isolated right ventricular failure, or progress to biventricular failure. Heart failure typically occurs in the fourth or fifth decade. In the report of Dalal et al. [6], heart failure occurred in one-quarter of patients who satisfied the criteria for diagnosis established by the task force and survived to the age of 56 years. Fontaine [13] reported that the annual incidence of death due to heart failure was 1%. The mechanism for failure is dilation of the right ventricle, thinning of its wall, and progressive loss of myocardial function because of reduction in functioning myocytes. Left ventricular dysfunction may also be due to a similar process of myocytic death and fibrofatty replacement, and an inflammatory response is often apparent.

18.5 Stratification of Risk

With the annual incidence of sudden death ranging from 1 per 1,000 affected in familial disease to 30 per 1,000 of probands at a tertiary referral centre, a tool for identification of those at risk who would benefit from protective therapy is highly desirable. Much of the currently available information has been obtained from retrospective analyses of discharge rates form defibrillators implanted in populations undergoing primary and secondary prevention. Whether *appropriate* therapy with an implanted defibrillator is a valid surrogate for aborted sudden cardiac death is a subject of ongoing debate.

Corrado et al. [14] reviewed the experience of 132 patients attending 23 centers, all but one in Italy, in whom defibrillators had been implanted. Patients had to fulfill a modification of the diagnostic criteria to be eligible for inclusion, needing to possess at least one major criterion, and not being admitted on the basis of four minor criterions. During a mean follow-up of 39 months, almost half had appropriate treatment, and one-quarter experienced ventricular fibrillation or flutter, which were considered to have likely been fatal in the absence of the device. On multivariate logistic regression analysis, independent predictors of ventricular fibrillation or flutter included a prior history of cardiac arrest or ventricular tachycardia with hemodynamic compromise, younger age, and involvement of the left ventricle. Programmed ventricular stimulation was of limited value in identifying those patients at risk.

In the reported experience from a single German center [15], of 273 patients who fulfilled the conventional diagnostic criterions, defibrillators were implanted in 60 patients, leading to successful resuscitation in over nine-tenths after cardiac arrest, documented sustained ventricular tachycardia, or syncope. Event-free survival from potentially life-threatening arrhythmias was 79%, 64%, 59%, and 56% after 1, 3, 5, and 7 years follow-up, respectively. Multivariate analysis identified extensive right ventricular dysfunction as an independent predictor of any *appropriate* discharge, but the only independent predictor of rapid and potentially fatal tachycardia or fibrillation was inducible fibrillation at electrophysiological studies.

A similar study of 42 patients in the US [16] reported a high incidence of appropriate discharge, occurring in over three-quarters of the patients over a mean of 42 months. Predictors of appropriate therapy included inducible tachycardia during an electrophysiological study, documentation of spontaneous ventricular tachycardia, male gender, and severe right ventricular enlargement, albeit that multivariate analysis showed only inducible tachycardia during the electrophysiological study to be a predictor. Another study [17] comparing those with devices implanted for primary as opposed to secondary prevention found that electrophysiological testing did not predict risk of discharge in those undergoing primary prevention. Overall, three-quarters of 55 patients who met the diagnostic criterions for the condition had an appropriate discharge from their device, leading the authors to conclude that patients who meet the diagnostic criteria should have devices implanted for primary and secondary prevention, regardless of the outcome of electrophysiological testing. Interestingly, the overall population studied included 12 patients who had *probable* disease, the features on investigation failing to fulfill the accepted diagnostic criteria. Electrophysiological studies were carried out on this subgroup showed that patients who had no inducible arrhythmia sustained without pharmacological provocation did not receive reveal discharges from their devices during follow-up.

Peters et al. [18] sought to identify risk factors for arrhythmia and cardiac arrest in a population without inserted devices. Global reduction in right ventricular systolic function, regional hypokinesia, and end-systolic or end-diastolic bulging were associated with an increased risk of cardiac arrest. In another series from France [5], all 21 patients who died of a cardiovascular cause had at least one episode of ventricular tachycardia originating from the left bundle branch. There were no deaths in the group in whom no tachycardia was documented. The presence of right ventricular failure, as well as documented tachycardia, trended toward a significantly increased risk of cardiovascular death.

Other potential indicators of increased risk include demonstration of delayed depolarization on the electrocardiogram, and late potentials on signal-averaged tracings. Turrini et al. [19] measured the variation in duration of the QRS complex in all leads in three groups, 20 victims of sudden death, 20 with sustained ventricular tachycardia, and 20 without significant arrhythmias, comparing them with 20 controls. They found a difference of 40 ms or more between the maximum and minimum duration of the QRS complexes recorded in any of the 12 leads was a strong predictor of risk. The detection of late potentials on the signal-averaged electrocardiogram is the surface counterpart of delayed or late potentials detected during endocardial or epicardial mapping. They are frequently found in patients with documented ventricular tachycardia, but lack specificity, being found in other settings, such as in the postmyocardial-infarction setting [20, 21]. The prevalence in arrhythmogenic right ventricular cardiomyopathy ranges from 50% to 80% [22, 23]. The variation possibly relating to severity of disease as a positive correlation has been found between late potentials and extent of right ventricular fibrosis, reduced right ventricular systolic function and significant morphological abnormalities on imaging, but not yet convincingly with risk of potentially fatal arrhythmia [24, 25].

The use of three-dimensional voltage mapping during electrophysiological studies is a potentially useful area for stratification, but data are limited at present. Corrado et al. [26] demonstrated that reduced and fractionated voltage signals correlated well with endomyocardial biopsy features of advanced familial disease. Correlation with risk of significant arrhythmia was statistically borderline, but further studies may confirm its value as an objective and reproducible risk marker. The presence of abnormal voltage maps also differentiated between classical disease with characteristic biopsy findings and phenocopies of the condition, such as sporadic disease associated with an inflammatory infiltrate and a more favorable arrhythmic outcome.

These studies examining prediction of risk have been performed in referral populations in major centers with an interest in electrophysiology. Limitations exist in applying these results to patients seen in a general cardiologic clinic, or indeed to services providing family screening. In all but one of the studies using implantable defibrillators, patients were only included if they fulfilled the diagnostic criteria, and in the multicentered study [14], an even more highly refined population was included. It is widely accepted, however, that reliance strictly on the diagnostic criteria will, by definition, exclude variants of the condition with left ventricular predominance, and incompletely penetrant disease in the setting of family screening, where risk of arrhythmia still undoubtedly exists. Larger, more inclusive prospective studies of populations with a broader phenotype are needed to further refine the stratification of risk. In addition, it could be argued that populations with desmosomal disease, this being made up of those confirmed to carry a disease-causing mutation in one of the five desmosomal genes, may have a different natural history to the approximately half of patients with a clinical diagnosis in whom no mutation can be identified. With further advances in genetic identification, perhaps gene-specific algorithms can be developed for predicting risk.

18.6 Treatment

Patients with proven or suspected disease are discouraged from participation in competitive sports or endurance training. Avoidance of stimulant recreational and therapeutic drugs is advisable. In those with symptomatic arrhythmia, therapy differs somewhat between American and European centers, with Europeans using pharmacologic, device, and interventional therapy, but centers in the United States leaning toward implantation of implantable defibrillators in those who meet the diagnostic criteria for the disease [16, 27]. The application of this approach to encompass those with a genetic diagnosis but who do not yet meet the diagnostic criteria would appear inappropriate.

18.7 Pharmacological Therapy

Pharmacological treatment (Table 18.1) is the first line of therapy for patients with symptomatic ventricular ectopy, or with hemodynamically well-tolerated ventricular arrhythmias. In the past, many agents have been used, including Vaughan–Williams Class I drugs, beta

blockers, Sotalol, Amiodarone, and Verapamil, and combinations of these drugs. Wichter et al. [28] evaluated the efficacy of these drugs in patients with spontaneous and inducible ventricular tachycardia, and found sotalol was the most efficacious (Table 18.2). In practice, both sotalol and amiodarone are used, although long-term side effects of amiodarone are a cause for concern. Both agents are also used in patients with defibrillators who have recurrent discharges or persistent sustained arrhythmias.

There is no place for the routine prescription of Class 1 drugs, either alone or in combination. Patients who are refractory to, or intolerant of, Sotalol or Amiodarone therapy should be referred early for nonpharmacological therapy, and more particularly for consideration of implantation of a cardioverter–defibrillator. In those patients who develop symptoms of heart failure, standard treatment with inhibitors of angiotensin-converting enzyme and/or angiotensin 2 receptor blocking agents, beta blockers, and diuretics, including spironolactone, are used, although data for efficacy in right ventricular failure is lacking. Anticoagulation may also be necessary, as both pulmonary and cerebral embolism are recognized complications [29].

18.8 Nonpharmacologic Therapy

18.8.1 Implantations of Automatic Cardioverter Defibrillators

Patients who have survived cardiac arrest, or have had hemodynamically unstable ventricular tachycardia are unsuitable for drug therapy alone. The role of implanted

Table 18.1 Efficacy of medication in patients with ventricular tachycardia

Drug	Those with inducible VT (%)	Those with noninducible VT (%)
Class Ia/b	5.6	0
Class Ic	12	17.4
Beta-blockers	0	28.6
Sotalol	68.4	82.8
Amiodarone	15.4	25
Verapamil	0	50
2 × Class I	0	0
Class I + B-blocker	0	0
Class I + sotalol	20	0
Class I + amiodarone *	50	50

VT = ventricular tachycardia (>30 s duration), NSVT = nonsustained VT (≥ 10 consecutive beats and <30 s duration), Pts = patients. All patients (n = 81) had ARVC or suspected ARVC and documented spontaneous VT or NSVT. During VT stimulation studies sustained VT was inducible in 42 patients and noninducible in 39 patients. * = not recommended for routine use.
Adapted from Wichter et al. [28]

Table 18.2 Indications for implantation of defibrillators

Definite

    Resuscitated Cardiac Arrest

    Hemodynamically unstable sustained ventricular tachycardia

    Unexplained syncope and major morphological abnormality on imaging

Probable

    Sustained tachycardia refractory to pharmacological therapy

    Sustained tachycardia and major morphological abnormality

    Nonspecific tachycardia and major morphological abnormality with symptoms

    Young age with major morphological abnormality

    Unexplained syncope with any feature on electrocardiogram or imaging

    LV ejection fraction less than 35%

    Task force criteria and significant presyncope

    Task force criteria and family history with more than one premature sudden death

Possible

    Task force criteria

    Family history with more than one premature sudden death and features of disease

    Sustained ventricular tachycardia

    Nonspecific tachycardia and young age

    Left ventricular involvement

    Extensive right ventricular involvement

    Features of disease with QRS dispersion greater than 40 ms

    Features of disease and late potentials on signal-averaged electrocardiogram

devices in secondary prevention is undisputed. The requirement for concomitant use of anti-arrhythmic therapy is usually determined by the individual circumstances. Patients with a single symptomatic episode who do not have an inducible sustained arrhythmia may be suitable for device therapy alone, whereas patients with recurrent episodes, and/or easily inducible sustained arrhythmia, should be considered for adjuvant pharmacological therapy, using Sotalol or Amiodarone. The fact that many of these patients are relatively young, and often have normal exercise capacity, means that most benefit from beta blockade to reduce the risk of inappropriate discharge from implanted devices.

The indications for, and efficacy of, implanted devices for primary prevention need to be evaluated prospectively. Although implantation may confer a survival benefit of up to half [30], potential complications should restrict its use to those in whom there is a positive ratio of benefit to risk. Apart from standard complications, which over a lifetime of revisions are not inconsequential, these are exacerbated by the condition itself, with scar tissue making satisfactory positioning of leads difficult, and mural thinning increasing risk of perforation. Lead-sensing problems may develop over time. The incidence of inappropriate discharge ranges from 10% to 23% [14, 15, 30]. Complications occurred in 62% of patients in one experience from a single center with a mean follow-up of 80 months, and 72% of these were classified as severe. Further advances in technology with development of

devices which are entirely extracardiac would be a significant advantage to this population.

18.8.2 Interventional Electrophysiology

Catheter ablation of ventricular-reentry circuits has been very successful in certain limited situations. Success rates of 60–90% have been reported, although relapses occur in up to 60%, probably due to development of new arrhythmic focuses as the disease progresses [8]. Previously, catheter ablation was only possible in those in whom tachycardia could be induced. Electroanatomical-voltage mapping has been used in some centers to identify likely areas of arrhythmogenesis [31]. Regions of low-voltage *scar*, and abnormal myocardium, were ablated with a success rate of 82% in the short term, although in this case series, a mean of 38 lesions were needed in each patient, which is a major cause for concern in the long term in an already thinned and fibrotic ventricle. Tachycardia recurred in 23%, 27%, and 47% of patients over 1, 2, and 3 years of follow-up, respectively. In general, ablative therapy should not be considered as a first-line treatment in patients with arrhythmia, and its main role should remain in patients with recurrent discharges from implantable devices who are not responsive to medication.

In extreme cases with refractory arrhythmia, surgical disconnection of the right ventricle has been performed, although this often led to refractory right ventricular failure after surgery due to loss of ventricular contraction. Multisite pacing has been used experimentally to address this problem [32]. Cardiac transplantation has a minor role to play in the management of advanced disease, both in the treatment of refractory right or biventricular failure, and, in extreme cases, for refractory ventricular arrhythmia.

18.8.3 Future Directions

Stem cell therapy does not look promising. Even in localized infarcts, early studies have disappointed. The diffuse nature of the pathological changes would render it challenging to deliver stem cells to areas of need. In addition, a major limitation of this therapy to date has been an inability to generate gap junctions, and perhaps consequently an increased risk of ventricular arrhythmia. This may in part be due to the source of stem cells used. Both studies involving skeletal myoblasts and those derived from the bone marrow have failed to elicit electrical coupling in the myocardium following implantation. Gene therapy is an attractive proposition, but probably speculative at this time.

Disease-modifying therapy is perhaps the most promising area for progress. Research groups are endeavoring to determine which factors influence the apparent penetrance of a gene—genetic, environmental, infective, and lifestyle factors are all potential contributors and may be amenable to therapeutic intervention to retard or prevent disease expression or progression. Better risk-stratification tools, most likely to be developed by sophisticated three-dimensional-mapping techniques will also improve the natural history of this condition.

References

1. Thiene G, et al. Arrhythmogenic right ventricular cardiomyopathy a still underrecognized clinical entity. Trends Cardiovasc Med. 1997;7(3):84–90.
2. Corrado D, et al. Does sports activity enhance the risk of sudden death in adolescents and young adults? J Am Coll Cardiol. 2003;42(11):1959–63.
3. Corrado D, Basso C, Thiene G. Arrhythmogenic right ventricular cardiomyopathy: diagnosis, prognosis, and treatment. Heart. 2000;83(5):588–95.
4. Corrado D, et al. Spectrum of clinicopathologic manifestations of arrhythmogenic right ventricular cardiomyopathy/dysplasia: a multicenter study. J Am Coll Cardiol. 1997;30(6):1512–20.
5. Hulot JS, et al. Natural history and risk stratification of arrhythmogenic right ventricular dysplasia/cardiomyopathy. Circulation. 2004;110(14):1879–84.
6. Dalal D, et al. Arrhythmogenic right ventricular dysplasia: a United States experience. Circulation. 2005;112(25): 3823–32.
7. Norman M, et al. Novel mutation in desmoplakin causes arrhythmogenic left ventricular cardiomyopathy. Circulation. 2005;112(5):636–42.
8. Corrado D, et al. Arrhythmogenic right ventricular cardiomyopathy: current diagnostic and management strategies. Cardiol Rev. 2001;9(5):259–65.
9. Gemayel C, Pelliccia A, Thompson PD. Arrhythmogenic right ventricular cardiomyopathy. J Am Coll Cardiol. 2001;38(7): 1773–81.
10. Aouate P, et al. [Holter and sudden death: value in a case of arrhythmogenic right ventricular dysplasia]. Arch Mal Coeur Vaiss. 1993;86(3):363–7.
11. Nava A, et al. Clinical profile and long-term follow-up of 37 families with arrhythmogenic right ventricular cardiomyopathy. J Am Coll Cardiol. 2000;36(7):2226–33.
12. Tabib A, et al. Circumstances of death and gross and microscopic observations in a series of 200 cases of sudden death associated with arrhythmogenic right ventricular cardiomyopathy and/or dysplasia. Circulation. 2003;108(24):3000–5.
13. Fontaine G, et al. Arrhythmogenic right ventricular dysplasia. Annu Rev Med. 1999;50:17–35.
14. Corrado D, et al. Implantable cardioverter-defibrillator therapy for prevention of sudden death in patients with arrhythmogenic right ventricular cardiomyopathy/dysplasia. Circulation. 2003;108(25):3084–91.
15. Wichter T, et al. Implantable cardioverter/defibrillator therapy in arrhythmogenic right ventricular cardiomyopathy: single-center experience of long-term follow-up and complications in 60 patients. Circulation. 2004;109(12): 1503–8.
16. Roguin A, et al. Implantable cardioverter-defibrillators in patients with arrhythmogenic right ventricular dysplasia/cardiomyopathy. J Am Coll Cardiol. 2004;43(10):1843–52.
17. Piccini JP, et al. Predictors of appropriate implantable defibrillator therapies in patients with arrhythmogenic right ventricular dysplasia. Heart Rhythm. 2005;2(11):1188–94.
18. Peters S, Reil GH. Risk factors of cardiac arrest in arrhythmogenic right ventricular dysplasia. Eur Heart J. 1995;16(1): 77–80.
19. Turrini P, et al. Dispersion of ventricular depolarization–repolarization: a noninvasive marker for risk stratification in arrhythmogenic right ventricular cardiomyopathy. Circulation. 2001;103(25):3075–80.
20. Breithardt G, Borggrefe M, Karbenn U. Late potentials as predictors of risk after thrombolytic treatment? Br Heart J. 1990;64(3):174–6.
21. Breithardt G, et al. Identification of patients at risk of ventricular tachyarrhythmias after myocardial infarction. Cardiologia. 1990;35 Suppl 1:19–22.
22. Blomstrom-Lundqvist C, et al. Quantitative analysis of the signal-averaged QRS in patients with arrhythmogenic right ventricular dysplasia. Eur Heart J. 1988;9(3):301–12.
23. Leclercq JF, Coumel P. Late potentials in arrhythmogenic right ventricular dysplasia. Prevalence, diagnostic and prognostic values. Eur Heart J. 1993;14(Suppl E):80–3.
24. Oselladore L, et al. Signal-averaged electrocardiography in familial form of arrhythmogenic right ventricular cardiomyopathy. Am J Cardiol. 1995;75(15):1038–41.
25. Turrini P, et al. Late potentials and ventricular arrhythmias in arrhythmogenic right ventricular cardiomyopathy. Am J Cardiol. 1999;83(8):1214–9.
26. Corrado D, et al. Three-dimensional electroanatomic voltage mapping increases accuracy of diagnosing arrhythmogenic

right ventricular cardiomyopathy/dysplasia. Circulation. 2005;111(23):3042–50.

27. Calkins H. Arrhythmogenic right-ventricular dysplasia/cardiomyopathy. Curr Opin Cardiol. 2006;21(1):55–63.

28. Wichter T, et al. Efficacy of antiarrhythmic drugs in patients with arrhythmogenic right ventricular disease. Results in patients with inducible and noninducible ventricular tachycardia. Circulation. 1992;86(1):29–37.

29. Sen-Chowdhry S, et al. Arrhythmogenic right ventricular cardiomyopathy: clinical presentation, diagnosis, and management. Am J Med. 2004;117(9):685–95.

30. Hodgkinson KA, et al. The impact of implantable cardioverter-defibrillator therapy on survival in autosomal-dominant arrhythmogenic right ventricular cardiomyopathy (ARVD5). J Am Coll Cardiol. 2005;45(3):400–8.

31. Verma A, et al. Short- and long-term success of substrate-based mapping and ablation of ventricular tachycardia in arrhythmogenic right ventricular dysplasia. Circulation. 2005;111(24): 3209–16.

32. Agarwal SC, et al. Pacing to restore right ventricular contraction after surgical disconnection for arrhythmia control in right ventricular cardiomyopathy. Pacing Clin Electrophysiol. 2005;28(10):1122–6.

Section 5
The Small Right Ventricle

Imaging the Hypoplastic Right Heart – How Small Is Too Small?

19

Norman H. Silverman

19.1 Introduction

The question of how small the right ventricle can be in order to be included in, or excluded from, the circulation is complex. There is no one answer that will provide a satisfactory answer in each and every case. Rather, this decision will require all the clinical and historical skills of the providers of care, involving multiple modalities of investigation. This chapter deals with the echocardiographic evaluation needed to assess the mode of treatment.

19.2 Methods for Assessing Right Ventricular Size

The problem of assessing the size of the hypoplastic right ventricle is more complicated than that for the hypoplastic left ventricle. For the left ventricle, it is an *all-or-none* phenomenon. For the right ventricle, however, there are three options. The ventricle may be large enough to support the entire pulmonary circulation, or it may be so small as to be excluded completely from the circulation, but by using a bidirectional Glenn anastomosis, there is also the option of the so-called *one-and-a-half ventricle repair* [1]. There are many factors other than size that are important in making this decision, depending not only on the measure of size, but also on ventricular function, compliance, valvar leakages and obstructions, timing (such as fetal presentation), presence of endomyocardial fibrosis or coronary arterial abnormalities, and several other factors [2, 3]. Because this is a complex issue, we must pay attention to the factors involved in decision making [4–7].

N.H. Silverman (✉)
Division of Pediatric Cardiology, Lucile Packard Children's Hospital, Stanford University Medical Center, 750 Welch Road – Suite 305, Palo Alto, California, 94304

19.3 Determinants of Right Ventricular Size

19.3.1 Assessment of the Tricuspid Annulus

Assessment of the tricuspid annulus using the z score, as described by Hanley and colleagues [8], is the first quantitative measurement for determining the utility of the right ventricle for a biventricular repair. These authors worked on the principle that the size of the tricuspid valve is closely correlated with that of the right ventricle. Measurement of the z score for the tricuspid valvar annular diameter, therefore, a simple measurement made by cross-sectional echocardiography, with one z value equal to 1 standard deviation from the mean, can serve as the primary decision maker for determining the adequacy of the size of the right ventricle. The authors further incorporated a hazard function to define risk for survival for their strategies. Their technique has become a standard for decision making as to whether or not the ventricle is too small (Fig. 19.1A). The problem, however, with all techniques having cutoff values is that they have less strength in the region of the cutoff than they do when the z values are further toward the extremes of the range.

Minich and colleagues [9] used the ratio of the annular diameters of the tricuspid and mitral valves as the determinant for deciding between univentricular and biventricular repair, arguing that this measurement is more precise than the z score (Fig. 19.1B). In their study, the group of patients in which it was possible to achieve successful as opposed to unsuccessful biventricular repairs had ratios of 0.8 ± 0.2 as opposed to 0.5 ± 0.1. Using a cutoff for the z-score of the tricuspid valve of more than -3, compared to a ratio between the valves of greater than 0.5, these authors found their ratio to be a better predictor for successful biventricular repair.

A.N. Redington et al. (eds.), *Congenital Diseases in the Right Heart*, DOI 10.1007/978-1-84800-378-1_19,
© Springer-Verlag London Limited 2009

(a)

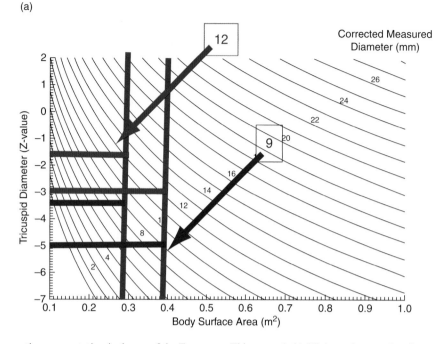

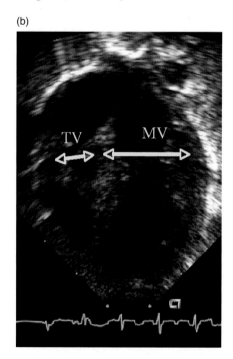

Fig. 19.1A A diagrammatic representation is shown of the Z scores of the tricuspid valve with respect to body surface area. The X axis is body surface area the Y axis is the tricuspid diameter z-value and the lines represent the different dimensions of the tricuspid valve

This figure is taken from the work of Hanley et al., (J Thorac Cardiovasc Surg 1993;105:406–23)

This example highlights valve annulus diameter of the tricuspid valve green: 12 mm and blue: 9 mm for body surface areas varying from 0.28 to 0.38 (m^2). Extrapolating from the body surface areas one can see that at 0.4 (m^2), the Z score is −5, whereas at 0.28 (m^2) the Z value is only −3.5 and for a valvar annulus of 12 mm at 0.38 (m^2) the z-values are −3 for the 0.38 (m^2) and −1.6 for a body surface of 0.28 (m^2)

(b)

Fig. 19.1B Is an example of the measurement of the tricuspid and mitral annuluses directly from a four-chamber apical view as used by Minich et al. [2].

The ratio of the mitral to tricuspid valves in these patients was always greater than 0.5:1 in patients who underwent a successful biventricular repair. Compared to a tricuspid valvar z-score of greater than –3, it appeared to be better predictor in their series for a biventricular repair

19.3.2 Area Planimetry and Ventricular Volume Measurement

In an earlier study [10] (Fig. 19.2), we had planimetered the area of the left and right ventricles in the four-chamber view, and found that if the area of the right ventricle was less than 0.45 of the left ventricle, attempted biventricular repair was unlikely to succeed.

Although these simple measurements ensure that observations can be made on a large number of patients, it seems that calculation of ventricular volume may provide a greater degree of predictive accuracy. Because of the shape of the right ventricle, however, there has been a reluctance to use measurements of volume, the argument being that the calculation is complicated. Because electronic methods are now incorporated into most modern ultrasonic machines, and into all offline systems for analysis currently available in North America, the operator would be required to perform only a simple planimetric tracing of the ventricular outline and a direct measurement of lengths, usually from biplane orthogonal images. We have used the method-of-disks measurement program that permits a summated biplane analysis of volume, designed for analysis of the left ventricle. For measuring the right ventricle, however, we used the diaphragmatic

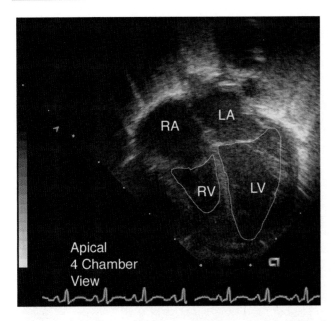

Fig. 19.2 In this figure, simple area measurements of the left and the right ventricle taken in the four-chamber view were used by Schmidt et al. for predicting the outcome of a biventricular repair. Ratios of greater than 0.45 of the right to the left ventricle were indicators of successful biventricular repair. In this apical four-chamber view the left atrium (LA), left ventricle (LV), right atrium (RA), and right ventricle (RV) are labeled. The planimetered areas of the two ventricles are indicated

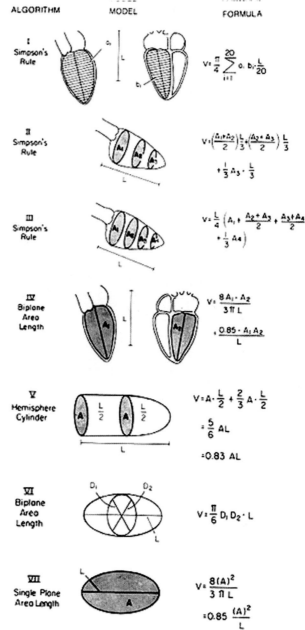

surface of the right ventricle to replace the plane of the mitral valve, and the pulmonary valve to replace the apex of the left ventricle. The common long axis then lies between the midpoint of the diaphragmatic surface of the right ventricle and the pulmonary valve (Figs. 19.3–19.5). Using subcostal imaging, and the biplane method-of-disks, which had been described in previous studies [11–13], we calculated right ventricular volumes in patients with various forms of hypoplastic right heart [10]. Our data indicated that, when the ventricular volume was greater than the 25th percentile of the normal range, a biventricular repair could have been undertaken successfully. A variety of methods have been used for measuring the left ventricle [14], but only a few are applicable to the right ventricle (Fig. 19.3).

Since our original description, it has become possible to obtain superior images, and also to enhance the tracing of ventricular outlines using Doppler color information. This latter factor is important, particularly in the presence of deep sinusoids, when tracing an endocardial outline is liable to exclude a substantial amount of the ventricular volume. This issue is also important to consider when doing echocardiographic studies, as with angiography, because after an operation, when there is regression of right ventricular hypertrophy, the volume of the ventricle appears to increase.

Fig. 19.3 This figure demonstrates various methods for calculating volumes of the left ventricle. The only plane that is suitable for the right ventricle is that using the biplane Simpson's rule method because of the different shapes of the right ventricle.
Method 1 is Simpson's rule method of disks.
Method 2 and Method 3 are Simpson's rule multiplanar short-axis imaging.
Method 4 a biplane area length method.
Method 5 is the hemisphere cylinder method or bullet method.
Method 6 a biplane area length method based on m mode or short/small dimensional measurements and Method 7 a single plane area length method.
The formulas for calculating these are shown in the right hand figure Figure taken from Silverman NH. Pediatric Echocardiography and published with permission of Lippincott – Williams Wilkins 1993

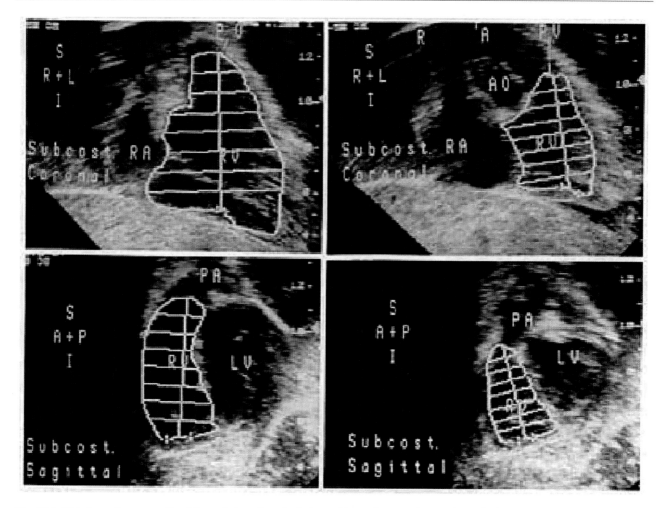

Fig. 19.4 This figure is an example of the technique for calculating biplane method of disks using octagonal planes from the subcostal coronal and sagittal planes, and shows the method of disks method used for calculating volumes in small right ventricles. The top left frame is a subcostal coronal view in diastole and top right is systole. The bottom frames are subcostal sagittal views in diastole and in systole with the comparative lines drawn

Note that an inverted method as for apical four-chamber imaging are from this ventricular logarithm is drawn using the pulmonary valve annulus as the apical point and the midpoint of the diaphragm as the equivalent of the coapted mitral valvar leaflets

Figure taken from Pediatric Echocardiography by Silverman and published with permission of Lippincott – Williams Wilkins;1993

Other techniques are available for calculating ventricular volume, including a biplane method based on four-chamber and short-axis views. Using this method, we calculated the volume from a summation of these two short-axis techniques, making possible a reasonable assessment of right ventricular volume and ejection fraction (Fig. 19.6). An echocardiographic method, based on the work of Levine and colleagues [15, 16], has proven to be accurate for the assessment of ventricular volume. This method uses the formula that volume is equal to two-thirds area multiplied by length. This measurement has recently been used for transesophageal assessment of right ventricular volume by Heusch and colleagues [17], modifying the formula such that volume is equal to two-thirds of area in the four-chamber projection multiple by length in the long axis of the ventricle, a possibility

for children as previously suggested by Denslow and Wiles [18].

Helbing and his colleagues [19, 20] and Lorentz [21] estimated right ventricular volume using magnetic resonance imaging, publishing standards for both the right and left ventricles. Resonance imaging is considered to be the gold standard for measuring volume, and thus provides a noninvasive opportunity to compare images of the right ventricle obtained by echo with those calculated by magnetic resonance imaging. In these studies, the correlation with echocardiography has proven reasonable. The comparisons made by Helbing and his associates [20] for echocardiographic volumes of the right ventricle determined by various methods with magnetic resonance imaging as the gold standard are shown in Table 19.1. They employed five different methods,

(a)

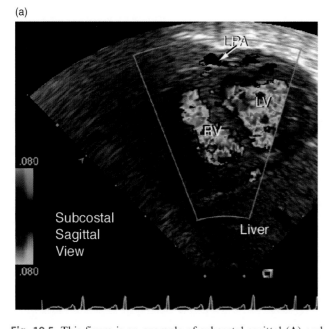

(b)

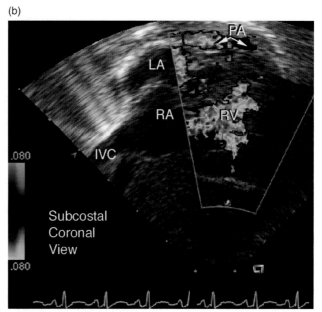

Fig. 19.5 This figure is an example of subcostal sagittal (A) and coronal (B) views of the right ventricle where color has been lowered to a very low Nyquist limit 0.80 to entirely fill the ventricle and aid the eye in seeking the ventricular outline for defining even the smallest ventricles

calculating volumes at end diastole and end systole. The methods are as follows.

The Monoplane Ellipsoid Approximation Method [21]:

$$VRV = 3/8\pi\{(Aap4)2/L\,ap4\} \qquad (19.1)$$

Where V RV is total right ventricular volume, Aap4 is the right ventricular area in the four-chamber view, and Lap4 is the distance from centre of the tricuspid valve to the apex, both determined in the apical four-chamber view.

The Monoplane Multiple-Slice Method [22]:

$$V\,RV = \sum_{n=1}^{20} \pi\ \{\ (Wn/2)2\}\ h, \qquad (19.2)$$

where the right ventricle, imaged from the apical four-chamber view, is assumed to consist of a stack of n, here where n is equal to 20, circular slices, with the width of each slice denoted. The W values, in effect the diameter of each slice, are measured perpendicular to the axis from the center of the tricuspid valve to the apex, halfway across the constant slice thickness (h).

The Modified Biplane Pyramidal Approximation Method [15]:

$$V\,RV = 2/3(Aap4\ ) (Ls) \qquad (19.3)$$

where Aap4 is the right ventricular area measured in the apical four-chamber view, and Ls, is the length from apex to pulmonary valve as measured in the subcostal view.

The Biplane Ellipsoid Approximation Method [23]:

$$V\,RV = \{0.849(Aap4,)2\},41 + \{0.849(Apsx)2/Lpsx\} \qquad (19.4)$$

where A is the right ventricular area, and Lap4 is the longest length, as measured in the apical four-chamber view, and Apex is the RV area, and Lp, the longest length, as measured in the parasternal short-axis view.

The Biplane Multiple-Slice Method [24]:

$$V\,RV = \sum_{n=1}^{20} 1/4\ \pi\ (Xn/2)(Yn/2)h, \qquad (19.5)$$

where the right ventricle is assumed to consist of a stack of n, here with n again equal to 20, elliptical slices with constant thickness. Xn is the width of the nth slice, halfway across the slice thickness, in the apical four-chamber view parallel to the axis from the center of the tricuspid valve to the apex, and Yn is the width of the nth slice in the parasternal short-axis view at the level of tricuspid valve and RV outflow tract, at a level corresponding to Xn Slice (Table 19.1; Fig. 19.7).

(a)

(c)

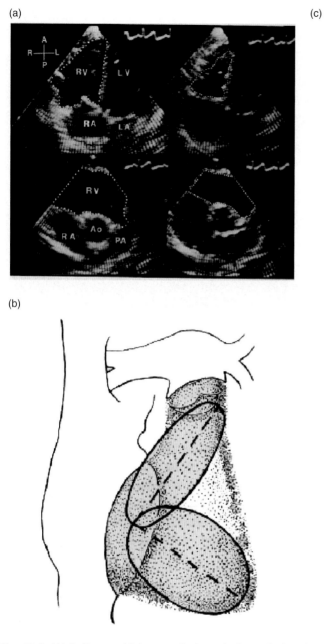

(b)

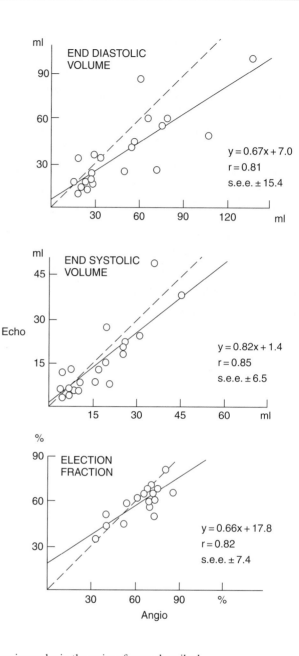

Fig. 19.6 (A) indicate a biplane method employing apical and parasternal short axis used for calculating the right ventricle and the concept of the synthesis of these planes is defined in (B). (C) indicate the end diastolic and systolic and ejection fractions related to angiography in the series of cases described

Published with permission of Silverman NH, Hudson S: Evaluation of right ventricular volume and ejection fraction in children by two-dimensional echocardiography. Pediatr Cardiol 1983;4:197–204

Helbing and his colleagues [25] also compared the volumes of the right ventricle calculated by angiographic methods with their method using resonance imaging, and further compared their measurements to those calculated for the right ventricle by others [26–28] (Table 19.2).

Other methods have provided interesting models for defining either ventricular function or right ventricular volume, such as volume equal to 2/3(A4ch)(DAD) [18].

This formula is derived from a difference-of-ellipsoids model of the right ventricle [15], and has recently been used for transesophageal assessment of right ventricular volume by Heusch and his colleagues [17], as discussed above.

Whereas two-dimensional methods allow reasonable quantification of the right ventricle, and may be adequate for assessing whether a ventricle can or cannot be used to support the pulmonary circulation

Table 19.1 Comparison of 2-Dimensional Echocardiographic and Magnetic Resonance Imaging (MRI) Right Ventricular Volumes in All Children Studied

	Manoplane Eilipsoid Apprax Method (n = 33)	Manoplane Multiple Slice Method (n = 33)	Biplone Pyramidal Apprax. Method (n = 17)	Biplane Ellipsoid Apprax. Method (n = 23)	Biplane Multiple Slice Method (n = 23)
EDV (ml)	46 ± 23	40 ± 23	72 ± 29	55 ± 26	55 ± 20
Mean diff. with MRI	46 ± 17	52 ± 17	14 ± 16	37 ± 23	37 ± 18
a*	50.5	57.4	21.5	62	48.1
b†	+0.90x	+0.86x	+0.89x	+0.54x	+0.80x
r	0.77	0.75	0.86	0.57	0.66
p Value	<0.001	<0.001	<0.001	0.004	0.001
ESV (ml)	19 ± 11	18 ± 11	32 ± 14	26 ± 13	27 ± 12
Mean diff. with MRI	14 ± 10	15 ± 10	−4 ± 7	9 ± 9	8 ± 8
a*	16.8	17.3	7.6	14.8	11.1
b†	+0.84x	+0.85x	0.64x	+0.77x	+0.89x
r	0.67	0.69	0.82	0.78	0.81
p Value	<0.001	<0.001	<0.001	<0.001	<0.001

See Text for Methods
*y intercept; †slope
Linear regression equation: (y = a + bx), where y – magnetic resonance imaging volume; x = echecordiographic volume.
See Statistics section for calculations of mean difference.
Date are expressed as mean ± SD
Apprax. = approximation, Diff. = difference, EDV = enddiestalic volume; ESV = end-systalic volume.

based on its size, three-dimensional method of volume as calculation by magnetic resonance imaging, computerized tomography, or three-dimensional echocardiography, offers a greater opportunity for accurate calculation [29].

19.4 Lessons Learned from the Left Heart

From a meta-analysis of patients with aortic stenosis surviving or dying after a biventricular repair, Hoffman [30] demonstrated that the minimal ventricular volume for a functioning left ventricle. He showed that patients with a left ventricle of less than $20\,ml/m^2$ of body surface area had an extremely low likelihood for survival (Fig. 19.8). This data was further elaborated on by considering heart rate and ejection fraction for determining a desired cardiac output. These data (Fig. 19.8b) show that, as the cardiac output increases with a particular ejection fraction, it is possible to predict the necessary left ventricular volume to ensure a cardiac output for which a univentricular repair would be adequate.

Although no such data exist for the right ventricle, the measurement of diastolic and stroke volumes, coupled with the opportunity for defining the size of the right ventricle and its ability to contract, provides additional quantitative assessment for the optimal surgical repair. Fortunately for situations involving the right ventricle, the alternative of using a bidirectional Glenn anastomosis has led to the opportunity of incorporating part of the right ventricle into the pulmonary circulation. This is sometimes termed the one-and-a-half ventricle repair. This philosophy for repair, in addition to its use in unbalanced atrioventricular septal defects, has been used for patients with Ebstein's malformation, as part of the double-switch procedure for corrected transposition, for those needing an arterial switch after Senning or Mustard procedures, as well as many other forms of complex congenital heart diseases.

19.5 Echocardiographic Modifiers for Right Ventricular Incorporation into the Circulation

19.5.1 Infundibular Obstruction

There are several other echocardiographic indicators that provide information about which ventricles cannot be incorporated into a biventricular circulation [31]. These

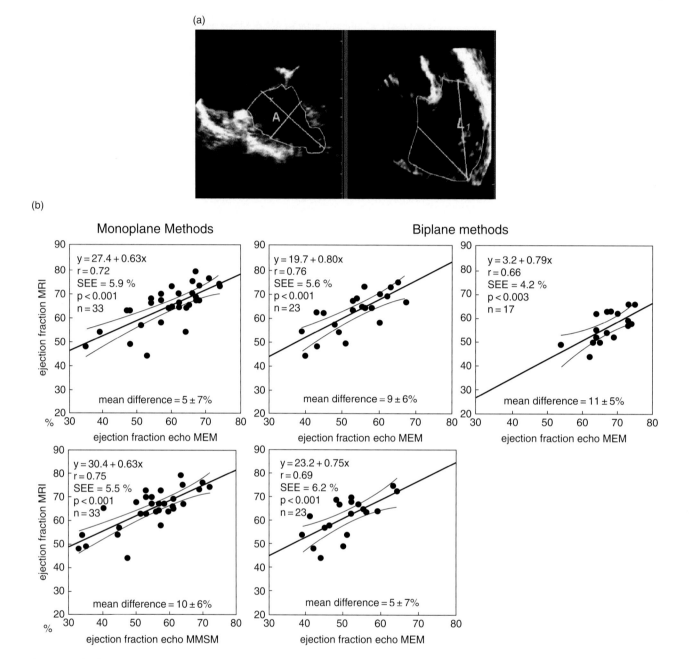

Fig. 19.7 (A) demonstrates a biplane method for calculating right ventricular volume using an area length method based on a transesophageal method from Heusch et al. involving a transesophageal four-chamber and transgastric view of the right ventricle
The volume is equal to 2/3 of the apical four chamber × the long axis view × the length (L1)
Published with permission of Cardiology in the Young (B) shows five graphs describing the relationship between calculations from magnetic resonance imaging [19] and the five methods mentioned in Table 19.1

include infundibular hypoplasia or total obstruction, which can be detected echocardiographically. Severe infundibular obstruction will require an outflow patch and, where possible, use of the ventricle in a one-and-a half or biventricular repair, based on ventricular size (Figs. 19.9 and 19.10).

19.5.2 Coronary Arterial Abnormalities

Coronary arterial abnormalities are found in many patients with this disorder. Freedom and his colleagues [2, 3] argued that there is probably no single group of congenitally malformed hearts where decisions about

Table 19.2 Comparison of results of this study with those of previously reported angiographic data

Reference	# of children	Ventricle	End Diastolic index	End Systolic index	Stoke Volume Index	EF
Graham[26]	16	Right	70	25	45	64
		Left	73	27	46	63
Thilenius[27]	17	Right	78	30	48	61
		Left	66	17	48	74
Fisher[28]	70	Right	64	25	39	61
		Left	59	19	40	68
Helbing[20]		Right	70 ± 9	21 ± 5	48 ± 7	70 ± 4
Age 6–15y	22	Left	67 ± 10	20 ± 5	47 ± 8	70 ± 6

Other methods have provided interesting models for defining either ventricular function or right ventricular volume. Vol = 2/3(A4ch)(DAD).

This formula is derived from a difference-of-ellipsoids model of the right ventricle. 19

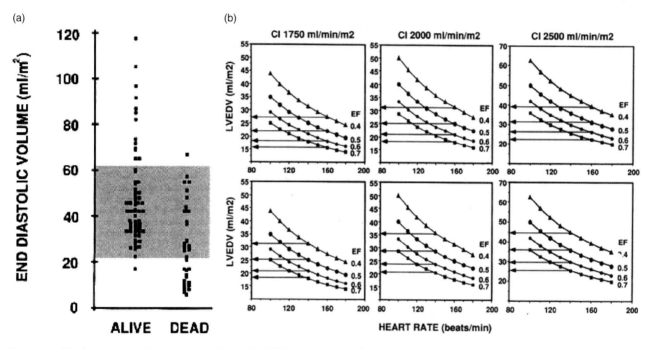

Fig. 19.8 (A) is an example of meta-analysis of defining the minimal functional volume for the left ventricle in patients who were either alive or dead as described by Hoffman in the *Cardiovascular Journal of Southern Africa* 1992;3:30–36. Although there was a scatter, almost no patient under 20 ml/m² of body surface area were alive after a repair of aortic stenosis in infants. (B) is the reconstruction of ejection fraction curves relating left ventricular end-diastolic volume on the abscissa to heart rate on the ordinate, in this group of neonates. The graphs represent cardiac indices of 1.75 l/min/m², 2 l/min/m², and 3 l/min/m², respectively. Using various ejection fractions it can be seen that as the heart rate decreases, from high levels on the top frames to low levels on the bottom frames, a greater stroke volume is required for each of these variables to pump the cardiac output from the left ventricle

delineation of the morphology and physiology of the coronary arterial circulation have more impact on ultimate survival. The abnormalities can occur at the origin, or within the distribution, of the coronary arteries. They may involve absence of the proximal course, with filling of the more distal circulation from the ventricles, termed a right ventricular-dependent coronary arterial circulation [32, 33]. There are varying degrees of ventriculo-coronary arterial connections, coronary arterial stenoses, and coronary-cameral communications. Many of these

abnormalities can be identified by echocardiography (Figs. 19.11–19.14) – even in the fetus (Fig. 19.12), particularly the ventriculo-coronary arterial connections [34, 35]. It is possible that, when the coronary arterial circulation is not derived from the aorta, a coronary arterial Doppler signal is monophasic, rather than the standard biphasic signal seen when the coronary artery is connected to the aorta (Fig. 19.14). Current technology for Doppler color flow is at least as sensitive as angiography for the definition of the ventriculo-coronary arterial connections,

(a)   (b)

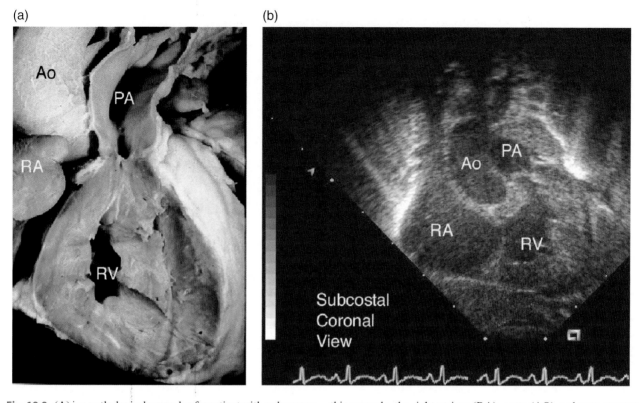

Fig. 19.9 (A) is a pathological example of a patient with pulmonary atresia and intact ventricular septum showing the diminutive size of the right ventricular cavity, the marked ventricular hypertrophy and near obliteration of the infundibulum of the right ventricle between the cavity and the main pulmonary artery above. (B) is an echocardiographic view showing a simulation of this projection. In this example, the right atrium (RA), aorta (AO), pulmonary artery (PA), and right ventricular cavity (RV) are shown. It is marked hypertrophy of the diminutive right ventricle with encroachment of the muscle into the outflow tract

The frame on the left was provided by courtesy of Robert Anderson

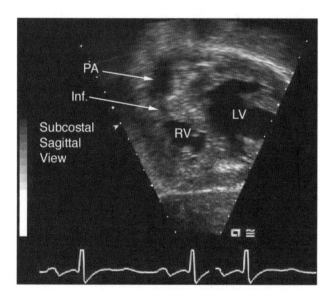

Fig. 19.10 This is a subcostal sagittal view showing marked infundibular hypoplasia (Inf) between the diminutive right ventricle (RV) and pulmonary artery (PA) The left ventricle (LV) posteriorly is seen to be of normal size by comparison with the cavity on the right side

but not for definition of right ventricular-dependent coronary arteries. As the importance of the ventricular-dependent coronary circulation is critical in decision making, but has not been validated by echocardiography, angiography is still required. Although right ventricular-dependent coronary arteries are found most frequently in the more severe forms of right ventricular-dependent coronary circulations, there are cases that are found with a larger right ventricle, making appropriate angiography mandatory.

Freedom and his associates [2, 3] examined the hearts of 39 pathological specimens from patients diagnosed during fetal life, three of whom died postnatally. Coronary arterial abnormalities were defined as nonconnection of the left or right coronary arteries to the aorta, ostial stenosis, marked tortuosity, dilation, and thickening or abnormal myocardial branching. Mild tortuosity, or myocardial bridging, was considered normal. The investigators measured the dimensions of the tricuspid valve, together with the inlet and outlet portions of the ventricles. They took particular note of Ebstein's malformation, tricuspid valvar dysplasia, and the

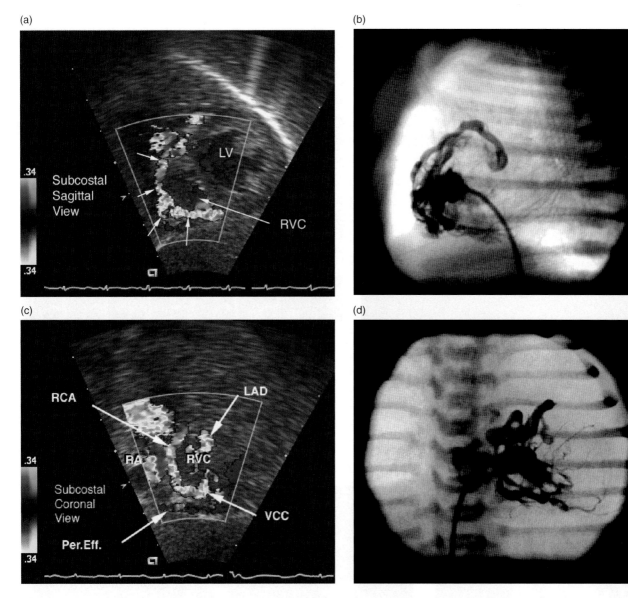

Fig. 19.11 This figure is an echocardiographic and angiographic comparison of ventricular coronary connections in the comparative subcostal sagittal view (A) with a lateral angiogram (B) and subcostal coronal view (C) with a frontal view (D) in a patient with pulmonary atresia, intact septum, and marked ventriculo-coronary connections. In the subcostal sagittal view (top left) only the right coronary artery is indicated by the presence of arrows and the connection with the right ventricular cavity (RVC) is seen. The right coronary artery (RCA) and the ventriculo-coronary connections (VCC) are shown. A small pericardial effusion (Per.Eff.) indicates the presence of a pericardial effusion which also fills with color and should not be confused with the coronary arterial morphology. In the frontal plane (bottom left) the right coronary artery (RCA) and left anterior descending (LAD) are also seen

presence or absence of the infundibulum. The dimensions of the right ventricle and tricuspid valves, and the gestational ages of the fetuses were compared to 14 of the 25 who had no abnormalities, using independent t-tests. The gestational ages were similar, at 21.9 as opposed to 21.1 weeks. The mean dimensions of the tricuspid valve, the median z-scores, and right ventricles were significantly smaller for those with coronary arterial abnormalities. A patent infundibulum was noted in 34 of 39 specimens. They concluded that over one-third of fetuses with pulmonary atresia and intact ventricular septum already exhibited coronary arterial abnormalities at the time of the mid-trimester. The presence of a patent infundibulum confirmed that atresia was an acquired process. Coronary arterial abnormalities are seen in half of those with hypoplastic right ventricles, but less frequently in the presence of well-developed ventricles, important information for those involved in counseling parents.

(a)

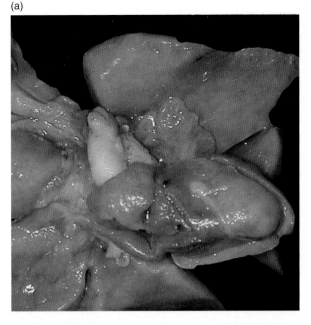

(b)

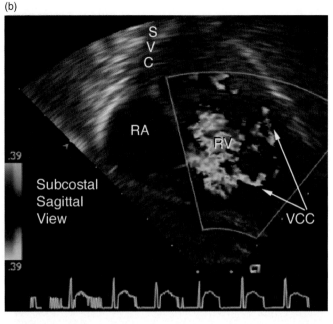

Fig. 19.12 This is an example of the fetal recognition of ventriculo-coronary connections (VCC) in an 18-week fetus with pulmonary atresia, intact ventricular septum, and ventricular coronary connections. (A) shows the pathologic specimen of the heart indicating the presence of an anterior descending coronary artery arising half-way down the ventricle and in no way connected to the aorta

(a)

(b)

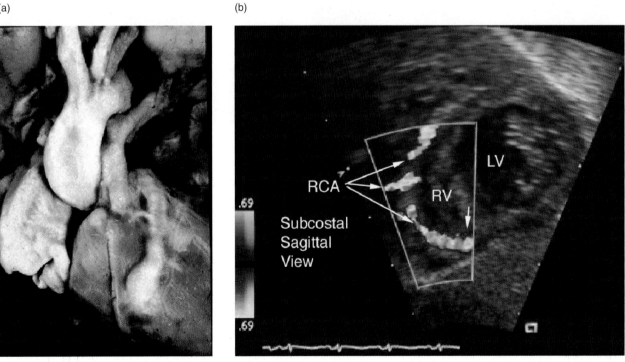

Fig. 19.13 This is a different example of the right coronary artery (RCA) filling from ventriculo-coronary connections through a diminutive right ventricle (RV). The image was taken in the subcostal sagittal view, the left hand frame is a frontal equivalent of this type of ventricular coronary connection

This pathological figure was provided courtesy of Robert Anderson

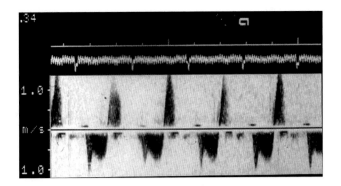

Fig. 19.14 This is a Doppler example of a flow in a coronary artery in a patient, such as the one shown above, and indicates the Doppler flow in this particular coronary artery. The coronary artery is imaged as shown in the section above and indicates flow toward the aorta in systole and flow into the ventricle in diastole. Such signals represent examples of patent coronary arteries without right ventricular-dependant coronaries in this example

19.5.3 Endocardial Fibroelastosis

Endocardial fibroelastosis is also important when considering potential repair. Although there was an inverse relationship between endocardial fibrosis and coronary arterial lesions [3], it was noted that many cases of milder hypoplasia had well-marked endocardial fibroelastosis. Freedom and his associates pointed out that the ventricle could exhibit a marked degree of subendocardial fibrosis, and even transmural fibrosis, as a result of ischemia. This is related to coronary arterial abnormalities, because the right ventricle contracts at suprasystemic pressures, and the mural stress and subendocardial areas are at greatest risk for lack of perfusion. Endocardial fibroelastosis, nonetheless, is much less common in the hypoplastic right than the left ventricle, and is patchy rather than diffuse (Fig.19.15).

(a)   (b)

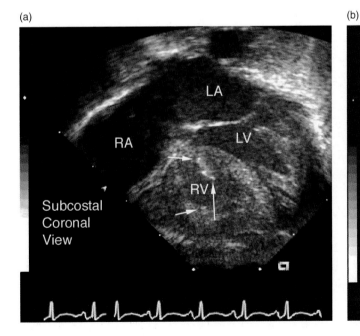

Fig. 19.15 These two examples of pulmonary atresia and intact ventricular septum show examples of unfavorable indications for repair. (A) taken in the subcostal coronal view, the arrows indicate areas of intense reflection of the endocardium indicating the presence of subendocardial fibrolastosis. (B) taken on the subcostal sagittal view shows a diminutive infundibulum although the pulmonary valve appears to dome, there was no forward flow, and there is in addition a diminutive cavity

19.5.4 Atrioventricular Septal Defects

In this lesion, echocardiographic evidence of the diminutive size of the ventricle has been derived from work on the left ventricle. D'Oliviera and colleagues [36] have helped determine whether, in atrioventricular septal defects, the right ventricle is of adequate size for inclusion as part of the circulation. Basing their observations of whether a particular hypoplastic right ventricle could be used in biventricular repair, they measured the atrioventricular valvar area according to the method of Cohen and colleagues [37] from the subcostal view, measuring the atrial chambers as shown in Fig. 19.16 (left), and the ratio of right to left ventricular lengths according to the method of Van Son et al. [38] and Phoon et al. [39] (Fig. 19.16 (right)). They graphed the ratio of ventricular

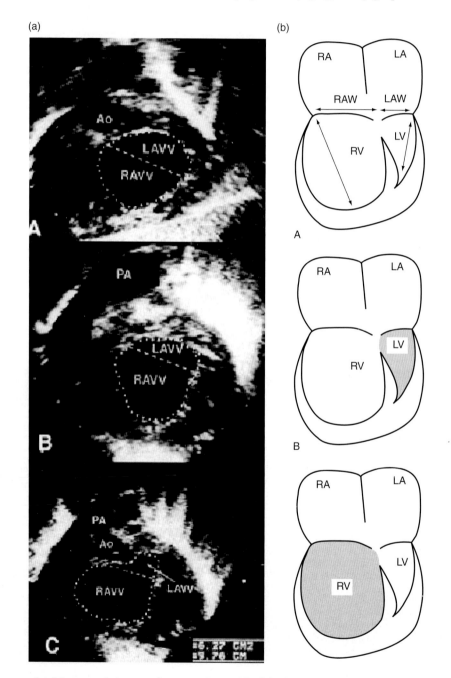

Fig. 19.16 This is an example of the two techniques used to assess the adequacy of the left ventricular atrioventricular valvar orifice in patients with unbalanced right-dominant atrioventricular septal defects. (A) is provided from Cohen et al. [37]. (B) is the diagram for the method of Phoon et al. [39] evaluating whether patients with right-dominant atrioventricular septal defects could undergo biventricular repair. In this method, the atrioventricular valvar orifices and long-axis length were measured to calculate the ventricular volume. These would be inversely related for a right dominant septal defect, and involve the consideration of bidirectional Glenn procedure

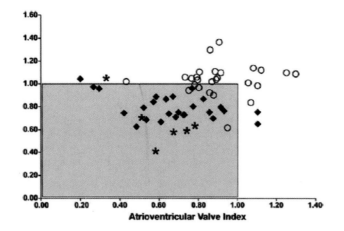

Fig. 19.17 RV/LV length ratio and AVVI are shown in the small/ BVR group (diamonds), the control/ BVR group (circles), and the SV palliation group (asterisks). Most patients in the small RV/BVR group are within the left and inferior quadrant (rectangle) defined by an RV/LV ratio and AVVI both less than one. Although two patients with a diagnosis of small RV had an AVVI of greater than one, they had among the lowest RV/LV ratios. Patients undergoing SV palliation had either a small AVVI small RV/LV ratio Printed from De Oliveira et al. [36], with permission

Table 19.3 Morphometric variable evaluated by echocardiography (n = 70)

Group	Small RV/BVR	Control/BVR	SV palliation	p value*
N (patients)	32	32	6	
RAVV area (cm²)	1.70 ± 1.14	2.92 ± 1.75	1.75 ± 0.62	.006
LAVV area (cm²)	2.58 ± 1.28	3.32 ± 2.31	2.75 ± 1.26	.03
AVVI (RAW/LAVV)	0.64 ± 0.26	0.92 ± 0.11	0.65 ± 0.08	<.001
RV length (cm)	2.81 ± 0.65	3.98 ± 1.30	1.98 ± 0.52	<.001
LV length (cm)	3.48 ± 0.74	3.88 ± 1.18	3.31 ± 1.22	.08
RV/LV length	0.80 ± 0.10	1.03 ± 0.13	0.62 ± 0.13	<.001

Values are presented as means standard error of the mean. *RV*, right ventricle; *BVR*, biventricular repair; *SV*, single ventricle; *RAVV*, right atrioventricular valve area; *LAVV*, left atrioventricular valve area; *AVVI*, atrioventricular valve index; *RV length*, right ventricular length from lateral aspect of annulus to apex; *LV length*, left ventricular length from annulus to apex; *RV/LV length*, right ventricle/left ventricle ratio. *P value (matched biventricular repair vs. control groups)
From De Oliveira et al. [36], with permission

lengths on the abscissa, and the ratio of area on the ordinate (Fig. 19.17). If the numbers were greater than unity, a biventricular repair seemed more likely, although the data did show minimal crossover. These data are listed in tabular form below in Table 19.3. Their series provides valuable information concerning the chances of incorporating the right ventricle into a biventricular repair, or whether to opt for a univentricular repair, or the one-and-a-half ventricular.

References

1. Van Arsdell GS. One and half ventricle repair. Semin Thorac Cardiovasc Surg. 2000;3:173–178.
2. Freedom RM. Wilson GJ. Endomyocardial abnormalities. In: Freedom RM, editor. Pulmonary atresia with intact ventricular septum. Mount Cisco, New York: Futura Publishing Company; 1989. p. 89–99 (Chapter 7).
3. Wilson GJ, Freedom RM, Koike K Perrin D. Coronary Arteries Anatomy and Histopathology. In: Freedom RM and Wilson GJ, editors. Pulmonary atresia with Intact Ventricular Septum. New York: Futura Publishing Company Mount Cisco; 1989. p 75–88 (Chapter 6).
4. Mainwaring RD, Lamberti JJ. Pulmonary atresia with intact ventricular septum: surgical approach based on ventricular size and coronary anatomy. J Thorac Cardiovasc Surg. 1993;106:733–8.
5. Reddy VM, McElhinney DB, Silverman NH, Marianeschi SM, Hanley FL. Partial biventricular repair for complex congenital heart defects: an intermediate option for complicated anatomy or functionally borderline right complex heart. J Thoracic Cardiovasc Surg. 1998;116:21–27.
6. Van Arsdell GS, Williams WG, Maser CM, et al. Superior vena cava to pulmonary artery anastomosis: an adjunct to biventricular repair. J Thorac Cardiovasc Surg. 1996;112:1143–9.
7. Van Arsdell GS. One and a half ventricle repairs. Semin Thorac Cardiovasc Surg. Pediatr Card Surg Annu. 2000;3:173–178.
8. Hanley FL, Sade RM, Blackstone EH, Kirklin JW, Freedom RM, Nanda NC. Outcomes in neonatal pulmonary atresia with

intact ventricular septum: a multiinstitutional study. J Thorac Cardiovasc Surg. 1993;105:406–23.

9. Minich LL, Tani LY, Ritter S, Williams RV, Shaddy RE, Hawkins JA. Usefulness of the preoperative tricuspid/mitral valve ratio for predicting outcome in pulmonary atresia with intact ventricular septum. Am J Cardiol. 2000;85:1325–1328.

10. Schmidt KG, Cloez J-L, Silverman NH. Changes of right ventricular size and function in neonates after valvotomy for pulmonary atresia or critical pulmonary stenosis and intact ventricular septum. J Am Coll Cardiol. 1992;19:1032–1037.

11. Trowitzsch E, Colan SD, Sanders SP. Global and regional right ventricular function in normal infants and infants with transposition of the great arteries after senning operation. Circulation. Nov 1985;72:1008–14.

12. Trowitzsch E, Colan SD, Sanders SP. Two-dimensional echocardiographic estimation of right ventricular area change and ejection fraction in infants with systemic right ventricle (transposition of the great arteries or hypoplastic left heart syndrome). Am J Cardiol. 1985;1153–7.

13. Trowitzsch E, Colan SD, Sanders SP. Two-dimensional echocardiographic evaluation of right ventricular size and function in newborns with severe right ventricular outflow tract obstruction. J Am Coll Cardiol. Aug 1985;6(2):388–93.

14. Silverman NH. Chapter 2. Quantitative methods to enhance morphhological information using ultrasound. Baltimore: Williams and Wilkings; 1993. 35–108.

15. Levine RA, Gibson TC, Aretz T, Gillam CD, Guyer DE, King ME, Weyman AE. Echocadiographic measurement of right ventricular volume. Circulation. 1984;69:497–505.

16. Gibson TC, Miller SW, Aretz T, Hardin NJ, Weyman AE. Method for estimating right ventricular volume by planes applicable to cross-sectional echocardiography: correlation with angiographic formulas. Am J Cardiol. 1985;55:1584–8.

17. Heusch A, Lawrenz W, Olivier Margarete, Schmidt KG. Cardiol Young. 2006;16:135–140.

18. Denslow S, Wiles HB. Right ventricular volumes revisited: a simple model and simple formula for echocardiographic determination. J Am Soc Echocardiogr. Sep 1998;11(9):864–73.

19. Helbing WA. Bosch HG, Maliepaard C, Rebergen SA, van der Geest RJ, Hansen B, Ottenkamp J, MD, Reiber JHC, de Roos A. Comparison of echocardiographic methods with magnetic resonanceImaging for assessment of right ventricular function in children. Am J Cardiol. 1995;76:589–594.

20. Lorenz CH. The range of normal values of cardiovascular structures in infants, children, and adolescents measured by magnetic resonance imaging pediatr cardiol. 2000;21:37–46.

21. Lange PE, Seiffert PA, Pices F, Wersel A, Onnasch DGW, Hahne HJ, Heintzen PH. Value of image enhancement and injection of contrast medium for right ventricular volume determination by two-dimensional echocardiography in congenital heart disease. Am J Cardiol. 1985;55:152–157.

22. Schiller NB, Shah PM, Crawford M, DeMaria A, Devereux R, Feigenbaum H, Gutgesell H, Reichek N, Sahn D, Schnittger J, Silverman N. Recommendations for quantitation of the left ventricle by two-dimensional echocardiography. J Am Soc Echocardiogr. 1989;2:358–367.

23. Silverman NH, Hudson S. Evaluation of right ventricular volume and ejection fraction in children by two-dimensional echocardiography. Pediatr Cardiol. 1983;4:197–204.

24. Ninomiya K, Duncan WJ, Cook DH, Olley PM, Rowe RD. Right ventricular ejection fraction and volumes after mustard repair: correlation of two dimensional echocardiograms and cineangiograms. Am J Cardiol. 1981;48:317–324.

25. Helbing WA, Rebergen SA, Maliepaard C, Hansen B, Ottenkamp J, Reiber JHC, de Roos A. Quantification of right ventricular function with magnetic resonance imaging in children with normal hearts and with congenital heart disease Am Heart J. 1995;130:828–37.

26. Graham TP, Jr., Jarmakani JM, Atwood GF, Canent RV Jr. Right ventricular volume determination in children: normal values and observations with volume or pressure overload. Circulation. 1973;47:144–53.

27. Thilenius OG, Arcilla RA. Angiographic right and left ventricular volume determination in normal infants and children. Pediatr Res. 1974;8:67–74.

28. Hiraishi S, DiSessa TG, Jamakani JM, Nakanishi T, Isabel-Jones JB, Friedman WF. Two-dimensional echocardiographic assessment of right ventricular volume in children with congenital heart disease. Am J Cardiol. 1982;50:1368–1375.

29. Nesser JH, Tkale KW, Patel AR, Masani ND, Niel J, Markt B, Pandian NG. Quantitation of right ventricular volume and ejection fraction by three-dimensional echocardiography in patients: comparison with magnetic resonance imaging and radionuclide ventriculography. Echocardiography. 2006;27:666–680.

30. Hoffman, JIE. Critical aortic stenosis in infancy: when is a hypoplastic left ventricle too small? Cardiovasc J of Southern Africa. 1992;3:30–36.

31. Pawade A, Capuani A, Penny DJ, Karl TR, Mee RB. Pulmonary atresia with intact ventricular septum: surgical management based on right ventricular infundibulum. J Card Surg. 1993;8:371–383.

32. Satou GM, Perry SB, Gauvreau K, Geva T. Echocardiographic predictors of coronary artery pathology in pulmonary atresia with intact ventricular septum. Am J Cardiol. 2000;85:1319–1324.

33. Freedom RM, Anderson RH, Perrin D. The significance of ventriculo-coronary arterial connections in the setting of pulmonary atresia with an intactventricular septum. Cardiol Young. 2005;15:447–468.

34. Maeno YV, Boutin C, Hornberger LK, et al. Prenatal diagnosis of right ventricular outflow tract obstruction with intact ventricular septum, and detection of ventriculocoronary connections. Heart. 1999;81:661–668.

35. Sandor GGS, Cook AC, Sharland GK, Ho YK, Potts JE, Anderson RH. Coronary arterial abnormalities in pulmonary atresia with intact ventricular septum diagnosed during fetal life. Cardiol Young. 2002;12:436–444.

36. De Oliveira NC, Sittiwangkul, McCrindle BW, Dipchand A, Yun T-J, Coles JG, Caldarone C, Williams William G, Van Arsdell GS. Biventricular repair in children with atrioventricular septal defects and a small right ventricle: anatomic and surgical considerations. J Thorac Cardiovasc Surg. 2005;130:250–7.

37. Cohen MS, Jacobs ML, Weinberg PM, Rychik J. Morphometric analysis of unbalanced common atrioventricular canal using two-dimensional echocardiography. J Am Coll Cardiol. 1996;28:1017–23.

38. Van Son JAM, Phoon CK, Silverman NH, Hass GS. Predicting feasibility of biventricular repair of right-dominant unbalanced atrioventricular canal. Ann Thorac Surg. 1997;63:1657–63.

39. Phoon CKL, Silverman NH. Conditions with right ventricular pressure and volume overload, and a small left ventricle: "Hypoplastic" left ventricle or simply a squashed ventricle? J Am Coll Cardiol. 1997;30:1547–1553.

The Small Right Ventricle—Who Should Get a Fontan?

20

Brian W. McCrindle

20.1 Introduction—Questions But No Easy Answers

The small right ventricle continues to be a subject of controversy in pediatric cardiology and pediatric cardiovascular surgery. Many questions regarding clinical management in this scenario have yet to be optimally resolved. There is, however, some general agreement regarding some preliminary answers to key questions:

1. *Who should get a Fontan procedure?* It could be agreed that patients with important hypoplasia or dysplasia of right-heart structures causing irreparable obstruction should be managed on a single ventricle pathway. This is particularly relevant in those settings where there is felt to be a lack of growth potential of those structures. An additional group of patients to be considered would be those who have right-ventricular dependence of the coronary artery circulation.
2. *Who should NOT get a Fontan?* Patients with associated abnormalities that will affect Fontan physiology may be contraindicated for this procedure. These include patients with important hypoplasia or obstruction in the pulmonary arterial and pulmonary venous systems. It would also include patients with impaired left ventricular function, which may have been influenced by the presence of severe coronary artery abnormalities or the presence of a hypertensive right ventricle and impaired interventricular interactions.
3. *Is some right ventricle better than no right ventricle at all?* It has been reported that poor outcomes with the Fontan procedure have been evident for those patients where the hypoplastic right ventricle has been incorporated into the Fontan pathway. However, this is in contrast to more recent studies that have defined a clear role for the 1½ ventricular type of repair in selected settings.
4. *Is the long-term functional status of the borderline patient better with biventricular repair or a Fontan procedure?* There is currently incomplete evidence to address this issue, although preliminary answer would suggest no.

20.2 What Lesions Are Associated with Right Ventricular Hypoplasia?

A number of congenital cardiac lesions are associated with important right heart hypoplasia or dysplasia. Tricuspid atresia is associated with important right heart hypoplasia, although little clinical controversy exists as patients are uniformly managed on a single ventricle pathway. Ebstein's anomaly of the tricuspid valve can present as a wide anatomic spectrum in terms of severity. The majority of patients are, however, managed on a biventricular pathway, with a few patients having the addition of a bidirectional cavopulmonary anastomosis. Atrioventricular septal defects (AVSD) can sometimes be associated with important right ventricular hypoplasia. The management of this lesion is complicated by the challenge of partitioning the common atrioventricular valve in this setting. The congenital lesions most commonly associated with a small right ventricle are critical pulmonary stenosis and pulmonary atresia and intact ventricular septum (PAIVS). The majority of patients with critical pulmonary stenosis undergo a biventricular repair. A much broader management spectrum is required for PAIVS. The focus of the subsequent discussion is on issues related to unbalanced AVSD and PAIVS.

B.W. McCrindle (✉)
Division of Cardiology, Department of Paediatrics, University of Toronto, The Hospital for Sick Children, Toronto, Ontario, Canada

A.N. Redington et al. (eds.), *Congenital Diseases in the Right Heart*, DOI 10.1007/978-1-84800-378-1_20,
© Springer-Verlag London Limited 2009

20.3 What Is the Impact of the Small Right Ventricle in the Management of Atrioventricular Septal Defect?

The small right ventricle in the setting of an AVSD remains an important management challenge. Adequacy of the right ventricle to support the pulmonary circulation must be carefully assessed. In addition, there are important challenges regarding partitioning of the common atrioventricular valve, which may render it more prone to the development of important regurgitation, which would be a challenge for maintenance of Fontan physiology.

De Oliveira and colleagues studied 38 patients, from a single institution, with AVSD and a small right ventricle [1]. They noted that 32 patients had biventricular repair, with four deaths and six reoperations. Of the six patients requiring reoperation, four had failed biventricular repair due to either severe restriction or right ventricular inadequacy. The remaining six patients had single ventricle palliation, with two deaths. The 32 patients who had biventricular repair were compared to a matched control group of balanced AVSD repair patients. Preoperative echocardiograms were analyzed in a blinded manner. The ratio of the long-axis length of the right ventricle to the left ventricle was calculated. In addition, an atrioventricular valve index was calculated as the ratio of the presumed area of the right versus the left atrioventricular valve that would be achieved along a theoretical partitioning plane of the common atrioventricular valve between the two septal defects. Figure 20.1 shows that, while there was some overlap, the patients with right

ventricular hypoplasia clearly fell into a quadrant characterized by a low right-to-left ventricular length ratio and a low atrioventricular valve index compared to those patients in the control (balanced) group. In addition to differentiating those patients with right ventricular hypoplasia, these indices also predicted outcomes. For patients with right ventricular hypoplasia who underwent biventricular repair, an atrioventricular valve index below 0.50 predicted reoperation for right ventricular inadequacy with 100% sensitivity and 95% specificity. In addition, this threshold also predicted operative death following repair with 75% sensitivity and 91% specificity. The authors concluded that the use of biventricular repair in the setting of AVSD and a small right ventricle requires careful echocardiographic quantitative assessment, with the atrioventricular valve index being a key predictor of adequacy. If biventricular repair is attempted in the setting of a small atrioventricular valve index, the authors recommended that atrial fenestration be utilized. Based on this report, it would appear that the adequacy of the right atrioventricular valve that can be achieved with repair is a key determinant of outcomes in this setting.

20.4 What Is the Impact of the Small Right Ventricle in the Setting of PAIVS?

20.4.1 How can Something so Small Cause so Much Grief?

Dr. Robert Freedom, who, throughout his career, had a strong interest in the issue of right heart hypoplasia in the setting of PAIVS, made the following assertion in an editorial published in 1992 [2]: "The reality of any single therapeutic maneuver providing therapeutic salvation is akin to a long-term ceasefire in those areas of the world devoured by genetic hatred: the ceasefire lasts only slightly longer (perhaps shorter) than the headline. For PAIVS, there have been many headlines. But the promise almost always falls short." Certainly many would argue that this quotation still bears a great deal of truth in the current era, both in terms of observations regarding world politics, but also management of PAIVS.

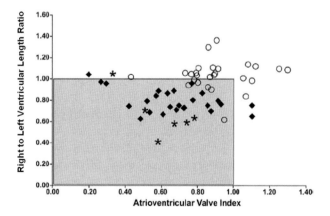

Fig. 20.1 Relationship of right ventricle to left ventricle length ratio and atrioventricular valve index for atrioventricular septal defect repair patients. Diamonds represent patients with small right ventricle who had biventricular repair, circles represent patients with balanced defects, and asterisks represent patients who had single ventricle palliation.
From De Oliveria et al. Biventricular repair in children with atrioventricular septal defects and a small right ventricle: anatomic and surgical considerations. J Thorac Cardiovasc Surg. 2005;130:250–257

20.4.2 What is the Anatomic Substrate for Patients with PAIVS?

While the anatomic substrate for PAIVS appears to follow a continuum, three broad groups can be identified. The first group is somewhat distinct and characterized by an enlarged thinned right ventricle and right atrium in the association with severe tricuspid valve dysplasia or Ebstein's malformation. The prognosis for these patients is extremely poor regardless of the management strategy adopted. The second group includes those patients where the right ventricle is well formed and relatively normal in size. There is a distinct inlet, trabecular zone, and outlet portion to the structure of the ventricle. It is likely that these patients form a spectrum with critical pulmonary stenosis, and the majority is managed along the biventricular repair pathway. The third group includes those patients characterized by a hypoplastic, hypertrophied right ventricle with a hypoplastic and sometimes mildly dysplastic tricuspid valve, often in the association with coronary artery abnormalities. The structure of the right ventricle is often disturbed, most prominently with severe attenuation of the trabecular zone and, less commonly, absence of the outlet zone. This group shows the greatest diversity in terms of severity, leading to the controversies regarding a selection of appropriate management pathway.

Daubeney and colleagues studied the range of morphology in a population-based study of PAIVS [3]. From 1991 to 1995 they identified 183 neonates from 18 institutions. The median Z score of the tricuspid valve was −5.2 from echocardiography and −1.6 related to normal pathology data. Of note, 4% of patients had a dilated right ventricle, all of whom had important tricuspid valve regurgitation. The right ventricular morphology was judged to be tripartite in 59%, bipartite in 33%, and unipartite in 8%. A number of associations were noted with a smaller Z score of the tricuspid valve. These included a smaller Z score of the right ventricular inlet, an abnormal angle with the ductus arteriosus in relationship to its communication with the aorta, the presence of coronary artery fistula and atresia, muscular atresia of the pulmonary outflow, presence of a uni- or bipartite right ventricle, the absence of tricuspid regurgitation, and the presence of higher right ventricular pressure. The coronary arteries were judged to be normal in 54%, with minor fistula in 21% and major fistula in 25%. Right ventricular dependence of the coronary artery circulation was felt to be present in 8%. Of note, one patient had a fistula from the right ventricle via the coronary arteries to the pulmonary arteries. The magnitude of coronary artery pathology was directly correlated with the degree of right ventricular hypoplasia. The authors also noted that coronary artery pathology can change over time, showing evidence of regression of fistula or progression to stenoses. All patients had confluent pulmonary arteries, with hypoplasia being noted in only 9%. Aortopulmonary collateral vessels were rare. Left

ventricular abnormalities occurred in 6%, with septal bowing into the left ventricular outflow tract causing obstruction. A trivial ventricular septal defect was noted in 7%.

Satou and colleagues studied 30 patients from 1991 to 1998 who all had echocardiography and angiography [4]. They noted the absence of coronary artery pathology in 30%, fistula only in 30%, fistula plus one right ventricular-dependent coronary artery in 20%, and fistula with two or more right ventricular-dependent coronary arteries in 20%. The Z score of the tricuspid valve was a strong correlate with the degree of coronary artery pathology. The presence of a Z score of the tricuspid valve at or below −2.5 predicted the presence of a right ventricular-dependent coronary artery with 100% sensitivity and 83% specificity. The Z score of the tricuspid valve was also a strong predictor of the eventual patient outcome regarding management state, with patients with more severe hypoplasia going on to having one and a half or single ventricle repairs.

Giglia and colleagues studied 82 patients from 1979 to 1990 and noted a coronary fistula in 23 patients, 16 of whom had right ventricular decompression as part of their management strategy. [5] Of those, seven patients with only coronary artery fistula who had decompression, all survived. Of six patients who demonstrated a single stenosis in the coronary artery, four survived; and for those three patients who had stenoses of both the right coronary artery and the left anterior descending branch, none survived. The authors concluded that "decisions regarding right ventricular decompression should be based, to a large extent, on coronary anatomy. [The results] do not indicate, however, that right ventricular outflow tract reconstruction is in fact warranted in all infants without right ventricular-dependent coronary circulation. Such a conclusion could only be based on studies demonstrating right ventricular growth regardless of right ventricular anatomy."

Given the correlations between the degree of right-sided hypoplasia and the presence of functional and coronary artery abnormalities, the anatomic substrate must be completely defined in the setting of PAIVS. The majority of the assessment can be determined through the use of echocardiography. Qualitative assessment must be accompanied by a careful quantitative assessment of right ventricular structures related to appropriate normal values. Functional assessment is also required. Additional imaging modalities may be of importance, particularly in the assessment of coronary artery abnormalities, where angiography remains the gold standard. However, improvements in imaging with MRI and CT may replace angiography for right heart and coronary artery assessment in the future. Given the fact that coronary artery abnormalities may regress or evolve over time, ongoing assessment remains important.

20.4.3 What is the relationship between anatomic substrate, management algorithm, and outcomes?

Given the broad spectrum of the anatomic substrate, management is concomitantly complex. The goal is to achieve optimal survival by appropriate patient selection for management pathways aimed at achieving a particular definitive end state. These end states may include biventricular repair, one and a half ventricular repair, single ventricle palliation or Fontan procedure, and primary heart transplantation. A large proportion of patients, however, will achieve these end states only after a period where they are in an intermediate state. Management prior to achievement of definitive end states may include early palliations. Various palliations that have been used include the placement of systemic to pulmonary arterial shunts, performance of right ventricular outflow tract procedures, atrial septostomy, and the creation of cavopulmonary connections. Substantial mortality and morbidity occurs for patients in these intermediate states.

Appropriate selection of the optimal management pathway should be based on a strategy accounting for right heart morphology and function. Yoshimura and colleagues reported outcomes of 45 neonates with PAIVS who had surgery from 1981 to 2002 [6]. The selection of initial palliation was based on an assessment of right ventricular morphology. The predominant early decision-making tool was the right ventricular development index, which incorporated measurements of the right ventricular volume, the tricuspid valve dimension and the dimension of the right ventricular outflow tract indexed to body surface area. Decision making for definitive repair rested on the right ventricular to tricuspid valve index, which incorporated the right ventricular volume and the tricuspid valve dimension. All patients underwent an initial valvotomy, with those patients with small right ventricular development indices additionally having a systemic-to-pulmonary artery shunt. Subsequent assessments of the right ventricle to tricuspid valve index informed decisions regarding definitive repair. Using this morphology-based management protocol, the authors noted a 5-year survival of 91% and 10-year survival of 82%. They concluded that the management protocol based on quantitative assessment of right ventricular morphology was associated with good outcomes.

Fenton and colleagues examined interim mortality in PAIVS by examining 35 infants who had an initial shunt procedure [7]. Right ventricular hypoplasia was noted in 22 patients, and was associated with one hospital death, five interim deaths, and one late death, for an overall survival of 64%. For the 13 patients judged to have two adequate ventricles, there was one hospital death and one late death, with an overall survival of 85%. Causes of the interim deaths are important to note. Two patients died of myocardial infarction, with a third patient with a single left coronary artery dying suddenly. The remaining two patients died from acute shunt thrombosis and obstruction. These findings indicate the precariousness of the intermediate state. It also provides justification for anticoagulation strategies in shunted patients and vigilant care for patients with coronary artery abnormalities.

The largest study of management strategy and outcomes for PAIVS patients was reported by Ashburn and colleagues on behalf of the Congenital Heart Surgeons Society. [8] From 1987 to 1997, 408 neonates were enrolled within 30 days of birth from 33 institutions. The median Z score of the tricuspid valve was −1.2, with 19% having right ventricular-dependent coronary artery circulation. There was a significant correlation between the Z score of the right ventricular size and the Z score of the tricuspid valve, the presence of coronary artery fistula and obstructions and right ventricular-dependent coronary circulation. Overall survival for the cohort at 5 years was 60%, with 79% survival for those patients born in 1997.

A competing risk analysis was performed for the end states of death before repair, biventricular repair, one and a half ventricular repair, Fontan procedure, and primary heart transplantation. The risk of death before achieving an end state was greatest at the time of initial admission then tapered rapidly to a constant risk. The achievement of biventricular repair appeared to occur at no particular specified time interval following admission. Several risk factors were independently associated with both early and late achievement of each of these end states. Patients were more likely to achieve early biventricular repair if the right ventricle and tricuspid valve were more normal in size and the left ventricular pressure was higher. They were more likely to achieve a biventricular repair later if they had more normal right ventricular and tricuspid valve sizes, a lesser degree of coronary artery fistula, and higher birth weight. Achievement of one and a half ventricular repair was predicted by higher right ventricular systolic pressure and more normal Z score of the tricuspid valve. A lower Z score of the tricuspid valve was the only anatomic predictor of single ventricle repair. Factors associated with early deaths before reaching a definitive end state included lower birth weight, severe tricuspid regurgitation, both lower and higher Z score of the tricuspid valve and the presence of an enlarged right ventricle. Factors associated with later deaths before reaching a definitive end state included a lower right to left ventricle systolic pressure ratio, the performance of a prior balloon atrial septostomy, and earlier date of admission.

Of note, in each of these analyses, there were selected institutions that, after adjustment for the significant factors, remained associated with the performance of certain types of repair. An analysis of these institution-specific outcomes based on tricuspid valve Z score and preferred management pathway is shown in Fig. 20.2. Institution Y was a high-risk institution for interim death across the range of tricuspid valve Z scores, with few patients achieving a definitive end state, and probably represents suboptimal management for patients in intermediate states. Institution L favored a biventricular repair for all except the more extreme values of

tricuspid valve Z score hypoplasia. This was associated with a particularly high risk of death for those patients with the smallest tricuspid valve Z scores. The graph for Institution T shows a preference for performing a Fontan procedure across the anatomic spectrum. The mortality appears to be much lower for those with smaller tricuspid valve Z scores but higher for those with larger Z scores, with very few patients achieving biventricular repair. Institution E shows a balanced approached, with Fontan procedure being performed on those patients with smaller tricuspid valve Z scores and biventricular repair performed for those with larger tricuspid valve Z scores. A Z score of −2 appears to be the cross-over point for achievement of these two end states. Of note, this institution had associated low mortality for patients with both small and large tricuspid valves. This indicates that a balanced management strategy based on quantitative assessment of the anatomic substrate can be associated with the greatest advantage in terms of survival.

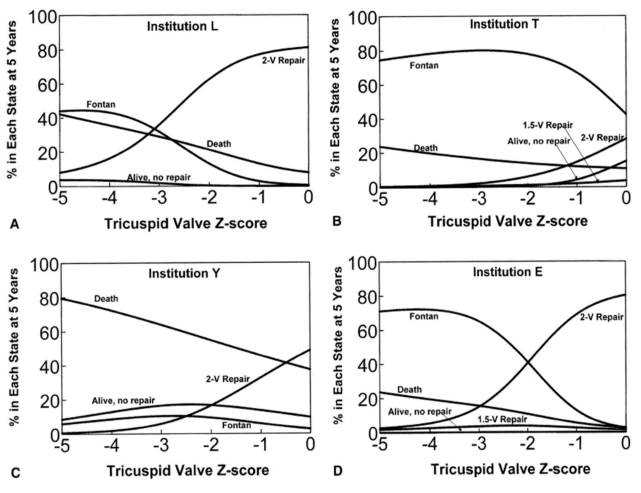

Fig. 20.2 Risk-adjusted competing-risks nomograms for individual institutions on the basis of morphologic spectrum of PAIVS. The predicted 5-year prevalences of end states (vertical axis) are plotted against tricuspid valve Z scores with commensurate adjustment of right ventricular size.
From Ashburn et al. Determinants of mortality and type of repair in neonates with pulmonary atresia and intact ventricular septum. J Thorac Cardiovasc Surg. 2004;127:1000–1008

20.4.4 Why is there a bias towards biventricular repair for borderline patients?

While it has been shown that institutions adopting a balanced approach to the management of PAIVS have excellent outcomes, there is a bias in many centers favoring management strategies to push the patient along toward a biventricular repair. This is based on a number of assumptions which have not been well supported from the current literature. The first assumption is that right heart structures will grow if the obstruction is relieved, particularly in response to changes in loading conditions. Humpl and colleagues studied 35 neonates with PAIVS enrolled from 1992 to 2000 [9]. Of the 20 patients who had single ventricle palliation, 13 had right ventricular-dependent coronary circulation, and 7 had a severely attenuated right ventricular cavity or infundibulum precluding a biventricular repair. The remaining 30 patients had an attempted radiofrequency-assisted perforation and balloon dilation of the pulmonary valve, with the procedure being successfully completed for 27 patients. For these 30 patients, there were 5 deaths, and 16 patients successfully achieved biventricular repair. Patients who achieved biventricular repair had significantly greater Z scores of the tricuspid valve and the right ventricular length and area. Measurements from serial echocardiograms were examined and showed that there was no change with increasing age regarding the Z score of the tricuspid valve diameter or of the right ventricular length. This is to say that hypoplasia persisted relative to the size of the patient with no evidence of any catch-up growth. There was no influence of management or effectiveness of management in relieving the obstruction on growth.

The second assumption that drives the bias toward biventricular repair is a feeling that functional outcomes will be better with a biventricular circulation than Fontan physiology. Sanghavi and colleagues examined 29 survivors with PAIVS born before 1997, 19 of whom had biventricular repair and 10 had Fontan procedure [10]. The two groups were similar with regard to age and gender. Abnormal aerobic capacity defined as peak oxygen consumption below 85% predicted was noted in 58% of the biventricular repair and 60% of the Fontan procedure patients. Figure 20.3 shows that the exercise capacity as indicated by the peak oxygen consumption and peak oxygen pulse was not significantly better in the biventricular repair patients compared to the Fontan patients. They did note that biventricular-repair patients had better chronotopic function and ventilatory efficiency. There was considerable variation and overlap between the exercise capacity between both groups, with no associated anatomic predictors noted. Predictors of abnormal aerobic capacity in the biventricular repair patients included an inability to increase their forward stroke volumes reflected by lower oxygen pulse, the presence of severe tricuspid regurgitation, and older age at the time of testing. The authors concluded that "…our data suggest that delaying Fontan completion by attempting to maintain a failing biventricular repair may ultimately cause long-term limitation to exercise function, perhaps because prolonged impaired oxygen delivery harms the myocardium."

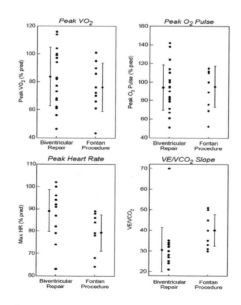

Fig. 20.3 Exercise parameters as a function of surgical anatomy for survivors with PAIVS.
From Sanghavi et al. Determinants of exercise function following univentricular versus biventricular repair for pulmonary atresia/intact ventricular septum. Am J Cardiol. 2006;97:1638–1643

Exercise capacity is only one aspect of functional status, and there is increasing interest regarding health-related quality of life assessment, and possible differences between biventricular and Fontan patients. Erkman-Joelsson examined 42 survivors with PAIVS in terms of their health-related quality of life [11]. They noted a few differences from a normal population, and no differences between patients who had biventricular repair versus Fontan procedure. There was a high level of psychosomatic complaints and a lower satisfaction with activities.

These assessments of exercise capacity and functional status are important, in that current management algorithms are driven by an emphasis on mortality with an unfounded bias toward biventricular repair based on presumed functional outcomes. Clearly further research is needed on a larger scale to determine the functional status and exercise capacity of these PAIVS patients and the influence of anatomic and management algorithms.

20.5 Who Should Get a Fontan?—Summary

Several issues become evident through appraisal of the recent literature. The decision regarding management should take into account initial anatomic and functional characteristics, with complete qualitative, quantitative, and functional ongoing assessment. The intermediate state is a precarious state, and if the patient is destined for a single ventricle pathway, the commitment should probably be made earlier. Finally, clinical decision making should not only be aimed at maximizing survival, but also ensuring optimal functional status and health-related quality of life.

References

1. De Oliveira NC, Sittiwangkul R, McCrindle BW, et al. Biventricular repair in children with atrioventricular septal defects and a small right ventricle: anatomic and surgical considerations. J Thorac Cardiovasc Surg. 2005;130(2):250–7.
2. Freedom R. How can something so small cause so much grief? Some thoughts about the underdeveloped right ventricle in pulmonary atresia and intact ventricular septum. J Am Coll Cardiol. 1992;19(5):1038–40.
3. Daubeney PE, Delany DJ, Anderson RH, et al. Pulmonary atresia with intact ventricular septum: range of morphology in a population-based study. J Am Coll Cardiol. 2002;39(10): 1670–9.
4. Satou GM, Perry SB, Gauvreau K, Geva T. Echocardiographic predictors of coronary artery pathology in pulmonary atresia with intact ventricular septum. Am J Cardiol. 2000;85(11): 1319–24.
5. Giglia TM, Mandell VS, Connor AR, Mayer JE Jr, Lock JE. Diagnosis and management of right ventricle-dependent coronary circulation in pulmonary atresia with intact ventricular septum. Circulation. 1992;86(5):1516–28.
6. Yoshimura N, Yamaguchi M, Ohashi H, et al. Pulmonary atresia with intact ventricular septum: strategy based on right ventricular morphology. J Thorac Cardiovasc Surg. 2003; 126(5):1417–26.
7. Fenton KN, Pigula FA, Gandhi SK, Russo L, Duncan KF. Interim mortality in pulmonary atresia with intact ventricular septum. Ann Thorac Surg. 2004;78(6):1994–8.
8. Ashburn DA, Blackstone EH, Wells WJ, et al. Determinants of mortality and type of repair in neonates with pulmonary atresia and intact ventricular septum. J Thorac Cardiovasc Surg. 2004; 127(4):1000–7.
9. Humpl T, Soderberg B, McCrindle BW, et al. Percutaneous balloon valvotomy in pulmonary atresia with intact ventricular septum: impact on patient care. Circulation. 2003;108(7): 826–32.
10. Sanghavi DM, Flanagan M, Powell AJ, Curran T, Picard S, Rhodes J. Determinants of exercise function following univentricular versus biventricular repair for pulmonary atresia/intact ventricular septum. Am J Cardiol. 2006;97(11): 1638–43.
11. Ekman-Joelsson BM, Berntsson L, Sunnegardh J. Quality of life in children with pulmonary atresia and intact ventricular septum. Cardiol Young. 2004;14(6):615–21.

Surgery for the Small Right Ventricle

Osman O. Al-Radi, Siho Kim, and Glen S. Van Arsdell

21.1 Introduction

Surgical solutions for congenital heart lesions traditionally fall into a single ventricle repair or a biventricular repair strategy. Ventricular size is the primary determinant of the surgical strategy. The degree of ventricular underdevelopment is a continuum, ranging from severely hypoplastic or nonexistent cavities to normal-sized cavities. Therefore, forcing a binary solution, single ventricle repair or biventricular repair, may not result in the best outcome. A more graded approach is considered.

Clearly, the systemic ventricle must be of adequate size and function to support a full survivable cardiac output against a normal systemic blood pressure. On the other hand, the pulmonary circulation may be left with no ventricular support, as is the case in the single ventricle Fontan circulation achieved by single ventricle repair strategies. That, however, is not without consequences. Decreased exercise tolerance, atrial arrhythmias, protein-losing entropathy (PLE), and late systemic ventricular failure are the most troubling adverse outcomes of single ventricle repair. It is hypothesized that incorporating a less than optimal ventricle into the pulmonary circulation may provide some physiologic benefit.

The most common impediments to biventricular repair are related to an inadequate ventricle—in this context, an inadequate right ventricle (RV). A suboptimal RV may be due to small size or inadequate function. In both cases the work load required of the RV can be reduced as much as 25–50% by performing a superior vena cava to pulmonary artery anastomosis along with biventricular repair [1]. This strategy is known as the one and a half ventricle repair (1 ½ ventricle repair) [1–4].

This chapter focuses on the problem of the small or inadequate RV (subpulmonary ventricle) and where it

may be appropriate to include it in the pulmonary side of the circulation. The pathological substrates, morphological, and functional criteria used to describe the RV, as well as the decision-making algorithm for the marginal patient is discussed. Additional issues that affect the surgical decision, including the anatomic and physiologic status of the pulmonary vasculature, the status of the atrioventricular valve, airway and chest wall anomalies, and associated anomalies are also considered.

21.2 What Is an Inadequate RV?

Once a certain threshold for right ventricular size is crossed, it becomes a diastolic compliance problem. The reduced compliance results in inadequate RV filling and reduced cardiac output. This leads to increased central venous pressure and a compensatory increase in heart rate. Alternatively, the RV may be of adequate size but deficient in terms of contractility. The poorly contractile RV is unable to maintain an adequate cardiac output, again resulting in an increase in central venous pressure and heart rate.

Either scenario may eventually lead to inadequate filling of the left (systemic) ventricle, thereby limiting systemic cardiac output and systemic blood pressure.

Defining the actual size threshold requires a discussion about how anatomic measurements are described in a standardized fashion.

21.2.1 Standardized Measurements

The size of the RV, or any anatomic measurement for that matter, may be expressed as a standardized value, known as the Z score. The Z score is the number of standard deviations (SDs) between the age-matched population mean and the observed value. For example, a Z score of −2 indicates that the observed value is 2 SD *below* the

O.O. Al-Radi (✉)
Department of Surgery, Hospital for Sick Children, , Toronto, ON, Canada

mean of a population of similar age. Moreover, since +2 and +3 SD happen to correspond with the 95th and 97th percentiles, a Z score of +2 and +3 indicate that the observed value is above the 95th and 97th percentiles, respectively [5]. Another method of presenting an anatomic measurement in a standardized fashion is indexed to the body surface area (BSA) in squared meter (m^2). The patient's BSA is obtained from standard tables using height and weight. The measured anatomic value is then divided by the BSA of the patient[5].

21.2.2 How Small Is Too Small?

In most cases estimation of RV size is based on indirect indicators. The most useful of which are tricuspid valve diameter, RV morphology, that is, unipartite, bipartite, or tripartite, and measured or estimated RV volume.

A detailed description of echocardiographic RV-assessment techniques is beyond the scope of this chapter. However, in summary, the RV size can be assessed echocardiographically by defining the dimension of the ventricle in the long and short axes, preferably in two orthogonal planes, the area of the ventricular cavity is then used to calculate the volume based on the geometric assumption that the ventricular cavity is cylindrical or conical in shape [6]. This measurement may be confounded by a malformed RV [7]. Nonetheless, several echocardiographic criteria have been described as tools to determine the adequacy of the RV. As seen in Table 21.1, a tricuspid valve diameter Z score of −2 to −5 indicated moderate RV hypoplasia, below −5 indicates severe RV hypoplasia. The importance of tricuspid valve diameter Z score was demonstrated in study by Hanley et al. of a multi-institutional cohort of patients with pulmonary atresia with intact ventricular septum (PA/IVS). Tricuspid valve diameter Z score was the only patientspecific risk factor for not receiving a biventricular repair [8]. Tabel 21.2 describes the values we currently use as indicators of how small an RV is adequate for biventricular repair or 1½ ventricle repair in the case of PA/IVS.

An RV without three distinct components, that is, unipartite or bipartite, is more likely to be smaller, less

compliant, and associated with a smaller tricuspid valve diameter, compared to a tripartite RV. Therefore, whether the RV is tripartite, bipartite, or unipartite is a useful overall indicator of the degree of hypoplasia.

Less-important echocardiographic indicators include RV/LV length ratio, and right to left atrioventricular valve ratio [9]. For the latter, a value > 0.5 is thought to indicate suitability for biventricular repair.

Direct assessment of the RV volume is theoretically ideal. Echocardiography, angiography, and magnetic resonance imaging (MRI) are the potential modalities for this measurement. Subjective assessment of RV volume by echocardiography and angiography is helpful; however, objective measurement with these methods frequently underestimates the size of the RV cavity. Recent advances in MRI have allowed direct measurement of RV volume. The threshold size for adequacy of the RV is not yet known. MRI also adds the possibility of functional assessment, including calculated forward flow through the tricuspid valve and PA, total cardiac output, extracardiac and intracardiac shunt volumes, and ejection fraction.

In critical aortic stenosis, a left ventricular volume less than 20 ml/m^2 is associated with poor outcomes due to inadequate cardiac output [10]. Extrapolating from this study and based on anecdotal cases, we currently regard an RV volume of more than 20 ml/m^2 to be adequate for biventricular repair or 1½ ventricle repair.

21.2.3 Physiologic RV Assessment

Systolic function of the RV is assessed qualitatively or semiquantitatively with echocardiography. Diastolic function is reflected by catheter measurements of end-diastolic pressure and CVP. These may not be accurate indicators if there are intracardiac shunts or tricuspid valve regurgitation. In the setting of PA/IVS and a borderline RV, occlusion of an ASD in the catheterization lab allows one to test the hemodynamic stability of a fully volume-loaded RV.

21.2.4 Pulmonary Vasculature

The anatomy of the pulmonary vasculature can be assessed by echocardiography, conventional or CT angiography, and MRI. Echocardiography is valuable for assessment of the RV outflow tract, the proximal pulmonary artery, and the pulmonary veins. The branch pulmonary arteries are not easily evaluated by echocardiography. CT angiography is the conventional method of studying branch pulmonary arteries as it provides excellent images and is

Table 21.1 Echocardiographic criteria used to assess the degree of RV hypoplasia

Criterion	RV hypoplasia		
	Mild	Moderate	Severe
RV components [28].	Tripartite	Bipartite	Unipartite
Apex formation	yes	no	no
Tricuspid valve diameter (z score) [22, 29, 30, 31].	>−2	−2 to −5	<−5

fast and readily available. MRI may also be used to assess branch pulmonary arteries. It has the added benefit of allowing for a calculation of flow to each lung. Conventional angiography provides excellent images and has the added benefits of the ability to measure pulmonary vascular resistance, test occlude atrial septal defects, and therapeutic pulmonary artery dilatation or stenting. The choice of modality generally depends on the specific case, institutional preference, and the need of therapeutic procedures.

21.3 The 1½ Ventricle Repair

The concept of incorporating an inadequate RV in the circulation, without giving it the burden of a full cardiac output is known as the 1½ ventricle repair (1½ ventricle repair). It was described by Billingsley et al. for PA/IVS [11]. The partial diversion of systemic venous return to the lung by creating a end-to-side anastomosis between the superior vena cava and the right pulmonary artery lessens the volume load on the RV by 25–50% [4]. Animal experiments showed that downsizing the RV to as low as 25% of normal resulted in survivable hemodynamics [4]. In a dog model, Ilbawi et al. recreated the Fontan circulation with the RV included in the Fontan circuit. They subsequently progressively reduced the size of the RV cavity by inflating a balloon in the RV. They demonstrated that as the RV size was progressively reduced, the heart rate increased. Down to the RV size 50% of normal, there was no change in the right atrial pressure and in the cardiac index. There was a modest drop in cardiac index at RV size 25% of normal, and an increase in RA pressure from 5 mm Hg at 50% of normal to 12 mm Hg at 25% of normal RV size.

Additionally, potential RV growth in the presence of pulsatile forward flow across the RV has been reported [12–15]. The long-term problems associated with the Fontan palliation, namely, protein-losing entropathy, persistent atrial arrhythmias, and progressive ventricular failure may be delayed or prevented by lessening the load on the dominant ventricle, and providing pulsatile pulmonary blood flow.

21.3.1 Classification of 1½ Ventricle Repair Based on Indication

A heterogeneous group of patients suffer from the clinical problem of an inadequate RV. We found it useful to classify the patients who underwent 1½ ventricle repair for inadequate RV into four groups. This was based on the indication for the repair [1]. The two major groups are

Table 21.2 Classification systems of repair based on indication

Group	Van arsdell	Mavroudis
A	Small pulmonary ventricle	Small right ventricle
B	Chronic RV dysfunction	Preoperative RV dysfunction
C	Facilitation of repair without size or functional problems in the RV	To facilitate biventricular repair
D	Acute RV dysfunction	To pressure unload the pulmonary ventricle in CCTGA, VSD, PS

CCTGA: Congenitally corrected transposition of the great arteries.
VSD: Ventricular septal defect.
PS: Pulmonary stenosis.

diastolic RV deficiency (small size), and systolic RV deficiency (reduced contractility). Mavroudis et al. adopted this classification with modification. Table 21.2 describes both these classifications and shows the difference between them. Here, we propose a simplified more general classification (Table 21.3).

Table 21.3 Simplified classification of repair based on indication

Group	Indication of repair	Example
A	Volume unload a small RV	PA/IVS
B	Volume unload a dysfunctional RV	Ebstein's anomaly
C	Facilitate biventricular repair/surgical convenience	Double switch with simplified atrial baffle
D	Pressure unload pulmonary ventricle	CCTGA + VSD + PS
E	Acute RV failure	post-biventricular repair with low output or desaturation

PA/IVS: Pulmonary atresia with intact ventricular septum.
CCTGA: Congenitally corrected transposition of the great arteries.
VSD: Ventricular septal defect.
PS: Pulmonary stenosis.

21.4 Congenital Anomalies Commonly Associated with an Inadequate RV

PA/IVS, and complete AVSD with a small RV are the most prevalent examples of diastolic RV dysfunction (small RV, group A). The most prevalent example of systolic RV dysfunction (Group B) is Ebstein's anomaly. Other entities are far less common.

21.4.1 Pulmonary Atresia with Intact Ventricular Septum (PA/IVS)

For infants with PA/IVS, tricuspid valve diameter, and RV-dependent coronary circulation are important factors that predict both overall outcome and suitability for biventricular repair. Traditionally, infants with PA/IVS in whom the RV size is judged to be too small to support a full cardiac output would undergo single ventricle repair. In a study of 51 patients with PA/IVS treated between 1971 and 1984, de Laval et al. described the outcomes of biventricular repair in infants with PA/IVS stratified by tricuspid valve diameter less than or more than the 99% lower confidence interval (Z score < -3). Of the ten patients with tricuspid valve Z score < -3 who had complete BVR eight died. Whereas of eighteen infants with tricuspid valve diameter Z score > -3, only 3 died [16, 17]. A multi–institutional Congenital Heart Surgeons Society (CHSS) study described the outcomes of infants with PA/IVS between 1987 and 1997. Of 404 infants 33% had undergone biventricular repair, 20% underwent single ventricle repair and 5% underwent 1 ½ ventricle repair, at 15 years after enrollment [18]. The limitations to biventricular repair and 1 ½ ventricle repair are continuously challenged. In the most recent published analysis of our outcomes from 1992 to 2000, Humple et al. showed that 53% had biventricular repair, 10% had 1 ½ ventricle repair, and only 10% were on an SVR track [19]. Fourteen patients with PA/IVS underwent repair at our institution between 1972 and 2003 (three included in above study). Two deaths occurred at 4 and 104 months of follow-up. Eleven of the remaining patients are in New York Heart Association (NYHA) class I, and one is in NYHA class II at last follow-up (unpublished data). Our current anatomic guidelines that direct the surgical strategy for PA/IVS are summarized in Table 21.4.

21.4.2 Unbalanced Atrioventricular Septal Defect (AVSD)

In most patients with complete AVSD, the two ventricles are of similar size and balanced. A subset of patients has a small RV that might be able to pump lesser than total systemic venous return to the lungs. Many infants having an AVSD also have trisomy 21 and its attendant respiratory problems potentially leading to increased pulmonary vascular resistance. Therefore, performing a cavopulmonary shunt to offload an anatomically

Table 21.4 Anatomic guidelines for repair of PA/IVS

Tricuspid valve z score	Pulmonary ventricular volume	Strategy
> -2	$> 80\%$	biventricular repair
-2 to -5	80–50%	1 ½ ventricle repair
-5 to -10	50–30%	1 ½ ventricle repair + ASD
< -10	$< 30\%$	single ventricle repair

small RV may not be a good option. De Olivera et al. described our approach to this population of patients and reported our results of a case match study where patients with AVSD with balanced ventricles were compared to patients with AVSD with a small RV [20]. Reducing the RV preload by leaving an atrial fenestration was felt to be important to the success of biventricular repair in the small RV group.

Others, however, have successfully used a 1 ½ ventricle-repair strategy in this setting. Alvarado et al. reported on the results for nine patients with small RV/AVSD and tricuspid valve Z score as small as -10 [21]. A preceding pulmonary artery band had been performed in over half of the cases thereby lessening the PVR issues. When the PVR is not in the range acceptable for single ventricle repair (PA diastolic pressure < 12 mm Hg) we prefer the use of biventricular repair with an adjustable ASD over 1 ½ ventricle repair.

21.4.3 Ebstein's Anomaly

Patients with Ebstein's anomaly have an enlarged dysfunctional RV. In this setting, 1 ½ ventricle repair is considered for systolic RV dysfunction (Group B) [1]. We have used the 1 ½ ventricle repair strategy in 28 patients with Ebstein's anomaly from 1965 to 2003. Three patients died at 0, 18, and 24 months postoperatively. The remaining patients were in NYHA class I or II at last clinical follow-up. Sarris et al. have reported the results of a multi-institutional study of 150 patients with Ebstein's anomaly. Seven patients underwent 1 ½ ventricle repair with no deaths, and only young age at operation was a risk factor for death in the entire group.

21.4.4 Transposition of the Great Arteries

Rare patients with simple transposition, VSD, and small RV may be treated by initial balloon atrial septostomy and pulmonary artery banding followed by an arterial switch and cavopulmonary anastomosis [1]. Patients with congenitally corrected TGA with a small morphologic RV may be treated by 1½ ventricle repair in the form of a double switch with a simplified atrial baffle and superior vena cava to pulmonary artery anastomosis [22].

21.5 Physiologic Testing, Adjustable ASD, and the 1¼ Ventricle Repair

The complex and heterogeneous nature of indications for 1½ ventricle repair leave the managing team with a degree of uncertainty about the suitability and success of 1½ ventricle repair versus biventricular repair or single ventricle repair. Every opportunity for physiologic testing and assessment should be utilized to aid in the decision making. Preoperative assessment of central venous pressure, diastolic RV pressure, pulmonary artery pressure, and MRI flow data are helpful in determining whether a cavopulmonary anastomosis is going to be tolerable. In general, 1½ ventricle repair requires the pulmonary vascular resistance (indirectly assessed by pulmonary artery pressure and RV diastolic pressure) to be low, in the same range as for a Fontan physiology of single ventricle repair. Intraoperative visual inspection of the anatomy, and the initial hemodynamic variables after separation form cardiopulmonary bypass assist in the decision to proceed with or accept biventricular repair, 1½ ventricle repair, 1½ ventricle repair + ASD, or to revert to single ventricle repair. A native or iatrogenic ASD should be left in all patients where the size or function of the RV is uncertain. A starting diameter of 4–5 mm is usually adequate to prevent perioperative low cardiac output. A purse string exteriorized outside of the heart on the posterolateral aspect of the RA may be used to adjust the ASD size. The desirable value for central venous pressure is below 12 mm Hg. Postoperatively in the ICU the ASD can be test occluded prior to chest closure. Later on the ASD may be test occluded in the catheterization laboratory with a balloon, and then device occluded if appropriate. The use of an adjustable ASD has been a valuable adjunct to biventricular repair in marginal patients [20, 23]. The temporary volume off-loading achieved has allowed the use of biventricular repair in patients who would otherwise undergo single ventricle repair, and reduced the risk of low cardiac output postoperatively. Similarly, some patients with moderate to severe RV hypoplasia undergoing repair may require such volume off-loading in the postoperative period to overcome the perioperative fluid over load state. When the ASD is left open indefinitely the final result may be called a 1¼ ventricle repair, as the pulmonary ventricle is bypassed by approximately three-quarters of the systemic venous return; half directly to the lungs via the SVC to PA connection, and a quarter via the ASD. At our institution, of the 115 patients who underwent 1½ ventricle repair 49 left the operating room with an ASD.

21.6 Midterm Results of 1½ Ventricle Repair

At our institution, 115 patients underwent 1½ ventricle repair for various indications between 1965 and 2003. The time-related survival from initial repair was 94%, 93%, 74%, and 66% at 1 month, 1, 10, and 20 years, respectively. The theoretical advantage of 1½ ventricle repair over single ventricle repair needs to be confirmed by valid clinical outcome analysis. As no studies of randomized or even comparable groups of patients are available, one is forced to examine studies that describe the outcomes of both strategies separately. This comparison is not suitable for reaching conclusions about the preferable strategy; however, it may set the stage for comparative studies to be commissioned.

In a recent analysis of medium to long-term results of single ventricle repair, Ono et al. reported an early death of rate 8% and long-term rate survival of 87% at 20 years [24]. Giannico et al. reported the results of extracardiac Fontan in 221 patients, survival at 15 years was 85% [25]. On the other hand, two recent reports of midterm results of the 1½ ventricle repair are available. Chowdhury et al. published in 2005, on 84 patients who underwent 1½ ventricle repair between 1990 and 2003 [26]. In patients who underwent an MRI, the end-diastolic RV volume indexed to BSA (RVEVVi) was 22 ± 2.2 ml/m^2. The operative mortality was 10.7%. The late mortality was 8%. With follow-up up to 14 years, time-related survival was 82% at 7 years. Clinical arrhythmia occurred in 15% of patients and 90% of patients were in NYHA heart failure class I or II. In 2003, Numata et al. published the results of 1½ ventricle repair for PA/IVS or PS with a small RV [27]. For 13 patients operated on between 1987 and 1999, the RVEDVi was 20–50% normal. The tricuspid valve diameter was 40–70% of normal. The mean follow-up was 10 years. There were no operative deaths. One late death occurred at 8 years and two patients were converted to Fontan circulation, with one death. Exercise testing revealed a maximum oxygen uptake (MVO$_{2 \, max}$) of 24.8 ± 4.9 ml, and anaerobic threshold of 16.6 ± 3.4 mls at 5 years. One patient developed PLE. In their conclusion, they expressed that they did not see an advantage for 1½ ventricle repair over single ventricle repair. Given that the patient populations are different it is difficult to make a direct comparison. However, from these contemporaneous recent reports, one might conclude that there is no gross difference between the outcomes of single ventricle repair and 1½ ventricle repair in patients selected for each strategy.

21.7 Summary

The main factors that play a role in deciding the operative strategy for an inadequate RV are size and function. An RV of size less than 30% of normal, or tricuspid valve Z score < -10 most likely necessitates single ventricle repair. Almost all patients with a tricuspid valve Z score of > -2 will be best served by a biventricular repair. Tricuspid valve Z score between -2 and -10 is a marginal area where many options are available, including the 1½ ventricle repair. In patients with Ebstein's anomaly, 1½ ventricle repair is considered for functional decompensation of the RV. The judicious use of preoperative imaging, intraoperative testing, and early postoperative hemodynamic monitoring aid in the decision making and ongoing assessment of these challenging patients.

References

1. Van Arsdell GS, W WG, Maser CM, Streitenberger KS, Rebeyka IM, Coles JG, Freedom, RM. Superior vena cava to pulmonary artery anastomosis: an adjunct to biventricular repair. J Thorac Cardiovasc Surg. 1996;112(5):1143–8; Discussion 1148–9.
2. Muster AJ, Z VR, Ilbawi MN, Backer CL, Duffy CE, Mavroudis C. Biventricular repair of hypoplastic right ventricle assisted by pulsatile bidirectional cavopulmonary anastomosis. J Thorac Cardiovasc Surg. 1993;105(1):112–9.
3. Gentles TL, K JF, Jonas RA, Marx GE, Mayer JE. Surgical alternatives to the Fontan procedure incorporating a hypoplastic right ventricle. Circulation. 1994;90(5 Pt 2):II1–II6.
4. Ilbawi MN, I FS, DeLeon SY, Kucich VA, Muster AJ, Paul MH, Zales VR. When should the hypoplastic right ventricle be used in a Fontan operation? An experimental and clinical correlation. Ann Thorac Surg. 1989;47(4):533–538.
5. Kouchoukos N, Eugene B, Doty D, Hanley F, Karp R. Cardiac Surgery Churchill Livingstone, 2003.
6. Silverman NH, M DB. Echocardiography of hypoplastic ventricles. Ann Thorac surg. 1998;66(2):627–33.
7. Graham TP, J JM, Atwood GF. & Canent RV. Right ventricular volume determinations in children. Normal values and observations with volume or pressure overload. Circulation. 1973;47(1):144–153.
8. Hanley FL, S RM, Blackstone EH, Kirklin JW, Freedom RM. & Nanda NC. Outcomes in neonatal pulmonary atresia with intact ventricular septum. A multiinstitutional study. J Thorac Cardiovasc Surg. 1993;105(3):406–23, 424–7; Discussion 423–4.
9. Minich LL, T LY, Ritter S, Williams RV, Shaddy RE, Hawkins JA.. Usefulness of the preoperative tricuspid/mitral valve ratio for predicting outcome in pulmonary atresia with intact ventricular septum. Am J Cardiol. 2000;85(11):1325–1328.
10. Hammon JW, L FM, Maples MD, Merrill WH, First WH, Graham TP, Bender HW. Predictors of operative mortality in critical valvular aortic stenosis presenting in infancy. Ann Thorac Surg. 1988;45(5):537–540.
11. Billingsley AM, L H, Boyce SW, George B, Santulli T, Williams RG. Definitive repair in patients with pulmonary atresia and intact ventricular septum. J Thorac Cardiovasc Surg. 1989;97(5):746–754.
12. Cobanoglu A, M MT, Pinson CW, Grunkemeier GL, Sunderland CO, Starr A. Valvotomy for pulmonary atresia with intact ventricular septum. A disciplined approach to achieve a functioning right ventricle. J Thorac Cardiovasc Surg. 1985;89(4):482–490.
13. Shaddy RES JE, Judd VE, McGough EC. Right ventricular growth after transventricular pulmonary valvotomy and central aortopulmonary shunt for pulmonary atresia and intact ventricular septum. Circulation. 1990;82(Suppl 5):IV157-IV163.
14. Graham TP, B HW, Atwood GF, Page DL, Sell CG. Increase in right ventricular volume following valvulotomy for pulmonary atresia or stenosis with intact ventricular septum. Circulation. 1974;50(Suppl 2):II69-II79.
15. de Leval M, B C, Stark J, Anderson RH, Taylor JF, Macartney FJ. Pulmonary atresia and intact ventricular septum: surgical management based on a revised classification. Circulation. 1982;66(2):272–280.
16. de Leval M, B C, Hopkins R, Rees P, Deanfield J, Taylor JF, Gersony W, Stark J, Macartney, FJ. Decision making in the definitive repair of the heart with a small right ventricle. Circulation. 1985; 2(3 Pt 2):II52–60.
17. Freedom R. How can something so small cause so much grief? Some thoughts about the underdeveloped right ventricle in pulmonary atresia and intact ventricular septum. J Am Coll Cardiol. 1992;19(5):1038–40.
18. Ashburn DAB, Eugene H, Wells Winfield J, Jonas, Richard A, Pigula, Frank A, Manning, Peter B; Lofland, Gary K, Williams, William G, McCrindle, Brian W, et al. Congenital Heart Surgeons Study. Determinants of mortality and type of repair in neonates with pulmonary atresia and intact ventricular septum. J Thorac Cardiovasc Surg. 2004;127(4):1000–7; Discussion 1007–8.
19. Humpl T, Björn S, McCrindle BW, Nykanen DG, Freedom RM, Williams WG, Benson LN. Percutaneous balloon valvotomy in pulmonary atresia with intact ventricular septum: impact on patient care. Circulation. 2003;108(7):826–832.
20. De Oliveira NCS, R., McCrindle BW, Dipchand A, Yun TJ, Coles JG. Caldarone C, Williams WG, Van Arsdell GS. Biventricular repair in children with atrioventricular septal defects and a small right ventricle: anatomic and surgical considerations. J Thorac Cardiovasc Surg. 2005;130(2):250–7.
21. Alvarado OS, N., McKay R, Boyd IM. Cavopulmonary connection in repair of atrioventricular septal defect with small right ventricle. Ann Thorac Surg. 1993;55(3):729–36.
22. Van Arsdell GSW, W.G., Freedom, RM. A practical approach to 1 1/2 ventricle repairs. Ann Thorac Surg. 1998;66(2):678–680.
23. Laks HP, J.M., Drinkwater DC, Jarmakani J, Isabel-Jones J, George BL, Williams RG. Partial biventricular repair of pulmonary atresia with intact ventricular septum. Use of an adjustable atrial septal defect. Circulation. 1992;86(Suppl 5):II159-II166.
24. Ono MB, Dietmar, Goerler, Heidi, Lange, Melanie; Westhoff-Bleck, Mechthild, Breymann, Thomas. Clinical outcome of patients 20 years after Fontan operation–effect of fe nestration on late morbidity. Eur J Cardiothorac Surg. 2006;30(6):923–929.
25. Giannico S, Fatma H, Amodeo A, Michielon G, Drago F, Turchetta A, Donato RD, Sanders SP. Clinical outcome of 193 extracardiac Fontan patients: the first 15 years. J Am Coll Cardiol. 2006;47(10):2065–2073.

26. Chowdhury UKA, B., Talwar S, Kothari SS, Saxena A, Singh R, Subramaniam GK, Juneja R, Pradeep KK, Sathia S, Venugopal P. One and one-half ventricle repair: results and concerns. Ann Thorac Surg. 2005;80(6):2293–300.

27. Numata SU, H., Yagihara T, Kagisaki K, Takahashi M, Ohuchi H. Long-term functional results of the one and one half ventricular repair for the spectrum of patients with pulmonary atresia/stenosis with intact ventricular septum. Eur J Cardiothorac Surg. 2003;24(4):516–20.

28. Goor DA, C.W.L. Congenital Malformations of the Heart: Grune & Stratton, 1975.

29. Bull CdL, M.R., Mercanti C, Macartney FJ, Anderson RH. Pulmonary atresia and intact ventricular septum: a revised classification. Circulation. 1982;66(2):266–272.

30. Patel RGF, R.M., Moes CA, Bloom KR, Olley PM, Williams WG, Trusler GA, Rowe RD. Right ventricular volume determinations in 18 patients with pulmonary atresia and intact ventricular septum. Analysis of factors influencing right ventricular growth. Circulation. 1980;61(2):428–440.

31. Zuberbuhler JRA, R.H. Morphological variations in pulmonary atresia with intact ventricular septum. Br Heart J. 1979;41(3):281–288.

Section 6
The Right Ventricle on the Intensive Care Unit

Mark A. Walsh and Tilman Humpl

22.1 Introduction

A postoperative increase of pulmonary artery pressures is usually a result of a combination of several factors, which may have different significance in the individual patient, but usually include pre-operative, intraoperative, and postoperative events (Fig. 22.1). Cardiopulmonary bypass invariably elevates pulmonary vascular resistance as a result of interrupted antegrade pulmonary blood flow. In the years that followed the introduction of cardiopulmonary bypass for congenital heart surgery, pulmonary hypertension was the leading cause of death in the postoperative period [1]. Increased survival in the current era can be attributed to improvements in preoperative, intraoperative, and postoperative conditions. The increasing trend toward earlier repair of congenital heart lesions has decreased both the incidence and severity of pulmonary hypertension [2]. In particular, with the introduction of nitric oxide, postoperative pulmonary hypertension is now a much less common indication for the use of extracorporeal mechanical support [3] However, retrospective studies have demonstrated significant associated morbidity, such as increased ventilation times, and a greater than twofold risk of prolonged intensive care stay [4].

In the absence of routine pulmonary artery pressure monitoring, the incidence of postoperative pulmonary hypertension is difficult to determine. In addition, many children will tolerate a rise in pulmonary artery pressures, with the pressures reverting to baseline without any treatment within weeks of surgery [5]. In the era of the first atrial switches for transposition of the great arteries, the early mortality was as high as 25%, with postoperative pulmonary hypertension being the leading cause of death [1]. Recent reports have suggested that the current incidence of clinically significant postoperative pulmonary hypertension is as low as 2% [2]. Lesions such as atrioventricular canal defects, truncus arteriosus, and total anomalous pulmonary venous drainage all have a higher incidence of pulmonary hypertension after cardiopulmonary bypass [5]. The pulmonary endothelial dysfunction that occurs in these lesions may be caused by either increased pulmonary blood flow or increased pulmonary endothelial wall stress [6].

In the postoperative period a combination of factors can combine to negatively impact right ventricular afterload, left ventricular preload and ventricular interdependence. It is important to distinguish between high pulmonary vascular resistance and pulmonary reactivity, with the former being associated with longstanding left-to-right shunts and the latter more often seen following cardiopulmonary bypass [7]. A pulmonary hypertensive crisis is often precipitated by a noxious stimulus causing a sudden increase in pulmonary arterial pressure, increased right ventricular afterload, decreased caval oxygen saturation, and decreased lung compliance [8]. The critical component of this condition is the fall in cardiac output, as apposed to the systemic right ventricular pressure per se [5]. In terms of treatment, vascular reactivity is more appropriately managed by limiting noxious stimuli, sedation, and paralysis. Increased pulmonary vascular resistance may be more appropriately managed with selective pulmonary vasodilators [5]. It remains unclear why airway resistance increases, however, it is a well-recognized phenomenon. It is possible that large reductions in pulmonary blood flow may result in the collapse of small caliber vessels which act as scaffolding for the respiratory bronchioles [9].

22.2 The Pulmonary Endothelium

Despite many technical refinements, cardiopulmonary bypass continues to induce a large systemic inflammatory response which peaks approximately 8 hours after

M.A. Walsh (✉)
Department of Critical Care Medicine, The Hospital for Sick Children, University of Toronto, Toronto, Canada

A.N. Redington et al. (eds.), *Congenital Diseases in the Right Heart*, DOI 10.1007/978-1-84800-378-1_22,
© Springer-Verlag London Limited 2009

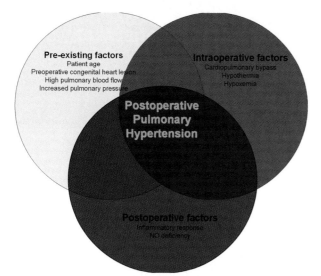

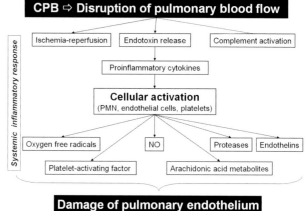

Fig. 22.2 Systemic inflammatory response to cardiopulmonary bypass

Fig. 22.1 Overlapping factors contributing to postoperative pulmonary hypertension. No: Nitric oxide

discontinuation (Fig. 22.2). Less appreciated is the fact that the pulmonary endothelium is the least protected of all organs and completely devoid of antegrade blood flow during cardiopulmonary bypass [10]. Ventilation of the lungs and perfusion of the pulmonary arteries during cardiopulmonary bypass have both been shown to reduce lung injury in the postoperative period [11]. Much of the ischemic injury occurs during reperfusion, which involves a complex cascade of interactions, including compliment activation, neutrophil migration, increased calpain activity, platelet activation, and nuclear factor kappa–beta activation [12, 13].

22.3 Endothelin-1

Endothelin-1 (ET-1) is a powerful vasoconstrictor released by the vascular endothelium which mediates smooth muscle proliferation, vascular remodeling, and inflammatory cascades [6]. Levels peak 3–9 h post-cardiopulmonary bypass and correlate with the rise in pulmonary arterial pressure, an effect which is more pronounced in patients with preexisting high pulmonary blood flow [14]. Several factors may be responsible for the rise in ET-1, such as interruption of normal blood flow, hypothermia, alveolar hypoxia, and components of the reperfusion injury as mentioned above [6].

Proendothelin is cleaved by membrane-bound, *endothelin-converting enzyme-1* to form ET-1, which acts on at least two different receptors. Endothelin-A receptors are found predominantly on vascular smooth muscle, and mediate the vasoconstrictor effects of ET-1. Endothelin-B receptors are found on the vascular endothelium and regulate the secretion of ET-1. They are also responsible for the vasodilatory effects of ET-1, releasing NO, and prostaglandin [15]. ET-1 is

both secreted and reabsorbed by the pulmonary endothelium in equilibrium, with approximately 50% of circulating ET-1 being recycled with one passage through the lungs. Elevated ET-1 levels following cardiopulmonary bypass may be due to reduced reabsorption, increased secretion, or a combination of both. Animal data has shown that high pulmonary blood effects to increase the number of ET-A receptors and causes a change in the locus of the ET-B receptor from the endothelium to the smooth muscle, both of which favor vasoconstriction [16]. There are various different types of ET-1 antagonists, with varying degrees of selectivity for A and B receptors. Blockage of the ET-A receptor following cardiopulmonary bypass significantly decreases pulmonary vascular resistance, with no additional effect from NO once ET-A blockade has occurred [14].

The delayed peak in ET-1 following cardiopulmonary bypass levels suggests that additional mechanisms such as decreased NO and increased thromboxane may be responsible for the immediate rise in pulmonary arterial pressure [17, 18]. The fact that NO donors only partially reverse cardiopulmonary bypass-induced pulmonary hypertension suggests an imbalance in the regulation of vascular tone with many mediators acting in unison to elevate pulmonary vascular resistance [19]. This would also explain the presence of nonresponders and the phenomenon of rebound pulmonary hypertension [20]. Prophylactic ET-1 blockade may be clinically beneficial in patients with a high preoperative risk profile. It is unlikely, however, that it would result in an acceptable risk–benefit ratio in all children undergoing cardiopulmonary bypass.

22.4 The Role of Nitric Oxide

The role of the endothelium in mediating vascular smooth muscle relaxation was first described by Furchgott and colleagues [21]. The endothelium was thought to secrete a relaxation factor which was subsequently identified as NO. It is produced in the pulmonary endothelium by NO synthase from the substrate L-arginine [22]. Acetylcholine acts on a muscarinic G_i-protein-linked receptor which elevates intracellular calcium, activating NO synthase [19]. NO then diffuses into the vascular smooth muscle-mediating relaxation by stimulating soluble guanylate cyclase to produce cyclic GMP [23]. The lack of endothelial-dependent relaxation of smooth muscle in response to acetylcholine following cardiopulmonary bypass may be related to be a dysfunctional G-protein-signaling process [24].

In the acute setting, the combination of NO and supplemental oxygen is more effective in treating a pulmonary hypertensive crisis than oxygen alone [23]. NO compares favorably with conventional strategies, such as hyperventilation and systemic pulmonary vasodilation, with treatment effects seen at 20–40 parts per million (ppm) [23]. NO improves lung compliance and decreases airway resistance, both of which are abnormal during a pulmonary hypertensive crises [8]. Studies have also shown a significant improvement in the alveolar–arterial gradient following inhaled NO because of its selective distribution to well-ventilated segments of lung tissue [25].

The use of routine prophylactic-inhaled NO has not been conclusively shown to reduce mortality or prevent a pulmonary hypertensive crisis. NO in select cases however is a very effective treatment and has contributed greatly toward improved survival [3]. NO donors serve to tip the complex balance of vasoactive mediators in favor of pulmonary vasodilation. This may however be only partially treating the underlying pathophysiology, as seen by the fact that NO donors only partially alleviate cardiopulmonary bypass-induced pulmonary hypertension.

22.5 Other Mediators

Prostacyclin is released by the endothelium and activates G-protein-linked smooth muscle cyclic AMP, mediating smooth muscle relaxation [26]. It has been shown that the action of acetylcholine and NO is influenced by prostacyclin and visa versa, suggesting an interdependence of both pathways [27]. Thromboxane A_2 is synthesized by cycloxygenase and causes smooth muscle vasoconstriction. It has a pronounced effect on the pulmonary vasculature, where it is mediates vasoconstriction in many different forms of pulmonary hypertension [28]. Both prostacyclin and thromboxane A_2 are elevated in children with increased pulmonary blood flow, particularly in the immediate postoperative period [29]. This imbalance is may be caused by endothelial injury post-cardiopulmonary bypass, although whether it is a mediator of the disease or a marker of endothelial dysfunction remains unclear.

Calpain is a calcium-activated serum protease, which has been shown to have a role in transmembrane signaling, cell differentiation, transcription, cytokine processing, and apoptosis [30]. In animal experiments, calpain inhibition following cardiopulmonary bypass has been shown to have a role in preventing endothelial dysfunction by attenuating the rise in ET-1 and preserving endothelial NO synthase activity [31]. Nuclear factor kappa–beta is a nuclear transcription factor which mediates many components of the inflammatory cascade. Calpain and inhibitor factor kappa beta modify this inflammatory response with calpain inhibitors attenuating nuclear factor kappa beta-induced reperfusion injury [32].

Inhibition of nuclear factor kappa beta has been shown to limit reperfusion injury in animal studies, with improved oxygenation, decreased pulmonary arterial pressure, and improved lung compliance in transplanted lungs. [13] Remote ischemic preconditioning is a novel process by which short periods of ischemia offer a protective effect against prolonged periods of ischemia to remote organs. The protective effect is dependent on inhibition of nuclear factor kappa beta. [33] Animal models of remote ischemic preconditioning have shown decreased airway resistance and increased pulmonary compliance following cardiopulmonary bypass [34].

Arginine vasopressin is a vasopressor which is sometimes used as an adjunct to other inotropic agents after cardiopulmonary bypass. In animal studies, low-dose vasopressin mediates pulmonary vasodilatation by acting on pulmonary endothelial V_1 receptors and releasing NO. Hypoxic pulmonary endothelium exhibits more pronounced vasodilation in response to arginine vasopressin, which may be due to an altered receptor-mediated process [35].

Recent years have seen increased research into *vascular endothelial growth factor (VEGF)*. VEGF acts as a central cytokine/growth factor and is primarily involved with angiogenesis. It has a profound effect on many functional aspects of the endothelium including NO synthesis, prostacyclin synthesis, and vascular permeability [36]. VEGF activates endothelial NO synthase via the tyrosine kinase and inositol triphosphate pathway [37]. Animal studies have shown increased levels of VEGF post-cardiopulmonary bypass, which correlate with increased lung permeability and decreased exhaled NO. The failure of VEGF to augment NO production may be related to either the deleterious effects of cardiopulmonary bypass on the endothelial cell membrane or a defect in endothelial NO synthase [24].

22.6 Therapeutic Approach

A comprehensive policy should be applied for patients at risk for postoperative pulmonary hypertension, including preoperative, intraoperative, and postoperative settings

- **Pre-operative**
  - Appropriate age at surgery
  - Ensure reactivity of pulmonary vasculature
- **Intra-operative**
  - Use of ultrafiltration
  - Avoid hypoxemia
- **Post-operative**
  - Exclude residual anatomic lesions
  - Leave/create atrial communication
  - Provide sedation/analgesia
  - Moderate hyperventilation/alkalosis
  - Pulmonary vasodilation (NO, PDE5 inhibitors)
  - Avoid alveolar hypoxemia

Fig. 22.3 Preventive measures to minimize postoperative pulmonary hypertension. No: Nitric oxide, PDE5: Phosphodiesterase 5

(Fig. 22.3). Most important for the initial postoperative management is the appropriate surveillance and limitation of any possible stimuli that might initiate a pulmonary hypertensive crisis. Although high ventilation pressures may be necessary to maintain a normal pH, high mean airway pressures negatively impact systemic venous return and increase right ventricular afterload. Pulmonary hypertension should be suspected when any stimulus causes a sudden decrease in cardiac output. Hyperventilation is commonly used in the treatment and prevention of pulmonary arterial hypertension [38]. Chang and colleagues pointed out that the effect of pH predominates over the effect of carbon dioxide in regulating pulmonary vascular resistance, which has important implications in determining the most efficacious therapeutic approach [39]. In the absence of a pulmonary artery catheter, central venous oxygen saturations will provide adequate monitoring of cardiac output [5]. Pressure tracings may reveal a high central venous pressure and cannon A waves from tricuspid regurgitation. Clinical features suggesting a sudden elevation in pulmonary artery pressures include tachycardia, agitation, and hypotension. Biochemical markers such as increased anaerobic metabolism and evidence of decreased end-organ perfusion may also indicate impaired cardiac output.

It is paramount to minimize potential triggers by maintaining an alkaline pH, normocapnia, normothermia, adequate sedation, and minimizing noxious stimuli. Factors that may adversely affect ventilation should be sought out and treated appropriately. Administration of 100% oxygen promotes pulmonary vasodilation and will correct hypoxic vasoconstriction of parenchymal origin if present [40]. Inhaled NO 20–40 parts per million is generally the first therapeutic intervention, with a rapid response seen in those who respond. Other potential

inhaled agents are iloprost (a prostacyclin derivative) and milrinone (a type 3 phosphodiesterase inhibitor). Iloprost has been shown to be as effective as NO, however, they do not act synergistically [41]. Iloprost [42] may be advantageous with less toxic side effects, easier mode of delivery, and the option of long-term treatment. Resistance to treatment suggests a residual, fixed anatomical lesion and should prompt further imaging [43].

The use of prophylactic intravenous milrinone following cardiopulmonary bypass may attenuate pulmonary hypertension by increasing smooth muscle cAMP in the pulmonary arteries [44]. It is a valuable adjunct to treatment in cases of impaired ventricular function where positive cardiac inotropy without pulmonary vasopressor activity is required. Animal models have demonstrated that inhaled milrinone causes less tachycardia, and less intrapulmonary shunting when compared to the intravenous form [45]. Hypoxia secondary to intrapulmonary shunting is a well-described phenomenon, whereby the use of a nonselective pulmonary vasodilator prevents hypoxic vasoconstriction in areas of impaired ventilation [40].

Cyclic GMP is one of the mediators of vasorelaxation in the pulmonary vascular bed and is catabolized by specific members of the phosphodiesterase family. The most widely studied of these is phosphodiesterase type 5A, which is abundant in the pulmonary vasculature [46]. Sildenafil is an inhibitor of phosphodiesterase type 5A, which is available in both oral and intravenous forms. It has been shown to attenuate hypoxic pulmonary hypertension when administered 1 h before the onset of hypoxia [47]. Some studies suggest that it is useful for weaning inhaled NO and to alleviate rebound pulmonary hypertension on withdrawal [48]. The intravenous form of sildenafil is a potent pulmonary vasodilator which is as effective as inhaled NO, also augmenting its effects with concomitant use. However, intravenous sildenafil when used at higher doses can cause systemic hypotension and hypoxia secondary to increased intrapulmonary shunting, an effect which is not reversed by inhaled NO [25].

The use of preoperative and intraoperative glucocorticoids has been associated with an improvement in cardiac and pulmonary function following cardiopulmonary bypass. Glucocorticoids suppress transcription and translation of inflammatory cytokines, and alter the expression of other proteins, such as endothelin-1 and inhibitor kappa beta [49]. Animal data has demonstrated that administration of glucocorticoids 6 h before and during cardiopulmonary bypass, decreases pulmonary edema, endothelin-1 levels, myeloperoxidase activity, and nuclear factor kappa beta activity [49]. More importantly, glucocorticoids administered 6 h before cardiopulmonary bypass completely prevented the subsequent rise in pulmonary vascular resistance. [49]

The use of modified ultrafiltration transiently improves hemodynamics, lung compliance, and pulmonary vascular resistance following cardiopulmonary bypass [50]. It remains unclear whether the improvement in pulmonary vascular resistance and lung compliance is related to the removal of excess fluid or the removal of proinflammatory cytokines [51]. The majority of studies are consistent in showing immediate improvements in pulmonary compliance and pulmonary vascular resistance however the effects are not sustained for longer than 12 h [52]. In addition, the magnitude of improved lung function and decreased pulmonary vascular resistance may depend on the method of ultrafiltration used [53].

22.7 Conclusion

Over the last decade we have seen a dramatic reduction in the amount of clinically significant postoperative pulmonary hypertension. Elevated pulmonary vascular resistance, however, continues to contribute significantly toward morbidity from cardiopulmonary bypass. Our understanding of the pathophysiology involved in the last decade has prompted the investigation of new therapeutic approaches, such as endothelin blockade, inhaled iloprost, and phosphodiesterase inhibitors. There are many more pathways involved in cardiopulmonary bypass-induced lung injury which have yet to be explored clinically. The focus of the future will no doubt focus on translating therapies based on the molecular genetics of the ischemia reperfusion injury into clinical useful treatments.

References

1. Champsaur GL, Sokol DM, Trusler GA, Mustard WT. Repair of transposition of the great arteries in 123 pediatric patients: early and long-term results. Circulation. 1973;47(5):1032–41.
2. Lindberg L, Olsson AK, Jogi P, Jonmarker C. How common is severe pulmonary hypertension after pediatric cardiac surgery? J Thorac Cardiovasc Surg. 2002;123(6):1155–63.
3. Goldman AP, Delius RE, Deanfield JE, de Leval MR, Sigston PE, Macrae DJ. Nitric oxide might reduce the need for extracorporeal support in children with critical postoperative pulmonary hypertension. Ann Thorac Surg. 1996;62(3):750–5.
4. Brown KL, Ridout DA, Goldman AP, Hoskote A, Penny DJ. Risk factors for long intensive care unit stay after cardiopulmonary bypass in children. Crit Care Med. 2003;31(1):28–33.
5. Bando K, Turrentine MW, Sharp TG, et al. Pulmonary hypertension after operations for congenital heart disease: analysis of risk factors and management. J Thorac Cardiovasc Surg. 1996;112(6):1600–7; discussion 7–9.
6. Beghetti M, Black SM, Fineman JR. Endothelin-1 in congenital heart disease. Pediatric Research. 2005;57:16R-20R.
7. Nyhan DP, Redmond JM, Gillinov AM, Nishiwaki K, Murray PA. Prolonged pulmonary vascular hyperreactivity in conscious dogs after cardiopulmonary bypass. J Appl Physiol. 1994;77(4):1584–90.
8. Schulze-Neick I, Werner H, Penny DJ, Alexi-Meskishvili V, Lange PE. Acute ventilatory restriction in children after weaning off inhaled nitric oxide: relation to rebound pulmonary hypertension. Intensive Care Med. 1999;25(1):76–80.
9. Schulze-Neick I, Penny DJ, Derrick GP, et al. Pulmonary vascular-bronchial interactions: acute reduction in pulmonary blood flow alters lung mechanics. Heart. 2000;84(3):284–9.
10. Allison RC, Kyle J, Adkins WK, Prasad VR, McCord JM, Taylor AE. Effect of ischemia reperfusion or hypoxia reoxygenation on lung vascular permeability and resistance. J Appl Physiol. 1990;69(2):597–603.
11. Suzuki T, Fukuda T, Ito T, Inoue Y, Cho Y, Kashima I. Continuous pulmonary perfusion during cardiopulmonary bypass prevents lung injury in infants. Ann Thorac Surg. 2000;69(2):602–6.
12. Redington AN. Protecting the heart and other organs after cardiac surgery: old problems, new solutions? Cardiol Young. 2004;14(2):182–91.
13. Ross SD, Kron IL, Gangemi JJ, et al. Attenuation of lung reperfusion injury after transplantation using an inhibitor of nuclear factor-kappaB. Am J Physiol Lung Cell Mol Physiol. 2000;279(3):L528–36.
14. Schulze-Neick I, Li J, Reader JA, Shekerdemian L, Redington AN, Penny DJ. The endothelin antagonist BQ123 reduces pulmonary vascular resistance after surgical intervention for congenital heart disease. J Thorac Cardiovasc Surg. 2002;124(3):435–41.
15. La M, Reid JJ. Endothelin-1 and the regulation of vascular tone. Clin Exp Pharmacol Physiol. 1995;22(5):315–23.
16. Reddy VM, Hendricks-Munoz KD, Rajasinghe HA, Petrossian E, Hanley FL, Fineman JR. Post-cardiopulmonary bypass pulmonary hypertension in lambs with increased pulmonary blood flow. A role for endothelin 1. Circulation. 1997;95(4):1054–61.
17. Adatia I, Barrow SE, Stratton PD, Miall-Allen VM, Ritter JM, Haworth SG. Thromboxane A2 and prostacyclin biosynthesis in children and adolescents with pulmonary vascular disease. Circulation. 1993;88(5 Pt 1):2117–22.
18. Lazor R, Feihl F, Waeber B, Kucera P, Perret C. Endothelin-1 does not mediate the endothelium-dependent hypoxic contractions of small pulmonary arteries in rats. Chest. 1996;110(1):189–97.
19. Schulze-Neick I, Penny DJ, Rigby ML, et al. L-arginine and substance P reverse the pulmonary endothelial dysfunction caused by congenital heart surgery. Circulation. 1999;100(7):749–55.
20. Atz AM, Adatia I, Wessel DL. Rebound pulmonary hypertension after inhalation of nitric oxide. Ann Thorac Surg. 1996;62(6):1759–64.
21. Furchgott RF, Zawadzki JV. The obligatory role of endothelial cells in the relaxation of arterial smooth muscle by acetylcholine. Nature. 1980;288(5789):373–6.
22. Palmer RM, Ferrige AG, Moncada S. Nitric oxide release accounts for the biological activity of endothelium-derived relaxing factor. Nature. 1987;327(6122):524–6.
23. Roberts JD, Jr., Lang P, Bigatello LM, Vlahakes GJ, Zapol WM. Inhaled nitric oxide in congenital heart disease. Circulation. 1993;87(2):447–53.

24. Serraf A, Aznag H, Baudet B, et al. Pulmonary vascular endothelial growth factor and nitric oxide interaction during total cardiopulmonary bypass in neonatal pigs. J Thorac Cardiovasc Surg. 2003;125(5):1050–7.

25. Stocker C, Penny DJ, Brizard CP, Cochrane AD, Soto R, Shekerdemian LS. Intravenous sildenafil and inhaled nitric oxide: a randomised trial in infants after cardiac surgery. Intensive Care Med. 2003;29(11):1996–2003.

26. Chen YF, Oparil S. Endothelial dysfunction in the pulmonary vascular bed. Am J Med Sci. 2000;320(4):223–32.

27. Kamper AM, Paul LC, Blauw GJ. Prostaglandins are involved in acetylcholine- and 5-hydroxytryptamine-induced, nitric oxide-mediated vasodilatation in human forearm. J Cardiovasc Pharmacol. 2002;40(6):922–9.

28. Cogolludo A, Moreno L, Bosca L, Tamargo J, Perez-Vizcaino F. Thromboxane A2-induced inhibition of voltage-gated K + channels and pulmonary vasoconstriction: role of protein kinase Czeta. Circ Res. 2003;93(7):656–63.

29. Adatia I, Barrow SE, Stratton PD, Ritter JM, Haworth SG. Effect of intracardiac repair on biosynthesis of thromboxane A2 and prostacyclin in children with a left to right shunt. Br Heart J. 1994;72(5):452–6.

30. Enns D, Karmazyn M, Mair J, Lercher A, Kountchev J, Belcastro A. Calpain, calpastatin activities and ratios during myocardial ischemia-reperfusion. Mol Cell Biochem. 2002;241(1–2):29–35.

31. Duffy JY, Schwartz SM, Lyons JM, et al. Calpain inhibition decreases endothelin-1 levels and pulmonary hypertension after cardiopulmonary bypass with deep hypothermic circulatory arrest. Crit Care Med. 2005;33(3):623–8.

32. McDonald MC, Mota-Filipe H, Paul A, et al. Calpain inhibitor I reduces the activation of nuclear factor-kappaB and organ injury/dysfunction in hemorrhagic shock. Faseb J. 2001;15(1):171–86.

33. Kharbanda RK, Mortensen UM, White PA, et al. Transient limb ischemia induces remote ischemic preconditioning in vivo. Circulation. 2002;106(23):2881–3.

34. Kharbanda RK, Li J, Konstantinov I, et al. Remote ischaemic preconditioning protects against cardiopulmonary bypass induced tissue injury - a preclinical study. Heart. 2006.

35. Evora PR, Pearson PJ, Schaff HV. Arginine vasopressin induces endothelium-dependent vasodilatation of the pulmonary artery. V1-receptor-mediated production of nitric oxide. Chest. 1993;103(4):1241–5.

36. Voelkel NF, Vandivier RW, Tuder RM. Vascular endothelial growth factor in the lung. Am J Physiol Lung Cell Mol Physiol. 2006;290(2):L209–21.

37. Shweiki D, Itin A, Soffer D, Keshet E. Vascular endothelial growth factor induced by hypoxia may mediate hypoxia-initiated angiogenesis. Nature. 1992;359(6398):843–5.

38. Wheller J, George BL, Mulder DG, Jarmakani JM. Diagnosis and management of postoperative pulmonary hypertensive crisis. Circulation. 1979;60(7):1640–4.

39. Chang AC, Zucker HA, Hickey PR, Wessel DL. Pulmonary vascular resistance in infants after cardiac surgery: role of carbon dioxide and hydrogen ion. Crit Care Med. 1995;23(3):568–74.

40. Schulze-Neick I, Hartenstein P, Li J, et al. Intravenous sildenafil is a potent pulmonary vasodilator in children with congenital heart disease. Circulation. 2003;108 Suppl 1:II167–73.

41. Rimensberger PC, Spahr-Schopfer I, Berner M, et al. Inhaled nitric oxide versus aerosolized iloprost in secondary pulmonary hypertension in children with congenital heart disease: vasodilator capacity and cellular mechanisms. Circulation. 2001; 103(4):544–8.

42. Fortier S, DeMaria RG, Lamarche Y, et al. Inhaled prostacyclin reduces cardiopulmonary bypass-induced pulmonary endothelial dysfunction via increased cyclic adenosine monophosphate levels. J Thorac Cardiovasc Surg. 2004;128(1): 109–16.

43. Beghetti M, Morris K, Cox P, Bohn D, Adatia I. Inhaled nitric oxide differentiates pulmonary vasospasm from vascular obstruction after surgery for congenital heart disease. Intensive Care Med. 1999;25(10):1126–30.

44. Hoffman TM, Wernovsky G, Atz AM, et al. Efficacy and safety of milrinone in preventing low cardiac output syndrome in infants and children after corrective surgery for congenital heart disease. Circulation. 2003;107(7):996–1002.

45. Lamarche Y, Malo O, Thorin E, et al. Inhaled but not intravenous milrinone prevents pulmonary endothelial dysfunction after cardiopulmonary bypass. J Thorac Cardiovasc Surg. 2005;130(1):83–92.

46. Rybalkin SD, Yan C, Bornfeldt KE, Beavo JA. Cyclic GMP phosphodiesterases and regulation of smooth muscle function. Circ Res. 2003;93(4):280–91.

47. Zhao L, Mason NA, Morrell NW, et al. Sildenafil inhibits hypoxia-induced pulmonary hypertension. Circulation. 2001; 104(4):424–8.

48. Atz AM, Wessel DL. Sildenafil ameliorates effects of inhaled nitric oxide withdrawal. Anesthesiology. 1999;91(1):307–10.

49. Pearl JM, Schwartz SM, Nelson DP, et al. Preoperative glucocorticoids decrease pulmonary hypertension in piglets after cardiopulmonary bypass and circulatory arrest. Ann Thorac Surg. 2004;77(3):994–1000.

50. Bando K, Turrentine MW, Vijay P, et al. Effect of modified ultrafiltration in high-risk patients undergoing operations for congenital heart disease. Ann Thorac Surg. 1998;66(3):821–7; discussion 8.

51. Pearl JM, Manning PB, McNamara JL, Saucier MM, Thomas DW. Effect of modified ultrafiltration on plasma thromboxane B2, leukotriene B4, and endothelin-1 in infants undergoing cardiopulmonary bypass. Ann Thorac Surg. 1999;68(4): 1369–75.

52. Mahmoud AB, Burhani MS, Hannef AA, Jamjoom AA, Al-Githmi IS, Baslaim GM. Effect of modified ultrafiltration on pulmonary function after cardiopulmonary bypass. Chest. 2005;128(5):3447–53.

53. Kirshbom PM, Page SO, Jacobs MT, et al. Cardiopulmonary bypass and circulatory arrest increase endothelin-1 production and receptor expression in the lung. J Thorac Cardiovasc Surg. 1997;113(4):777–83.

Ventilatory Management of the Failing Right Heart

23

Desmond Bohn

The development in our knowledge and understanding of cardiovascular and respiratory physiology has tended to proceed along parallel lines. However, many of the texts on cardiac physiology have tended to underestimate the major hemodynamic changes that occur during the transit of blood through the thoracic cavity from the venous to the arterial side of the circulation. Since the heart and lungs share the same body cavity, changes in pleural pressure associated with either spontaneous or mechanical ventilation have important effects on preload or afterload of both ventricles. With the development of intensive care and in particular positive pressure ventilation (PPV), we now have a greater appreciation that the heart and lungs are more than two independent but connected systems, and events that occur in either organ will impact on the other. In congenital heart disease this is best exemplified in obstructive right heart disease and palliated single ventricle with cavopulmonary shunts.

23.1 Ventilation and Cardiac Function in the Normal Heart

Perhaps the easiest way to begin to understand the fundamentals of the complex interaction between the systemic and pulmonary circulations within the thorax is to use a model of two pumps connected in series, enclosed within a chamber where the pressure is constantly changing. The reservoir for the filling of the right heart lies partly outside the thorax and is consequently subject to atmospheric or intra-abdominal pressure (eg. the inferior vena cava), whereas some of the large venous connections (eg. the superior vena cava) are intrathoracic

and subject to pleural pressure. On the other hand, the reservoir for left heart filling (the pulmonary circulation) and the systemic pumping chamber lie entirely within the thorax, although the pump ejects against a high impedance which is largely extrathoracic (systemic vascular resistance). Since pleural pressure is constantly changing during the respiratory cycle, it follows that the resulting fluctuations in intrathoracic pressure will affect the output from the pump by altering preload or filling on the right side and afterload or ejection on the left side.

The interaction between respiratory and cardiac function is a complex one with major differences occurring under conditions of spontaneous or positive pressure respiration. These are illustrated in Fig. 23.1, which shows hemodynamic pressure changes during ventilation. The dashed lines represent the inspiratory phase of the respiratory cycle. During spontaneous breathing, pleural pressure becomes negative during inspiration, increasing the pressure gradient for venous return, transmural right atrial pressure (Pra_{tm}) rises and right ventricular stroke volume (SV_{RV}) increases. Coincidently, there is a transient fall in left ventricular stroke volume (SV_{LV}), which is then augmented within a couple of cardiac cycles. The reasons suggested for this include the pooling of blood in the pulmonary circulation due to lung expansion, right heart filling causing a change in left ventricular diastolic compliance or increased afterload on the left ventricle due to negative intrathoracic pressure. Positive inspiratory pressure on the other hand leads to a fall in Pra_{tm} as the rise in intrathoracic pressure decreases the gradient for venous return, filling of the atrium is impeded, and SV_{RV} falls, but there is a phase lag before this reduction is seen in the left heart. As intrathoracic pressure increases there is a very transient rise in SV_{LV} due to either reduced afterload on the LV or enhanced flow from pulmonary capillaries to the LA associated with the increase in intrathoracic pressure. This is more than offset by the subsequent fall in SV_{LV} as right-sided events become predominant.

D. Bohn (✉)
The Department of Critical Care Medicine, The Hospital for Sick Children, 555 University Ave, Toronto, Ontario, M5G 1X8
e-mail: desmond.bohn@sickkids.ca

A.N. Redington et al. (eds.), *Congenital Diseases in the Right Heart*, DOI 10.1007/978-1-84800-378-1_23,
© Springer-Verlag London Limited 2009

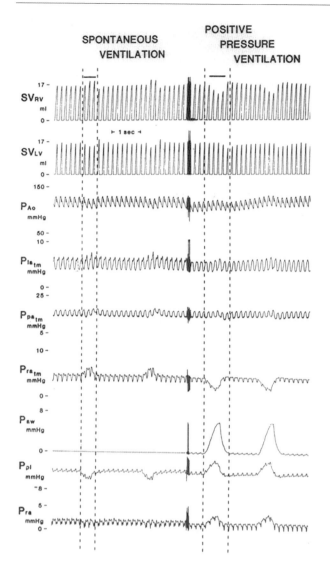

SPONTANEOUS VENTILATION

POSITIVE PRESSURE VENTILATION

Fig. 23.1 Changes in hemodynamics associated with spontaneous and positive pressure ventilation (PPV) in the normal human
The area between the dashed lines represents the inspiratory phase. The reduction in pleural pressure during spontaneous inspiration increases right atrial filling and the right atrial pressure rises, together with right ventricular stroke volume. There is a simultaneous fall in left ventricular stroke volume. During PPV, as right heart filling decreases, LV stroke volume rises. For a more detailed explanation see text.
From Pinsky MR: Cardiopulmonary Interactions in Cardiopulmonary Critical Care, 2nd edition. Dantzker DR ed. WB Saunders Philadelphia 1991

Cournaud in 1948 published one of the classic physiological studies on cardiopulmonary interactions, in which he demonstrated that positive pressure respiration (delivered by face mask) in normal subjects resulted in a fall in cardiac output due to decreased venous filling of the right heart [1]. Furthermore, he was able to show a relationship between the level of mean airway pressure (MAP) pressure and the fall in cardiac output, the lower MAP the lesser the effect. These fundamental observations are as relevant today as they were 50 years ago when approaching ventilation in patients with right heart dysfunction.

23.2 Ventilation and Total Cavopulmonary Connections

Understanding the relationship between ventilation and cardiac function is of fundamental importance in the management of patients with single ventricle physiology and cavopulmonary connections. In this type of reconstruction, pulmonary blood flow occurs predominantly during diastole and is highly preload dependent. PPV used in the post operative period, particularly when used with positive end-expiratory pressure (PEEP,) impedes venous return and has an adverse effect on cardiac output [2]. Indeed, in his original paper describing the operation of atriopulmonary connection for tricuspid atresia, Fontan made the comment that "respiratory assistance should be stopped early because positive pressure prevents venous return" [3].

Important new insights into that have improved our understanding of the cardiorespiratory physiology and how ventilation can change hemodynamics have come from a series of investigations done by Redington and colleagues at the Royal Brompton Hospital. In a series of patients with left atrial isomerism studied remotely following total cavopulmonary anastomosis, they showed that there is significant augmentation of the pulmonary blood flow Doppler signal during the inspiratory (negative pleural pressure) phase of spontaneous respiration [4] (Fig. 23.2). The application of a Valsava maneuver resulted in complete obliteration of the pulmonary blood flow, while the large negative pleural pressure produced by a Mueller maneuver gave rise to augmentation of the signal. Penny [5] in a study on patients with a Fontan circuit found a 35% augmentation of pulmonary blood flow during the inspiratory phase of spontaneous respiration breathing.

The implication from these studies is that positive intrathoracic (pleural) pressure impedes pulmonary blood flow, while negative pressure increases it. The logical next step was to compare negative pressure breathing with PPV in patients with cavopulmonary anastomosis. The device used to deliver negative pressure ventilation was a Hayek oscillator, which is a cuirass respirator enclosing the chest and upper abdomen and delivers a continuous negative pleural pressure. In a series of studies, the authors demonstrated when they applied positive and negative extrathoracic pressure to Fontan patients that while positive pressure resulted in retrograde blood flow away from the lungs, negative extrathoracic pressure increased pulmonary blood flow, and therefore cardiac output [6, 7]. These studies were extended by Shekerdemian and colleagues, where conventional PPV in intubated patients was compared with continuous negative pleural pressure

Fig. 23.2 The effect of changes in intrathoracic pressure on pulmonary blood flow in patients following total cavopulmonary connection measured by Doppler. During the Mueller maneuver (top), the flow signal is augmented, while during the Valsalva (lower) it decreases
From Redington AN: Pulmonary blood flow after total cavopulmonary shunt. Br Heart J. 1991;65:213

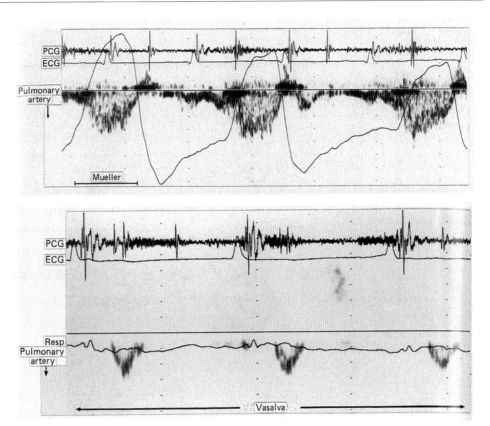

delivered by the Hayek oscillator [8]. Positive and negative pressure ventilation was compared in 18 post-Fontan patients (nine acute postoperatively and nine convalescent during cardiac catheterization). They again found that switching to NPV was associated with a significant increase in PBF (54%), SvO$_2$, and stroke volume, and that this improvement was maintained over an extended period. Attempts have also been made to see if high-frequency, low tidal-volume ventilation would confer any benefit on cardiac output following the Fontan operation. Meliones compared high-frequency jet ventilation (HFJV) with conventional ventilation (CMV), patients being ventilated to the same PaCO$_2$ levels (27 mmHg) [9]. This was achieved with a 50% lower MAP on jet ventilation and this resulted in a 25% increase in cardiac output and a 59% reduction in pulmonary vascular resistance. In a second study where high-frequency oscillatory ventilation (HFOV) was compared with CMV at similar (low) MAPs, no difference in cardiac output or PVR was found [10].

23.3 Ventilation and Obstructive Right Heart Lesions

Patients who undergo surgical reconstruction of obstructive right heart lesions constitute another group where changes in intrathoracic pressure have important effects on venous

return and PBF. These would include patients with tetralogy of Fallot and pulmonary atresia. Diastolic right ventricular dysfunction is a common finding following surgical repair of severe right ventricular outflow tract obstruction and is characterized by a pulsed Doppler signal showing antegrade pulmonary artery flow during atrial systole accompanied by retrograde flow in the superior vena cava [11, 12]. This is due to the fact that right ventricular end-diastolic pressure exceeds pulmonary artery diastolic pressure due to the stiffness of right ventricle. There is premature opening of the pulmonary valve and the RV acts as a passive conduit between the right atrium and the pulmonary artery (Fig. 23.3). In a study by Cullen [13] of postoperative tetralogy patients, half had this feature and those that did had a higher incidence of ascites and pleural effusions and longer durations of ICU stay. He also made the important observation that during the inspiratory phase of PPV the Doppler signal of antegrade flow in the pulmonary artery was obliterated, and there was a decrease in the flow signal across the tricuspid valve (Fig. 23.4). This again gives rise to speculation that NPV might actually improve cardiac output and PBF in children following biventricular repairs. In an initial study, Shekerdemian and colleagues compared positive with negative pressure in otherwise healthy children undergoing catheterization and PDA closure with seven children in ICU who had undergo biventricular repair of CHD [14]. They found that NPV was associated with a significant increase in

Fig. 23.3 Pulmonary artery
Doppler flow (A) in a patient
with tetralogy of Fallot and
restrictive RV physiology
demonstrating antegrade PA
diastolic flow (arrow). The effect
of PPV on trans-tricuspid
(middle panel B) and pulmonary
artery (lower panel B) Doppler
flow. During the inspiratory
phase of PPV there is diminution
of peak velocity flow and the
obliteration of antegrade
diastolic flow
*From Cullen S: Characterisation
of right ventricular diastolic
performance after complete repair
of tetralogy of Fallot Circulation.
1995;91:1782*

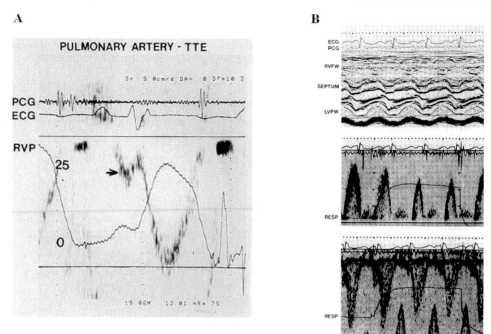

cardiac output in the postoperative patients. They further conducted a series of acute studies in 11 patients after repair of tetralogy or the Fontan operation [15]. Patients were switched from positive pressure to negative pressure ventilation for 15-min periods, while cardiac output, PBF, and oxygen consumption were measured by the Fick equation and mass spectrometry. NPV was associated with a 46% increase in PBF, a 48% increase in stroke volume, and a 4.6% increase in SVO2. Similar to the extended studies in the Fontan patients, they did a series of short-term (15 min) and extended trials of NPV in 23 children who had undergone repair of tetralogy, eight of whom had restrictive right ventricular physiology [16]. These patients were characterized by antegrade diastolic pulmonary artery flow and had a more significant degree of metabolic acidosis compared with their nonrestrictive peers. By the end of 45 min of NPV, pulmonary blood flow had increased by 67% in the group as a whole but interestingly the improvement trend was lower in the restrictive group. The beneficial effect was lost when patients were switched back to PPV.

23.4 Implications for Postoperative Management

What are the implications of these studies using negative pressure ventilation for the postoperative management of patients with Fontan and tetralogy with restrictive right ventricular physiology? It is unlikely that negative pressure ventilation will become a standard method for postoperative respiratory support. All these studies were done with patients intubated, anesthetized, and on pressure-support ventilation. The device requires a significant amount of expertise to efficiently operate in the postoperative period and cannot be used unless the sternum is intact. However, these studies do demonstrate an important physiological principle, that is, that all other things being equal spontaneous breathing is a preferred option over PPV in this patient group. The goal should be early weaning and the reestablishment of spontaneous breathing progressing toward early extubation [17] on the assumption that this would have a beneficial effect on venous return and pulmonary blood flow, echoing the comments made by Fontan himself 35 years ago [3]. Our postoperative management strategy is to leave postoperative Fontan and tetralogy patients intubated but start short-acting sedative/analgesic infusions in the operating room prior to transfer to ICU. If there are no bleeding complications, rhythm disturbances, or other factors that would preclude early extubation, sedation is discontinued, and patients are extubated within 6–8 h of returning from the operating room. If low cardiac output or other postoperative complications prevent this plan from being implemented, then a ventilation strategy based on minimizing mean airway pressures would seem logical.

It should also be borne in mind that, with increased numbers of children with single ventricle lesions surviving

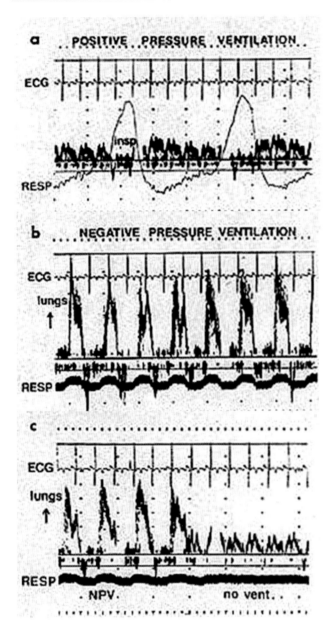

Fig. 23.4 The effect of (a) positive and (b) negative pressure ventilation in a patient after the Fontan operation. During the positive pressure inspiration antegrade pulmonary artery flow is lost, while there is a marked increase during negative pressure inspiration. The augmentation of pulmonary blood flow was lost when the negative pressure cuirass was removed (c)
From Shekerdemian LS: Negative-pressure ventilation improves cardiac output after right heart surgery. Circulation. 1996;94[suppl II] II-49

the third-stage reconstruction and into adulthood, there are important messages to be learned from these studies by practitioners administering anesthesia to patients with Fontan physiology, namely, the importance of maintaining adequate filling pressures and using low intrathoracic pressure ventilation [18].

23.5 Ventilation and the Bidirectional Superior Cavopulmonary Anastomosis (BCPS)

A second group of patients where there have been important new insights into cardiopulmonary interactions are those following the bidirectional cavopulmonary shunt operation (BCPS), performed as a second-stage reconstruction for single ventricle lesions. In this operation, the superior vena cava is disconnected from the right atrium and anastomosed to the pulmonary artery. This places the cerebral and pulmonary circulations in series. Pulmonary blood flow is dependent on venous return from the head, neck, and upper limbs. Oxygenation depends on an adequate transpulmonary pressure gradient between the SVC and the pulmonary capillaries. Typically, the postoperative systemic saturation is in the region of 80%. For patients in whom saturations fail to reach the expected level after the BCPS, the diagnostic algorithm is outlined in Table 23.1.

Having excluded the anatomical causes that may be responsible, the traditional therapeutic approach has been, having ensured an adequate filling (right atrial) pressure, to assume that this is a downstream problem due to an increased pulmonary vascular resistance and to attempt to reduce it by inducing an alkalosis with hyperventilation, with or without inhaled nitric oxide (iNO). However, there is little evidence to show that iNO has any beneficial effect on pulmonary vascular resistance following a BCPS as measured by an increase in SvO_2, PaO_2, or SaO_2, despite a minor decrease in Pa pressure [19]. There is also the possibility that the increase in mean airway pressure associated with hyperventilation may actually result in an increase in pulmonary vascular resistance. One might also draw the conclusion that the problem does not lie downstream from the pulmonary artery, and the focus should shift to in the inflow side of the cavopulmonary connection. Bradley and colleagues reasoned that since hyperventilation by lowering the $PaCO_2$ actually results in a decrease in cerebral blood flow, this might adversely effect pulmonary blood flow and oxygen delivery [20]. They studied a series of 13 postoperative

Table 23.1 Causes of hypoxemia following BCPS

Cyanosis with elevated (>18 mm Hg) SVC (PA) pressure
• High underlying PVR
• Kinking or distortion of SVC/PA anastomosis
Cyanosis with *normal* SVC (PA) pressure
• Decompressing venous collaterals
• Pulmonary arteriovenous malformations
• Baffle leak (hemi-Fontan)
• Pulmonary parenchymal disease

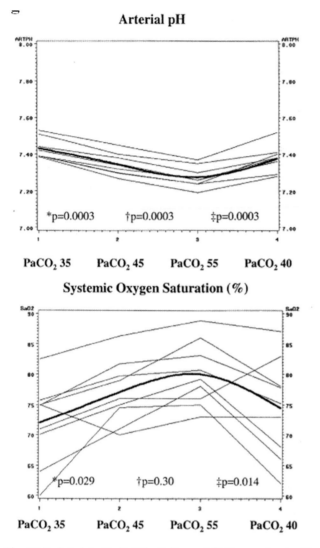

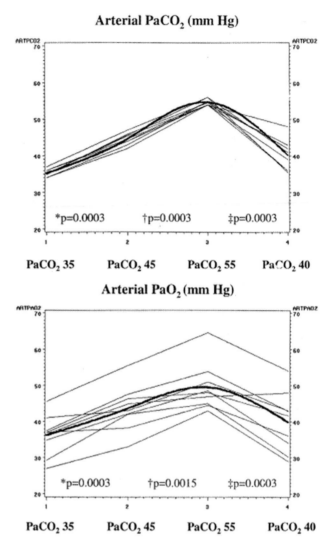

Fig. 23.5 Arterial pH, PaCO₂, SaO₂, and PaO₂ associated with various levels of hypercarbia in nine patients following BCPS
The lines represent individual patients, while the bold line indicates the mean value

From Hoskote A. The effects of carbon dioxide on oxygenation and systemic, cerebral and pulmonary vascular hemodynamics after bidirectional superior cavopulmonary anastomosis. J Am Coll Cardiol. 2004;44:1501

BCPS patients (nine hemi-Fontan patients). Hyperventilation was induced by increasing the respiratory rate while keeping the tidal volume constant. The PaCO₂ fell from 50 mmHg to 33 mmHg, while pH increased from 7.38 to 7.5. This resulted in a fall in PaO₂, SaO₂, and an increase in upper body a-vDO₂. In addition, they measured cerebral blood flow velocity by transcranial Doppler and showed that this decreased with hyperventilation. These findings reversed when patients were changed back to baseline ventilation. The proposed mechanism was an alkalosis-induced cerebral vasoconstriction resulting in lower SVC blood flow. They then reasoned that, since hyperventilation decreased PBF, hypoventilation might actually improve it. In a second series of studies, they induced hypercabia by decreasing the ventilator rate and compared this with a metabolic alkalosis induced by

bicarbonate and ventilation to baseline normocarbia [21]. Hypoventilation resulted in improved systemic saturation, PaO₂, reduced a-vDO₂, and increased cerebral blood-flow velocity. Metabolic alkalosis resulted in no significant change compared with baseline ventilation. In both these studies, mean airway pressure changed with the increases and decreases in ventilator rate.

These studies left unanswered whether the improvements in oxygenation whether hypercarbia improves oxygenation and O₂ delivery by increasing total cardiac output or by selectively increasing CBF. There was also the issue of what effect the change in mean airway pressure might have had in Bradley's studies. These issues were addressed in a study by Hoskote where hypercarbia was induced by the addition of CO₂ to the inspiratory gas flow of the ventilator, while other parameters were unchanged

Transcranial A V O₂ difference

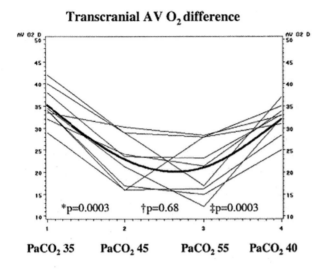

NIRS - Tissue Oxygenation Index

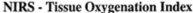
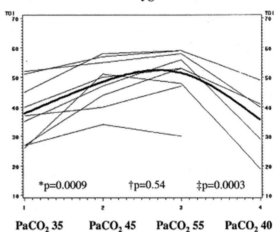

Transcranial Doppler Peak velocity (cm/sec)

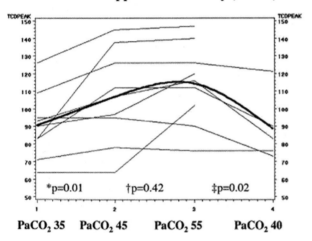

Transcranial Doppler Mean velocity (cm/sec)

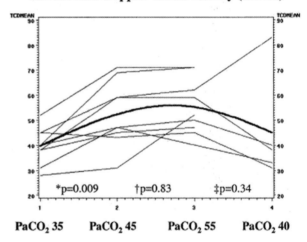

Fig. 23.6 Transcranial arteriovenous oxygen difference, NIRS tissue oxygen index, peak transcranial Doppler velocity, and mean transcranial Doppler velocity at various levels of hypercarbia *From Hoskote A. The effects of carbon dioxide on oxygenation and systemic, cerebral and pulmonary vascular hemodynamics after bidirectional superior cavopulmonary anastomosis. J Am Coll Cardiol. 2004;44:1501*

[22]. CBF was measured by near-infrared spectroscopy and transcranial Doppler, and blood samples were obtained from a jugular venous bulb, PA, and femoral catheters. Patients were studied at PaCO₂ levels of 35, 45, 55 mmHg and then on return to 40 mmHg. Arterial PaO₂, SaO₂, cerebral oxygen saturation and systemic oxygen delivery increased at PaCO₂ levels of 45 mmHg and 55 mmHg compared with 35 mm Hg (Figs. 23.5 and 23.6). This beneficial effect was lost when PaCO₂ levels returned to 40 mmHg. Furthermore, hypercarbia resulted in reduced oxygen consumption and decreased arterial lactate concentrations in this patient group [23]. It can be concluded from these studies that hypercarbia post-BCPS improves both cardiac output and cerebral blood flow and that hypocarbia has the opposite effect.

23.6 Implications for Postoperative Management

These studies suggest that the traditional approach to hypoxemia after BCPS of using hyperventilation is not only ineffective, but may be harmful. The management algorithm for postoperative hypoxemia in these patients should include a diligent search to exclude anatomical obstruction in at the level of the cavopulmonary anastomosis and a bubble study to exclude decompressing venous collaterals. The optimum ventilation strategy is moderate hypercarbia (PaCO₂ 55 mmHg) with a pH in the region of 7.35, proceeding to early extubation with the expectation that the combination of spontaneous respiration and hypercarbia will augment PBF.

23.7 Summary

The optimal ventilatory management of patients with right heart failure or single ventricle physiology requires a fundamental understanding of the physiological principles that govern the interaction between breathing and circulation. Emphasis needs to be placed on the importance of the potential for adverse hemodynamic effects of positive intrathoracic pressure, and how negative pleural pressure and hypercarbia can enhance cardiac output and pulmonary blood flow rather than the traditional approaches to PPV and normal blood-gas values.

References

1. Cournand A, Motley H, Werko L, Richards D. Physiological studies of the effect of intermittent positive pressure breathing on cardiac output in man. Am J Physiol. 1948;152: 162–74.
2. Williams DB, Kiernan PD, Metke MP, Marsh HM, Danielson GK. Hemodynamic response to positive end-expiratory pressure following right atrium-pulmonary artery bypass (Fontan procedure). J Thorac Cardiovasc Surg. Jun 1984;87(6): 856–61.
3. Fontan F, Baudet E. Surgical repair of tricuspid atresia. Thorax. May 1971;26(3):240–8.
4. Redington AN, Penny D, Shinebourne EA. Pulmonary blood flow after total cavopulmonary shunt. Br Heart J. Apr 1991;65(4):213–7.
5. Penny DJ, Redington AN. Doppler echocardiographic evaluation of pulmonary blood flow after the Fontan operation: the role of the lungs. Br Heart J. Nov 1991;66(5): 372–4.
6. Penny D, Hayek Z, Reawle P, Rigby M, Redington A. Ventilation with external high frequency oscillation around a negative baseline increases pulmonary blood flow after the Fontan operation. Cardiol Young. 1992;2:277–80.
7. Penny DJ, Hayek Z, Redington AN. The effects of positive and negative extrathoracic pressure ventilation on pulmonary blood flow after the total cavopulmonary shunt procedure. Int J Cardiol. Jan 1991;30(1):128–30.
8. Shekerdemian LS, Bush A, Shore DF, Lincoln C, Redington AN. Cardiopulmonary interactions after Fontan operations: augmentation of cardiac output using negative pressure ventilation. Circulation. Dec 2 1997;96(11):3934–42.
9. Meliones JN, Bove EL, Dekeon MK, Custer JR, Moler FW, Callow LR, et al. High-frequency jet ventilation improves cardiac function after the Fontan procedure. Circulation. Nov 1991;84 Suppl 5:III364–8.
10. Kornecki A, Shekerdemian LS, Adatia I, Bohn D. High-frequency oscillation in children after Fontan operation. Pediatr Crit Care Med. Apr 2002;3(2):144–7.

11. Kisanuki A, Tei C, Otsuji Y, Natsugoe K, Kawazoe Y, Arima S, et al. Doppler echocardiographic documentation of diastolic pulmonary artery forward flow. Am J Cardiol. Mar 1 1987;59(6):711–3.
12. Redington A, Penny D, Rigby M, Hayes A. Antegrade diastolic pulmonary arterial flow as a marker of right ventricular restriction after complete repair of pulmonary atresia with intact ventricular septum and critical pulmonary valve stenosis. Cardiol Young. 1992;2:382–6.
13. Cullen S, Shore D, Redington A. Characterization of right ventricular diastolic performance after complete repair of tetralogy of Fallot. Restrictive physiology predicts slow postoperative recovery. Circulation. Mar 15 1995;91(6): 1782–9.
14. Shekerdemian LS, Bush A, Lincoln C, Shore DF, Petros AJ, Redington AN. Cardiopulmonary interactions in healthy children and children after simple cardiac surgery: the effects of positive and negative pressure ventilation. Heart. Dec 1997;78(6):587–93.
15. Shekerdemian LS, Shore DF, Lincoln C, Bush A, Redington AN. Negative-pressure ventilation improves cardiac output after right heart surgery. Circulation. Nov 1 1996;94 Suppl 9:II49–55.
16. Shekerdemian LS, Bush A, Shore DF, Lincoln C, Redington AN. Cardiorespiratory responses to negative pressure ventilation after tetralogy of fallot repair: a hemodynamic tool for patients with a low-output state. J Am Coll Cardiol. Feb 1999;33(2):549–55.
17. Shekerdemian LS, Penny DJ, Novick W. Early extubation after surgical repair of tetralogy of Fallot. Cardiol Young. Nov 2000;10(6):636–7.
18. Hosking MP, Beynen FM. The modified Fontan procedure: physiology and anesthetic implications. J Cardiothorac Vasc Anesth. Aug 1992;6(4):465–75.
19. Adatia I, Atz AM, Wessel DL. Inhaled nitric oxide does not improve systemic oxygenation after bidirectional superior cavopulmonary anastomosis. J Thorac Cardiovasc Surg. Jan 2005;129(1):217–9.
20. Bradley SM, Simsic JM, Mulvihill DM. Hyperventilation impairs oxygenation after bidirectional superior cavopulmonary connection. Circulation. Nov 10 1998;98 Suppl 19:II372–6; discussion II6–7.
21. Bradley SM, Simsic JM, Mulvihill DM. Hypoventilation improves oxygenation after bidirectional superior cavopulmonary connection. J Thorac Cardiovasc Surg. Oct 2003;126(4): 1033–9.
22. Hoskote A, Li J, Hickey C, Erickson S, Van Arsdell G, Stephens D, et al. The effects of carbon dioxide on oxygenation and systemic, cerebral, and pulmonary vascular hemodynamics after the bidirectional superior cavopulmonary anastomosis. J Am Coll Cardiol. Oct 6 2004;44(7):1501–9.
23. Li J, Hoskote A, Hickey C, Stephens D, Bohn D, Holtby H, et al. Effect of carbon dioxide on systemic oxygenation, oxygen consumption, and blood lactate levels after bidirectional superior cavopulmonary anastomosis. Crit Care Med. May 2005;33(5):984–9.

24.1 Introduction

Acute right heart dysfunction in the perioperative period following orthotopic heart transplantation is a long-recognized occurrence that contributes significantly to early post-transplant mortality and to intermediate and long-term survival [21, 23, 25, 26, 33]. Reported early postoperative mortality ranges from 14% to 26% [14, 26, 45, 46]. The cause of death is multifactorial and include both donor and recipient factors [Fig. 24.1]. Most commonly, it results from a donor heart impaired by the sequelae of brain death and ischemia-reperfusion injury, and not prepared for the increased afterload of pulmonary hypertension (PHT) and increased pulmonary vascular resistance (PVR) in the recipient. Understanding the issues from both the donor and recipient perspectives is important in order to maximize donor-organ usage and optimize recipient outcomes. Management strategies have evolved over time.

24.2 The Effect of RV Function on LV Function and Cardiac Output

The normal right ventricle (RV) has multiple anatomic and physiologic characteristics that differentiate it from the left ventricle (LV). However, the RV and LV are highly interdependent physiologically, partly due to the *shared* interventricular septum. RV failure results in dilation, ischemia, and decreased contractility. Shift of the interventricular septum toward the LV and decreased pulmonary blood flow leads to underfilling of the LV and the clinical scenario of decreased cardiac output [29]. Concurrent underperfusion of the coronary circulation further aggravates the right ventricular dysfunction and a vicious cycle ensues [22, 29]. Clinically, in the acute post-heart transplant patient, this manifests as an elevated central venous pressure and signs of decreased cardiac output including systemic hypotension that is refractory to, and often worsened, by fluid administration. Echocardiography demonstrates decreased right ventricular contractility with dilatation and varying degrees of tricuspid regurgitation [7].

24.3 What Contributes to RV Failure? [Fig. 24.1]

Figure 24.1 illustrates some of the contributing factors to right heart failure post-heart transplant. The adaptive mechanisms of the RV are not well suited to large increases in pressure. The energy efficiency related to ejection during pressure decline in the RV is lost in the face of increased afterload related to high pulmonary pressure or resistance. The effect of positive pressure ventilation on stroke volume, without and with normalization of preload, is well described, as is the impact of cardiopulmonary bypass on RV contractility. There is data from the International Society of Heart Lung Transplantation illustrating adverse outcomes from a lower donor to recipient weight ratio in the face of PHT. Even the effect of LV contraction (LV systolic function) on pressure generated in the RV an impact the clinical scenario in the early post-transplant period. Heart rate and preload are also critical in the postoperative phase.

From a donor perspective, the donor heart was accustomed to *low* or normal afterload and suddenly is faced with the PHT in the recipient (see below). Ischemia and reperfusion can significantly affect the function of both ventricles. But the bigger issues, from a donor perspective, are the effects of brain death.

A.I. Dipchand (✉)
Department of Paediatrics, Hospital for Sick Children, Toronto, ON, Canada

A.N. Redington et al. (eds.), *Congenital Diseases in the Right Heart*, DOI 10.1007/978-1-84800-378-1_24,
© Springer-Verlag London Limited 2009

What contributes to RV failure?

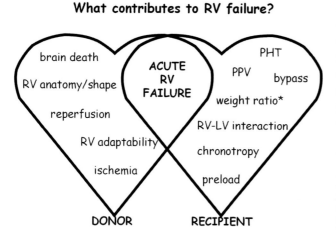

Fig. 24.1 Factors contributing to right ventricular dysfunction in the early post-transplant period LV, left ventricle; PHT, pulmonary hypertension; PPV, positive pressure ventilation; RV, right ventricle.* donor to recipient weight ratio

24.4 Impact of Brain Death

Understanding the potential effects of brain death is important clinically as it relates to (1) management of the potential organ donor with acute intracranial hypertension, (2) determination of the appropriate timing for the assessment of organ function, and (3) recognition of the potential for functional recovery and allowing time for recovery and reassessment in an organ donor.

Brain death is characterized by a unique set of physiologic responses which have varying and temporal effects on cardiac function. Acute brain death is associated with a transient massive catecholamine release or *autonomic storm*—both systemically and at the neuronal level [32, 36, 39, 41]. This is subsequently followed by significant acute right ventricular dilation and dysfunction within minutes of the acute rise in intracranial pressure [30, 34]. The magnitude of catecholamine released and the extent of myocardial injury depends on the rate of rise of intracranial pressure [41]. The cardiac dysfunction that follows is related in part to catecholamine-related myocardial injury *but* is amenable with time and appropriate intervention to functional recovery, therefore allowing for successful organ donation [18, 34]. However, it may also play a role in the early postoperative right ventricular dysfunction seen post transplant [Fig, 24.2b] [8, 48].

The reported frequency of echocardiographic myocardial dysfunction in brain-dead patients ranges from 10% to 42% [15, 19, 20]. In the largest study involving 66 brain dead patients, the presence of myocardial dysfunction could not be predicted by clinical characteristics, including etiology of brain death, time from brain injury to brain death, or need for press or support [15]. Myocardial

dysfunction was both segmental and global. Pathology demonstrated varying degrees of contraction band necrosis, a characteristic feature of neurogenic myocardial dysfunction. There was poor correlation between echocardiographic dysfunction and pathologic findings, suggesting that despite segmental wall motion abnormalities, pathologic abnormalities may be mild or absent and the myocardium may not be irreversibly damaged.

There is a well-described cardiovascular response to brainstem ischemia [8, 34, 39]. Animal experiments clearly demonstrate hypertension and bradycardia, followed by a hyperdynamic state (tachycardia and elevated cardiac output) of varying duration [8, 18, 30, 39]. Using a load-independent index in a canine brain-death model, Bittner demonstrated significant systolic biventricular dysfunction following brain death, which was more prominent in the right ventricle (37% decrease) compared with the left (22% decrease) [Fig. 24.2b]. There was a concurrent progressive increase in right ventricular end-diastolic volume. There was no evidence of myocardial ischemia or dysfunction of the β-adrenergic receptor system as possible contributory factors to the ventricular dysfunction. In fact, there was upregulation of the β-adrenergic receptor system evidenced by increased β-adrenergic receptor density, increased isoproterenol-stimulated adenylate cyclase activity, and increased sensitivity to isoproterenol. In a cohort of 40 pigs, Ryan demonstrated sympathetic storm leading to transient cardiac dysfunction that was reversible and associated with an absence of troponin release (supportive of lack of cell necrosis) [39]. In a similar pig model, Mertes demonstrated an early impaired LV contractility and a deleterious effect of rapid volume infusion on hemodynamic status [31].

In humans, White compared 10 donor hearts with dysfunction with 13 without dysfunction, and demonstrated less maximum net tension response and net contractile response to isoproterenol in RV myocardium [48]. As with Bittner, White did not demonstrate a decreased number of total β-adrenergic receptors, he did demonstrate abnormalities in receptor coupling manifested as a decrease in isoproterenol-mediated stimulation of adenylyl cyclase, a rightward shift of the isoproterenol-adenylyl cyclase dose-response curve, and a reduced β-receptor agonist-binding affinity [48]. This was felt to be consistent with desensitization to β-agonist stimulation and myocardial damage due to catecholamine storm. Finally, White used creatine kinase measurements to assess the amount of remaining viable myocardium and found no difference between the two groups, and hypothesized the possibility of myocardial recovery in the group with dysfunction.

Following the autonomic storm, a normo- to hypotensive state ensues characterized by impaired cardiac inotropy and chronotropy, impaired vascular tone, and reduced

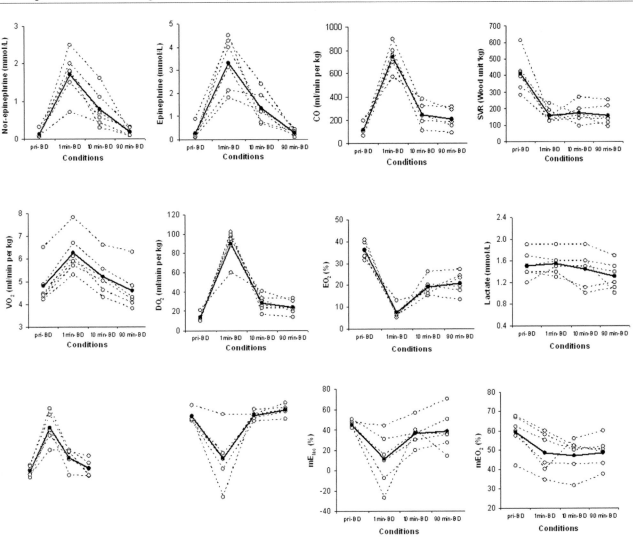

Fig. 24.2a Data obtained from six pigs: there is an initial catecholamine surge following brain death with an increase in cardiac output and decrease in systemic vascular resistance. Cardiac output then decreases back toward normal with systemic vascular resistance remaining low. This may explain the clinical observations in brain-dead patients and have implications for management of the donor. Oxygen consumption increased, but this was compensated for by an even greater increase in oxygen delivery. Oxygen extraction decreased and lactate remained low. Oxygen consumption and delivery subsequently decreased over the next 90 min. dP/dT max increased at 1 min followed by a decrease and subsequent return to baseline. Overall, systemic aerobic metabolism appeared adequate but data supported an imbalance in myocardial oxygen transport

cardiac output [30, 37]. In a pig model, Li demonstrated a significant and persistent fall in systemic vascular resistance, and a significant increase in oxygen consumption with an accompanying greater increase in oxygen delivery [Figure 24.2a]. Despite these findings, systemically there was evidence of impaired myocardial metabolism. Appropriate donor management, in this scenario, is imperative in order to optimize cardiac function and facilitate organ donation. Therapy should be directed toward restoration of intravascular volume and appropriate support of the myocardium and vascular system to ensure optimal cardiac output [40]. Detailed discussion about the optimal management of the organ donor is published elsewhere [40]. However, with

optimal management and time, unacceptable or marginal donor organs may have significant recovery of function demonstrable both clinically and by echocardiography, allowing for successful heart transplantation. The unknown factor is, despite functional recovery, the extent of microscopic ischemic myocardial damage that may contribute to acute post-transplant graft dysfunction—particularly the right ventricle.

In a human study looking at a load-independent index of right ventricular systolic and diastolic function in brain-dead donors, marked abnormalities of RV function were demonstrated.[personal communication, A. Redington, 2006] Donor hearts were significantly more dilated

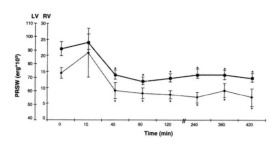

Graph showing systolic right (RV, {blacksquare}) and left ventricular (LV, {diamondsuit}) myocardial performance measured by preload-recruitable stroke work (PRSW) before (0) and after induction of brain death in 17 animals

Fig. 24.2b Significant systolic biventricular dysfunction following brain death; more prominent in the right ventricle (37% decrease) compared with the left (22% decrease)

with a lower end-systolic pressure–volume relationship (ESPVR), reflecting a reduced contractile state. With inotropic stimulation, there was no change in ESPVR but a paradoxical increase in RV end-diastolic volume–RV dilatation in the face of increased preload, an observation that has clinical implications for the management of these patients in the early postoperative period.

Both animal studies and human experience support dynamic changes in echocardiographic systolic function following brain death. Systolic dysfunction evidenced early following brain death may persuade medical personnel to forego organ transplantation. However, as noted above, there is potential for improvement. The role for serial echocardiography is supported by the literature. Kono demonstrated improvement and even resolution of segmental wall motion abnormalities over time in 12 patients with subarachnoid hemorrhage [27]. Utilizing low-dose dobutamine stress echocardiography, he then demonstrated that patients with dobutamine-responsive wall motion abnormalities normalized their ventricular function prior to death [28].

The response to brain death is of deterioration in ventricular function with the RV myocardium more affected than the LV. There is potential for functional recovery with appropriate and intensive monitoring and intervention. Repeat echocardiography is essential to reassess suitability for organ donation. Both animal and human models, despite functional recovery, provide evidence for myocardial insult and/or susceptibility to dysfunction in the acute postoperative period due to the physiologic changes resulting from progressing through brain death.

24.5 Pulmonary Hypertension and Risk Following Heart Transplant

From a recipient perspective, the major risk factor contributing to right heart dysfunction in the postoperative period is PHT. In 1971, Griepp and colleagues first

documented elevated pulmonary vascular resistance (PVR) as a risk factor for early death post-transplant from acute right heart failure [21]. Bourge reported acute RV failure associated with elevated preoperative or intraoperative PVR in 16% of early deaths post-heart transplant [9]. In a large cohort from Columbia, acute right-sided failure was responsible for 17% of the deaths within 30 days post-transplant [16]. Finally, PHT or right heart failure was the reported cause of death within 90 days post-transplant in 26% in a large cohort from Stanford, which corresponded to an overall mortality rate due to PHT or right heart failure of 3.3% (10/301). A further 10 patients (3.3%) had significant postoperative complications related to PHT and right heart failure [14]. Elevated PVR has consistently been a risk factor for death in multiple single and multicenter analyses [Fig. 24.3] [25]. A linear relationship has been described between PVR and mortality [Fig. 24.4] [23, 25].

The mechanism and degree of the PHT has implications for predicting the success or failure of the transplanted heart. All 20 patients who either died or had significant postoperative issues with PHT and right heart failure in the Stanford series had a PVR > 2.5 Wood units (WU) [14]. Murali reported a 15.4%, 0–2 day mortality rate, and 19.2%, 7-day mortality rate in patients with a transpulmonary gradient (TPG) of >15 mmHg (compared to 4.3% and 6.4%, respectively) [33]. In the study by Bourge, the 1-month mortality rate for patients with a pretransplant PVR >4 was 19% compared with 7.4% with PVR < 4 WU. Similar 30-day mortality figures from Columbia were

ADULT HEART TRANSPLANTATION

Kaplan-Meier Survival by PVR   (Transplants: 1/2000-6/2003)

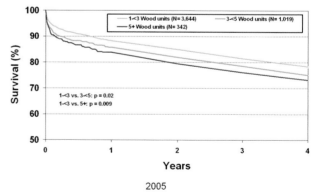

2005

Fig. 24.3 Kaplan Meier survival curves associated with increasing PVR Reprinted from International Society of Heart and Lung Transplantation, 24:945–982, David O. Taylor MD, Leah B. Edwards PhD, Mark M. Boucek MD, Elbert P. Trulock MD, Mario C. Deng MD, Berkeley M. Keck MPH and Marshall I. Hertz MD, Registry of the International Society for Heart and Lung Transplantation: Twenty-second Official Adult Heart Transplant Report–2005 Copyright 2005, with permission from Elsevier

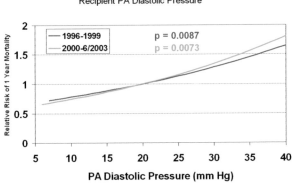

ADULT HEART TRANSPLANTS (1/1996-6/2003)
Risk Factors for 1 Year Mortality
Recipient PA Diastolic Pressure

Fig. 24.4 The relationship between PA diastolic pressure and risk of 1 year mortality Reprinted from International Society of Heart and Lung Transplantation, 24:945–982, David O. Taylor MD, Leah B. Edwards PhD, Mark M. Boucek MD, Elbert P. Trulock MD, Mario C. Deng MD, Berkeley M. Keck MPH and Marshall I. Hertz MD, Registry of the International Society for Heart and Lung Transplantation: Twenty-second Official Adult Heart Transplant Report–2005 Copyright 2005, with permission from Elsevier

5.1% and 17.7% for a PVR of <2 WU and >3 WU, respectively. The corresponding PVR indexed for body surface area (PVRi) numbers were 5.7% and 18.0% for PVRi of <4 WU × m² and >7 WU × m² [13]. In general, increased PVR (>4 WUs) and/or PVRi or a trans-pulmonary gradient of more than 15 mmHg are considered a relative contraindication to Tx.

Not all series report an adverse outcome with PHT. The largest series from Germany reported 400 patients in whom 83 had elevated PVR with no increase in 2-day, 30-day, 3-month, or late mortality [44]. In a cohort reported by Erickson, preoperative systolic pulmonary artery pressure (PAP), PVR, and PVRi were not predictive of 1-month, 6-month, or 1 year mortality [16]. Finally, 119/145 patients in the Stanford series with a PVR of >2.5 WU survived the early post-operative period [14].

The parameters deemed to be important to delineate prior to heart transplantation remain controversial, but include PVR, PVR indexed (PVRi), systolic PAP, and TPG [13, 16, 43]. Whether or not these hemodynamics are *fixed* or *reactive* is also felt to be of variable significance. In reality, these indices are useful for risk assessment, though no one test can accurately predict outcome [16]. The situation can be complicated by the fact that determination of pulmonary resistance is imprecise, especially in infants with complex congenital heart disease [5, 6].

Early registry data from the Transplant Cardiologists Research Database demonstrated higher PVR as a risk factor for death in the pediatric population (age <16 years) [9]. In a review of their single-center experience, Bando et al. reported an elevated transpulmonary

gradient (>15 mmHg) and elevated PVRi (>4 WU-m²) as significant preoperative risk factors for death in their early experience (fourfold greater mortality) with only elevated trans-pulmonary gradient being significant in their later experience [5].

In one of the earliest pediatric series, Addonizio, et al. reported on six patients with resting elevation of PVR ranging from 7 to 15. Five underwent transplantation following demonstration of a decrease in PVR with nitroprusside infusion (range 4–5.5) with four long-term survivors [2].

Addonizio subsequently compared PVR and PVRi values with clinical course post-Tx in 82 patients ranging in age from 4 to 61 years [1]. Systolic pulmonary artery pressure did not distinguish patients at risk as greater than 50% who had a pressure of over 50 mmHg. PVRi identified patients at risk better than PVR. Thirty-three percent of patients with a PVRi of >6 units developed right ventricular failure with a mortality of 15%. No patient with a PVRi of <6 units developed RV failure. The results also confirm that high PVR is not an absolute contraindication to transplantation as 28/33 patients with a PVRi of >6 and 10/12 patients with a PVRi of >9 were successfully transplanted, although at a higher risk of RV failure (40%) and mortality (15%).

Gajarski reported the outcomes in eight patients with a mean PVRi of 11.5 WU × m² which was reactive to vasodilator testing. Mortality was 12% (1/8). In the seven survivors, PVRi decreased to 3.3 WU × m² by the time of the first biopsy (approximately 10 days post-transplant) [17].

The infant population either with congenital heart disease predisposing to systemic pulmonary pressures (duct-dependent single ventricle physiology) or cardiomyopathy has a low incidence of significant postoperative complications from PHT. Bailey reported a single death from PHT in a group of 139 consecutive infant transplants up to 12 months of age [4].

It is important to define the presence or absence of fixed versus reactive PHT [1, 2, 10, 14]. Data from Columbia described a nearly fourfold increase in incidence of 30-day mortality in patients with fixed PHT [13]. Even those patients with reversible PHT retrospectively had an increase in 30-day mortality compared with transplant recipients without preoperative PHT. Conversely, seven pediatric patients reported by Gajarski with very high PVRi (mean 12.3 WU × m² which might prompt certain centers to exclude these patients from heart transplantation) were all reactive (mean 3.9 WU × m² with vasodilator testing) with six of the seven surviving. Costard-Jackle reported 3-month mortality figures in 293 patients in whom reversibility was assessed with nitroprusside. Those patients in whom the PVR could not be reduced

Pulmonary Hypertension

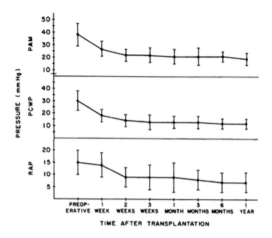

Time course for remodelling in 24 patients post-Tx w PHT

Fig. 24.5 Following heart transplantation, the elevated pulmonary artery pressure and/or pulmonary vascular resistance is expected to fall toward normal, though the degree and time course varies

to less than 2.5 WU with or without systemic hypotension had a higher 30-day mortality rate (33.3% vs. 3.8%), with a higher rate of death due to right heart failure (13.9%) [14].

Following heart transplantation, the elevated PAP and/or PVR is expected to fall toward normal, though the degree and time course varies. Bhatia et al. prospectively followed a cohort of 24 adult heart transplant recipients for 1 year post-Tx to assess the time course for changes in pulmonary arterial pressures and donor RV remodeling. [Figure 24.5] Right and left heart filling pressures declined in parallel, reaching their nadir at 2 weeks post-Tx. PVR was normal in the majority (80%) at 1 year post-Tx. Right ventricular size was increased on day 1 and even larger at 1 month post-Tx, returning to immediate postoperative values by 1 year post-Tx. Tricuspid regurgitation, which was present in 67% immediately post-Tx, improved with time (36% at 1 year) [7]. In a larger, retrospective series, Bourge reported normalization of pulmonary hemodynamics by 1 week post-Tx [10]. In the small pediatric cohort reported by Gajarski, the mean PVRi dropped from 11.5 to 3.3 WU × m^2 by 10 days post-transplant [17].

Looking at more long-term survival, Erickson, et al. despite showing no difference in 30-day mortality based on TPG or PVR, and PVRi demonstrated higher 6- and 12-month mortality in patients with a trans-pulmonary

gradient > 12 mmHg (24% and 36%) versus <12 mmHg (5%) [16]. There was a corresponding slow and gradual increase in probability of death for increasing PVR and PVRi without a clear cutoff.

There is no threshold hemodynamic values beyond which RV failure is certain. Conversely, there are no values below which RV failure is avoidable. Therefore, it is up to each center to define guidelines or make patient-specific decisions regarding eligibility for heart transplantation.

24.6 Other

Normal preoperative PVR does not rule out the potential for increased PVR and acute RV failure after heart transplantation. Cardiopulmonary bypass in and of itself has been shown to lead to an increase in PVR, primarily due to complement activation and the release of inflammatory mediators [42]. Organ preservation techniques may have a deleterious effect on ventricular function, with the right ventricular myocardium more susceptible to transient preservation-induced injury.

24.7 Management

There is no one approach to dealing with acute RV failure after transplant [43]. The goal is to provide adequate support of the transplanted heart permitting time for recovery. The overall approach should be to dilate pulmonary vasculature and decrease PVR while maintaining systemic blood pressure and coronary perfusion. Important interventions include reducing preload to the distended and ischemic RV, reducing RV afterload or PVR, optimizing coronary perfusion by maintaining systemic blood pressure, and optimizing myocardial oxygen delivery while minimizing oxygen consumption. Table 24.1 gives an overview of the approach to management.

Pharmacologic pulmonary vasodilation is a cornerstone of therapy and has evolved over the last 15 years. Studies looking at pharmacotherapy for PHT and right heart failure post-transplant have been nicely summarized by Stobierska-Dzierzek [43]. Sodium nitroprusside and nitroglycerin are longstanding agents used to produce pulmonary vasodilatation. There were several early reports in the early to mid-1990s of successful treatment of acute right heart failure post-heart transplant with prostaglandin E$_1$ (PGE$_1$) [3, 47]. The Loma Linda infant experiences reported the routine use of postoperative prostaglandin infusion for 7–10 days in all infants with pretransplant duct-dependent diagnoses [4].

Table 24.1 Approach to treatment of RV failure post-heart transplant

- Optimize coronary perfusion (systemic blood pressure)
  - Inotropic support (dobutamine, isoproterenol, milrinone)
  - Pulmonary vasodilators (reduce RV afterload - see below)
  - Chronotropy (heart rate) – pacing, isoproterenol
- Reduce preload to distended and ischemic RV
  - Limit fluid
  - If systemic blood pressure/cardiac output does not respond to fluid admin (with increased RAP) would suggest that further volume replacement is NOT warranted
- Reduce RV afterload – PVR
  - 100% O_2 (pulmonary dilation)
  - pharmacologic vasodilation
    - prostaglandins
      - prostaglandin E_1
      - prostacyclin
    - beta-sympathomimetics
      - isoproterenol (nonselective beta-agonist)
        - positive inotrope/chronotrope
        - pulmonary and peripheral vasodilation
      - dobutamine (beta-agonist)
    - phosphorylase III inhibitors
      - milrinone
    - nitro compounds (nitroglycerin, sodium nitroprusside)
    - alpha-adrenolitics (tolazoline, hydralazine)
    - adenosine
  - inhaled NO
  - optimize LV function (see above)
- Optimize stroke volume: treat arrhythmias, ensure AV synchronous rhythm
- Ventilatory management
  - Increased tidal volume, optimal PEEP
  - Early extubation
  - Intubated, ventilated, and sedated ± paralyzed for severe elevation of PVR
- Mechanical assist
  - RVAD
  - Interarterial balloon pump
  - ECMO

Bauer et al. reported a strategy to prophylactically manage all patients for right heart failure prior to coming off cardiopulmonary bypass with PGE_1 and alkalinization in the post-transplant period with good results. Successful use of prostacyclin was reported in several series over a similar time period [24, 35].

Milrinone has been shown in an animal model to be an effective means to improve right ventricular dysfunction and pulmonary vascular efficiency after heart transplantation in the setting of chronic pulmonary hypertension. Milrinone is both a positive inotrope and a pulmonary vasodilator [12].

The earliest report of inhaled nitric oxide (NO) for the management of right heart failure post-transplant was in 1993. Williams subsequently reported the successful use in five patients, all of whom failed treatment with nitroprusside and prostacyclin; all survived to hospital discharge [49]. Kieler-Jensen and colleagues examined the roles of sodium nitroprusside, prostacyclin, PGE_1, and NO on hemodynamics and right heart function post-heart transplant. Systemic and pulmonary vascular resistance were lowest with prostacyclin, but NO was the only selective pulmonary vasodilator that resulted in increased cardiac output and no change in systemic vascular resistance [24].

Isoproterenol, a nonselective beta-agonist that is both a positive inotrope and chronotrope also results in pulmonary vasodilatation, making it a preferred choice for an inotropic agent post-transplant. Alpha-agonists are often needed to balance the peripheral vasodilatation and resultant systemic hypotension related to the above-mentioned vasodilatory drugs, the majority of which have peripheral vasodilatory effects as well.

There are reports in the literature of successful mechanical support for a failing right ventricle, despite therapeutic maneuvers as outlined above and in Table 24.1. Consideration must be given to choice of device and optimal timing of insertion [38, 43, 45, 46].

24.8 Summary

Acute right heart dysfunction following heart transplantation contributes significantly to post-transplant mortality. Most commonly, it results from a donor heart impaired by the sequelae of brain death and ischemia-reperfusion injury and not prepared for pulmonary hypertension and increased pulmonary vascular resistance in the recipient. The resultant right heart failures manifests with signs of low cardiac output. There are issues from both the donor and recipient perspectives. The cardiac dysfunction that follows brain death is amenable to functional recovery, given appropriate management, allowing for successful organ donation. With regard to the recipient, it is clear that there are no threshold hemodynamic values beyond which RV failure is certain, and no values below which RV failure is avoidable. Therefore, it is up to each center to define guidelines or make patient-specific decisions regarding eligibility for heart transplantation. Management strategies have evolved over time, but with a consistent goal of pulmonary vasodilatation while maintaining systemic blood pressure and coronary perfusion.

References

1. Addonizio LJ, Gersony WM, Robbins RC, Drusin RE, Smith CR, Reison DS, Reemtsma K, Rose EA. Elevated pulmonary vascular resistance and cardiac transplantation. Circulation. 1987;76(Suppl V):V–52.
2. Addonizio LJ, Gersony WM, Rose EA. Cardiac transplantation in children with increased pulmonary vascular resistance. Am Heart J. 1986;112:647. [Abstract]
3. Armitage JM, Hardesty RL, Griffith BP. Prostaglandin E1: an effective treatment of right heart failure after orthotopic heart transplantation. J Heart Transplant. 1987;6:348–51.
4. Bailey LL, Gundry SR, Razzouk AJ, Wang N, Sciolaro CM, Chiavarelli M. Bless the babies: one hundred fifteen late survivors of heart transplantation during the first year of life. J Thorac Cardiovasc Surg. 1993;105:805–15.
5. Bando K, Konishi H, Komatsu K, Fricker FJ, del Nido PJ, Francalancia NA, Hardesty RL, Griffith BP, Armitage JM. Improved survival following pediatric cardiac transplantation in high-risk patients. Circulation. 1993;88[part2]:218–223.
6. Bauer J, Dapper F, Demirakca S, Knothe C, Thul J, Hagel KJ. Perioperative management of pulmonary hypertension after heart transplantation in childhood. J Heart Lung Transplant. 1997;16:1238–47.
7. Bhatia SJ, Kirshenbaum JM, Shemin RJ, Cohn LH, Collins JJ, Di Sesa VJ, Young PJ, Mudge GH, Sutton MG. Time course of

resolution of pulmonary hypertension and right ventricular remodeling after orthotopic cardiac transplantation. Circulation. 1987;76:819–826.
8. Bittner H, Chen E, Milano CA, Kendall SWH, Jennings RB, Sabiston DC, Van Trigt P. Myocardial β-adrenergic receptor function and high-energy phosphates in brain death-related cardiac dysfunction. Circulation. 1995;92:472–478.
9. Bourge RC, Naftel DC, Costanzo-Nordin MR. Kirklin JK, Young JB, Kubo SH, Olivari MT, Kasper EK. Pretransplantation risk factors for death after heart transplantation: a multiinstitutional study. J Heart Lung Transplant. 1993;12:549–62.
10. Bourge RC, Kirklin JK, Naftel DC, White C, Mason DA, Epstein AE. Analysis and predictors of pulmonary vascular resistance after cardiac transplantation. J Thoracic Cardiovasc Surg. 1991;101:432–45.
11. Boucek MM, Edwards LB, Keck BM, Trulock EP, Taylor DO, Hertz MI. Registry of the International Society of Heart and Lung Transplantation: eighth official pediatric report – 2005. J Heart Lung Transplant. 2005;24:968–82.
12. Chen EP, Bittner HB, Davis RD, Van Trigt P. Hemodynamic and inotropic effects of milrinone after heart transplantation in the setting of pulmonary hypertension. J Heart Lung Transplant. 1998;17:669–678.
13. Chen JM, Levin HR, Michler RE, Prusmack CJ, Rose EA, Aaronson KD. Reevaluating the significance of pulmonary hypertension before cardiac transplantation: determination of optimal thresholds and quantification of the effect of reversibility on perioperative mortality. J Thorac Cardiovasc Surg. 1997;114(4):627–34.
14. Costard-Jackle A, Fowler MB. Influence of preoperative pulmonary artery pressure on mortality after heart transplantation: testing of potential reversibility of pulmonary hypertension with nitroprusside is useful in defining a high risk group. J Am Coll Cardiol. 1992;19:48–54.
15. Dujardin KS, McCully RB, Wijdicks, EFM, Tazelaar HD, Seward JB, McGregor CGA, Olson LJ. Myocardial dysfunction associated with brain death: clinical, echocardiographic, and pathologic features. JHLT 2001;20:350–7.
16. Erikson KW, Costanzo-Nordin MR, O'Sullivan J, Johnson MR, Zucker MJ, Pifarre R, Lawless CE, Robinson JA, Scanlon PJ. Influence of preoperative transpulmonary gradient on late mortality after orthotopic heart transplantation. J Heart Transplant. 1990;526–37.
17. Gajarski RJ, Towbin JA, Bricker JT, Radovancevic B, Frazier OH, Price JK, Schowengerdt KO, Denfield SW. Intermediate follow up of pediatric heart transplant recipients with elevated pulmonary vascular resistance index. J Am Coll Cardiol. 1994;23:1682–7.
18. Galinanes M, Hearse DJ. Brain death-induced impairment of cardiac contractile performance can be reversed by explantation and may not preclude the use of hearts for transplantation. Circ Res. 1992;71:1213–1219.
19. Gallardo A, Anguita M, Franco M, et al. The echocardiographic findings in patients with brain death. The implications for their selection as heart transplant donors. Rev Esp Cardiol. 1994;47:604–8.
20. Gilbert EM, Kreuger SK, Murray JL, et al. Echocardiographic evaluation of potential cardiac transplant donors. J Thorac Cardiovasc Surg. 1988;95:1003–7.
21. Griepp RB, Stinson EB, Dong Jr E, Clark DA, Shumway NE. Determinants of operative risk in human heart transplantation. Am J Surg. 1971;122:192–197.
22. Guyton AC, Lindsey AW, Gilluly JJ. The limits of right ventricular compensation following acute increase in pulmonary circulatory resistance. Circ Res. 1954;11:326–332.

23. Hosenpud JD, Bennett LE, Keck BM, Boucek MM, Novick RJ. The Registry of the International Society for Heart and Lung Transplantation: Seventeenth Official Report – 2000. J Heart Lung Transplant. 2000;19:909.

24. Kieler-Jensen N, Lundin S, Ricksten S-E. Vasodilator therapy after heart transplantation: effects of inhaled nitric oxide and intravenous prostacyclin, prostaglandin E1, and sodium nitroprusside. J Heart Lung Transplant. 1995;14:436–43.

25. Kirklin JK, Naftel DC, Kirklin JW, Blackstone EH, White-Williams C, Bourge RC. Pulmonary vascular resistance and the risk of heart transplantation. J Heart Transplant. 1988;7:331–6.

26. Kirklin JK, Naftel DC, McGiffin DC, McVay RF, Blackstone EH, Karp RB. Analysis of morbid events and risk factors for death after cardiac transplantation. J Am Coll Cardiol. 1988;II:917–24.

27. Kono T, Morita H, Kuroiwa T, Onaka H, Takatsuka H, Fujiwara A. Left ventricular wall motion abnormalities in patients with subarachnoid hemorrhage: Neurogenic stunned myocardium. JACC 1994;24:636–40.

28. Kono T, Nishina T, Morita H, Hirota Y, Kawamura K, Fujiwara A. Usefulness of low-dose dobutamine stress echocardiography for evaluating reversibility of brain death-induced myocardial dysfunction. Am J Cardiol. 1999;84:578–82.

29. Lee FA. Hemodynamics of the right ventricle in normal and disease states. Cardiol Clin. 1992;10:59–67.

30. Li J, Konstantinov IE, Shimizu M, Cai S, Redington AN. Systemic and myocardial oxygen transport responses to brain death in pigs. 2006. In press.

31. Mertes PM, El Abassi K, Jaboin Y, Burtin P, Pinelli G, Carteaux JP, Burlet C, Boulange M, Villemot JP. Changes in hemodynamic and metabolic parameters following induced brain death in the pig. Transplantation. 1994;58:414–418.

32. Mertes PM, Burtin P, Carteaux JP, Jaboin Y, Dopff C, Pinelli G, Villemot JP, Burlet C, Boulange M. Brain death and myocardial injury: role of cardiac sympathetic innervation evaluated by in vivo interstitial microdialysis. Transp Proc. 1994;26:231–232.

33. Murali S, Kormos RL, Uretsky BF, Schechter D, Reddy S, Denys BG, Armitage JM, Hardesty RL, Griffith BP. Preoperative pulmonary hemodynamics and early mortality after orthotopic cardiac transplantation: the Pittsburgh experience. Am Heart J. 1993;126:896–902.

34. Novitzky D. Detrimental effects of brain death on the potential organ donor. Transp Proc. 1997;29:3770–3772.

35. Pascual JMS, Fiorelli AI, Bellotti GM, Stolf NAG, Jatene AD. Prostacyclin in the management of pulmonary hypertension after heart transplantation. J Heart Transplant. 1990; 644–51.

36. Powner DJ, Hendrich A, Nyhuis A, Strate R. Changes in serum catecholamine levels in patients who are brain dead. J Heart Lung Transplant. 1992;11:1046–53.

37. Pratschke J, Wilhelm MJ, Kusaka M, Hancock WW, Tilney NL. Activation of proinflammatory genes in somatic organs as a consequence of brain death. Transp Proc. 1999;31:1003–1005.

38. Radovancevic B, Nakatani T, Frazier OH, Moncrief C, Vega J, Haupt H, Duncan JM. Mechanical circulatory support for perioperative donor heart failure. ASAIO Transactions. 1989;35:539–541.

39. Ryan JB, Hicks M, Cropper JR, Garlick SR, Kesteven SH, Wilson MK, Feneley MP, Macdonald PS. Functional Evidence of reversible ischemic injury immediately after the sympathetic storm associated with experimental brain death. JHLT. 2003;22: 922–928.

40. Shemie SD, Ross H, Pagliarello J, Baker AJ, Greig PD, Brand T, Cockfield S, Keshavjee S, Nickerson P, Rao V, Guest C, Young K, Doig C, on behalf of the Pediatric Recommendations Group: Organ management in Canada: recommendations of the Forum on Medical Management to Optimize Donor Organ Potential. Can Med Assoc J. 2006;174(6):S13–S30.

41. Shivalkar B, Van Loon J, Wieland W, Tjandra–Maga TB, Borgers M, Plets C, Flameng W. Variable effects of explosive or gradual increase of intracranial pressure on myocardial structure and function. Circulation. 1993;87:230–9.

42. Smith WJ, Murphy MP, Appleyard RF, Rizzo RJ, Aklog L, Laurence RG, Cohn LH. Prevention of complement-induced pulmonary hypertension and improvement of right ventricular function by selective thromboxane receptor antagonism. J Thorac Cardiovasc Surg. 1994;107:800–6.

43. Stobiersak-Dzierzek B, Awad H, Michler RE. The evolving management of acute right-sided heart failure in cardiac transplant recipients. J Am Coll Cardiol. 2001;38:923–931.

44. Tenderich G, Koerner MM, Stuettgen B, Mirow N, Arusoglu L, Morshuis M, Bairaktaris A, Minami K, Koerger R. Pre-existing elevated pulmonary vascular resistance: long-term hemodynamic follow-up and outcome of recipients after orthotopic heart transplantation. J Cardiovasc Surg. 2000;41: 215–19.

45. Tenderich G, Koerner MM, Stuettgen B, Hornik L, Mirow N, Morshuis M, Mannebach H, Minami K, Koerfer R. Does pre-existing elevated pulmonary vascular resistance (transpulmonary gradient >15 mmHg or >5 Wood) predict early and long-term results after orthotopic heart transplantation? Transp Proc. 1998;30:1130–1131.

46. Tenderich G, Koerner MM, Stuettgen B, Minami K, El-Banayosy A, Arusoglu L, Mirow N, Wlost S, Gromzik H, Kleesiek K, Meyer H, Koerfer R. Mechanical circulatory support after orthotopic heart transplantation. Int J Artif Organs. 1998;21:414–416.

47. Vincent JL, Carlier E, Pinsky MR, Goldstein J, Naeije R, Lejeune P, Brimioulle S, Leclerc JL, Kahn RJ, Primo G. Prostaglandin E$_1$ infusion for right ventricular failure after cardiac transplantation. J Thorac Cardiovasc Surg. 1992;103: 33–9.

48. White M, Wiechmann RJ, Roden RL, Hagan MB, Wollmering MM, Port JD, Hammond E, Abraham WT, Wolfel EE, Lindenfeld J, Fullerton D, Bristow MR. Cardiac β-adrenergic neuroeffector systems in acute myocardial dysfunction related to brain injury. Evidence for catecholamine-mediated myocardial damage. Circulation. 1995;92:2183–2189.

49. Williams TJ, Salamonsen RF, Snell G, Kaye D, Esmore DS. Preliminary experience with inhaled nitric oxide for acute pulmonary hypertension after heart transplantation. J Heart Lung Transplant. 1995;14:419–23.

25.1 Echocardiographic Assessment of RV Function

Imaging of the right ventricle by b-mode echocardiography has notoriously been difficult. In order to assess right ventricular (RV) ejection fraction, the end-diastolic and end-systolic volume need to be measured. As the RV shape is very complex, none of the formulas to measure RV volume and calculate RV ejection fraction from cross-sectional (b-mode) images has stood the test of time [1]. With the advent of three-dimensional (3D) echocardiography it has been possible accurately to calculate right ventricular (RV) volumes. We have validated 3D echocardiographic measurements of RV volume *in vitro* [2] and *in vivo* [3] and have applied it clinically in patients with tetralogy of Fallot [4]. Recent developments in 3D echocardiography have made the method a lot less time consuming and thus expanded its clinical applicability (Fig. 25.1). Unfortunately RV ejection fraction is a poor index of ventricular contractile function because it is very load dependent. Loading conditions are abnormal or widely variable in many patients with congenital heart defects, so the use of any ejection-phase index to determine RV function in congenitally malformed hearts is questionable.

Simple alternative methods to assess RV function like the myocardial performance (TEI) index may be applied independent of RV shape but have similar limitations as ejection fraction with regard to load dependency [5].

Furthermore, many patients with congenitally malformed hearts have abnormal regional RV function on top of a reduced global dysfunction.

Myocardial Doppler which is based on sampling myocardial velocities anywhere along the ventricular wall has the potential to (1) assess global function independent of RV shape and (2) to assess regional wall motion [6].

Doppler myocardial imaging (DMI)-derived peak systolic and diastolic velocities, strain and strain rate have emerged as useful tools to quantify regional ventricular function [6–8]. Their utility to assess global function is limited, like most single-beat ejection-phase indices by both pre- and afterload dependency [9, 10]. However, they have greatly facilitated the assessment of regional ventricular function [7] and have led to new clinical insights [6]. For the assessment of global function, measurements of myocardial contraction during the isovolumic period are likely to be more robust than ejection phase-based indices. One of the most common measured isovolumic indices remains dP/dt_{max} which can only be assessed by invasive techniques [11]. Previous myocardial Doppler studies have assessed myocardial velocities during isovolumic contraction or so-called pre-ejection [12]. The peak myocardial velocity during isovolumic contraction, measured in the posterior wall of a short-axis section, changed appropriately with m-mode-derived ejection fraction changes during dobutamine infusion. The lack of further pharmacologic manipulation with negative intotropic drugs, a lack variation of pre- or afterload, and the use of ejection fraction as the index of contractility to which velocities were compared to make interpretation of these data difficult.

Ten years ago, the acceleration of the endocardium was measured using an accelerometer sensor mounted on a pacemaker lead [13]. An almost linear increase of endocardial acceleration during an infusion with dobutamine was detected [13]. More importantly, these studies found that peak endocardial acceleration occurred during isovolumic contraction rather than during the ejection phase [14]. Recently, endocardial acceleration assessment was also used to detect acute myocardial ischemia during percutaneous transluminal coronary angioplasty [15].

M. Vogel (✉)
Kinderherz-Praxis. Leopoldstr. 27, D-80802 Munich, Germany, and Department of Paediatric and Congenital Cardiology, German Heart Center, Muenchen, Lazarettstr. 36, D-80336 Munich, Germany

A.N. Redington et al. (eds.), *Congenital Diseases in the Right Heart*, DOI 10.1007/978-1-84800-378-1_25,
© Springer-Verlag London Limited 2009

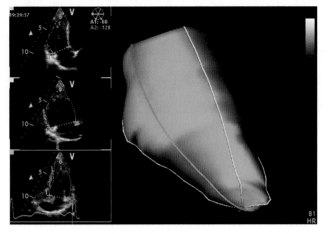

Fig. 25.1 3D reconstruction of the RV in patient with repaired tetralogy. The RV endocardial border is manually traced in 3 different Echocardiographic planes (*left side*) and the computer calculates and reconstructs the volume (*right side*)

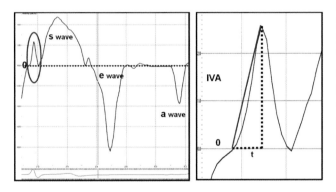

Fig. 25.2 Measurement of IVA (IsoVolumicAcceleration) from the myocardial Doppler tracing. The mean acceleration is calculated from the maximal velocity during isovolumic contraction divided by the time from zero line crossing to peak velocity

Myocardial Doppler allows for noninvasive measurement of acceleration during isovolumic contraction. If the peak myocardial velocity is known, and temporal resolution is adequate, the calculation of the acceleration during isovolumic contraction (IVA) is straightforward (Fig. 25.2). This measurement has been tested by our group in a variety of experimental and clinical settings.

25.2 Validation of IVA as an Index of Contractile Function

We used myocardial Doppler to measure the acceleration of the myocardium during isovolumic contraction (IVA), after we had noticed that the ventricular myocardial

velocity during isovolumic contraction increased more markedly than the peak systolic velocity during dobutamine stress evaluation of contractile reserve in adults with congenital heart disease.

Subsequently we validated experimentally IVA as an index of contractile function, comparing it to myocardial acceleration, and velocities measured during the ejection phase [16]. For the purpose of these experiments we chose a 15–17 kg closed-chest pig model, which offered the best compromise between good echocardiographic windows and neck vessel diameters suitable for insertion of six and seven French catheters. As the independent index of contractility for comparison of DMI data, we used pressure–volume analysis, derived by conductance catheter, to measure endsystolic (Ees), and maximal elastance (Emax) in the LV and RV, respectively [17, 18]. Our studies confirmed that small changes in contractile function during beta blockade (esmolol) or beta-receptor stimulation (dobutamine) can be detected by measuring IVA. Importantly, changes in pre- and afterload in a physiological range did not affect IVA, while the DMI-derived ejection phase indices were all influenced significantly by these changes. To some extent therefore ejection indices, such as peak systolic velocities and strain or strain rate, offer little advantage over ejection/shortening fraction in terms of assessing ventricular performance. Conversely, IVA represents a robust measurement of LV or RV contractile function with a sensitivity approaching or exceeding those indices traditionally measured using invasive techniques [19].

25.3 Clinical Validation of IVA to Assess RV Function

We have applied IVA to the evaluation of myocardial disease in right ventricular disease. In the clinical validation study, we addressed the important problem of evaluating contractile function in patients with a morphologic right ventricle supporting the systemic circulation. In patients with complete transposition of the great arteries who have been treated with atrial redirection procedures, such as the Mustard or the Senning operation, the right ventricle remains the systemic ventricle. Some of these patients develop systemic ventricular dysfunction as early as the second or third decade of life. We assessed the contractile reserve of the right ventricle supporting the systemic circulation in 12 clinically well patients with transposition of the great arteries and a Mustard or Senning operation. Under beta-receptor stimulation by dobutamine (10 mcgs/kg/min for 10 min) we analyzed conductance-catheter-derived pressure–volume relations, to assess endsystolic elastance (Ees), and measured IVA simultaneously. Both parameters of contractile function increased significantly during beta stimulation, demonstrating that IVA can detect changes in contractile function in the human [21]. There was a considerable variety in the contractile reserve of the systemic RV in asymptomatic patients with complete transposition of the great arteries following the Mustard or Senning operation [21]. Patients with a good contractile reserve, that is, an increase of IVA or Ees of 200% or more continued to do well clinically, while among the four patients with little change of IVA or Ees, one patient subsequently died, one had to be listed for transplantation, and one was transplanted successfully. In the future, assessment of the contractile reserve may be used as additional clinical information to predict long-term outcome.

After IVA was validated in patients, the normal values of IVA from infancy to adulthood in a database of 272 volunteers were established. IVA was measured in the basal, midventricular, and apical segment of the RV, the ventricular septum, and the LV lateral wall. Our data demonstrate that IVA, and therefore ventricular contractile function, is age dependent in both ventricles. We found the highest IVA in the second decade of life, that is, between ages 10 years and 20 years, with a progressive decline of IVA in each following decade. Thus, age-appropriate control values have to be used in clinical studies. IVA is generally higher in the RV than in the LV. This, in keeping with experimental data, shows that RV twitch velocities *in vitro* exceed those of the LV. While establishing this database of normal values, we also have assessed interobserver variability. The Bland–Altman curves of limits of agreement between two observers for measurement of IVA are very similar to those of measurement of peak systolic velocities and other manually measured echo-Doppler parameters.

25.4 Clinical Studies of IVA in Congenital Heart Disease

Patients with tetralogy of Fallot have an excellent outcome of initial surgical repair in the current area. However, pulmonary regurgitation as a common sequela of surgical corrections leads to a progressive dilatation of the right ventricle with subsequent right ventricular dysfunction, wall motion abnormalities, and abnormal electrical de- and repolarization resulting in an increased risk of sudden, unexpected, premature cardiac death [4, 22, 23]. We examined 124 patients with tetralogy of Fallot and measured IVA, systolic myocardial velocities, and strain/strain rate in the longitudinal axis of both the right and left ventricle. IVA was lower in all tetralogy patients compared to normals and correlated with the severity of

pulmonary regurgitation (PR), whereas systolic velocities, strain, and strain rate, while being abnormally low, failed to correlate with severity of PR. Significantly, patients with severe PR had a high incidence of tricuspid regurgitation which by altering RV load makes it difficult to apply load-dependent ejection phase indices and may be an explanation for the fact that IVA and not myocardial systolic velocities or strain detected a reduced contractile function, especially in those patients with PR who also had tricuspid regurgitation. Thus, the study in the tetralogy patients demonstrates well the clinical need for a less load-dependent index like IVA in patients in whom an abnormal contractile function may be masked by significant changes in loading conditions caused by severe atrioventricular valve regurgitation.

In patients with thalassemia, we found a high number of wall motion abnormalities in those patients who had an abnormal iron loading diagnosed by magnetic resonance imaging. Regional dysfunction in this patient group likewise affected global function and IVA was significantly lower in those with abnormal than in those with normal wall motion [24].

Atrial septal defect (ASD) closure by an Amplatzer device results in acute volume unloading of the RV and is a good clinical model to assess load dependency of indices of ventricular function. Myocardial velocities and IVA were measured before and immediately following ASD closure in 39 patients in the cardiac catheterization laboratory. While systolic-myocardial velocities in the right ventricle fell immediately after ASD closure, IVA remained unchanged, confirming our previous experimental findings of a load independency of IVA in a physiological range [25].

Pauliks et al. also assessed various myocardial Doppler-derived functional parameters to test their ability to detect acute allograft rejection in 65 children following heart transplantation. They found that of all tissue Doppler-derived data, IVA was the most sensitive parameter to prospectively detect transplant rejection [26].

25.5 Measurement of IVA and Current Limitations

When measured using the currently available software, IVA is a measurement of the average rate of acceleration during isovolumic contraction. The potential for online measurement of peak IVA clearly exists, however. We have also used the raw digital data available from system fiVe (GE Vingmed) to derive an instantaneous peak acceleration curve, which behaves in a similar way to the manually measured average myocardial acceleration.

Fig. 25.3 Simultaneous RV pressure curve (*light blue*) and myocardial Doppler tracing (*white*). The onset of IVA is just at the time of initial pressure build-up before the pulmonary valve opens

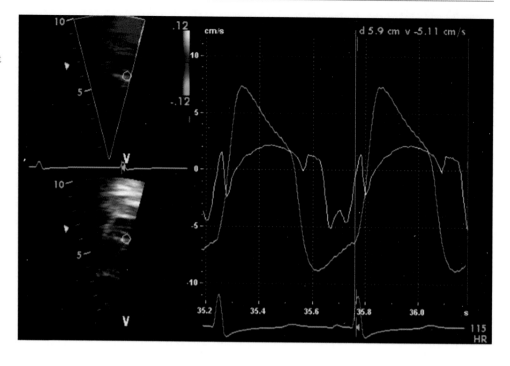

Furthermore, using the Vivid seVen ultrasound scanner (GE Vingmed) with inputted micromanometer ventricular pressure recordings, we can compare the timing of IVA and the ventricular pressure signal. In this way, we confirmed that IVA starts at the onset of ventricular-pressure rise and reflects a very early systolic event (**Fig.** 25.3). This observation may partially explain the load independence of IVA, the timing of which is occurring at a point of minimal diastolic or systolic load.

We have predominantly assessed that contractile function in the longitudinal axis as the angle of interrogation of the Doppler beam is not optimal in echocardiographic views commonly used to assess radial function. The analysis of longitudinal function may be superior to indices derived from the LV short axis as longitudinal fibers start to shorten before radial fibers and are the first to be affected by myocardial ischemia. We have found that IVA is higher in the basal segments and decreases with sampling toward the apex in a similar fashion as DMI-derived myocardial velocities. Thus, different ranges of normal values of IVA are required for different segments of the heart when comparing normal values to disease. As others, we usually assessed function in the basal, midventricular, and apical segment of the respective chamber placing the sample volume for Doppler interrogation at the base of each of the three segments. Measurement of IVA has only become possible because of the high frame rate achieved by currently available ultrasound technology. The duration of IVA is in the range of 10–40 milliseconds (ms), thus even with the high frame rates used in our studies (130–250 frames per second), data were acquired only every 4–6 ms, that is, 2–10 frames

were acquired during isovolumic acceleration. With recent hardware developments, such as Vivid seVen (GE Vingmed), frame rates of up to 350 frames per second can be achieved but the machine settings still require careful adjustment with regard to depth and sector width to achieve these very high frame rates. Like all Doppler measurements, IVA, myocardial velocities, and the myocardial velocity-derived one-dimensional strain are angle dependent. This angle dependency is exemplified when comparing data acquired by transthoracic echocardiogrphy to those acquired by the transesophageal technique [27]. While Bland–Altman plots showed comparable data for both methods in normally positioned hearts, we found significant differences in malpositioned hearts when the angle of Doppler interrogation cannot be optimally aligned to the myocardium [27]

25.6 2D Strain

To overcome this limitation of influence of insonation angle on Doppler-derived myocardial acceleration and velocities, the new method of two dimensional (2D) strain has been developed. 2D strain is not angle dependent, because it is not based on Doppler-derived data. Instead, this technique is based on tracking of radiofrequency image patterns. This allows for estimating the velocity vector. For each pixel in the b-mode image, angle-independent velocity estimation is performed by selecting a search pattern around that pixel in one frame. The new technique has

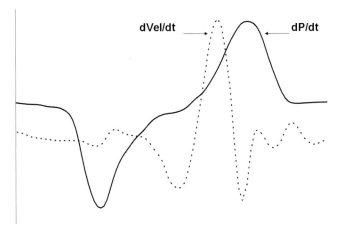

Fig. 25.4 Basal RV velocities and IVA from the 2-D strain dataset (*left side*) and myocardial Doppler tracing (*right side*) from the same patient. IVA is identical and peak S wave and e wave velocities are similar with the exception of a biphasic s wave. Note that in diastole while e wave velocities are very similar the a wave velocity is lower in the myocardial Doppler trace

recently been validated in tissue-mimicking phantoms [28], in animal experiments [29], and in humans with normal hearts [30]. From the 2D strain, data set myocardial velocities can be derived, but unlike Doppler-based data these derived velocities are completely angle independent. **Figure** 25.4 demonstrates a 2D strain image of a right ventricle acquired from a subcostal and four-chamber view, both at a different angle. The myocardial velocities and IVA derived from those data sets are virtually identical, although they have been obtained by completely different methods. The fact that the velocity from the 2D strain data set acquired in the subcostal view is identical to the Doppler-derived velocity in the apical four-chamber view (at an optimal Doppler angle) is a proof of the angle independency of 2D strain and indirectly validates this new method.

For patients with congenital disease measurement of IVA and myocardial velocities either by Doppler interrogation or RF signal-based 2D strain offers new insights into RV contractile function and for the first time allows assessment of systolic function independent of RV shape and position.

References

1. Helbing WA, Bosch HG, Maliepaard C, Rebergen SA, van der Geest RJ, Hansen B, Ottenkamp J, Reiber JH, de Roos A. Comparison of echocardiographic methods with magnetic resonance imgaging for assessment of right ventricular function in children. Am J Cardiol. 1995;76:589–594.
2. Vogel M, White P, Redington A. In vitro validation of right ventricular volume measurement by 3-dimensional echocardiography. British Heart J. 1995;74:460–463.
3. Vogel M, Gutberlet M, Dittrich S, Hosten N, Lange PE. Comparison of transthoracic three-dimensional echocardiography with magnetic resonance imaging in the assessment of right ventricular volume and mass. Heart. 1997;78:127–130.
4. El Rahman MY, Abdul-Khaliq H, Vogel M, Alexi-Meskishvili V, Lange PE. Relation between right ventricular enlargement, QRS Duration, and right ventricular function in patients with tetralogy of Fallot and pulmonary regurgitation after surgical repair. Heart. 2000;84:416–420.
5. Cheung MM, Smallhorn JF, Redington AN, Vogel M. The effects of changes in loading conditions and modulation of inotropic state on the myocardial performance index: comparison with conductance catheter measurements. Eur Heart J. 2004;25:2236–2242.
6. Sutherland GR, Stewart MJ, Groundstroem KW et al. Color Doppler myocardial imaging: a new technique for the assessment of myocardial function. J Am Soc Echocardiography. 1994;7:441–458.
7. Gorcsan J 3rd, Strum DP, Mandarino WA, Gulati VK, Pinsky MR. Quantitative assessment of alterations in regional left ventricular contractility with color-coded tissue Doppler echocardiography. Comparison with sonomicrometry and pressure-volume relations. Circulation. 1997;95:2423–2433.
8. Abraham TP, Nishimura RA, Holmes DR, Belohlavek M, Seward JB. Strain rate imaging for assessment of regional myocardial function. Results from a clinical model of septal ablation. Circulation. 2002;105:1403–1406.
9. Greenberg NL, Firstenberg MS, Castro PL, Main M, Travaglini A, Odabashian JA, Drinko JK, Rodriguez LL, Thomas JD, Garcia MJ. Doppler-derived myocardial systolic strain rate is a strong index of left ventricular contractility. Circulation. 2002;105:99–105.
10. Oki T, Fukuda K, Tahara T et al. Effect of acute increase in afterload on left ventricular regional wall motion velocity in healthy subjects. J Am Soc Echocardiogr. 1999;12:476–483.
11. Kass DA, Maughan WL, Guo ZM, Kono A, Sunagawa K, Sagawa K. Comparative influence of load versus inotropic states on indices of ventricular contractility: experimental and theoretical analysis based on pressure-volume relationships. Circulation. 1987;76:1422–1426.
12. Pellerin D, Berdeaux A, Cohen L, Guidicelli JF, Witchitz S, Veyrat C. Pre-ejectional left ventricular wall motions studied on conscious dogs using Doppler myocardial imaging: relationships with indices of left ventricular function. Ultrasound Med Biol. 1988;24:1271–1283
13. Rickards AF, Bombardini T, Corbucci G, et al. An implantable intra-cardiac accelerometer for monitoring myocardial contractility. The multicenter PEA study group. PACE. 1996;19:2066–2071.
14. Bongiorni MG, Soldati E, Arenta G, et al. Local myocardial contractility related to endocardial acceleration signals detected by transvenous pacing lead. PACE. 1996;19: 1682–1688.
15. Theres HP, Kaiser DR, Neslon SD, Glos M, Leuthold T, Baummann G, Sowelam S, Sheldon TJ, Stylos L. Detection of acute myocardial ischemia during percutaneous transluminal coronary angioplasty by endocardial acceleration. Pacing Clin Electrophysiol. 2004;27:621–625.
16. Vogel M, Schmidt R, Kristiansen S, Cheung M, White PA, Sorensen K, Redington AN: Validation of myocardial acceleration during isovolumic contraction as a novel non-invasive index of right ventricular contractility: Comparison with ventricular pressure-volume relations in an animal model. Circulation. 2002;105:1693–1699.
17. White PA, Chatuverdi RR, Shore D et al. Left ventricular parallel conductance during cardiac cycle in children with congenital heart disease. Am J Physiol. 1997;273:H295–302.

18. Brookes CIO, White PA; Bishop A, et al. Validation of a new intraoperative technique to evaluate load-independent indices of right ventricular performance in patients undergoing cardiac operations. J Thorac Cardiovasc Surg. 1998;116:468–476.

19. Vogel M, Schmidt MR, Kristiansen SB, Cheung M, White PA, Sorensen K, Redington AN. Non-invasive assessment of LV force-frequency relationships using tissue Doppler derived isovolumic acceleration: Validation in an animal model. Circulation. 2003;107:1651–1655.

20. Cheung MM, Li J, White PA, Smallhorn JF, Redington AN, Vogel M. Doppler tissue echocardiography: can transesophageal echocardiography be used to acquire functional data. J Am Soc Echocardiogr. 2003;16:732–737.

21. Vogel M, Derrick G, White PA, Cullen S, Aichner H, Deanfield JD, Redington AN. Systemic ventricular function in patients with transposition of the great arteries after atrial repair: a tissue Doppler and conductance catheter study. J Am Coll Cardiol. 2004;43:100–106.

22. Vogel M, Sponring J, Cullen S, Deanfield JE, Redington AN. Regional wall motion and abnormalities of electrical depolarisation and repolarisation in patients after surgical repair of tetralogy of Fallot. Circulation. 2001;103:1669–1673.

23. Frigiola A, Redington AN, Cullen S, Vogel M. Pulmonary regurgitation is an important determinant of right ventricular contractile dysfunction in patients with surgically repaired tetralogy of Fallot. Circulation. 2004; SuppI 110:I53–57.

24. Vogel M, Anderson LJ, Holden S, Deanfield JE, Pennell D, Walker JM. Tissue Doppler echocardiography in patients with thalassaemia detects early myocardial dysfunction related to myocardial iron overload. Eur Heart J. 2003;24:113–119.

25. Pauliks LB, Chan KC, Chang D, Kirby KS, Logan L, DeGroff CG, Boucek MM, Valdez-Cruz LM. Regional myocardial velocities and isovolumic contraction acceleration before and after device closure of atrial septal defects: a color tissue Doppler study. Am Heart J. 2005;150:294–301.

26. Pauliks LB, Pietra BA, deGroff CG, Kirby KS, Knudson OA, Logan L, Boucek MM, Valdez-Cruz LM. Non-invasive detection of acute allograft rejection in children by tissue Doppler imaging: myocardial velocities and myocardial acceleration during isovolumic contraction. J Heart Lung Transplant. 2005; Suppl 24:S239–243.

27. Cheung MM, Li J, White PA, Smallhorn JF, Redington AN, Vogel M. Doppler tissue Echocardiography: can trans-esophageal echocardiography be used to acquire functional data? J Am Soc of Echocardiography. 2003;16:6732–737.

28. D'hooge J, Konofagou E, Jamal F, Heimdal A, Barrios L, Bijnens B, Thoen J, Van de Werf F, Sutherland GR, Suetens P. Two-dimensional myocardial strain rate measurements of the human heart in vivo. IEEE Trans Ultrason Ferroelectr Freq Control. 2002; 49:281–286.

29. Langeland S, D'Hooge, Claessens T, Claus P, Verdonck P, Suetens P, Sutherland GR, Bijnens B. RF-based two-dimensional cardiac strain estimation: a validation study in a tissue-mimicking phantom. IEEE Trans Ultrason Ferroelectr Freq Control. 2004;51:1537–1546.

30. Langeland S, D'Hooge J, Wouters PF, Leather A, Claus P, Bijnens B, Sutherland GR. Experimental Validation of a new ultrasound method for the simultaneous assessment of radial and longitudinal myocardial deformation independent of insonation angle. Circulation. 2005;112: 2157–2162.

Acute Right Ventricular Failure

Steven M. Schwartz

Differences in anatomy and physiology between the right ventricle (RV) and left ventricle (LV) can be vitally important when treating the patient with acute heart failure. Although the success of the Fontan operation for palliation of single ventricle lesions in pediatric patients is an example that pulmonary blood flow does not require a pulsatile cardiac chamber to provide mechanical impetus, a failing RV in a two-ventricle circulation places a burden on the heart not present in the single ventricle circulation. Evidence of this principle abounds: acute RV failure from right coronary infarction, pulmonary embolus, pulmonary artery hypertension, or secondary to LV failure is associated with significant mortality [1–3]. Furthermore, failure to recognize the presence of RV dysfunction as a cause of heart failure and low cardiac-output risks neglecting essential aspects of treatment, or misapplication of therapy that while beneficial for the failing LV may further impair the failing RV.

26.1 Pathophysiology of RV Failure

Understanding the basic geometry of the RV yields insight into the way the RV adapts to various disease states. Despite similarity to the LV in terms of functioning as a blood pump, the RV is distinctly designed to serve as a conduit from the right atrium to the pulmonary artery. The compliance of the thin-walled chamber allows effective emptying of the right atrium during diastole, and maintenance of low right atrial and central venous pressure (CVP). Systole consists of contraction of the free wall toward the septum fueled by transversely oriented fibers

within the anterior wall of the RV, and then twisting of the septum; the consequence of spirally aligned fibers in this part of the heart [4]. Compliance of the chamber during systole prolongs and minimizes pressure rise [5].

One of the consequences of the geometric arrangement of the ventricles is the way in which ventricular–ventricular interactions develop as the RV dilates. In the short axis, the LV is circular, reflective of a bullet shape in three dimensions, whereas the RV forms a crescent around the anterior surface of the heart. Both ventricles are constrained by the pericardium, which puts a finite limit on the degree to which ventricular dilation can be tolerated without an accompanying rise in intracavitary diastolic pressure [6]. Given the normal shapes and relationships of the ventricles with respect to one another, the ventricular septum is normally bowed toward the RV. When RV diastolic pressure becomes higher than LV diastolic pressure, the ventricular septum shifts toward the LV impairs LV filling, and raises left atrial pressure. This puts an additional hemodynamic burden on the already failing RV, since increased left atrial pressure ultimately increases the amount of pressure the RV needs to generate for complete ejection. Although severe dilation of the LV may impair RV filling [7], failure of the LV alone is not usually accompanied by the same degree of adverse effects on RV function and physiology because the natural position of the ventricular septum is maintained, and because maintaining a high CVP to ensure RV filling in this situation does not increase afterload stress on the LV. When RV failure occurs in the context of LV failure, RV volume overload is an important cause of impaired cardiac output.

In addition to the geometric differences between the RV and LV, there are important physiologic differences as well. The normal RV pressure–volume curve is triangular in shape (Fig. 26.1) unlike the more rectangular LV pressure–volume curve [8]. This difference is accounted for by a relative lack of isovolumic contraction and relaxation times in the RV. The normally low afterload of the RV and the high compliance of the outflow portion of the

S.M. Schwartz (✉)
Head, Division of Cardiac Critical Care Medicine, Associate Professor of Paediatrics, University of Toronto, Departments of Critical Care Medicine and Paediatrics Divisions of Cardiac Critical Care Medicine and Cardiology, The Hospital for Sick Children, 555 University Ave., Toronto, M5G 1X8, Canada
e-mail: steven.schwartz@sickkids.ca

A.N. Redington et al. (eds.), *Congenital Diseases in the Right Heart*, DOI 10.1007/978-1-84800-378-1_26,
© Springer-Verlag London Limited 2009

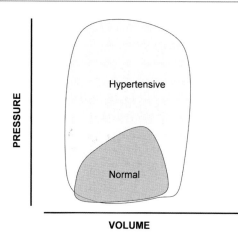

Fig. 26.1 Schemetic pressure–volume loops from the normal right ventricle and hypertensive right ventricle. Note how the shape chauges from a trapezoidal or triangular shape to a square or rectangular shape. Coincidentally the area subtended by the loop (reflecting stroke work) increases

ventricle allow ejection to begin almost instantaneously after the onset of contraction and proceed through pressure decline so that there is near complete emptying of the ventricle by the end of systole and the ejection time of the RV, thus spans the entire period of systole. An important consequence of this relationship is that even small increases in RV afterload begin to make the RV pressure–volume curve begin to resemble the normal LV pressure–volume curve, with isovolumic contraction and relaxation times becoming more prominent [9] (Fig. 26.1). Ejection fraction is reduced, although stroke volume may be maintained due to RV dilation [10], and the thin-walled RV may handle this new physiology quite poorly.

Increased RV afterload can also adversely affect RV function because it impedes RV coronary blood flow. Coronary flow to the RV occurs in both systole and diastole, so that the flow pattern in the right coronary artery resembles the flow pattern in the aorta (Fig. 26.2). As RV pressure increases, RV coronary flow becomes more like LV flow, occurring predominantly in diastole. Since the pressure-loaded RV has increased oxygen demands because of the need to generate more pressure and the appearance of isovolumic contraction and relaxation times, there is further impairment of RV function. This can lead to low cardiac output, which in turn leads to hypotension, further decreasing coronary perfusion pressure. The combination of pulmonary artery hypertension and systemic hypotension can therefore have an additively detrimental effect on perfusion of the RV muscle.

These aspects of RV anatomy and physiology may explain why sudden changes in loading conditions like pulmonary artery hypertensive crises or acute contractile dysfunction can result in life-threatening compromise of cardiac output. When an afterload stress is placed on the

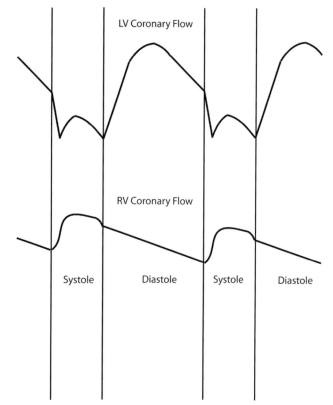

Fig. 26.2 Coronary flow patterns in the right and left ventricles. Coronary flow in the left ventricle (upper tracing) occurs predominantly in diastole. In contrast, coronary flow in the lower-pressure right ventricle occurs mostly in systole. RV = right ventricle; LV = left ventricle

RV, the alterations in contractile performance and perfusion lead to acute ventricular dilatation and regurgitation of the tricuspid valve. Tricuspid insufficiency places a further volume stress on the RV and limits antegrade flow which is ultimately the source of LV inflow and thus cardiac output. The decrease in LV filling and output, coupled with increasing RV dilatation exacerbates unfavorable ventricular interactions. A vicious cycle develops in which pressure and volume stresses on the RV becomes greater and greater, and RV function becomes more and more compromised as the cardiac output declines. Cardiovascular collapse rapidly ensues unless effective intervention is instituted.

26.2 Recognition of Acute RV Failure

Since treatment of acute heart failure is often about treating low cardiac output more so than it is about specific heart-failure therapy, and because there are no RV-specific inotropic agents, the distinction between acute RV failure and acute LV failure may seem somewhat academic. Because effective treatment of acute RV failure often requires treatment of the precipitating cause and because certain strategies commonly used for the treatment of low cardiac output affect the RV and LV differently, distinguishing acute RV failure from acute LV failure is of significant clinical importance.

Proper recognition of acute RV failure as the cause of low cardiac output depends on identification of certain characteristic hemodynamic patterns and a high index of clinical suspicion. Two of the most common scenarios in which acute RV failure occurs in the adult population, pulmonary embolus and right coronary artery infarction, are rare in the pediatric population. The association of pulmonary hypertension and RV failure with acute lung injury is frequently considered, but is rare in pediatric practice. The most common cause of acute RV failure in pediatric patients is pulmonary artery hypertension, most often as a consequence of congenital heart disease, and most commonly presenting surgery involving cardiopulmonary bypass. There are two specific aspects of congenital heart repairs that make sudden increases in pulmonary vascular resistance likely to occur in the early postoperative period. The first is that these types of repairs often involve septation of the atria or ventricles and therefore diminish or eliminate the possibility of right-to-left shunting of blood as a response to a sudden rise in pulmonary vascular resistance. Instead, RV failure and low cardiac output become manifest. The second reason that pulmonary hypertensive events are more likely to occur in the immediate postoperative period is that injury of the pulmonary endothelium occurs during cardiopulmonary bypass. The pulmonary endothelium receives its nutritive blood flow from the pulmonary circulation. During bypass, this circulation is absent, even though the rest of the body, including the bronchial arteries, is well perfused. Following bypass, the ability of the endothelium to regulate the production of nitric oxide and endothelin is deranged, and pulmonary vasoconstriction is often the result [11, 12].

Acute RV failure should thus be considered as a potential cause of low cardiac output in at-risk patients. Specific predisposing factors for postoperative pulmonary hypertension include high preoperative resistance from a long-standing ventricular or great artery level left-to-right shunt, mitral valve disease, or left ventricular failure with left atrial hypertension. Operations that tend to be associated with these risk factors include repair of truncus arteriosus, repair of aortopulmonary window, repair of cor-triatriatum, mitral valve repair or replacement (particularly for mitral stenosis), or cardiac transplantation. Ventricular septal defect where there is preexisting pulmonary vascular disease or atrioventricular canal repair in patients with Trisomy 21 can also be associated with postoperative pulmonary hypertension. Neonates undergoing repair or palliation using cardiopulmonary bypass are also potentially at increased risk because of the vasoactive capacity of the neonatal pulmonary vasculature.

Acute RV failure can also occur in the setting of long-standing LV failure because of severe LV dilation, development of associated pulmonary hypertension secondary to left atrial hypertension, or simply because of diffuse cardiac muscle disease that affects the RV and LV simultaneously. Acute RV failure should be considered in patients with chronic LV failure who experience a sudden decompensation not accounted for by changes in LV function. Echocardiographic assessment of RV pressure and clinical testing of therapy designed to lower pulmonary resistance may be necessary to identify this problem.

Perhaps the most common finding in low cardiac output secondary to acute RV failure is a high CVP. Elevated CVP is not specific for RV failure, since LV failure with severe dilatation or very-high left atrial pressure can also cause a rise in CVP. Nevertheless, a low CVP makes acute RV failure very unlikely. When there is low cardiac output and concomitant evidence of elevated pulmonary artery pressure out of proportion to the degree of left atrial hypertension (when present), it is strongly suggestive of RV failure as a contributing cause for the low cardiac output. It should be noted that the onset of a pulmonary hypertensive event may not be heralded by an acute rise in pulmonary artery pressure. The most apparent hemodynamic event may be decrease in systemic arterial pressure with no change in pulmonary artery pressure. This phenomenon occurs because cardiac output decreases as pulmonary resistance increases. The increased resistance maintains pulmonary artery pressure despite the decrease in blood flow, but lack of systemic vasoconstriction to the same degree results in systemic hypotension. In other words, when monitoring pulmonary artery pressure in a patient at risk for a pulmonary hypertensive event, one must look at changes in the ratio of pulmonary artery to systemic artery pressure. An increase in this ratio in the setting of signs of a decrease in cardiac output should be considered the result of an acute increase in pulmonary resistance and failure of the RV.

When RV failure occurs in the presence of a residual atrial or ventricular communication, cardiac output is often preserved albeit at the expense of systemic saturation. It is important to understand that atrial level shunts are driven by the relative compliance of the two ventricles. Therefore, increases in pulmonary artery pressure will not lead to a right-to-left atrial shunt until the degree of RV failure is such that RV end-diastolic pressure becomes higher than LV end-diastolic pressure. A ventricular level shunt, on the other hand, will present with cyanosis when the RV systolic pressure exceeds LV systolic pressure. In the event that the communication is not restrictive to pressure, the relative ventricular compliance (atrial shunt) or vascular resistance (ventricular shunt) will determine the direction of blood flow. When there are no patent atrial or ventricular communications, there is no opportunity for a right-to-left shunt to preserve cardiac output. If the RV is not well prepared to handle the hemodynamic effects of pulmonary vasoconstriction, or when RV filling is impeded by diastolic dysfunction, acute RV failure, and low cardiac output ensue, usually without associated cyanosis unless there is coexisting lung disease or ventilation–perfusion mismatch.

Bedside diagnosis of acute RV failure can be aided by assessing the response to relatively simple maneuvers designed to treat RV failure or its underlying causes. In the pediatric population this generally means using hyperventilation, 100% oxygen, and/or nitric oxide to acutely lower pulmonary resistance. When this is effective, the improvement in hemodynamics can be almost immediate [13, 14], with a decrease in CVP and pulmonary artery pressure and/or rise in systemic arterial pressure and even the acute appearance of urine output in a previously oliguric or anuric patient. Nitric oxide can also effectively prevent further pulmonary hypertensive events [15], although currently cost makes prophylactic use of the drug prohibitive except in the highest-risk circumstances. When there is doubt as to the contribution of RV failure or the need to apply specific therapy to treat the causes of acute RV failure, further modes of investigation are needed. Specifically, echocardiography and/or cardiac catheterization may be necessary.

26.3 Treatment of Acute RV Failure

Once there is recognition that a patient has acute RV failure, treatment must be directed at the underlying cause, and cardiovascular and respiratory support must be adjusted insofar as possible so that RV preload is optimized, afterload is minimized, and contractility is enhanced. This may require departures from the approach normally used to treat acute LV failure, so that biventricular disease with an important component of RV failure (cardiomyopathy with pulmonary hypertension, for example) requires frequent reassessment to verify improvement in RV function has not been accompanied by reduction in LV function.

One of the most important ways in which treatment of low cardiac output due to RV failure differs from treatment of low cardiac output caused by LV failure is in the way in which positive-pressure mechanical ventilation

affects ventricular loading. Ventricular-wall tension is determined by the law of Laplace, which states that tension = (pressure × radius)/(2 × wall thickness). Pressure in this equation refers to the ventricular transmural pressure, which is intracavitary pressure minus intrathoracic pressure. As intrathoracic pressure increases, ventricular transmural pressure, and thus wall tension decreases so long as intracavitary pressure does not increase even more. When intrathoracic pressure is changed from negative to positive, LV intracavitary pressure remains unchanged, or it may even decrease due to changes in circulating catecholamines, diminished work of breathing and sedation. The net effect on LV transmural pressure, and thus wall stress, is often a significant reduction. This is one of the underpinnings for the use of positive pressure ventilation in the treatment of cardiogenic shock. The transition from negative-pressure to positive-pressure ventilation has a more complex effect on the RV. Positive pressure still increases intrathoracic pressure, which would, in the absence of any other hemodynamic change, reduce afterload. The important aspect of the introduction of positive airway pressure with regard to RV afterload, however, is that positive-pressure ventilation can increase intracavitary pressure. The important principles governing the relationship of airway pressure to RV afterload are that pulmonary vascular resistance accounts for a substantial part of the afterload on the RV, and that the lowest pulmonary resistance occurs at functional residual capacity. When the lungs are relatively healthy, and pulmonary compliance is normal, positive pressure applied to the airways is easily transmitted to the pulmonary vasculature, raising effective pulmonary vascular resistance and increasing afterload on the RV. Clinically, this can occur when a person with normal lung compliance is placed on positive-pressure ventilation with anything more than minimal pressure. When there is lung disease, the relationship between airway pressure and pulmonary vascular resistance is muddied, with lung volume becoming the important intermediary. When the airway pressure is high enough to cause over-distention of the lungs, or of large lung segments, pulmonary resistance and RV afterload will be increased. On the other hand, low lung volume can also increase RV afterload by inducing atelectasis and collapse of pulmonary vessels, and can further increase pulmonary resistance because of hypoxia and ventilation–perfusion mismatch. Thus, it is apparent that using positive-pressure mechanical ventilation in the context of a failing RV is governed by the effect of positive-pressure ventilation on the RV, which requires one to have a sense of whether or not the lung compliance and pulmonary parenchyma are normal. Frequent reassessment of lung volume and clinical correlation of different ventilator settings with indicators of cardiac output, systemic perfusion, and oxygen delivery are often necessary.

Volume status is another aspect of management of low cardiac output that is both vitally important and potentially hazardous in the presence of a failing RV. Although much of this chapter has dealt with the issue of systolic RV failure, the most commonly encountered type of RV failure in pediatrics is RV diastolic failure. This is characterized by the presence of restrictive RV physiology in which the RV is preload dependent and maintenance of cardiac output may require a supranormal CVP [16, 17]. Because hydrostatic forces favor third spacing of fluids when the CVP is high, administration of large amounts of intravenous fluids becomes necessary to maintain the CVP and cardiac output. Third-space losses then contribute to accumulation of peripheral edema, ascites, and pleural effusions [16]. Unless the peritoneal and thoracic cavities are well drained, extravascular fluid collections can impair maintenance of appropriate lung volumes, and thus impart a deleterious effect on oxygenation and ventilation. Hypoxia and respiratory acidosis combined with atelectasis from compression of lung tissue by pleural fluid or limited excursion of the diaphragm can raise pulmonary vascular resistance and place an additional afterload stress on the already struggling RV. Furthermore, the dilated, high-pressure RV can impair LV efficiency via ventricular–ventricular interactions. Renal blood flow may be compromised as a consequence of increasing intraperitoneal pressure, leading to decreased renal perfusion pressure, oliguria, and inability to manage fluid balance. Essential to any strategy designed to break this cycle of high CVP, third-space fluid losses, and low cardiac output with impending respiratory and renal failure is that the RV must be able to fill and provide cardiac output at a more physiologic pressure. Creation of an ASD when one does not exist may allow maintenance of LV filling via a right-to-left atrial shunt, and also decrease the amount of volume that the RV needs to handle. Drainage of pleural and peritoneal spaces can help maintain oxygenation and ventilation at appropriately low airway pressure and also maintain renal perfusion. The use of negative-pressure ventilation may have very favorable hemodynamic effects [18, 19]. Postoperative patients may benefit from delayed sternal closure or reopening of the sternotomy in the critical care unit. Since the RV is the anterior ventricle, this maneuver can allow the RV to expand beyond the plane of the sternum and thus effectively improve compliance. Delayed sternal closure is most likely to be effective; therefore, in situations where high RV-filling pressure is partly driven by a dilated and dysfunctional RV rather than a small and hypertrophied RV since the latter is less likely to be compressed by the anterior chest wall.

When RV systolic function is poor, it is important to maintain a low CVP. In pediatric practice, the relative frequency of RV diastolic failure requiring volume loading often leads to the erroneous belief that volume loading is the appropriate strategy for RV systolic failure as well. This problem may be compounded because clinical presentations of RV systolic and diastolic failure are quite similar. History, underlying disease state, and echocardiography may be required to differentiate these entities, but the distinction is vital to institution of appropriate fluid management. When RV contractility is compromised, high CVP impedes, rather than enhances cardiac output, and the adverse effects of high RV-filling pressure on cardiac output that occur even in normal hearts are magnified. Acute volume unloading to relieve a high CVP can occasionally improve cardiac output rather rapidly. Although not well described in the literature, anecdotal experience suggests that removal of aliquots of 2–3 ml/kg of blood at a time, accompanied by close monitoring of blood pressure and clinical indicators of cardiac output can sometimes lower CVP and simultaneously increase cardiac output. Again, maintaining low afterload on the RV is crucial and can be accomplished by minimizing ventilator pressure, maintaining functional residual capacity at end expiration and imaging to rule out any residual anatomic RV outflow obstruction.

Because of the importance of systolic coronary blood flow for perfusion of the RV, maintenance of systolic blood pressure is important in RV failure. Unfortunately, increased systemic resistance and blood pressure adds afterload to the LV, so that this principle may not be realistically applicable when the contractility of both ventricles is more or less equally impaired. Nevertheless, when the situation suggests that the underlying cause of low cardiac output is RV failure, and restoration of RV function might improve LV output as well, use of alpha-adrenergic agonists or other vasoconstricting agents, such as vasopressin, may be beneficial. Since RV failure in pediatrics is often seen after relief of RV-outflow obstruction, it is important to determine if the substrate for dynamic obstruction remains postoperatively. In the event that there is still significant subpulmonary muscle, use of vasoactive drugs with beta-adrenergic activity may worsen the situation. When there is no concern regarding the RV outflow tract, use of beta-adrenergic agonists can acutely enhance RV function and relieve symptoms of low cardiac output, just as in LV failure. Milrinone and levosimendan have nonselective pulmonary vasodilating properties [20, 21]. Dobutamine, and more so epinephrine, also show benefit in animal models of right-heart failure [22]. Although there have not been studies of the long-term effects of beta-adrenergic stimulation in RV failure, it is reasonable to assume that they have the same detrimental effects as is seen in LV failure. As such, limitation of the drugs to the symptomatic patient or those with transient RV failure (such as, after repair of congenital heart disease) is probably wise.

Many studies have shown that the development of acute RV failure in the setting of preexisting LV failure is associated with a particularly poor prognosis and must be treated aggressively. RV ejection fraction is an independent predictor of survival or need for transplant in patients with established LV failure [23–25]. Even after implantation of an LV-assist device, RV dysfunction can remain an important problem that, without treatment, can limit survival to transplant [26, 27]. When there is evidence of restrictive filling in the LV, acute RV volume unloading improves LV diastolic function and cardiac output [28, 29]. Use of pulmonary vasodilators in this situation should be undertaken, recognizing the possibility of acute pulmonary edema in the event that pulmonary resistance is decreased without any relief of left atrial hypertension [30, 31]. Nevertheless, pulmonary vasodilators can improve cardiac output and heart-failure symptoms in some patients [32].

When medical support of the patient with acute RV failure is ineffective, mechanical circulatory support may be used. Although there are a variety of devices and techniques for supporting the failing LV, some may be better than others for the failing RV. The most commonly used type of mechanical support for acute RV failure has been the right ventricular-assist device, frequently employed in post-transplant RV failure [33, 34]. Although this technique is effective, more recent data suggests that biventricular support with extracorporeal membrane oxygenation may be more effective than right ventricular assist device alone [35], although conclusions from this study are limited by the use of historical rather than contemporary controls. Interestingly, in a porcine model of ischemic RV failure, use of an intra-aortic balloon pump was associated with a marked increase in stroke volume [36]. These results emphasize the importance of restoration of coronary flow in improving RV systolic performance. The degree to which this might be applicable to pediatric practice is unclear.

In addition to mechanical devices, there are also surgical/interventional options for patients with chronic RV failure but preserved RV function. Creation of an atrial septal defect can allow for decompression of the right heart and adequate filling of the left, albeit at the cost of systemic saturation. This principle is commonly taken advantage of in pediatric patients in that when postoperative RV dysfunction is expected, it is usual to leave the foramen ovale patent at the time of surgery. There is also a report of the creation of a bidirectional cavopulmonary anastamosis for acute RV failure following myocardial infarction in an adult [37]. This practice is also used in pediatrics for the patient with a small but not miniscule RV when a bidirectional cavopulmonary anastamosis is combined with closure of the atrial septal defect in the so-called "one and a half ventricle" repair.

26.4 Conclusion

Acute RV failure must be distinguished from LV failure because of important differences between the ventricles in terms of geometry, physiology, coronary flow, and the differential effects of common modes of therapy. Furthermore, RV failure often has a specific inciting cause that may be amenable to treatment. Positive-pressure mechanical ventilation and volume loading of the RV must be repeatedly and critically assessed. In general, these are treatment modalities where less is better in the setting of acute systolic RV failure. When a patient with RV failure has a simultaneously failing LV, consideration should be given as to whether or not volume unloading, decrease in mechanical ventilatory support, or increased systemic blood pressure via systemic vasoconstriction will result in improved RV function, geometrically beneficial ventricular–ventricular interactions, and ultimately improved cardiac output and oxygen delivery. Mechanical support, either univentricular or biventricular, may allow time to obtain resolution of the underlying impetus for RV failure and can result in a favorable outcome.

References

1. Cohn JN, Guiha NH, Broder MI, Limas CJ. Right ventricular infarction. Clinical and hemodynamic features. Am J Cardiol. 1974;33(2):209–14.
2. Jacobs AK, Leopold JA, Bates E, et al. Cardiogenic shock caused by right ventricular infarction: a report from the SHOCK registry [see comment]. J Am Coll Cardiol. 2003;41(8):1273–9.
3. Vieillard-Baron A, Schmitt JM, Augarde R, et al. Acute cor pulmonale in acute respiratory distress syndrome submitted to protective ventilation: incidence, clinical implications, and prognosis [see comment] [erratum appears in Crit Care Med 2002 Mar;30(3):726]. Crit Care Med. 2001;29(8):1551–5.
4. Buckberg GD, Group R. The ventricular septum: the lion of right ventricular function, and its impact on right ventricular restoration. Eur J Cardio-Thorac Surg. 2006;29 Suppl 1:S272–8.
5. Stephanazzi J, Guidon-Attali C, Escarment J. Fonction ventriculaire droite: bases physiologiques et physiopathologiques. Annales Francaises d Anesthesie et de Reanimation. 1997;16(2):165–86.
6. Visner MC, Arentzen CE, O'Connor MJ, Larson EV, Anderson RW. Alterations in left ventricular three-dimensional dynamic geometry and systolic function during acute right ventricular hypertension in the conscious dog. Circulation. 1983;67(2):353–65.

7. Taylor RR, Covell JW, Sonnenblick EH, Ross J Jr. Dependence of ventricular distensibility on filling of the opposite ventricle. Am J Physiol. 1967;213(3):711–8.

8. Redington AN, Gray HH, Hodson ME, Rigby ML, Oldershaw PJ. Characterisation of the normal right ventricular pressure-volume relation by biplane angiography and simultaneous micromanometer pressure measurements. Br Heart J. 1988;59(1):23–30.

9. Redington AN, Rigby ML, Shinebourne EA, Oldershaw PJ. Changes in the pressure–volume relation of the right ventricle when its loading conditions are modified. Br Heart J. 1990;63(1):45–9.

10. Matthay RA, Arroliga AC, Wiedemann HP, Schulman DS, Mahler DA. Right ventricular function at rest and during exercise in chronic obstructive pulmonary disease. Chest. 1992;101 Suppl 5:255S–62S.

11. Komai H, Adatia IT, Elliott MJ, de Leval MR, Haworth SG. Increased plasma levels of endothelin-1 after cardiopulmonary bypass in patients with pulmonary hypertension and congenital heart disease. J Thorac Cardiovasc Surg. 1993;106(3):473–8.

12. Wessel DL, Adatia I, Giglia TM, Thompson JE, Kulik TJ. Use of inhaled nitric oxide and acetylcholine in the evaluation of pulmonary hypertension and endothelial function after cardiopulmonary bypass. Circulation. 1993;88(5 Pt 1):2128–38.

13. Adatia I, Atz AM, Jonas RA, Wessel DL. Diagnostic use of inhaled nitric oxide after neonatal cardiac operations. J Thorac Cardiovasc Surg. 1996;112(5):1403–5.

14. Miller OI, Celermajer DS, Deanfield JE, Macrae DJ. Very-low-dose inhaled nitric oxide: a selective pulmonary vasodilator after operations for congenital heart disease. J Thorac Cardiovasc Surg. 1994;108(3):487–94.

15. Miller OI, Tang SF, Keech A, Pigott NB, Beller E, Celermajer DS. Inhaled nitric oxide and prevention of pulmonary hypertension after congenital heart surgery: a randomised double-blind study [see comment]. Lancet. 2000;356(9240):1464–9.

16. Cullen S, Shore D, Redington A. Characterization of right ventricular diastolic performance after complete repair of tetralogy of Fallot. Restrictive physiology predicts slow postoperative recovery. Circulation. 1995;91(6):1782–9.

17. Mercat A, Diehl JL, Meyer G, Teboul JL, Sors H. Hemodynamic effects of fluid loading in acute massive pulmonary embolism.[see comment]. Crit Care Med. 1999;27(3): 540–4.

18. Shekerdemian LS, Bush A, Shore DF, Lincoln C, Redington AN. Cardiorespiratory responses to negative pressure ventilation after tetralogy of fallot repair: a hemodynamic tool for patients with a low-output state. J Am Coll Cardiol. 1999;33(2):549–55.

19. Shekerdemian LS, Schulze-Neick I, Redington AN, Bush A, Penny DJ. Negative pressure ventilation as haemodynamic rescue following surgery for congenital heart disease. Intens Care Med. 2000;26(1):93–6.

20. Chang AC, Atz AM, Wernovsky G, Burke RP, Wessel DL. Milrinone: systemic and pulmonary hemodynamic effects in neonates after cardiac surgery. Crit Care Med. 1995;23(11):1907–14.

21. Stocker CF, Shekerdemian LS, Norgaard MA, et al. Mechanisms of a reduced cardiac output and the effects of milrinone and levosimendan in a model of infant cardiopulmonary bypass. Crit Care Med. 2007;35(1):252—9.

22. McGovern JJ, Cheifetz IM, Craig DM, et al. Right ventricular injury in young swine: effects of catecholamines on right ventricular function and pulmonary vascular mechanics. Pediatr Res. 2000;48(6):763–9.

23. de Groote P, Millaire A, Foucher-Hossein C, et al. Right ventricular ejection fraction is an independent predictor of survival in patients with moderate heart failure. J Am Coll Cardiol. 1998;32(4):948–54.

24. Frey B, Hulsmann M, Berger R, Zuckermann A, Stanek B, Pacher R. Right ventricular ejection fraction predicts urgent need for heart transplantation. Transplant Proc. 1997;29(1–2):592.

25. Ghio S, Gavazzi A, Campana C, et al. Independent and additive prognostic value of right ventricular systolic function and pulmonary artery pressure in patients with chronic heart failure. J Am Coll Cardiol. 2001;37(1):183–8.

26. Kavarana MN, Pessin-Minsley MS, Urtecho J, et al. Right ventricular dysfunction and organ failure in left ventricular assist device recipients: a continuing problem. Ann Thorac Surg. 2002;73(3):745–50.

27. Morgan JA, John R, Lee BJ, Oz MC, Naka Y. Is severe right ventricular failure in left ventricular assist device recipients a risk factor for unsuccessful bridging to transplant and post-transplant mortality. Ann Thorac Surg. 2004;77(3):859–63.

28. Atherton JJ, Moore TD, Lele SS, et al. Diastolic ventricular interaction in chronic heart failure [see comment]. Lancet. 1997;349(9067):1720–4.

29. Atherton JJ, Moore TD, Thomson HL, Frenneaux MP. Restrictive left ventricular filling patterns are predictive of diastolic ventricular interaction in chronic heart failure [erratum appears in J Am Coll Cardiol 1998 Mar 1;31(3):744]. J Am Coll Cardiol. 1998;31(2):413–8.

30. Argenziano M, Dean DA, Moazami N, et al. Inhaled nitric oxide is not a myocardial depressant in a porcine model of heart failure [see comment]. J Thorac Cardiovasc Surg. 1998;115(3):700–8.

31. Bocchi EA, Bacal F, Auler Junior JO, Carmone MJ, Bellotti G, Pileggi F. Inhaled nitric oxide leading to pulmonary edema in stable severe heart failure. Am J Cardiol. 1994;74(1):70–2.

32. Moraes DL, Colucci WS, Givertz MM. Secondary pulmonary hypertension in chronic heart failure: the role of the endothelium in pathophysiology and management. Circulation. 2000;102(14):1718–23.

33. Barnard SP, Hasan A, Forty J, Hilton CJ, Dark JH. Mechanical ventricular assistance for the failing right ventricle after cardiac transplantation. Eur J Cardio-Thorac Surg. 1995;9(6):297–9.

34. Odom NJ, Richens D, Glenville BE, Kirk AJ, Hilton CJ, Dark JH. Successful use of mechanical assist device for right ventricular failure after orthotopic heart transplantation. J Heart Transplant. 1990;9(6):652–3.

35. Taghavi S, Zuckermann A, Ankersmit J, et al. Extracorporeal membrane oxygenation is superior to right ventricular assist device for acute right ventricular failure after heart transplantation. Ann Thorac Surg. 2004;78(5):1644–9.

36. Nordhaug D, Steensrud T, Muller S, Husnes KV, Myrmel T. Intraaortic balloon pumping improves hemodynamics and right ventricular efficiency in acute ischemic right ventricular failure. Ann Thorac Surg. 2004;78(4):1426–32.

37. Kunihara T, Dzindzibadze V, Aicher D, Schafers HJ. Bidirectional cavopulmonary shunt for acute right ventricular failure in an adult patient. Ann Thorac Surg. 2004;78(3):1066–8.

27.1 Heart Failure as a Biventricular Disease

The clinical recognition of right ventricular dysfunction as a part of the syndrome of heart failure dates to the Hippocratic writings of the third century BC, where the description "The abdomen fills with water, the feet and legs swell, the shoulders, clavicles, chest and thighs melt away" first appears. Numerous early classical physicians [1] went on to contribute to the understanding of heart failure as a biventricular phenomenon, including Arataeus of Capadoccia (describing *Cor pulmonale*), Galen (who nevertheless failed to recognize the existence of the pulmonary circulation), and Ibn an-Nafis , a physician in Cairo writing in the twelfth century (who did recognize it) [2]. Eventually in 1669, Lower [3] formulated a definition of heart failure, and in 1674 Mayow [4] observed that mitral stenosis appeared to obstruct blood flow through the lungs, with the result that the right ventricle became dilated. In 1832, James Hope proposed the *backward failure hypothesis* [5] to account for the hydropic consequences of heart failure, stating that "when a ventricle fails to empty its contents, blood accumulates, and pressure rises in that ventricle and in the venous system emptying into it". Much later still, early in the twentieth century, Mackenzie [6] proposed the "forward-failure" hypothesis emphasizing systemic and renal underperfusion as a feature of heart failure.

Given this historical recognition, has the phenomenon of right ventricular dysfunction following upon left ventricular failure been described in the modern era? Direct hemodynamic measurements of patients with advanced left heart failure reveal that right atrial pressure (and therefore right ventricular-filling pressure) is significantly elevated [7]. Importantly there is also a direct relationship between right atrial and pulmonary capillary wedge pressures in these patients. Furthermore, there is good evidence of right ventricular remodeling occurring as a consequence of isolated disease of the left ventricle. This was described by Hirose et al. [8] who performed serial electron beam CT scans of asymptomatic patients following angiographically proven left ventricular anterior wall infarction. The authors demonstrated a progressive increment in both left *and* right ventricular volumes after the index event, apparently related to altered filling rates of both of the ventricles, and unrelated to changes in intrinsic systolic contractile function of the left ventricle.

Subsequent studies have detailed the presence of altered right ventricular and central hemodynamics, as well as diminished right ventricular contractile function in chronic left ventricular failure: Spinarova et al. [9] described the difference between patients with symptomatic left ventricular failure with diminished right ventricular function (quantified by tricuspid annular velocity) versus those with only left ventricular dysfunction. It was evident that those patients with diminished right ventricular function also had abnormal loading of the right ventricle, with higher filling pressures, higher pulmonary vascular resistance, and evidence of right ventricular remodeling, despite having a similar left ventricular ejection fraction to those with isolated LV dysfunction. This implies that altered loading conditions may result in right ventricular dysfunction in some, but not all patients with left ventricular failure.

27.2 The Importance of RV Dysfunction in Heart Failure

What then is the relevance of right ventricular dysfunction in the presence of left ventricular failure? DiSalvo [10] has shown retrospectively by multivariate analysis, that in patients with advanced left ventricular failure, right ventricular function during exercise (as determined by

P.F. Kantor (✉)
Department of Paediatrics, Hospital for Sick Children, Toronto, ON, Canada

radionuclide angiography) was able to predict survival over a period of 3 years following transplant listing. In this series of 65 patients, right ventricular ejection fraction (RVEF) of greater than 35% at exercise was *the only* independent predictor of event-free survival by a proportional hazards analysis. In contrast, more recognized indices of cardiac function, like resting cardiac index, maximal oxygen consumption, left ventricular ejection fraction (LVEF) at rest, or incremental increase in left or right ejection fraction by >5% on exercise were *not* predictive of survival on univariate or multivariate analysis.

In a subsequent prospective series of 205 patients with moderate symptomatic heart failure, DeGroote and co-authors [11] noted that an RVEF of <25% was highly predictive of a lower event-free survival (59%) over a median follow-up duration of 2 years, as compared to equivalent patients with better-preserved right ventricular function. More recently, others have demonstrated that both load-dependent (tricuspid annulus velocity), and load-independent (isovolumic acceleration) myocardial Doppler indices of right ventricular function appear to be predictive of survival in patients with chronic stable left ventricular failure [12].

It would appear from these data that a case can be made both for the existence and the relevance of right ventricular failure occurring secondarily to left ventricular dysfunction. Does this secondary right ventricular dysfunction represent a form of left–right ventricular–ventricular interaction?

27.3 Ventricular Interaction in Heart Failure

Ventricular interaction, as described originally in 1910 by Bernheim [13], was a theory purporting that pathologic left ventricular hypertrophy and failure might result in a reduction in right ventricular diastolic function. In 1914, Henderson and Prince later noted that progressive right ventricular pressure and volume loading could also result in diminished left ventricular ejection partly attributed to pericardial constraint [14]. Thus the concept of ventricular interaction has long been appreciated, especially in the context of heart failure. A concise definition of ventricular interaction, articulated by Santamore would be "forces transmitted from one ventricle to the other ventricle through the myocardium and pericardium, independent of neural, humoral and circulatory effects" [15]. In this respect, one should confine the concept to those effects that occur by direct transmural (i.e., septal) force transmission or volume displacement, rather than *series effects* of altered pulmonary vascular resistance and pressure or volume loading of the right ventricle.

Diastolic ventricular interaction has been well described in open-chest experimental models perhaps most elegantly by Weber and colleagues [16], wherein an increase in ventricular pressure results in diastolic septal shift with altered diastolic pressure and filling-volume relationship for the contralateral ventricle. Hence, a supraphysiologic rise in right-sided venous return should result in a corresponding decrease in left-sided filling volume and an increase in left-sided filling pressures *in vivo*. While this effect is immediate and reflected by transseptal pressure and septal position in experimental models [17], the threshold for its occurrence in clinical heart failure with an intact pericardium was unclear.

In the clinical setting, most hemodynamic data are acquired in the context of advanced heart failure, frequently at pretransplant assessment [7]. There is clearly an association between elevated left ventricular and elevated right ventricular filling pressures, and a reduction in systemic venous return (following diuretic therapy) results in improved symptoms, and perhaps in an *improved* pressure–volume relation, for both ventricles.

Atherton and colleagues [18] have studied patients with stable chronic heart failure, and an ejection fraction of less than 35%. The authors demonstrated that the application of lower body suction (−30 mmHg) for 5 min resulted in an expected decrease in right ventricular diastolic volume, and small but significant *increase* in left ventricular end-diastolic volume, (which did not occur in control patients) with no change in atrial filling pressures (Fig. 27.1). Subsequently, Bleasdale and colleagues [19] have demonstrated that the immediate effect of inferior caval vein occlusion in spontaneously breathing patients

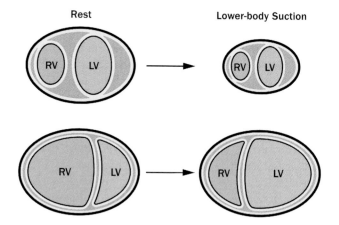

Fig. 27.1 Schematic representation of changes in ventricular volumes that occur during acute volume unloading such as that produced by application of lower-body suction **A**: Normal individuals. **B**: Direct diastolic ventricular interaction in heart failure patients with pericardial constraint. RV = right ventricle; LV = left ventricle.
Adapted from [18]

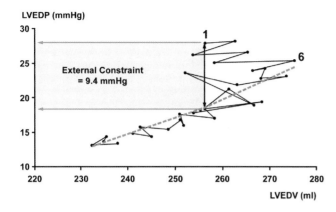

Fig. 27.2 An example of instantaneous end-diastolic pressure-volume measurements during IVC occlusion of a patient with significant external (i.e., right ventricular) constraint. This acute reduction in RV volume removes external constraint to LV filling from the RV and pericardium. "During this intervention, the LVEDP is progressively reduced over several beats. For each beat, the relation between LVEDP and LVEDV was assessed. In the absence of external constraint, IVC occlusion gradually reduces both LVEDP and LVEDV, with the values progressing downward and leftward along a single end-diastolic pressure–volume relation. In contrast, in severe heart failure, when marked external constraint is present, LVEDV initially (for a few beats) increases as LVEDP falls. Only after the external constraint has been removed do the pressure–volume values move down and to the left. Number markers represent successive beats after IVC occlusion."
Adapted from [19]

with heart failure is an immediate increment in left ventricular volume for the same filling pressure (Fig. 27.2).

27.4 When and How Does Clinically Relevant Left–Right Ventricular Interaction Result?

There is clear evidence that the volume status of the right ventricle has become a liability to the patients described above. It is not clear, however, whether this volume loading of the right ventricle has occurred by virtue of the chronic fluid retention seen in left ventricular failure, or whether right ventricular remodeling and dysfunction has in fact occurred as a direct myofiber or interventricular effect of a failing left ventricle on the susceptible right ventricle.

If one examines the situation of isolated, asymptomatic left ventricular diastolic dysfunction, as occurs in patients with left ventricular hypertrophy due to systemic hypertension, one finds that there are indeed subtle direct effects of the left ventricle on right ventricular diastolic function [20, 21]. In these patients, diastolic-filling indices, and longitudinal diastolic tissue velocity of the right ventricle closely mirror those of the left ventricle,

with similar (albeit load-dependent) features of delayed relaxation. In the situation of established systolic dysfunction, it is clear from several cross-sectional studies [9–12] that right ventricular function is significantly impaired in a sizeable proportion if not a majority of adult patients with chronic heart failure. The following factors have been identified as being relevant to the pathogenesis of secondary right ventricular failure in these (predominantly adult) populations. Figure 27.3A–E indicates a theoretical construct of ventricular pressures, septal positions, and empirical ventricular interactions in various phenotypes of heart failure.

27.5 Pressure Overload of the Right Ventricle

Increased right ventricular afterload results in right ventricular hypertrophy, which is traditionally considered to be compensatory and beneficial to the maintenance of normal ventricular systolic wall stress. However, in humans with idiopathic pulmonary hypertension [22], there is a substantial *rise* in right ventricular wall stress, regardless of the degree of compensatory hypertrophy attained (Fig. 27.3B). Furthermore there is a close inverse relationship between right ventricular ejection fraction, and right ventricular wall stress, demonstrating that deteriorating right ventricular function in the face of increased afterload is inevitable.

In the case of chronic left ventricular failure, as reported by Ghio et al. in a large single-center experience of adult patients with congestive heart failure of mixed etiology [23], an elevated pulmonary arterial pressure (mean > 20 mmHg) was demonstrated in approximately 60%. A close correlation was evident between the mean pulmonary arterial and the pulmonary capillary wedge pressures in these patients ($r = 0.8$). Also, a reasonable inverse correlation was found between mean pulmonary arterial pressure and right ventricular ejection fraction (RVEF). In this, and other studies, mortality was by far the highest in patients with both low RVEF, and an elevated pulmonary arterial pressure suggesting that these two variables together may be a good indicator of end-stage left ventricular failure. Drazner and co-workers have demonstrated similar findings in an even larger multicenter study of patients during assessment for possible cardiac transplant [7]. In 1,000 adult patients who underwent right heart catheterization, the following data emerged: systolic pulmonary arterial pressure was elevated (mean of 52 ± 16 mmHg) and varied in direct proportion to the pulmonary capillary wedge pressure ($r = 0.79$). This suggested that elevated right-sided systolic pressure was determined primarily by left-sided filling pressure, and not by the presence of

Patterns of Ventricular Interaction in Heart Failure

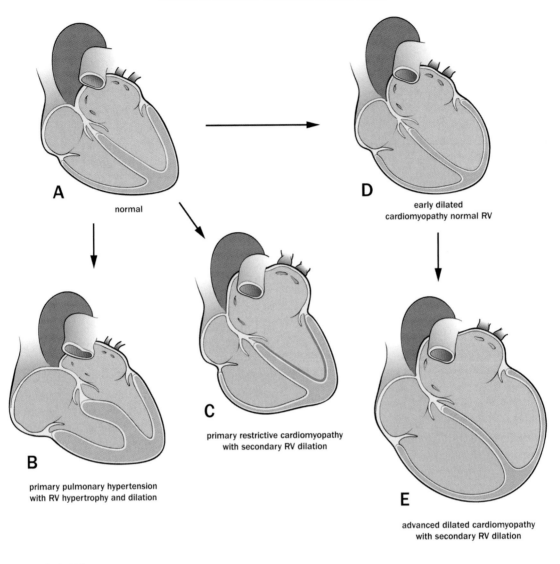

© 2007 SickKids Graphic Centre

Fig. 27.3 Illustrations of recognizable patterns of biventricular failure with important ventricular–ventricular interactions. **A.** normal: neutral position of atrial septum, ellipsoid left ventrical, and trapezoid right ventricle. **B.** right ventricular pressure overload as a result of pulmonary: hypertension. Dilated and hypertrophied right ventricle, compromising left ventricular diastolic filling. **C.** Primary restrictive cardiomyopathy with massive dilation of the left atrium, and secondary compromise of right ventricular systolic function. **D.** Dilated cardiomyopathy with predominant left ventricular involvement. Left ventricular remodeling has occurred, and ventricular septal position is neutral, revealing early equalization of transseptal diastolic pressure. Right ventricular function is preserved. **E.** Advanced dilated cardiomyopathy: left ventricular systolic function is severely compromised. Right ventricular filling pressure and systolic pressure are significantly elevated, and right ventricular remodeling has occurred through several possible mechanisms (see text). Left ventricular filling is also compromised by external constraint from the right ventricle, with associated left bundle branch block distorting septal position

parenchymal lung disease. As would be expected, these patients also had elevated right-sided preload, with right atrial filling pressures of 12 ± 7 mmHg (Fig. 27.3D). Interestingly, the concordance rate of elevated right atrial with elevated pulmonary wedge pressure was around 80%, right ventricular ejection fraction was not, however, measured in this study.

Acquired restrictive physiology of the left ventricle is not uncommon in adult populations, where it may occur in the context of amyloidosis, hemochromatosis, and other systemic conditions. Primary (sarcomeric origin) restrictive cardiomyopathy is an uncommon disease more frequently noted in children or young adults. However, in both cases, a chronic and severe elevation of LV end-diastolic pressure results in the restriction of late diastolic mitral inflow, with LA dilatation and chronic pulmonary venous hypertension. While such patients frequently have a pulmonary capillary wedge pressure in the range of 25–30 mmHg, they infrequently demonstrate any fixed elevation of pulmonary vascular resistance. Nonetheless, PA and RV pressure is frequently elevated, and over a number of years RV dilatation and systolic dysfunction can be demonstrated (Fig. 27.3C). An ominous sign in such patients is the progressive elevation of RV diastolic pressure, and clinical features of RV dysfunction, including pleural effusions and ascites. Thromboembolic complications and arrhythmic sudden death are also well-recognized clinical sequelae in this context, but the contribution of the RV to these events is unclear.

27.6 Volume Overload of the Right Ventricle

It has been noted that the prognosis for patients with heart failure is worse if both ventricles are congruently dilated (Fig. 27.3E), and better if the right ventricular dimension is less than that of the left ventricle [24]. In a small single-center experience, Lewis et al. [25] noted that the survival of children with biventricular dilation in nonischemic cardiomyopathy was significantly worse than in those who had a smaller right ventricular dimension. This survival disadvantage was also associated with more severe mitral and tricuspid regurgitation in these subjects.

As is the case in left ventricular disease, right ventricular chamber remodeling can occur as a result of several processes. Ischemic damage to the septum and inferior wall of the left ventricle can be associated with right ventricular volume enlargement. Progressively elevated pulmonary arterial pressure may result in pulmonic or tricuspid valve insufficiency. A cardiomyopathic process may involve both left and right ventricle with tissue damage and apoptosis distributed variably. Regarding the latter, aside from the classic scenario of arrhythmogenic right ventricular dysplasia, right ventricular involvement may be particularly pronounced in cases of iron overload cardiomyopathy resulting from thallassemia major [26]. In this condition, left ventricular failure is typically accompanied by profound right ventricular diastolic dysfunction in the presence of a normal pulmonary vascular resistance.

27.7 Altered Right Atrial and Right Ventricular Flow Dynamics

Diastolic function of the right ventricle is compromised when right ventricular hypertrophy and elevated preload and afterload occur. Detailed MRI assessment of right ventricular systolic and diastolic filling rates suggests that right atrial reservoir function increases as a result of impaired right ventricular diastolic function, and that right atrial contractile function (late diastolic filling) compensates in order to maintain the same ventricular preload [27]. Resting cardiac output remains unchanged in the short term, but during hemodynamic stress, or during exercise, reduced right ventricular filling occurs, corresponding to a decrease in cardiac output.

The effect of elevated right ventricular and right atrial diastolic pressure, transmitted to the coronary sinus may also result in an impediment to effective coronary perfusion pressure as would be assumed from a vascular waterfall model of coronary flow [28, 29]. By the same token, it is clear that a simple arithmetic assessment of effective perfusion pressure across the coronary bed by extrapolation from diastolic arterial and coronary sinus pressure is seriously flawed [29]. The effects of both elevated left ventricular diastolic pressure on coronary flow distribution, and the possibility of regional cross-talk between left and right ventricular coronary beds remain unresolved. Some authors have described a substantial redistribution of coronary flow occurring in the presence of massively elevated coronary sinus pressure [30], but such reports are anecdotal, and the physiologic mechanisms for regional ventricular coronary flow distribution remains to be described.

27.8 Sympathetic, Endocrine and Paracrine Effects of Right Ventricular Failure

The right heart is intrinsic to the regulation of intravascular volume during normal homeostasis. Baroreceptors are present in both right and left atrial chambers, and function in the autoregulation of intravascular volume: first, they respond immediately to increasing filling pressure by a reflex inhibition of sympathetic tone, resulting in vasodilation. Second, they suppress the nonosmotic production of arginine–vasopressin from the hypothalamus and pituitary gland (The Henry–Gauer reflex), and as a result, renal tubular collecting duct V2 receptors are inactivated, allowing aquaresis to proceed. Third, they regulate the local production of atrial natriuretic peptide, which has the effect of increasing glomerular filtration rate, and sodium excretion from the proximal tubule. In addition, the local production of renin is inhibited, further potentiating vasodilation.

An additional mechanism of recruiting renal water and sodium excretion is via the secretion of the natriuretic peptides atrial natriuretic peptide (ANP) (produced by atrial tissue), and brain natriuretic peptide (BNP) (by ventricular tissue). BNP production has similar effects to atrial natriuretic peptide production, resulting in increased urinary water and sodium loss, as well as vasodilation. One might assume therefore that increased preload on the right atrium or ventricle, under conditions of diminished ventricular ejection will result in vasodilation, increased glomerular blood flow, filtration, natriuresis, and aquaresis. These three effects, however, are subject to the more powerful feedback loop of arterial baroreceptors, which respond to lower mean arterial pressure by stimulating adrenergic drive, vasopressin production, and also renin and angiotensin production. The presence of nondilute urine in most patients with heart failure suggests that the arterial arm predominates in this feedback loop [31]. In the presence of compensated LV systolic failure, without volume overload, Brain natriuretic peptide levels remain mildly elevated. Then if sudden volume overload occurs, Brain natriuretic peptide levels climb dramatically, although there may be no remarkable change in either LV systolic function or in mean arterial pressure, but rather a change in central venous filling pressure. The latter suggests that right ventricular and atrial level receptors, which reflect diastolic function, also have a pivotal role in regulating intravascular volume once LV failure has occurred; however, this is unproven.

Some data [32] have been generated which supports the concept of differential Brain natriuretic peptide levels in association with either predominantly right or left ventricular dysfunction (Fig. 27.4). There are also data that support a differential expression of local Angiotensin II receptors, matrix metalloproteinases, and indeed Brain natriuretic peptide production in the RV versus the LV depending on the loading conditions of each ventricle [33].

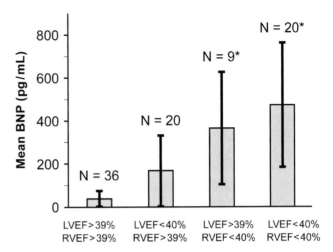

Fig. 27.4 Among patients with RVEF >40%, no significant Brain natriuretic peptide difference was found between patients with or without additional left ventricular systolic dysfunction ($P = 0.51$). Among patients with LVEF <40%, plasma Brain natriuretic peptide levels were significantly higher in patients with RVEF <40% than in patients with RVEF > 40% ($P = 0.004$) whereas age, renal function, clinical findings, ventricular volumes, LVEF, or medication were not significantly different. Adapted from [32]

heterogeneity result in diminished left ventricular function?" (to which the answer remains to be defined)

27.9 Electromechanical Coupling of the Right Heart

It has been evident for some time that the presence of unabated pulmonary insufficiency of whatever cause will ultimately result in right ventricular failure [34] Redington et al. have coined the phrase mechano-electrical interaction [35] in describing the interaction that exists within the right ventricle between mechanical dysfunction and electrical perturbation. In patients with postoperative right ventricular dysfunction, there is a direct qualitative association between regional right ventricular tissue Doppler velocity inhomogeneity and the extent of QRS duration lengthening, as well as QRS, QT, and JT interval dispersion [36]. Numerous questions arise from this important observation, including: "Does mechanical and electrical heterogeneity within a ventricle progress with worsening dysfunction? " (to which the answer is likely yes), and "Does right ventricular

27.10 Hemodynamic Implications of Right Ventricular Dysfunction for the Left Ventricle

For intravascular volume to remain stable, each ventricle must eject all the blood that it receives from the other ventricle. Thus, a progressive decline in RV stroke volume after the onset of LV failure is in some respects, a necessary adaptation: a hypertrophied RV with a relatively preserved stroke volume may contribute to the occurrence of acute pulmonary edema with sudden changes in LV systolic function, leading to a rise in pulmonary capillary hydrostatic pressure in the face of sustained RV stroke volume. The limits of tolerance of the alveolar capillary endothelium to wide swings in hydrostatic pressure may be overwhelmed if the RV does not decrease its ejection fraction.

The alternate side of this *double-edged sword*, is seen with progressive dilation of the right ventricle: as it adapts to the scenario of left ventricular systolic, and eventual diastolic failure, a reduction in right ventricular stroke volume coexists with increased venous pressure, and may result in a combination of adverse sequelae: (Fig 27.5) systemic venous congestion, elevated systemic vascular

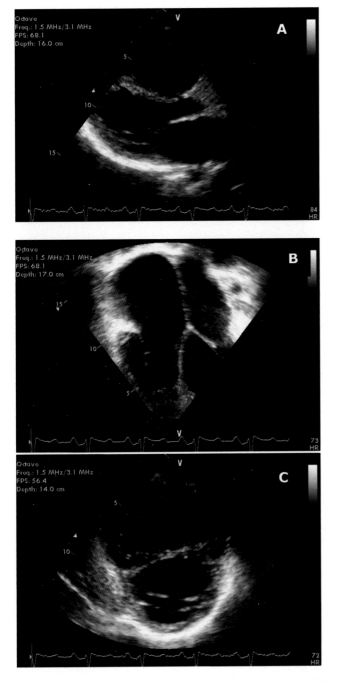

Fig. 27.5 Echocardiographic images of a 15-year-old patient with end-stage dilated cardiomyopathy (post-anthracycline exposure). There has been significant right ventricular remodeling, with a loss of tricuspid valve coaptation, severe tricuspid regurgitation, and right ventricular failure. Notice the septal position in long-axis (**A**) and short-axis (**C**) views, and massive atrial enlargement in the four-chamber view (**B**). These suggest that right ventricular failure is likely to compromise left ventricular diastolic filling and cardiac output

27.11 Closing the RV–LV Loop: Ventricular Interaction and Biventricular Failure

The latter question is intriguing, and may help to explain the observation noted since the 1970s [38] that numerous patients with right ventricular dysfunction following surgical repair of right ventricular outflow tract obstruction go on to develop late left ventricular failure. Early work in the clinical and experimental setting of acute pulmonary embolism, and right ventricular pressure and volume overload showed as a proof of concept that there is an adverse left ventricular diastolic interaction conferred by a shift in septal position [39, 40]. Subsequent echocardiographic and MRI studies of patients with primary right ventricular dysfunction (following the repair of congenital heart lesions) have demonstrated subtle abnormalities in left ventricular filling as well as left ventricular systolic function [41, 42]. The precise mechanism that results in this secondary left ventricular dysfunction is not yet clear. Possible candidate pathways include: abnormal septal position and left ventricular diastolic filling [43, 44], abnormal electrical synchrony of the septum resulting from left bundle branch block [19], and abnormal myofibril function, involving fibers shared by both ventricles.

In patients with established combined ventricular dysfunction as a result of primary right ventricular disease, the relationship between right and left ventricular ejection fraction as determined by MRI is relatively strong, with an *r* value of 0.67 [45]. Not surprisingly, the incidence of sudden arrhythmic death in patients with left ventricular dysfunction secondary to right ventricular disease is approximately *fivefold* higher than in those with normal left ventricular function [46]. One plausible explanation for this phenomenon is that the electrical dispersion that occurs in the right ventricular dysfunction has a direct influence on left ventricular function: this interventricular conduction block has previously been shown to impact exercise performance in patients with postoperative disease of the right ventricle [47]. There is also good evidence from detailed MRI-derived flow data that abnormal septal motion is the primary mechanism for impaired diastolic filling of the left ventricle following right ventricular failure [48]. Recent data from our institution [24] and from others [19] suggests that multisite pacing which reverses interventricular septal activation delay in patients with RV dysfunction may improve left ventricular contractile performance and resting cardiac output.

27.12 Summary

Traditional views that heart failure manifests itself clinically as either *forward* failure or *backward* failure (*series ventricular interaction*) may have decreased the appreciation that

resistance, and increased right ventricular diastolic volume. Will further impairment of LV filling via direct right-to-left ventricular interaction then result in a further progression of left ventricular failure? [37].

both normal and failing ventricles are directly codependent (*parallel ventricular interaction*). The distinct roles of the right and the left ventricle in the pathogenesis of heart failure can now be more accurately dissected by means of invasive hemodynamic studies, real-time noninvasive imaging, intracardiac electrophysiologic studies, and tissue genomic profiling. The overall picture that emerges is one of ventricular interaction during heart failure in which the function of the right ventricle can decline after left ventricular failure has occurred, and vice versa. This implies an interdependence of right and left ventricular hemodynamics, and that disease of the one ultimately leads to dysfunction of the other as well.

Regardless of these concepts, patients with right ventricular and left ventricular diseases are at considerably higher risk for death than those with left ventricular disease alone. The progression of right ventricular failure following left ventricular dysfunction is likely to be heralded by several specific events, such as:

- chronic elevation of LV diastolic pressure resulting in elevated pulmonary arterial pressure;
- chronic volume loading of the right ventricle as a result of pulmonary and tricuspid valvular insufficiency, and right ventricular remodeling;
- electrical dyssynchrony of septal motion due to the effects of adverse mechano-electrical coupling;
- loss of shared contractile fibers between the two ventricles;
- the override of the right ventriclular neurohormonal response by that of increased arterial baroreceptor-mediated signaling; and
- specific disease involvement of the right ventricular matrix and contractile elements.

To date, there has been little investigation into the possible role of coronary flow redistribution in the pathophysiology of secondary right ventricular dysfunction. Important recent data support the concept that reversal of right ventricular and septal electrical and mechanical dyssynchrony can benefit LV function, and contribute to the reversal of disease progression in these patients

References

1. Riegger E. History of heart failure (including hypertension). Z Kardiol. 2002;91(Suppl 4):IV/60–IV/63.
2. Meyerhof M. Ibn an-Nafis (XIIIth Cent.) and his theory of the lesser circulation. Isis. 1935;23:100–20
3. Lower R. Tractatus de Corde. London: Allestry, 1669.
4. Mayow J. Tractatus Quinque Medico-Physici, 1674
5. Hope JA. Treatise on the disease of the heart and great vessels. London, Churchill, 1832
6. Mackenzie J. Disease of the heart, (3rd edn). London: Oxford University Press, 1913.
7. Drazner MH, Hamilton MA, Fonarow G, Creaser J, Flavell C, Stevenson L. Relationship between right and left-sided filling pressures in 1000 patients with advanced heart failure. J Heart Lung Trans. 1999;18:1126–32.
8. Hirose K, Reed JE, Rumberger JA. Serial changes in left and right ventricular systolic and diastolic dynamics during the first year after an index left ventricular Q wave myocardial infarction. J Am Coll Cardiol. 1995;25:1097–104.
9. Spinarova L, Meluzin J, Toman J, Hude P, Krejci J, Vitovec J. Right ventricular dysfunction in chronic heart failure patients. Eur J Heart Fail. 2005;7:485–9.
10. Di Salvo TG, Mathier M, Semigran MJ, Dec GW. Preserved right ventricular ejection fraction predicts exercise capacity and survival in advanced heart failure. J Am Coll Cardiol. 1995;25:1143–53.
11. De Groote P, Millaire A, Foucher-Hossein C, Nugue O, Marchandise X, Ducloux G, et al. Right ventricular ejection fraction is an independent predictor of survival in patients with moderate heart failure. J Am Coll Cardiol. 1998;32:948–54.
12. Meluzin J, Spinarova L, Hude P, Krejci J, Kincl V, Panovsky R, et al. Prognostic importance of various echocardiographic right ventricular functional parameters in patients with symptomatic heart failure. J Am Soc Echocardiogr. 2005;18:435–44.
13. Bernheim E. De L'asystoleveineuse dans l'hypertrophe du Coeur gauche par stenose concomitante du ventricule droit. Rev de Med. 1910;30:785 (cited by deBono D, The Lancet. 1997;349:1712).
14. Henderson Y, Prince AL. The systolic discharge and the pericardial volume. Am J Physiol. 1914;36:116.
15. Bove AA, Santamore WP: Ventricular interdependence. Prog Cardiovasc Dis. 1981;23:365–388.
16. Weber KT, Janicki JS, Shroff S, Fishman AP. Contractile mechanics and interaction of the right and left ventricles. Am J Cardiol. 1981;47:686–95.
17. Kroeker CA, Shrive NG, Belenkie I, Tyberg JV. Pericardium modulates left and right ventricular stroke volumes to compensate for sudden changes in atrial volume. Am J Physiol—Heart Circ Physiol. 2003;284(6):H2247–54.
18. Atherton JJ, Moore TD, Lele SS, Thomson HL, Galbraith AJ, Belenkie I, et al. Diastolic ventricular interaction in chronic heart failure. Lancet. 1997;349:1720–24.
19. Bleasdale RA, Turner MS, Mumford CE, Steendijk P, Paul V, Tyberg JV, et al. Left ventricular pacing minimizes diastolic ventricular interaction, allowing improved preload-dependent. Systol Perf Circ. 2004;110:2395–400
20. Chakko S, de Marchena E, Kessler KM, Materson BJ, Myerburg RJ. Right ventricular diastolic function in systemic hypertension. Am J Cardiol. 1990;65:1117–20.
21. Cicala S, Galderisi M, Caso P, Petrocelli A, D'Errico A, de Divitiis O. et al. Right ventricular diastolic dysfunction in arterial systemic hypertension: analysis by pulsed tissue Doppler [Journal Article]. Eur J Echocardiogr. 2002;3: 135–42
22. Quaife RA, Chen MY, Lynch D, Badesch DB, Groves BM, Wolfel E, et al. Importance of right ventricular end-systolic regional wall stress in idiopathic pulmonary arterial hypertension: a new method for estimation of right ventricular wall stress. Eur J Med Res. 2006;11:214–20.
23. Ghio S, Gavazzi A, Campana C, et al. Independent and additive prognostic value of right ventricular systolic function and pulmonary artery pressure in patients with chronic heart failure. J Am Coll Cardiol. 2001;37:183–8.
24. Redington AN. Pathophysiology of right ventricular failure. Seminars in thoracic and cardiovascular surgery. Pediatr Card Surg Ann. 2006;9:3–10.
25. Lewis AB. Prognostic value of echocardiography in children with idiopathic dilated cardiomyopathy. Am Heart J. 1994;128:133–6.

26. Hahalis G, Manolis AS, Apostolopoulos D, Alexopoulos D, Vagenakis AG, Zoumbos NC. Right ventricular cardiomyopathy in beta-thalassaemia major. Eur. Heart J. 2002;23(2): 147–56.

27. Gaynor S, Maniar HS, Bloch JB, Steendijk P, Moon MR. Right atrial and ventricular adaptation to chronic right ventricular pressure overload. Circulation. 2005;112[Suppl I]:I212–8.)

28. Kazmaier S, Hanekop G-G, Grossmann M, Dörge H, Götze K, Schöndube F, et al. Instantaneous diastolic pressure–flow relationship in arterial coronary bypass grafts. Eur J Anaesthesiol. 2006;23:373–9.

29. Dole WP, Richards KL, Hartley CJ, Alexander GM, Campbell AB, Bishop VS. Diastolic coronary artery pressure–flow velocity relationships in conscious man. Cardiovasc Res. 1984;18: 548–54.

30. Verma S. Coronary sinus flow reversal in congestive heart failure detected during biventricular pacing. J Interv Card Electrophysiol. 2005;14:45–9.

31. Schrier RW, Abraham WT. Hormones and hemodynamics in heart failure. N Eng J Med. 1999;341:577–86.

32. Mariano-Goulart D, Eberle MC, Boudousq V, Hejazi-Moughari A, Piot C, Caderas de Kerleau C, et al. Major increase in brain natriuretic peptide indicates right ventricular systolic dysfunction in patients with heart failure. Eur J Heart Fail. 2003 Aug;5(4):481–8.

33. Bolger AP, Sharma R, Li W, Leenarts M, Kalra PR, Kemp M, et al. Neurohormonal activation and the chronic heart failure syndrome in adults with congenital heart disease. Circulation. 2002;106(1):92–9.

34. Shimazaki Y. Blackstone EH. Kirklin JW. The natural history of isolated congenital pulmonary valve incompetence: surgical implications. Thorac Cardiovasc Surg. 1984;32:257–9.

35. Vogel M, Sponring J, Cullen S, Deanfield JE, Redington AN. Regional wall motion and abnormalities of electrical depolarization and repolarization in patients after surgical repair of tetralogy of Fallot. Circulation. 2001;103(12): 1669–73.

36. Chow PC, Liang XC, Lam WW, Cheung EW, Wong KT, Cheung YF. Mechanical right ventricular dysynchrony in patients after atrial switch operation for transposition of the great arteries. Am J Cardiol. 2008;15(101):874–81.

37. Morris-Thurgood J, Frenneaux MP. Diastolic ventricular interaction and ventricular diastolic filling. Heart Fail Rev. 2000;5:307–23.

38. Related Articles, Links Garson A Jr, Nihill MR, McNamara DG, Cooley DA. Status of the adult and adolescent after repair of tetralogy of Fallot. Circulation. 1979;59:1232–40.

39. Belenkie I, Dani R, Smith ER, Tyberg JV. Effects of volume loading during experimental acute pulmonary embolism. Circulation. 1989;80:170–88.

40. Jardin F, DuBourg O, Guéret P, Delorme G, Bourdarias J-P. Quantitative two-dimensional echocardiography in massive pulmonary embolism: emphasis on ventricular interdependence and leftward septal displacement. J Am Coll Cardiol. 1987;10: 1201–6.

41. D'Andrea A, Caso P, Sarubbi B, D'Alto M, Giovanna Russo M, Scherillo M, et al. Right ventricular myocardial activation delay in adult patients with right bundle branch block late after repair of Tetralogy of Fallot. Eur J Echocardiogr. 2004;5: 123–31.

42. Geva T, Sandweiss BM, Gauvreau K, Lock JE, Powell AJ. Factors associated with impaired clinical status in long-term survivors of tetralogy of Fallot repair evaluated by magnetic resonance imaging. J Am Coll Cardiol 2004;43:1068–74.

43. Santamore WP, Dell'Italia LJ. Ventricular interdependence: significant left ventricular contributions to right ventricular systolic function. Progr Cardiovasc Dis. 1998; 40: 89–308.

44. Janicki JS. Influence of the pericardium and ventricular interdependence on left ventricular diastolic and systolic function in patients with heart failure. Circulation. 1990;81(2 Suppl.) III15–20.

45. Davlouros P, Kilner PJ, Hornung TS, Li W, Francis JM, Moon JC, et al. Right ventricular function in adults with repaired tetralogy of Fallot assessed with cardiovascular magnetic resonance imaging: detrimental role of right ventricular outflow aneurysms or akinesia and adverse right-to-left ventricular interaction. J Am Coll Cardiol. 2002;40:2044–52.

46. Ghai A, Silversides C, Harris L, Webb GD, Siu SC, Therrien J. Left ventricular dysfunction is a risk factor for sudden cardiac death in adults late after repair of tetralogy of Fallot. J Am Coll Cardiol. 2002;40:1675–80.

47. D'Andrea A, Caso P, Sarubbi B, D'Alto M, Giovanna Russo M, Scherillo M, et al. Right ventricular myocardial activation delay in adult patients with right bundle branch block late after repair of Tetralogy of Fallot. Eur J Echocardiogr. 2004;5:123–31.

48. Gan CT, Lankhaar JW, Marcus JT, Westerhof N, Marques KM, Bronzwaer JG, et al. Impaired left ventricular filling due to right-to-left ventricular interaction in patients with pulmonary arterial hypertension. Am J Physiol—Heart Circ Physiol. 2006:290(4):H1528–33.

Section 7
Tetralogy of Fallot

Tetralogy of Fallot: Managing the Right Ventricular Outflow

Glen S. Van Arsdell, Tae Jin Yun, and Michael Cheung

The first complete repair of tetralogy of Fallot (TOF) was reported by Lillehei in 1955 [1]. The diagram from that initial publication (Fig. 28.1) illustrates primary closure of the ventricular defect (VSD) and resection of parietal and septal muscle bundles via a generous ventriculotomy approach. Survival was a remarkable six of ten patients. While the initial cross-circulation technique of circulatory support was soon abandoned for the developing heart–lung machine, the fundamental approach for repair of TOF remained the same for the ensuing 25–30 years or more: the VSD was closed through a generous

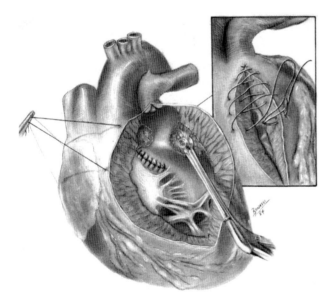

Fig. 28.1 An illustration from Lillehei's original publication of repairing tetralogy of Fallot. Note the generous ventriculotomy and parietal and septal muscle bundle resection. A ventriculotomy for VSD closure was the standard for 40 or more years and continues to be used by some today

ventriculotomy and complete or near-complete relief of right ventricular outflow obstruction was achieved. It was not until Edmunds [2], in 1976, reported transatrial closure of the VSD in TOF that an evolving change in strategy for repairing TOF began. It had been generally thought, through the 1980s and even early 1990s, that *repair* of TOF was curative and that the consequences of a transannular patch (TAP) and ventriculotomy for VSD closure were minimal. In the ensuing decades we have learned that repaired TOF is really just a palliated disease—albeit a good palliation. Near-certain death from cyanosis has been traded for a definable incidence of right heart failure, atrial arrhythmias, ventricular arrhythmias, and sudden death.

Following is a brief synopsis of late-outcomes data, a delineation of current options for repair of TOF and a presentation of a strategy that may yield better long-term palliation for TOF. The identified strategy is based on a transatrial closure of the VSD, three component management of the right ventricular outflow (RVOT), a presumption that the annulus may be preserved, and a functional assessment of the RVOT performance before proceeding to a transannular patch. The hypothesis is that for equivalent anatomy, a mixed lesion of moderate stenosis and associated pulmonary insufficiency is superior to near-complete relief of obstruction and free pulmonary insufficiency. That is to say that an associated hypertrophy signal caused by some stenosis may be protective of the dilation signal caused by pulmonary insufficiency, thereby enhancing long-term ventricular performance.

28.1 Known Outcomes for Repaired Tetralogy of Fallot

In 1993, the Mayo Clinic reported 30-year outcomes for 163 survivors of TOF repairs performed between 1955 and 1960 [3]. Survival was 87% with survival in the

G.S. Van Arsdell (✉)
Department of Paediatrics, Hospital for Sick Children, Toronto, ON, Canada

A.N. Redington et al. (eds.), *Congenital Diseases in the Right Heart*, DOI 10.1007/978-1-84800-378-1_28,
© Springer-Verlag London Limited 2009

normal control group being 96%. Late sudden death occurred in 6%. There was a subgroup of patients in whom a statistically significant higher survival occurred—those with a high RV/LV pressure ratio.

The group from Munich reported up to 35-year follow-up on 490 patients operated between 1958 and 1977 [4]. Included patients in the late follow-up analysis were those that survived more than 1 year. A 3.1% incidence of late sudden death was identified. They also identified a subset of patients, with an RV/LV pressure ratio greater than 0.7, that appeared to have a superior survival of 94.4% as compared to the others of 83.7%.

The early and late potential problems with a transannular patch were clearly defined by Kirklin [5] who reported on a series of 814 repaired TOF patients operated between 1967 and 1986 and followed for up to 20 years. Operative mortality was 4.1% for those repaired with a transannular patch versus 1.4% for those having annulus preservation. At 20 years following repair, their data predicted a 7% incidence of reoperation, for right-ventricular problems in those patients having a transannular patch. Overall 20-year survival was 88% (including operative outcome). The early and late problems of a transannular patch have been documented by us and others.

In an effort to understand the importance of pulmonary insufficiency, Kirklin's group also summarized an interesting group of patients who had native pulmonary valve regurgitation and otherwise normal hearts [6]. Their findings were that those free of symptoms of right heart failure dropped from about 90% at 25 years of age to less than 50% at 50 years of age. Essentially, right heart dilation from free pulmonary insufficiency, even in the non-TOF setting, was not benign like had been originally thought.

28.2 Late Mechanical and Electrical Findings in Repaired Tetralogy of Fallot

In a 1995 publication analyzing echocardiographic and ECG findings, Redington's group [7] identified that restrictive physiology (defined by antegrade flow in the pulmonary artery during atrial contraction) was protective of the cardiothoracic ratio and duration of the QRS complex. Those having restriction had a QRS duration of 129 ms and a cardiothoracic ratio (CTR) of 0.51. Those lacking restrictive physiology had a QRS duration of 157 ms and a CTR of 0.54. Patients found to have ventricular tachycardia had an even longer QRS duration, often of greater than 199 ms. A QRS duration of greater than 180 ms was found to be 100% sensitive for sudden death or ventricular tachycardardia in their relatively small cohort.

28.3 Implications of Late Follow-Up Data

Late follow-up data correlating surgical outcomes to anatomy has shown that free pulmonary insufficiency (transannular patch) is a marker of need for reintervention related to a dilating ventricle. The echocardiographic and electrical findings demonstrate that a ventricle that is large (too compliant) and that does not have restrictive physiology is prone to abnormal electrical conductance. A prolonged QRS duration has been shown to be a marker for risk of ventricular tachycardia and sudden death.

Early treatment strategy for TOF included a generous ventriculotomy and liberal use of a transannular patch. These had the consequence of broad free pulmonary insufficiency and a large noncontractile RV outlet. Based on what we presently know, is it any surprise that what was once thought to be a good repair, actually predicts ventricular dilation and the later potential for arrhythmia's and sudden death? That is to say, free pulmonary insufficiency causes RV dilation with ensuing tricuspid valve regurgitation which leads to right atrial dilation and eventual atrial arrhythmias. A dilating RV begins to function poorly and develops a prolonged QRS which is associated with ventricular arrhythmias and sudden death.

The question then becomes, can a surgeon alter strategy such that the late complications of repaired TOF can be mitigated? Clues to that possibility are provided in the late outcome data from the Mayo Clinic and Munich where a higher RV/LV pressure ratio was associated with improved long-term survival.

28.4 Evolving Surgical Strategy

28.4.1 Transatrial VSD Closure with Small Transannular Patch

As noted, the cardiac repair technique remained much the same as originally described, until Edmunds [2] published a report of transatrial repair of TOF in 1976. In 1981, Kawashima reported a series of transatrial closure of ventricular septal defects with appropriate associated resection of right ventricular muscle bundles [8]. Karl and Mee followed that report with a large series of transatrial/transpulmonary repair of TOF [9]. In their series, the VSD was closed via an atriotomy, the muscle resection was performed through atrial and pulmonary windows, and most had a limited transannular patch as a means of dealing with the right ventricular outflow obstruction. The transannular incision was not large enough to use as a means of closing the VSD. Early survival was outstanding with an operative mortality of 0.5% for 366 patients. Freedom from reoperation at 5 years was 95%. This type of surgical strategy illustrates that not all transannular patches are the same—some are large enough to use for VSD closure and some are insufficient for that purpose but large enough to adequately relieve obstruction.

The characteristics of the above studies were that surgical strategy was being altered to provide a solution for tetralogy of Fallot without being as radical with the right ventricular incisions and muscle resection. Acceptance of this less-radical approach is not uniform, that is, some still perform transventricular closure and utilize a high incidence of transannular patch.

28.4.2 Transventricular VSD Closure with Annulus Preservation

Yasui took a somewhat different strategy and focused on preserving the pulmonary annulus while achieving VSD closure via a ventriculotomy [10]. In his series of patients operated between 1981 and 1990, he was able to achieve a 79% annulus preservation rate. In follow-up of these patients it was reported that RV pressures fell with time and that there appeared to be disproportionate growth of

the pulmonary annulus once the infundibular obstruction was relieved. Absolute outcome for this strategy was also excellent with mortality, in that series of children repaired at an average age of 3.1 years, being 0.7%—well below what was achieved for conventional approaches at the time.

What is clear from the above is that there are differing surgical strategies. How these strategies impact late ventricular function has not fully been resolved but suggestions of impact on late outcomes are present.

28.5 Spectrum of Disease and Its Relation to Postrepair RVOT Gradient

The presentation of simple TOF (nonpulmonary atresia variety) varies in severity from that of pink tetralogy (minimal outflow obstruction) to near-complete obstruction of the RVOT. In addition to the intrinsic anatomy, surgical repair strategy partially determines whether there will be free pulmonary insufficiency (PI) and no outflow gradient or varying degrees of PI and outflow obstruction. The ventricles of late follow-up repaired TOF with severe PI can appear quite different than those of pulmonary atresia-type TOF where a conduit has been implanted (see Fig. 28.2). The failure mode of the conduit is that of obstruction, which progresses over years, thereby resulting in ventricular hypertrophy. Systolic function is usually preserved but the hypertrophy can impact diastolic compliance—something that may be favorable in late repaired TOF. By contrast, late follow-up of TOF with free PI and a dilating ventricle, we see

Fig. 28.2 Illustration of the ventricle in a failing conduit with stenosis being the pathology. Note the ventricle is not dilated and the RV has hypertrophy. There is retention of systolic function. These characteristics are in contradistinction to late RV failure in TOF where there is systolic dysfunction and marked ventricular dilation

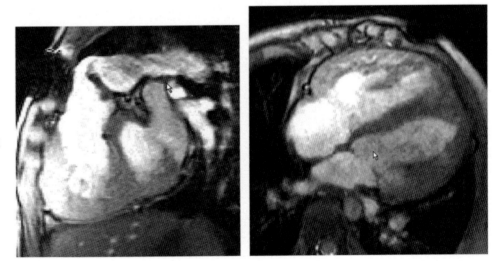

systolic failure and too much diastolic compliance. We know from the Redington late follow-up data [7], that of the two scenarios, poor diastolic compliance with restrictive physiology is the better choice.

Reports in the literature show a varying use of TAP from 20% to 80%. Clearly, the best surgical option for TOF is to create an unobstructed or nearly unobstructed RV outflow with pulmonary competence—essentially a normal ventricle. Unfortunately, the spectrum of RVOT anatomy allows for that scenario perhaps only 20% of the time. We also know from those who have pushed the limits of annulus preservation, and reported it, that at least 20% of the time a transannular patch is required.

We and others have hypothesized that leaving a gradient in the RVOT, rather than performing a transannular patch, will allow for some ventricular hypertrophy that will lessen diastolic compliance, and thereby protect the ventricle from significant dilation. Long-term ventricular performance will be enhanced. Epidemiologic evidence to support this hypothesis lies with those long-term follow-up reports of improved survival in those having a higher RV/LV pressure ratio [3, 4].

28.6 Managing the RV Outflow: Three Components

The right ventricular outflow tract can be divided into three components: the infundibular outlet chamber, the *pulmonary annulus*, and the pulmonary artery. While there is no true pulmonary annulus, we use the term to refer to the area bounded by the confluence of the RV outlet muscle and the pulmonary valve leaflets.

In an analysis of a series of 185 consecutive TOF patients operated by three surgeons, we calculated indexed sizes for each of the three outlet components on a graph (z values). All three components had nonuniform z values. The infundibular chamber size was consistently smaller than the pulmonary valve indexed size. The main pulmonary artery was also smaller but to a lesser extent. The fact that each of the components is different suggests that they should be treated individually. Figure 28.3 demonstrates differing infundibular chamber sizes.

Surgeons have, by observation and creation of nomograms, evaluated the adequacy of the *pulmonary annulus* at the time of repair. This approach has been somewhat nebulous and has led to the widely variable reported incidence of use of a transannular patch. Surgeons with

Fig. 28.3 The infundibular chamber of three different patients. The volume in the chamber is variable between patients and does not absolutely correlate with the pulmonary annulus size, thus warranting treatment as a separate entity

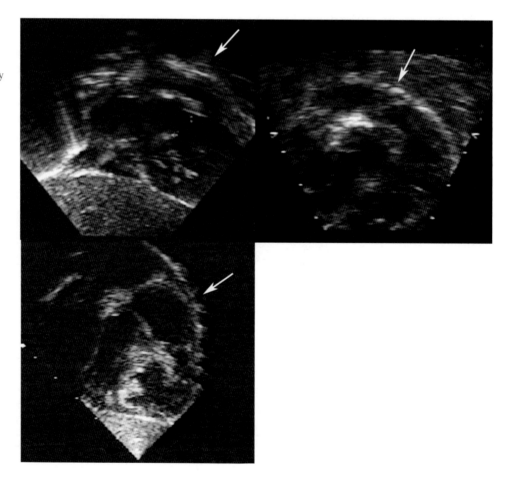

a bias for little or no obstruction had a high incidence of TAP, and conversely, those willing to work with a marginal outlet accepting a higher gradient had a lower incidence of TAP.

The data on our own patients demonstrated that the predictability of need for TAP was most closely correlated to the pulmonary annulus size. The main pulmonary artery size can be enlarged and has generally been of only secondary consideration with regard to decision making. On the other hand, when we broke out the component of the infundibular chamber and treated it as a separate entity to the pulmonary annulus, the infundibular chamber size and or augmentation of the chamber size were predictors of a higher incidence of successful preservation of the pulmonary annulus. Treating the outlet as components can therefore favorably impact the incidence of pulmonary annulus preservation.

28.7 Testing an Annulus Preservation Hypothesis

We reviewed a series of 185 patients evaluated over a 6-year time frame where in one surgeon performed an annulus preservation strategy described below, and two surgeons performed mostly conventional transventricular repair. The two strategies were then compared. For the annulus preservation strategy, a transatrial/transpulmonary muscle release and resection was performed in the region of the parietal band. The infundibular septum was thinned, where it appeared to be obstructive, and the major septal band was preserved (Fig. 28.4). A decision was made to place an infundibular patch if the infundibular chamber appeared to be smaller than the pulmonary annulus or if by impression it was excessively small (Fig. 28.5). In 10% of patients the annulus was so small that an attempt at preservation of the pulmonary annulus was abandoned, that is, there was a direct proceeding to a mini-transannular patch. For the most part we have chosen to use a polytetroflouroethylene patch for the infundibular and transannular patches in order to preclude late dilation of the patch as can be seen with autologous pericardium.

A functional physiologic test of the adequacy of the repaired RVOT was achieved after weaning from cardiopulmonary bypass. Revisions to the RVOT were then made as necessary based on pressure measurements and echocardiographic findings. Those having RV to systemic pressure ratios of greater than 0.75 were generally revised to either an addition of an infundibular patch, if not already placed, or a limited transannular patch, as in the Karl, Mee technique. It should be noted that, in general, the infundibular incisions made were not large enough for a VSD closure to occur through that route, that is, it is a limited incision.

Of the 118 patients treated with an annulus preservation strategy, 80% were successfully preserved. One half had a transatrial transpulmonary repair alone and an

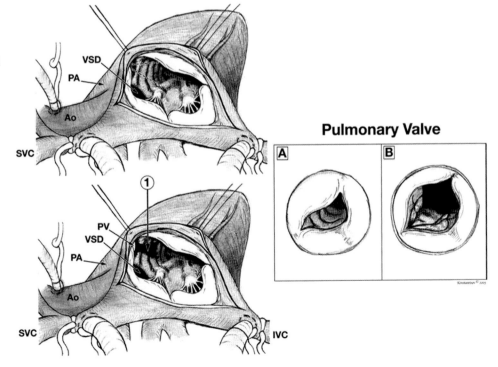

Fig. 28.4 Transatrial/ transpulmonary resection of muscle bundles. In this case the major septal band is preserved, the parietal band is released and thinned, the infundibular septum is thinned where appropriate

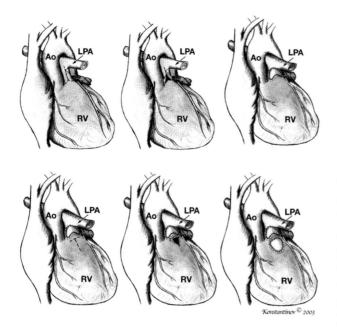

Fig. 28.5 The top panel illustrates the finished external view of the heart in a transatrial/transpulmonary repair of TOF. This was achieved in our experience in about 50% of TOF repaired in the first year of life. The lower panel illustrates the addition of an infundibular patch that increases the infundibular chamber volume. A number of these were performed after a functional failure of a transatrial/transpulmonary repair alone. Note that the ventricular incision is generally not of adequate size for a transventricular VSD closure

additional 25–30% received an infundibular patch with annulus preservation. In the conventional group, the TAP rate was 50%. Interestingly, intraoperative revision of the procedure was required in 16% of the annulus preservation group. One might think this to be relatively high except that in the conventional repair the revision rate was 10%. There was no mortality with the annulus preservation strategy.

28.8 Is It Surgical Strategy or Is It the Anatomy?

In an effort to ensure that the different incidence of TAP was not simply because of differing anatomy, an echocardiographic-based anatomic-propensity matching was performed to find matching patients between the two surgical strategies. Thirty-five anatomically equivalent patients in each arm were identified. Even with the propensity matching, the discrepancy in the incidence of TAP was still present between the two surgical strategies indicating that it was not the anatomy that yielded the lower use of a TAP.

The intraoperative and midterm follow-up data on these propensity-matched patients revealed similar gradients, ICU stays, and ventricular size demonstrating that no harm was caused by the increased annulus preservation strategy.

28.9 Marginal Patients

The question of benefit to the patient, for the additional effort required, in an annulus preservation strategy needs to be answered. Based on reports in the literature it appears that regardless of surgical strategy, 20% of all patients require a TAP and 20% do not. It is the middle 60% of patients where surgical strategy may impact outcomes. We identify that middle 60% as the marginal anatomy. In order to increase the numbers for statistical power, we performed a second analysis on the entire cohort of 185 patients.

A regression equation that predicted the probability of a TAP in the 118 annulus-preservation-strategy patients was created. The equation was then applied to the entire cohort of 185 patients and used to identify, in each patient, the probability of having a TAP irregardless if one was performed. The marginal patients were identified and defined as those with either a greater than 20% or less than 20% probability of a TAP, that is, the middle 60%. A total of 107 patients fell into the marginal anatomy category. In those patients, the annulus was preserved in 55 and a TAP was performed in 52. An analysis of the preoperative anatomy showed that there was a slight difference in the z value of the pulmonary annulus for those receiving a TAP (z of –6 vs. –5.2).

Outcomes analysis showed that those having annulus preservation had significantly lower inotropic scores and better SVC saturations in the early recovery phase. Those that did not have a TAP had a measured intraoperative RVOT gradient that was higher: 19 mmHg versus 12 mmHg. These findings of a poorer postoperative clinical course for those having a TAP are consistent with other presentations in the literature.

28.10 Midterm Outcomes for the Marginal Patients

Interestingly, follow-up echocardiography on the above marginal patients at 17 months revealed that the RVOT gradient difference between those having annulus preservation and those receiving a TAP had resolved. Perhaps importantly, however, a difference in the jet width of pulmonary insufficiency was present with those having annulus preservation showing a narrower jet –8 mm versus 13 mm. In an attempt to measure physiologic adaptation, midcavity RV and LV size was measured. The absolute RV size was smaller in those patients receiving annulus preservation as was the RV/LV ratio –0.5 versus 0.65.

Other supporting evidence that modifications in repair of TOF improve outcomes can be seen in a comparison of a change of practice by a single surgeon. Bove and colleagues [11] reported on a transatrial/transpulmonary-repair strategy using a minimal transannular patch versus a more conventional transventricular repair. Ten-year follow-up revealed that the transatrial repair yielded a smaller RV size, a better CTR, a shorter QRS duration, as well as less ventricular ectopy.

Evidence in our series and the Bove series suggests that long-term outcome of TOF can be impacted by surgical strategy.

28.11 Reoperations in Tetralogy of Fallot

28.11.1 Operations for Obstruction

One of the concerns of preserving more pulmonary annuli and leaving a higher RVOT gradient is the potential need for reoperation due to obstruction. Not surprisingly, there were some patients from the above noted 118 patients having the annulus-preservation strategy that subsequently developed RV pressures that were too high. Four patients (3%) required reintervention from 3 months to 3 years following the initial repair. Of those, one required a transannular patch, one was successfully treated with balloon intervention, and two had repeat RVOT muscle resection.

28.11.2 Operations for Pulmonary Insufficiency

Late right ventricular failure in TOF has been managed by implantation of a pulmonary valve—in the Toronto practice, a bioprosthesis. However, not all patients have an improvement in ventricular function or RV volume. One of the interesting findings in those undergoing a late pulmonary valve replacement has been the finding of disproportionate enlargement or even aneurysmal dilation of the RVOT. This may be related to a pericardial patch that has dilated with time or native RVOT that is now dilating scar caused by infundibular coronary

branch ischemia from the initial operation. This noncontractile area contributes to poor ventricular ejection. One of the present strategies proposed by Del Nido [12] is to remodel the RVOT to minimize this noncontractile area much as one would treat a left ventricular aneurysm with surgical remodeling. In essence, this is ventricular volume-reduction surgery that minimizes the noncontractile area and likely lessens RV wall stress. Quantitative data on this strategy has yet to be presented; however, anecdotal evidence is that of a disproportionate improvement in right ventricular performance as compared to pulmonary valve implant alone for similar anatomy.

28.12 Summary and Conclusions

Late follow-up of TOF has revealed a concerning incidence of right ventricular failure and sudden death. The failing right ventricle appears to be associated with pulmonary insufficiency and the resultant dilated poorly contractile right ventricle. Late follow-up studies have also shown that those patients having right ventricular restrictive physiology and a higher RV/LV pressure ratio have a higher survival. Retention of some stenosis in the right ventricular outflow tract may limit the jet width of pulmonary insufficiency and provide a protective hypertrophy signal that diminishes the deleterious effects of pulmonary insufficiency.

Reports in the medical literature show a varying incidence of the use of a transannular patch from 20% to 80%. In numerous studies, a TAP has been associated with less favorable outcomes. We hypothesized that for equivalent anatomy surgical strategy determines the incidence of use of TAP. We showed this to be true in an analysis of a contemporary cohort operated by three surgeons employing a conventional versus an annulus-preservation strategy. Management of the RVOT is key to an annulus-preservation approach. It consists of three separate components that we have shown to be of varying z values within a single individual. Managing the RVOT as three separate components such as infundibular chamber, pulmonary annulus, and pulmonary artery allow a higher rate of annulus preservation. Medium-term follow-up has shown that the resulting pulmonary insufficiency jet width in annular preservation patients is smaller than in those having a TAP and that right ventricular performance is improved as measured by the RV/LV ratio.

The findings that surgical strategy impacts the probability of employing a TAP are encouraging, in that more patients may be repaired in a manner that predicts favorable long-term right ventricular function.

References

1. Lillehei C. Walton, Cohen Morley, Warden Herbert E, Read Raymond C, Aust Joseph B, DeWall Richard A, Varco Richard L. Direct vision intracardiac surgerical correction of the tetralogy of Fallot, pentalogy of Fallot and pulmonary atresia defects. Ann Surg.142(3):418–445.
2. Edmunds Henry L, Saxena Naresh C, Friedman Sydney, Rashkind William J, Dod Paul F. Transtrial repair of tetralogy of Fallot. Surgery. 80(6):681–688.
3. Murphy JG, Gersh BJ, Mair DD, Fuster V, McGoon MD, Ilstrup DM, McGoon DC, Kirklin JW, Danielson GK. Long-term outcome in patients undergoing surgical repair of tetralogy of Fallot. New England J Med. Aug 26 1993;329:593–599.
4. Nollert G, Fischlein T, Bouterwek S, Bohmer C, Klinner W, Reichart B. Long-term survival in patients with repair of tetralogy of Fallot: 36-year follow-up of 490 survivors of the first year after surgical repair. J Am Coll Cardiol. 1997;30:1374–1383.
5. Kirklin JK, Blackstone EH, Milano A, Pacifico AD. Effect of transannular patching on outcome after repair of tetralogy of Fallot. Ann Thorac Surg. Jul 1989;48:783–791.
6. Shimizaki Y, Blackstone EH, Kirklin JW. The natural history of isolated congenital pulmonary valve incompetence: surgical implications. Thorac Cardiovasc Surg. Aug 1984;32(4):257–9.
7. Gatzoulis Michael A, Till Jan A, Somerville Jane, Redington Andrew N. Mechanoelectrical interaction in tetralogy of Fallot: QRS prolongation relates to right ventricular size and predicts malignant ventricular arrhythmias and sudden death. Circulation. 1995;92:231–237.
8. Kawashima Y, Kitamura S, Nakano S, Yagihara T. Corrective surgery for tetralogy of Fallot without or with minimal right ventriculotomy and with repair of the pulmonary valve. Circulation. Aug 1981;64(2 Pt 2):II147–53.
9. Karl TR, Sano S, Pornviliwan S, Mee RB. Tetralogy of Fallot: favorable outcome of nonneonatal transatrial, transpulmonary repair. Ann Thorac. Surg. Jul 1992;54:903–907.
10. Yasui H, Nakamura Y, Kado H, Yonenaga K, Aso T, Sunagawa H, Kanegae Y, Tominaga R, Tokunaga K. Preservation of the pulmonary valve during intracardiac repair of tetralogy of Fallot. J. Cardiovasc Surg (Torino). Sep–Oct 1992;33(5):545–53.
11. Atallah-Yunes Nader, Kavey Rae-Ellen, Bove Edward, Smith Frank, Kvesclis Daniel, Byrum Craig, Gaum Winston. Postoperative assessment of a modifiend surgical approach to repair of tetralogy of Fallot. Circulation. Nov 1996; 94 Suppl 9:pII–22–26.
12. del Nido, Pedro J. Surgical management of right ventricular dysfunction late after repair of tetralogy of Fallot: right ventricular remodeling surgery. Seminars in Thoracic and Cardiovascular Surgery. 2006;29–34.

Restrictive Right Ventricular Physiology: Early and Late Effects

Andrew N. Redington

The effects of restrictive diastolic physiology have long been recognized as an important part of left heart disease. Poor left ventricular compliance, or its reciprocal increased myocardial stiffness, may be a primary disease of the myocardium (restrictive cardiomyopathy) or occur as a secondary phenomenon in the setting of other cardiomyopathies, or cardiovascular diseases. The understanding of right ventricular restrictive disease has been hampered by an inability to demonstrate its presence, in the intact heart. This is because of the unique pressure–volume characteristics of the subpulmonary right ventricle (see Chapter 3). However, during the past decade, several techniques have been shown to provide a qualitative assessment of right ventricular diastolic physiology, and the importance of abnormal right ventricular compliance is increasingly understood. In this chapter, our understanding of right ventricular restrictive physiology in tetralogy of Fallot will be discussed.

29.1 Recognition of Abnormal Right Ventricular Compliance

The trapezoidal nature of the normal right ventricular pressure–volume relationship reflects its low hydraulic impedance. As discussed in Chapter 3, this leads to poorly defined isovolumic periods and ejection occurring almost continuously throughout right ventricular pressure rise and fall. Clearly, ejection from any ventricle will occur when its pressure exceeds that of the diastolic pressure in the vascular bed to which it is connected, and in the normal pulmonary circulation, this approximates to 10 mmHg. Thus, ejection from the right ventricle occurs early during right ventricular pressure rise, and continues

during right ventricular pressure decline. Because of this, the concepts developed for understanding left ventricular diastolic compliance are not valid for the right ventricle. In the left ventricle, the slope of the end-diastolic pressure volume relationship (derived from a family of pressure–volume loops) is a robust measure of the passive characteristics of the left ventricle at end diastole [1]. Furthermore, several Doppler characteristics have been described as surrogates for this abnormal pressure and volume relationship, in the beating heart [2, 3]. Under these circumstances, the description of ventricular compliance requires knowledge of both the change in pressure, and change in volume, of the ventricle, instantaneously. In clinical practice, inflow Doppler is used as a surrogate for the change in volume, and this is best combined with a surrogate of ventricular pressure rise, such as the apex cardiogram, or the demonstration of flow patterns in the pulmonary veins [3]. Thus, reduced blood flow through the mitral valve at end diastole, in combination with a prominent A-wave on the apex cardiogram, or retrograde flow in the pulmonary veins during atrial systole, implies a poorly compliant left ventricle. A prerequisite of pressure–volume analysis, or Doppler flow analysis, is a closed system, that is, that the aortic valve is closed, and changes occurring within the ventricle therefore reflect muscle mechanics. This cannot be considered always the case in the normotensive right ventricle. If right atrial pressure rises above the level of the pulmonary artery diastolic pressure, then transtricuspid flow will be transmitted to the pulmonary artery (Fig. 29.1), rather than translating to right ventricular filling. This clearly will undermine the interpretation of transtricuspid flow characteristics as an index of ventricular compliance, and negates the validity of pressure–volume analysis, because the RV is not *closed* at end diastole. Nonetheless, this ability of the right atrial pressure to exceed right arterial diastolic pressure does provide for a surrogate measurement of ventricular compliance. Using Doppler echocardiography, these pressure transients equate to abnormal

A.N. Redington (✉)
Department of Cardiology, Hospital for Sick Children, Toronto, ON, Canada

A.N. Redington et al. (eds.), *Congenital Diseases in the Right Heart*, DOI 10.1007/978-1-84800-378-1_29,
© Springer-Verlag London Limited 2009

Fig. 29.1 Monitoring screen illustrating the postoperative physiology of restrictive physiology in an infant after repair of tetralogy on the cardiac intensive care unit. Note the pulmonary artery pressure (PAP—*blue*) and the right atrial pressure (RAP—*yellow*). There is a transient rise in RAP above diastolic PAP which generates antegrade PA flow recorded by Doppler (Inset box). The phasic elevation of PAP above RAP abolishes the antegrade flow, and is due to the effects of positive pressure ventilation

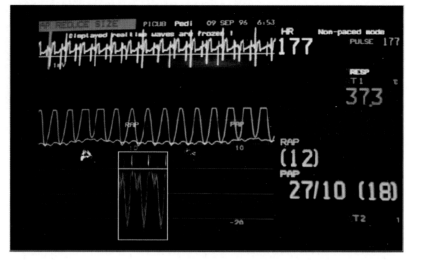

blood-flow patterns in the main pulmonary artery at end diastole. Essentially, when the resistance to right ventricular filling (increased stiffness) is greater that the resistance to pulmonary artery filling, there will be antegrade diastolic flow in the pulmonary artery, coincident with atrial systole.

We first described this Doppler phenomenon in congenital heart disease in patients with pulmonary atresia with intact ventricular septum, after complete repair [4]. The presence of gross right ventricular hypertrophy, small RV cavity volumes, and fibrosis are well described in these patients, and the majority of them display restrictive right ventricular physiology on the basis of the persistence of antegrade diastolic flow in the pulmonary artery coincident with a true systole. Subsequently, this physiology has been described in many forms of right heart disease, particularly, however, in tetralogy of Fallot [5, 6]. Its physiologic implications and secondary effects will be detailed later.

While the presence of antegrade diastolic flow represents a useful marker of poor right ventricular compliance, there are many caveats to its interpretation. The generation of this flow depends on pressure transients of just 1–2 mmHg (Fig. 29.1). Thus, small changes in pulmonary vascular resistance, right contractile properties, or preload, can all markedly influence the presence and extent of antegrade pulmonary arterial diastolic flow. Loss of atrial systole or changes in PR interval and other abnormalities of ventricular preload are also likely to modify its appearance. In tetralogy of Fallot, there is usually free pulmonary incompetence. There must, therefore, be a complicated relationship between right ventricular filling as a result of pulmonary incompetence and right ventricular filling across the tricuspid valve. It would be a surprise therefore if restrictive physiology were not more common in those patients with markedly increased

preload. Finally, the transient nature of antegrade diastolic flow, particularly in regard to heart–lung interactions, is vitally important. In our original descriptions, the definition of restrictive physiology was made on the basis of antegrade diastolic flow occurring throughout the inspiratory and expiratory phases of respiration. In the normal circulation, a small amount of antegrade diastolic flow, with reopening of the pulmonary valve in late diastole, has been described during vigorous inspiration (generating a low intrathoracic pressure, lower than the right atrial pressure during that phase) [7]. Techniques that average blood flow across the respiratory cycle may therefore overdiagnose the presence of restrictive physiology. This is particularly the case in magnetic resonance evaluations, where pulmonary blood-flow characteristics are averaged from many cardiac and respiratory cycles [8]. Furthermore, in regard to magnetic resonance assessment, the site of blood flow measurement may be crucial. Clearly, it is normal for the ventricle to receive flow in atrial systole. After repair of tetralogy of Fallot, the definition of the ventriculoarterial junction is poorly defined. If a magnetic resonance flow measurement is made proximal to the main pulmonary artery, then flow within it will be physiologic and normal, during atrial systole. Indeed, during our early clinical studies of restrictive physiology, it became apparent that antegrade diastolic flow could sometimes be seen in the right ventricular outflow tract, but not in the branch pulmonary arteries, whereas in those with clear-cut restrictive physiology, antegrade diastolic flow was measurable throughout the pulmonary vascular tree.

These latter observations are important, given some of the disparate data using Doppler and magnetic resonance imaging (MRI) techniques [6, 8]. This will be discussed in more detail later.

Fig. 29.2 Chest radiographs and magnetic resonance images from two patients late after transannular patch repair of tetralogy of Fallot. The patient on the left has a nonrestrictive RV, and has gross dilation of the RV and is symptomatic. The patient illustrated in the right panel has restrictive RV physiology. Despite decades of *free* pulmonary regurgitation, the cardiothoracic ratio and RV size are normal. This patient had a normal exercise tolerance on cardiopulmonary testing

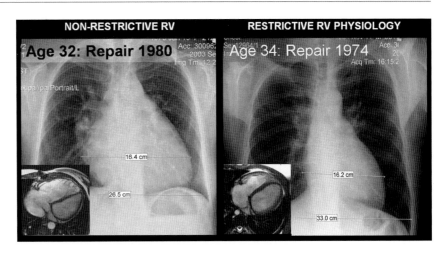

29.2   The Effects of Restrictive Physiology in Tetralogy of Fallot

Early implications: The surgical repair of tetralogy of Fallot represents one of the success stories of contemporary congenital cardiac surgery. Nonetheless, albeit with decreasing frequency, there is a significant incidence of postoperative low cardiac output syndrome and cardiovascular collapse after repair. Indeed, postoperative tetralogy represented the second most common reason for postoperative extracorporeal membrane oxygenation in the late 1990s [9]. Even today, many patients suffer a slow postoperative recovery, with evidence of a raised central venous pressure, a low cardiac output, fluid retention, pleural effusion, and ascites. In the absence of significant residual ventricular septal defect, obstructive lesions, etc., it is very likely that such a patient will have restrictive right ventricular physiology. Indeed, we demonstrated that tetralogy patients with antegrade diastolic flow in their pulmonary arteries in the immediate postoperative period were characterized by signs of low cardiac output and fluid retention [9]. This is usually a transient phenomenon, lasting 2–5 five days, and correctly treated need not represent a major hemodynamic burden. Correct treatment relies upon the understanding of the determinants and features of restrictive physiology. As discussed above, antegrade diastolic flow reflects a series of interdependent boundary conditions. While it is a manifestation of adverse hemodynamics, its presence reflects a beneficial pattern of blood flow. Antegrade diastolic flow not only contributes to the total antegrade flow within the pulmonary artery (and therefore cardiac output), but also limits diastolic regurgitation, further augmenting total forward cardiac output. Its presence therefore should be encouraged and sustained. Maintenance of sinus rhythm,

adequate right atrial filling, and lowering the pulmonary vascular resistance are all crucial to the management of such patients. As discussed in Chapter 23, one of the most important determinants of total pulmonary resistance in such patients is the mean airway pressure. Vigilant attention to this can make major differences to cardiac output in patients with restrictive right ventricular physiology. Essentially, the lower the mean airway pressure the higher the cardiac output. This is most manifest when negative intrathoracic pressure ventilation is maintained, either by early encouragement of normal respiration, or with the negative pressure ventilator that we described as a physiological tool over a decade ago. Cardiac output under these circumstances may be 10–30% higher than with intermittent positive-pressure ventilation [10, 11].

The cause of restrictive physiology is not fully understood. Initially thought to be a direct consequence of hypertrophy itself, the detailed demographic and anthropomorphic analyses failed to demonstrate any relationship to outcomes. Chaturvedi et al. used sequential measurements of cardiac troponin and other biomarkers during and after surgical repair. Those patients destined to display restrictive physiology in the intensive care unit had greater troponin released from their myocardium at the time of aortic cross-clamp removal. All other measurements of an adverse hemodynamic milieu appeared to be secondary phenomena, and occurred later in the postoperative course. The implication, therefore, is that poor myocardial protection leads to increased myocardial damage (manifest by this early increased troponin release), and the generation of restrictive physiology. While, as discussed above, this has important adverse consequences in the immediate postoperative period, paradoxically, restrictive physiology may be beneficial in the later postoperative follow-up of these patients.

Late implications: In the mid-1990s, Gatzoulis et al. showed that the presence of restrictive physiology (again manifest at antegrade diastolic flow in the pulmonary arteries) in the late follow-up of tetralogy patients conferred a benefit overall [6]. Those with a stiff, poorly compliant right ventricle failed to have the normal (adverse) remodeling, and therefore had a smaller heart on their chest radiograph (Fig. 29.2), smaller right ventricular dimensions by echocardiography, and interestingly, improved exercise tolerance, presumably because of the limiting effects of restrictive physiology on pulmonary incompetence, a key determinant of exercise function [12]. Subsequently, our understanding of the relationship between the QRS duration and right ventricular size evolved. Nonetheless, it was noted early-on that those patients with restrictive physiology had a shorter QRS duration and ultimately we found a reduced risk of ventricular arrhythmia [13]. The relationship between QRS duration, right ventricular size (no matter what its determinants), and arrhythmia risk is now well established [14–16].

It should be remembered that not all patients with restrictive physiology have a normal sized or only mild right ventricular dilatation. Clearly, restrictive physiology as a manifestation of poor ventricular compliance can occur at any stage of remodeling of a right ventricle. Our early data, obtained in patients operated on late in life, often with extreme right ventricular hypertrophy, represents one end of this physiologic spectrum. It is entirely possible for a ventricle to demonstrate restrictive physiology, even though (and perhaps because) it is dilated. This has led to some confusion in the literature. As mentioned above, the definition of restrictive physiology (while almost certainly reflecting a spectrum of disease) must be borne in mind when applying alternative techniques for its diagnosis. Magnetic resonance assessment of pulmonary blood flow, if used for the diagnosis of restrictive physiology, must take account of the anatomic and physiologic determinants of antegrade diastolic flow. Thus, ideally, it should be measured in the distal main pulmonary artery or proximal branch pulmonary arteries, and take account of respiratory variations rather than average-flow patterns over many respiratory cycles (something that is rarely done in magnetic resonance studies).

What is clear, however, is that the lack of restrictive physiology allows for continuing right ventricular remodeling (and therefore dilatation) in response to a chronic ventricular preload. Progressive right ventricular dilatation can be expected under those circumstances. If the ventricle becomes restrictive early in its natural history, then right ventricular dilatation will be limited, and functional outcome is likely to be improved (at least in the median term).

It is interesting to speculate, therefore, that some of the so-called advantages of improved myocardial-preservation techniques, earlier operation to avoid hypertrophy and fibrosis, and a relatively high transannular patch rate when corrective surgery for tetralogy of Fallot is performed in early infancy [17, 18], may have adverse outcomes in a counter-intuitive way. Preservation of the integrity of the right ventricular myocardium may delay the onset of restrictive physiology, and allow for a greater degree of right ventricular dilatation in response to free pulmonary incompetence. It is already apparent that later cohorts of surgically repaired patients do not have the 30–40% incidence of restrictive physiology described by Gatzoulis et al. in his study of adult patients [6], operated upon in a much earlier era. It will be interesting to see how the results of contemporary surgery will be impacted by an understanding of this physiology. Given the nature of the effects of pulmonary incompetence, the results of such studies will not be known for three or four decades, however.

References

1. Bourdillon PD, Lorell BH, Mirsky I, Paulus WJ, Wynne J, Grossman W. Increased regional myocardial stiffness of the left ventricle during pacing-induced angina in man. Circulation. 1983 Feb;67(2):316–23.
2. Klein AL, Hatle LK, Taliercio CP, Taylor CL, Kyle RA, Bailey KR, et al. Serial Doppler echocardiographic follow-up of left ventricular diastolic function in cardiac amyloidosis. J Am Coll Cardiol. 1990 Nov;16(5):1135–41.
3. Klein AL, Tajik AJ. Doppler assessment of pulmonary venous flow in healthy subjects and in patients with heart disease. J Am Soc Echocardiogr. 1991 Jul–Aug;4(4):379–92.
4. Redington AN, Rigby ML, Hayes A, Penny D. Right ventricular diastolic function in children. Am J Cardiol. 1991 Feb 1;67(4):329–30.
5. Cullen S, Shore D, Redington A. Characterization of right ventricular diastolic performance after complete repair of tetralogy of Fallot. Restrictive physiology predicts slow postoperative recovery. Circulation. 1995 Mar 15;91(6):1782–9.
6. Gatzoulis MA, Clark AL, Cullen S, Newman CG, Redington AN. Right ventricular diastolic function 15 to 35 years after repair of tetralogy of Fallot. Restrictive physiology predicts superior exercise performance. Circulation. 1995 Mar 15; 91(6):1775–81.
7. Gibbs JL, Wilson N, Witsenburg M, Williams GJ, Goldberg SJ. Diastolic forward blood flow in the pulmonary artery detected by Doppler echocardiography. J Am Coll Cardiol. 1985 Dec;6(6):1322–8.
8. Helbing WA, Niezen RA, Le Cessie S, van der Geest RJ, Ottenkamp J, de Roos A. Right ventricular diastolic function in children with pulmonary regurgitation after repair of tetralogy of Fallot: volumetric evaluation by magnetic resonance velocity mapping. J Am Coll Cardiol. 1996 Dec;28(7):1827–35.
9. Bartlett RH. Extracorporeal life support registry report 1995. ASAIO J. 1997 Jan–Feb;43(1):104–7.

10. Shekerdemian LS, Shore DF, Lincoln C, Bush A, Redington AN. Negative-pressure ventilation improves cardiac output after right heart surgery. Circulation. 1996 Nov 1;94(9 Suppl):II49–55.

11. Shekerdemian LS, Bush A, Shore DF, Lincoln C, Redington AN. Cardiorespiratory responses to negative pressure ventilation after tetralogy of fallot repair: a hemodynamic tool for patients with a low-output state. J Am Coll Cardiol. 1999 Feb;33(2):549–55.

12. Wessel HU, Cunningham WJ, Paul MH, Bastanier CK, Muster AJ, Idriss FS. Exercise performance in tetralogy of Fallot after intracardiac repair. J Thorac Cardiovasc Surg. 1980 Oct;80(4):582–93.

13. Gatzoulis MA, Till JA, Somerville J, Redington AN. Mechanoelectrical interaction in tetralogy of Fallot. QRS prolongation relates to right ventricular size and predicts malignant ventricular arrhythmias and sudden death. Circulation. 1995 Jul 15;92(2):231–7.

14. Gatzoulis MA, Till JA, Redington AN. Depolarization-repolarization inhomogeneity after repair of tetralogy of Fallot. The substrate for malignant ventricular tachycardia? Circulation. 1997 Jan 21;95(2):401–4.

15. Berul CI, Hill SL, Geggel RL, Hijazi ZM, Marx GR, Rhodes J, Walsh KA, Fulton DR. Electrocardiographic markers of late sudden death risk in postoperative tetralogy of Fallot children. J Cardiovasc Electrophysiol. 1997 Dec;8(12):1349–56.

16. Abd El Rahman MY, Abdul-Khaliq H, Vogel M, Alexi-Meskishvili V, Gutberlet M, Lange PE. Relation between right ventricular enlargement, QRS duration, and right ventricular function in patients with tetralogy of Fallot and pulmonary regurgitation after surgical repair. Heart. 2000 Oct;84(4):416–20.

17. Reddy VM, Liddicoat JR, McElhinney DB, Brook MM, Stanger P, Hanley FL. Routine primary repair of tetralogy of Fallot in neonates and infants less thanthree months of age. Ann Thorac Surg. 1995 Dec;60(6 Suppl):S592–6.

18. Pigula FA, Khalil PN, Mayer JE, del Nido PJ, Jonas RA. Repair of tetralogy of Fallot in neonates and young infants. Circulation. 1999 Nov 9;100(19 Suppl):II157–61.

30.1 Introduction

This chapter offers thoughts on pulmonary regurgitation, especially on the altered, pathophysiological role of pulmonary arterial compliance when there is free or almost free regurgitation. Although arterial compliance helps to limit the ventricular afterload when the outflow valve is competent, it may play a detrimental role, exacerbating regurgitation, when there is no effective pulmonary valve. Table 30.1 offers some suggested measurements and definitions relevant to pulmonary regurgitation.

Andrew Redington has, with collaborators, contributed important insights relating to the factors, besides incompetence of the valve itself, relevant to the assessment of pulmonary regurgitation [1–3]. This chapter assumes knowledge of this work, addressing aspects which, on the basis of cardiovascular magnetic resonance imaging experience, I believe should also be recognized and investigated further.

30.2 Pulmonary Arterial Compliance in the Absence of an Effective Pulmonary Valve

In the absence of an effective pulmonary valve, the compliance or capacitance (see definitions, Table 30.1) of the pulmonary arteries and their branches not only contributes to regurgitation, but also is arguably the sole available source of regurgitation. The only other theoretical contributor of regurgitant volume would be reversal of flow at pulmonary microvascular level, which would require a period of reversed pressure gradient across the microvessels. It remains unproven, but

it seems unlikely that pulmonary venous pressure would exceed pulmonary arterial pressure to any significant degree in the cardiac cycle. In a sense, therefore, the pulmonary microvascular resistance takes on a valve-like role, serving as a threshold of no return, in this context [4].

In a patient with free pulmonary regurgitation, the volume equivalent to that ejected by the right ventricle will be propelled forward, effectively escaping across the threshold of the microvessels *except* for the volume that is accommodated by pulmonary arterial compliance or capacitance. The word *capacitance* helps to convey the relevance of capacity or size as well as elasticity. In early diastole, it is the elastic recoil of the pulmonary arteries that delivers blood back through an incompetent pulmonary valve. If there is no reversal of flow at pulmonary microvascular level, the regurgitant volume comes from the compliance of the pulmonary arterial tree and nowhere else, and the more voluminous and elastic the arteries then the greater their capacity to deliver regurgitant volume. Theoretically, and on the basis of comparisons of flow and pulmonary arterial expansion seen in different patients, pulmonary arterial compliance is at least as important as right ventricular compliance in exacerbating regurgitation in the absence of an effective valve.

It is relevant that some patients born with tetralogy of Fallot, with smaller than normal pulmonary arteries, are likely to have lower than normal pulmonary artery compliance, while other patients may have unusually large and compliant arteries, for example, those born with absent pulmonary valve syndrome, or those who have developed poststenotic dilatation or otherwise dilated, but low-pressure pulmonary arteries. Kang et al. found a weak correlation between the cross-sectional area of the proximal right or left branch pulmonary artery and the regurgitant volume in the same vessel ($R^2 = 0.221$, $P = 0.027$) in 22 patients studied 3–16 years after repair of tetralogy of Fallot [5]. This could be explained by the

P.J. Kilner (✉)
Cardiovascular Magnetic Resonance Unit, Royal Brompton Hospital and Imperial College, London, UK

A.N. Redington et al. (eds.), *Congenital Diseases in the Right Heart*, DOI 10.1007/978-1-84800-378-1_30,
© Springer-Verlag London Limited 2009

Table 30.1 Pulmonary regurgitation: some suggested measurements, definitions and notes

Regurgitant orifice size: This crucial variable is hard to measure, but one approach is to visualize forward and reversed flow using in-plane magnetic resonance velocity mapping, then to measure the cross sectional area of the regurgitant jet in a through-plane velocity map located to transect the jet immediately beneath the level of the valve, if present. Problems include the difficulty of defining valve level in the absence of a valve, and the effects of flow separation past angulations or distortions of the pulmonary trunk

Free pulmonary regurgitation: Pulmonary regurgitation can be regarded as free when there is neither effective valve action nor any fixed stenosis of the outflow tract. Fixed outflow tract stenosis resists forward flow and diastolic reversed flow, so limiting otherwise free regurgitation

Pulmonary regurgitant volume: The volume of diastolic reversed flow measured at the level of the RV–PA junction, for example, by through-plane magnetic resonance velocity mapping

Pulmonary regurgitant fraction: Pulmonary regurgitant volume expressed as a percentage of the forward flow volume. If the forward flow, at the RV-PA junction, includes late diastolic forward flow, then the total forward flow may be slightly more than the RV stroke volume

Compliance or capacitance: Volume change of an elastic-walled compartment per unit of pressure change. This may refer to elastic vessels, or to a relaxed ventricle, where it is harder to quantify. Using cross-sectional area and pressure measurements, *in vivo* estimates of vascular compliance assume no change of vascular length

Vascular resistance: (mean) pressure loss divided by (mean) flow rate across a vascular bed. Attempted measurements of phasic variations of vascular resistance during pulsatile flow would be complicated by the inertia of blood and the compliance of vascular walls. Normal pulmonary vascular resistance is reported to be widely distributed along the arterial and venous branches as well as the microvessels. The microvessels nevertheless account for a significant part of the total pulmonary vascular resistance and compliance

Vascular impedance: The total opposition to vascular flow. When flow is continuous, impedance is the same as resistance, but when pulsatile, there is an additional component of 'inertance', caused by the inertia of the parts of the blood mass that are being accelerated. Resistance resists flow, while inertance opposes *changes* of flow rate. These changes will be steeper than normal in the presence of regurgitation. Momentum is directional, however, and forward momentum in systole will help to carry blood forward into branches in early diastole. But inertance is lower in shorter, wider, more compliant tubes, and so it is a smaller consideration in the pulmonary than the systemic arteries

regurgitant volume being related to the capacitant volume of the vessel and its branches.

The contribution of pulmonary arterial compliance to pulmonary regurgitation remains hard to confirm clinically, however, as there are always several interacting variables. While regurgitant fraction or regurgitant volume, and local arterial expansion, can be measured by magnetic resonance, other variables are harder to quantify, notably the compliance versus stiffness of the right ventricle, the failure of coaptation of the pulmonary valve itself, the compliance of the smaller arterial branches, and the pulmonary vascular resistance and its changes through a cardiac cycle [6].

Branch pulmonary artery stenosis and/or elevated pulmonary microvascular resistance are probably among the most potent exacerbators of pulmonary regurgitation, but pulmonary arterial compliance may be equally important as a compounding factor. Furthermore, the locations of compliances relative to resistances matter. A fixed resistance, for example, a suture line or conduit, *proximal* to most of the arterial compliance can be expected to limit otherwise free regurgitation, while elevated resistance distal to the compliant pulmonary trunk has been shown to exacerbate regurgitation [2].

30.3 Factors Upstream of a Regurgitant Pulmonary Valve

Pathophysiological considerations on the upstream side of a regurgitant pulmonary valve should begin well upstream, with function of the left ventricle. The work of the left ventricle dominates the circulation as a whole, more so than usual when the pulmonary valve is incompetent and right ventriclular function is impaired. Doppler echocardiographic evidence of late diastolic forward flow in the distal pulmonary trunk through the whole respiratory cycle has been taken to represent restrictive right ventricular physiology [3]. Magnetic resonance flow studies, acquired over a period of free breathing or during an expiratory breath hold, do not register the variation with breathing. As I understand it, however, the late diastolic forward flow that is usually found by magnetic resonance in the pulmonary trunk when there is no effective pulmonary valve results indirectly from work of the left ventricle, maintaining systemic venous return until atrial systole adds a peak of pressure and forward flow through a full, conduit-like right ventricle. An in-breath would presumably boost venous return to the right atrium, partly by compression of the abdominal venous reservoir. A right ventricle becomes full and conduit-like more readily if it is small and thick-walled or otherwise incompliant, whereas more blood is needed to refill a large, compliant RV cavity with a high stroke volume. But either type of right ventricle can be associated with late diastolic forward pulmonary flow. According to my mind *full* would be a more appropriate description of the RV than *restrictive* in these circumstances, when, in late diastole, the dynamics of the circulation as a whole temporarily simulate those of a Fontan circulation. This state—forward pulmonary flow maintained indirectly by left ventricular work—tends to limit the amount of regurgitation relative to forward pulmonary flow. This moderator of pulmonary regurgitation will be more effective when the LV is functioning vigorously and the RV is impaired, but less effective, allowing more regurgitation, if the RV has preserved contractile function but contractility of the LV is impaired. The latter may further exacerbate PR through elevation of left atrial and pulmonary venous pressure.

On the subject of the echocardiographic regurgitant index described by Wei Li [7] the index (expressing the length of the diastolic regurgitant period relative to the whole length of diastole) was found to have a useful but by no means perfect relation to pulmonary regurgitant fractions measured by magnetic resonance. The index complements other echocardiographic approaches to assessment of pulmonary incompetence, all of which have limitations. Unsurprisingly, cases can be found which do not accord with the usual trend, and there are several possible reasons for this, on the downstream as well as the upstream side of an incompetent pulmonary valve.

30.4 Regurgitant Fraction or Volume?

Andrew Redington has argued that indexed regurgitant volume is a more telling comparative clinical measurement than regurgitant fraction [3]. Each needs to be considered in context, however, relative to upstream and downstream variables. Although I can see the value of indexed regurgitant volume and will add it to the measurements I record, I would not want to discard the familiar and immediately comprehensible regurgitant fraction. Both can be measured by magnetic resonance velocity mapping through a plane transecting the proximal pulmonary trunk. Free pulmonary regurgitation is typically associated with a regurgitant fraction of about 40%, although it can vary between about 25% and 65%, depending on combinations of upstream and downstream factors, as discussed. The regurgitant volume is a measure of the amount of blood delivered back to the RV by the elasticity of the pulmonary

arteries, representing the volume load on the right ventricle that is potentially correctable by valve replacement. The regurgitant fraction is expressed relative to the total forward flow. Both measurements may, theoretically at least, decrease slightly in later stages if there is progressive dysfunction of the RV.

30.5 Concluding Thoughts

Hopefully the above descriptions make theoretical sense, even if supporting clinical data is lacking. This may in part be due to the difficulty of distinguishing cause and effect among several interdependent variables.

The main conclusion is that in patients with pulmonary regurgitation, it is not sufficient to grade the regurgitation as *mild*, *moderate*, or *severe*. The incompetence of the valve itself should be described, on the basis of careful imaging and flow measurement, as mild, moderate, *almost free*, or *free*, reserving *severe* for the occasional case where the regurgitant fraction exceeds 50% due to exacerbating factors downstream. The regurgitant fraction and (normalized) regurgitant volume should be measured. Any exacerbating or alleviating factors, beyond incompetence of the valve itself, should also be characterized. Of particular relevance, in the absence of an effective valve, are the size and compliance of the pulmonary arteries, and the presence and location, relative to the compliance, of any arterial stenoses.

Unfortunately, these considerations extend rather than alleviate the challenge of deciding if and when to replace a regurgitant pulmonary valve, but that is no reason to ignore or discount them!

References

1. Gatzoulis MA, Clark AL, Cullen S, Newman CG, Redington AN. Right ventricular diastolic function 15 to 35 years after repair of tetralogy of Fallot. Restrictive physiology predicts superior exercise performance. Circulation. Mar 15 1995;9;1:1775–81.
2. Chaturvedi RR, Kilner PJ, White PA, Bishop A, Szwarc R, Redington AN. Increased airway pressure and simulated branch pulmonary artery stenosis increase pulmonary regurgitation after repair of tetralogy of Fallot. Real-time analysis with a conductance catheter technique. Circulation. 1997;9;5:643–9.
3. Redington AN. Determinants and assessment of pulmonary regurgitation in tetralogy of fallot: practice and pitfalls. Cardiol Clin. 2006;2;4:631–9.
4. Kilner PJ. Pulmonary resistance in cardiovascular context. Int J Cardiol. 2004;97 Suppl 1:3–6.

5. Kang IS, Redington AN, Benson LN, Macgowan C, Valsangiacomo ER, Roman K, Kellenberger CJ, Yoo SJ. Differential regurgitation in branch pulmonary arteries after repair of tetralogy of Fallot: a phase-contrast cine magnetic resonance study. Circulation. 2003;10;7:2938–43.

6. Presson RG, Jr., Baumgartner WA, Jr., Peterson AJ, Glenny RW, Wagner WW, Jr. Pulmonary capillaries are recruited during pulsatile flow. J Appl Physiol. 2002; 9;2:1183–90.

7. Li W, Davlouros PA, Kilner PJ, Pennell DJ, Gibson D, Henein MY, Gatzoulis MA. Doppler-echocardiographic assessment of pulmonary regurgitation in adults with repaired tetralogy of Fallot: comparison with cardiovascular magnetic resonance imaging. Am Heart J. 2004;14;7:165–72.

Nicholas Collins and Louise Harris

Surgical repair of tetralogy of Fallot can be reliably performed with the expectation of low operative mortality, excellent long-term survival [1–4] and quality of life [5]. Late complications following repair relate to right ventricular dysfunction, arrhythmia, and the risk of sudden cardiac death. As the risk of sudden death appears to increase with late follow-up, it is apparent that appropriate identification of those at risk for adverse outcomes will remain an integral component of the management of patients with repaired tetralogy of Fallot [6, 7].

Despite advances in our understanding of the late complications to be anticipated in patients with previous tetralogy of Fallot repair, as well as an appreciation of the risk factors associated with sudden cardiac death, prediction in any given individual remains problematic. Optimal management for this patient population would be to identify those at risk and intervene before the development of malignant arrhythmia as sudden cardiac death may be the first manifestation of ventricular arrhythmia for many patients [8]. This goal, however, remains elusive [9].

The incidence of sudden death following operative repair has been estimated as up to 6% in long-term follow-up [1], with the risk in patients having previously undergone tetralogy repair believed to be the result of the interaction between right ventricular dysfunction and the concomitant electrical perturbations predisposing to arrhythmia [10]. Prevention of these sequelae remains the objective in the ongoing surveillance and management of these patients [11, 12].

The mechanism of sudden death in tetralogy of Fallot is believed to be multifactorial. In a population-based evaluation of patients who died suddenly late after congenital heart surgery, Silka et al. identified arrhythmic death to be the most common cause in tetralogy of Fallot but sudden death secondary to both circulatory and heart failure events was also observed in this patient cohort [6]. The mechanism of arrhythmic death is believed to be largely the consequence of ventricular tachycardia (VT) (Fig. 31.1) and ventricular fibrillation [8, 13–16], supported by electrophysiologic studies demonstrating inducible monomorphic ventricular tachycardia in patients with repaired tetralogy of Fallot [17]. However, bradycardia secondary to complete heart block may account for some of the mortality in these patients [18–21]. In the study by Silka, agonal rhythm due to complete heart block was the first rhythm observed in 2 of 11 patients dying suddenly and both patients had preexisting conduction deficits [6].

The mechanism of sustained ventricular tachycardia in the patient with tetralogy of Fallot is believed to be primarily reentrant. Intraoperative electrophysiologic mapping has demonstrated reentrant circuits originating from the right ventricular outflow tract [22], with typical associated structural abnormalities seen in these patients including the presence of right ventricular outflow tract aneurysms [23] and pulmonary regurgitation [17]. Electrophysiologic studies have also shown arrhythmia originating from the right ventricular inflow adjacent to the interventricular septum [24] and site of prior ventriculotomy [25]. Supportive evidence for reentry as the mechanism of ventricular tachycardia includes intraoperative demonstration of fractionated potentials and continuous activity [25] as well as induction of the arrhythmia by premature stimuli and entrainment of ventricular tachycardia during electrophysiologic study [26].

While the ventriculotomy scar [27] and ventricular septal defect patch are purported to provide anatomic barriers around which the circuit can reenter, other studies have demonstrated functional block with critical delays in activation in areas without visible scar as the mechanism for reentry [22]. Consistent with this, fibrosis surrounding isolated bundles of myocardial cells has been observed histologically in tetralogy of Fallot [28, 29] in a manner analogous to the border zone of myocardial

N. Collins (✉)
Toronto General Cardiac Centre for Adults, University Health Network, Toronto, ON, Canada

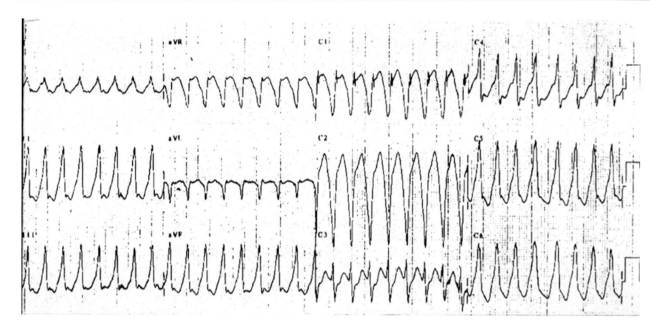

Fig. 31.1 Sustained monomorphic ventricular tachycardia of Left bundle branch block morphology in a patient late after repair of teralogy of Fallot

(a)   (b)

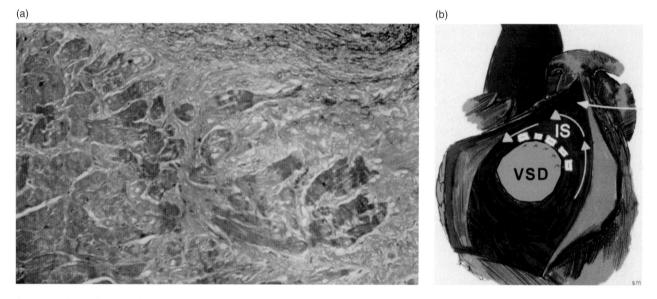

Fig. 31.2 The substrate for ventricular tachycardia in tetralogy of Fallot. Histologic examination from the margin of the right ventricular outflow tract aneurysm removed at surgery, reveals myocardial fibers interspersed with fibrosis in a manner analogous to that observed in the scar of myocardial infarction

infarction and may provide the necessary substrate for reentry (Fig. 31.2).

In addition to the substrate described above, susceptibility to ventricular tachycardia and fibrillation is also determined by right ventricular function and long-term volume overload [30]. The effect of chronic pulmonary regurgitation, subsequent right ventricular dilatation, and fibrosis [31] must also be taken into account as potential triggers for tachyarrhythmia and will be discussed further in this chapter.

31.1 Risk Stratification

Large, randomized, prospective trials have demonstrated the survival benefit of prophylactic implantable defibrillator insertion in patients with ischemic and nonischemic left ventricular dysfunction for the prevention of sudden cardiac death [32, 33]. Risk stratification in these populations has largely been based upon reduction in left ventricular ejection fraction and more recently, T-wave alternans has emerged as a potentially important predictor of risk [34]. There are, at present, no comparable trials upon which to base decisions regarding management of patients with congenital heart disease and specifically those with previous tetralogy of Fallot repair. Much of our knowledge and current clinical practice is based on retrospective studies of relatively small sample size. From these, a number of risk factors for arrhythmia and sudden death have been identified in the patient with previous tetralogy of Fallot repair. This chapter will explore these factors with respect to the timing and nature of the initial surgery, electrophysiological parameters, and the hemodynamic and structural sequelae following repair [23, 35, 36].

31.2 Timing and Nature of Initial Surgery

The timing and nature of corrective surgery for patients with tetralogy of Fallot has an important influence on future arrhythmogenic potential. While previous palliative surgery, particularly with a prior Potts or Waterston shunt [1, 4, 37], may be associated with an increased risk of ventricular tachycardia and sudden death, older age at the time of initial repair has proved to be a robust predictor of risk for late ventricular arrhythmia [35, 38–40]. More than a decade ago, Deanfield [18] and colleagues demonstrated increasing frequency and complexity of ventricular arrhythmias detected by ambulatory monitoring, with increasing age at repair and duration of follow-up. Similarly, at electrophysiologic study, Chandar et al. [41] in a multicenter study, observed that inducibility of ventricular arrhythmias—both nonsustained and sustained, monomorphic and polymorphic ventricular tachycardia—increased with increasing age at repair and follow-up, an observation that has more recently been confirmed by Khairy and co-authors [42]. This suggests there may be progressive changes in the myocardial substrate as a function of the underlying congenital condition and long-standing cyanosis that cannot be fully reversed by subsequent repair.

In addition, the surgical technique employed at the time of repair also influences the risk of future arrhythmia. Previous ventriculotomy has been demonstrated to be associated with an increased risk of ventricular tachycardia and sudden cardiac death, as well as right ventricular dysfunction and severity of pulmonary regurgitation [43]. Inducible ventricular tachycardia originating from the region of the previous ventriculotomy has been demonstrated at electrophysiologic study. More recent utilization of a transatrial surgical approach has been shown to decrease the risk of subsequent ventricular arrhythmia and right ventricular dilatation [44] without concomitant

increase in atrial arrhythmia [43]. The fact that avoidance of a ventriculotomy reduces the risk of late arrhythmia reinforces the concept that multiple factors contribute to the development of tachyarrhythmia in these patients. Additional surgical factors which have been identified as increasing the risk of future arrhythmia include the use of a transannular [37] or right ventricular patch [39] for relief of right ventricular outflow obstruction. Postoperative pulmonary regurgitation is inevitable, and the subsequent propensity to tachyarrhythmia may reflect the interaction between the consequent chronic pulmonary regurgitation and right ventricular dilatation.

The presence of transient heart block persisting greater than 3 days after surgical repair also confers an increased risk of sudden death [19, 21]. This presumably relates to damage to the conducting system incurred at the time of surgery, with complete heart block implicated in sudden death. Conduction abnormalities noted on the surface ECG, most commonly, right bundle branch block with left anterior hemiblock and prolongation of the PR interval, support injury to the conducting system with subsequent complete heart block as a potential mechanism for sudden death [45, 46]. Of note, injury to the conduction system has been demonstrated using both atrial and ventricular approaches to repair [47]. With advances in surgical techniques, damage to the conduction system should be minimized in the current surgical era.

31.3 Electrophysiologic Predictors of Sudden Death

Abnormalities of right ventricular conduction noted on the surface ECG have a demonstrated association with sudden death, and as such the surface ECG is a simple, noninvasive test that can provide important insight into arrhythmic risk. These ECG changes have been ascribed to the so-called mechano-electrical interaction between right ventricular dilatation and hypertrophy secondary to chronic pulmonary regurgitation, and disordered conduction.

The duration of the QRS complex is well recognized as a marker for arrhythmia propensity [10, 35], with evidence that prolongation of the QRS reflects not only increased right ventricular volume but also decreasing right ventricular ejection fraction and increased left ventricular mass [48]. In their initial study, Gatzoulis et al. [10] found a QRS duration $\geq$ 180 ms to be a sensitive predictor of sustained ventricular tachycardia and sudden death in an adult cohort of previously repaired tetralogy of Fallot patients with a mean duration of follow-up of >2 decades. QRS duration $\geq$ 180 ms had a sensitivity of

100% and a specificity of 95%. A more recent larger multicenter study by the same author [35] not only affirmed the value of QRS duration as a sensitive predictor of VT and sudden death but also identified rate of change of QRS duration as a marker for increased risk of ventricular arrhythmia. Those patients with a rapid progression in QRS duration were at increased risk of developing ventricular tachycardia or sudden death [35]. Finally, the utility of monitoring of the QRS interval may also be reflected in the stabilization [49] and possible reduction [50] in QRS duration that has been observed after pulmonary valve replacement in concert with reduction in right ventricular volume. That pulmonary valve replacement may be associated with decreased arrhythmic risk [50] and may be accompanied by electrical and mechanical reverse remodeling, reinforces the ability of the QRS duration to provide a noninvasive marker of risk.

While abnormalities of depolarization within the right ventricle in tetralogy of Fallot are reflected in QRS prolongation, abnormalities of repolarization as measured by QT dispersion, have also been observed. QT dispersion >60 ms is an additional risk factor for sudden death and in a study, when combined with QRS duration > 180 ms, had a sensitivity of 98% and specificity of 100% in identifying patients with sustained VT [51]. QT dispersion was unrelated to the presence of RBBB and remains predictive independent of right ventricular volume [51, 52].

In addition to the standard 12-lead ECG, a number of other noninvasive electrophysiologic parameters used to predict risk in other patient populations, have been examined for their ability to predict increased risk of ventricular arrhythmia and sudden death in tetralogy of Fallot. In contrast to the studies in ischemic and dilated cardiomyopathy, the number of subjects studied is often small, and the ability of these various measures to prospectively determine risk, inconclusive. The signal-averaged ECG (SAECG) as a predictor of risk is of uncertain benefit in this patient population. While the filtered QRS duration as measured by SAECG is associated with increased risk, no significant association with malignant arrhythmias was observed for other standard SAECG parameters. Specifically, high-frequency, low-amplitude signal duration (HFLA) and root mean square (rms) of the mean voltage of the terminal portion of the QRS (rms), both measurements of delayed conduction, were not significantly different in those with and without malignant arrhythmias [53]. Perturbations of autonomic nervous regulation, as measured by heart rate variability and baroreflex sensitivity, are of value in predicting risk in ischemic heart disease and have been examined in tetralogy of Fallot. Both of these measures are significantly reduced in tetralogy of Fallot [54, 55] and diminished heart-rate variability correlates with increased right ventricular size and QRS duration

[54]. Data on the utility of these indices to predict risk are lacking. Microvolt T-wave alternans testing, a recent addition to risk stratification in ischemic cardiomyopathy, has been studied in limited fashion in tetralogy of Fallot [56] and its role in risk prediction in this population has yet to be defined.

While ventricular ectopy on ambulatory ECG monitoring may be associated with inducible ventricular tachycardia [41, 57] in tetralogy of Fallot, the ability of ambulatory monitoring to predict risk appears limited. Ventricular ectopy and nonsustained ventricular tachycardia are commonly encountered with ambulatory monitoring and long-term follow-up of patients with ectopy on Holter monitoring reveals that this does not necessarily imply adverse clinical outcome [58, 59]. Atrial arrhythmia is common following tetralogy of Fallot repair with an incidence of up to 30–40% [60]. In addition to the significant associated morbidity [61], development of atrial arrhythmias in this population may also portend a poor prognosis. Follow-up of patients with atrial arrhythmia has been demonstrated to be associated with an increased risk of heart failure, ventricular arrhythmia, and death [61].

There have been a number of studies [41, 42, 57, 62] over the years addressing the utility of the electrophysiologic study (EPS) for risk stratification of patients with repaired tetralogy of Fallot, but the data have yielded mixed results and the role of EPS in asymptomatic patients remains controversial. The discordance in outcomes between studies may be attributable, in part, to the differences in the patient populations studied, the definition of a positive study, the relatively small sample sizes, and relatively low frequency of ventricular tachycardia and sudden death events. While prolongation of QRS duration has been shown to correlate with both risk of ventricular arrhythmia and inducibility of monomorphic ventricular tachycardia, the predictive value of a positive electrophysiologic study has been variable [62, 63]. The yield of EPS in asymptomatic patients remains low, with positive studies noted in approximately 10% of patients [41, 57]. Several studies have suggested a negative EPS confers a favorable prognosis, with a low risk of ventricular arrhythmia and sudden death during follow-up [42, 63]. Of note, however, in one multicenter retrospective study, all five patients who experienced sudden death had negative electrophysiologic studies for inducible ventricular tachycardia [41]. A more recent retrospective multicenter study [42] found not only inducible, sustained, monomorphic ventricular tachycardia, but also inducible, sustained, polymorphic ventricular tachycardia to be important predictors of subsequent events. These authors concluded that sustained polymorphic VT enhanced the predictive accuracy of the EP study with an overall sensitivity of 77% and minimal impact on specificity, and should therefore not be disregarded as a nonspecific finding. The complexity of the role of electrophysiological testing is reinforced by data suggesting that ventricular ectopy on Holter monitoring may be associated with inducible ventricular tachycardia [41, 57].

31.4 Hemodynamic and Structural Sequelae Following Repair as Predictors of Risk

An important advance in the long-term management of patients with repaired tetralogy of Fallot has been the appreciation of the contribution of chronic pulmonary regurgitation and subsequent right ventricular dilatation to ventricular arrhythmia [23, 35]. Chronic right ventricular volume overload and associated right ventricular dilatation contribute to impairment of right ventricular function. This is in turn associated with abnormal conduction within the right ventricle, reflected in prolongation of the QRS duration late after surgical repair, and subsequent propensity to arrhythmia [64]. Of note, it appears that it is the maladaptive response of the right ventricle to chronic pulmonary regurgitation, rather than the severity of pulmonary regurgitation *per se*, that dictates outcome. In an early study of mechano-electrical interaction, those patients with so-called restrictive right ventricular physiology, had a narrower QRS, smaller cardiothoracic ratio and lower likelihood of ventricular arrhythmias [10]. This is supported by data showing that the pulmonary regurgitant fraction alone does not correlate with clinical outcome [48]. An important benefit of pulmonary valve replacement, with associated cryoablation, has been a decrease in the risk of subsequent arrhythmia [50]. More recently, a reduction in right ventricular parameters [65] has been demonstrated with percutaneous pulmonary valve replacement, with reduction in ventricular arrhythmia hopefully a future benefit. Additional structural abnormalities of the right ventricle documented to predispose to ventricular tachycardia include right ventricular outflow tract aneurysmal dilatation [22] and the presence of right ventricular outflow tract akinesis [11].

Further evolution in the understanding of mechanisms of tachyarrhythmia and outcome has recently focused on the important interaction between the left and right ventricles in tetralogy of Fallot. Left ventricular dysfunction, which correlates with right ventricular impairment, has been demonstrated to be an independent risk factor for impaired functional status [48] and is associated with an increased risk of sudden cardiac death when assessed in combination with QRS prolongation [48, 66]. Impairment of left ventricular function in tetralogy of Fallot is

multifactorial but has recently been attributed, in part, to left ventricular dyssynchrony in the setting of RBBB [67].

The ability of these hemodynamic and structural abnormalities to predict risk of sudden cardiac death in tetralogy of Fallot has been assessed noninvasively using echocardiographic and magnetic resonance imaging (MRI) techniques.

Right ventricular dimension, function, and volume can be readily assessed by standard echocardiographic techniques. As described above, increasing right ventricular dimension and decreasing right ventricular function are associated with increased risk of sudden cardiac death and the probability of ventricular tachycardia or sudden cardiac death increases progressively with increases in right ventricular end-diastolic volume [68]. However, no specific value for right ventricular volume or function has been identified as predictive of risk. A left ventricular ejection fraction of <40% by visual assessment on echocardiography has been identified as an additional predictor of sudden cardiac death risk in tetralogy of Fallot [66]. In this retrospective single-center study, left ventricular dysfunction when combined with QRS duration ≥180 ms, had a positive and negative predictive value for sudden cardiac death of 66% and 93%, respectively.

The more recent innovation of tissue Doppler-derived strain has identified left ventricular dyssynchrony in association with a reduction of global and regional left ventricular function in this patient population [67] but its value in risk stratification has yet to be studied.

MRI has contributed to our ability to identify those at risk of ventricular tachycardia by facilitating improved anatomic assessment of the right ventricle, including identification of right ventricular outflow tract aneurysms and right ventricular akinesis. MRI also permits accurate assessment of both left and right ventricular size, volume, and function, as well as severity of pulmonary regurgitation. Studies utilizing MRI have identified a threshold right ventricular volume, beyond which regression of right ventricular dilatation is less likely following pulmonary valve replacement [69]. There are no comparable MR data of right ventricular volume and its relation to ventricular arrhythmia and sudden cardiac death. However, the application of MRI techniques to the assessment of risk in tetralogy of Fallot continues to evolve. Recently, the MRI technique of late gadolinium enhancement, a marker of myocardial fibrosis, has been found to correlate with ventricular dysfunction and functional class in tetralogy of Fallot, with the extent of fibrosis within the right ventricle significantly associated with clinical arrhythmia [31].

There is little doubt that our understanding of the mechanisms that contribute to the risk of sudden cardiac death in patients with tetralogy of Fallot repair has improved and continues to evolve. There are, however, outstanding issues yet to be addressed. Despite the optimism engendered by recent progress, our ability to accurately predict those individuals of the increasingly large cohort of survivors most at risk remains limited. Even though there are extensive studies of hemodynamic and electrophysiologic parameters addressing this problem using a wide variety of techniques, it is clear that no single risk factor is likely to emerge as sufficiently predictive. A scoring system, derived from a composite of different risk factors, may hold the greatest promise for the identification of those at highest risk. Then, having identified those at risk, there must be effective management strategies for risk reduction in these patients. For the tetralogy of Fallot patient, this will include measures directed at both hemodynamic and electrophysiologic perturbations. That the risk of ventricular tachycardia and sudden death may be moderated by appropriately timed pulmonary valve replacement is a promising advance in the management of these patients. The implantable cardioverter-defibrillator (ICD) is of proven benefit in the secondary prevention of aborted sudden cardiac death [70]. Whether the results of trials demonstrating similar benefit in primary prevention for patients with dilated and ischemic cardiomyopathies [32, 33], can be extrapolated to this patient cohort is unknown but possible. Other evolving therapeutic strategies offer promise for the future. These include catheter ablation for ventricular tachycardia and percutaneous valve replacement, while cardiac resynchronization therapy may potentially be of benefit in the patient with substantial biventricular dysfunction [71].

References

1. Murphy JG, Gersh BJ, Mair DD, Fuster V, McGoon MD, Ilstrup DM, McGoon DC, Kirklin JW, Danielson GK. Long-term outcome in patients undergoing surgical repair of tetralogy of Fallot. N Engl J Med. 1993;329(9):593–9.
2. Fuster V, McGoon DC, Kennedy MA, Ritter DG, Kirklin JW. Long-term evaluation (12 to 22 years) of open heart surgery for tetralogy of Fallot. Am J Cardiol. 1980;46(4):635–42.
3. Horneffer PJ, Zahka KG, Rowe SA, Manolio TA, Gott VL, Reitz BA, Gardner TJ. Long-term results of total repair of tetralogy of Fallot in childhood. Ann Thorac Surg. 1990;50(2):179–83; discussion 183–5.
4. Katz NM, Blackstone EH, Kirklin JW, Pacifico AD, Bargeron LM, Jr. Late survival and symptoms after repair of tetralogy of Fallot. Circulation. 1982;65(2):403–10.
5. Norgaard MA, Lauridsen P, Helvind M, Pettersson G. Twenty-to-thirty-seven-year follow-up after repair for Tetralogy of Fallot. Eur J Cardiothorac Surg. 1999;16(2):125–30.
6. Silka MJ, Hardy BG, Menashe VD, Morris CD. A population-based prospective evaluation of risk of sudden cardiac death after operation for common congenital heart defects. J Am Coll Cardiol. 1998;32(1):245–51.
7. Williams RG, Pearson GD, Barst RJ, Child JS, del Nido P, Gersony WM, Kuehl KS, Landzberg MJ, Myerson M, Neish SR and others. Report of the National Heart, Lung, and Blood Institute Working Group on research in adult congenital heart disease. J Am Coll Cardiol. 2006;47(4):701–7.
8. Dunnigan A, Pritzker MR, Benditt DG, Benson DW, Jr. Life threatening ventricular tachycardias in late survivors of surgically corrected tetralogy of Fallot. Br Heart J. 1984;52(2):198–206.
9. Saul JP, Alexander ME. Preventing sudden death after repair of tetralogy of Fallot: complex therapy for complex patients. J Cardiovasc Electrophysiol. 1999;10(9):1271–87.
10. Gatzoulis MA, Till JA, Somerville J, Redington AN. Mechanoelectrical interaction in tetralogy of Fallot. QRS prolongation relates to right ventricular size and predicts malignant ventricular arrhythmias and sudden death. Circulation. 1995;92(2):231–7.
11. Davlouros PA, Karatza AA, Gatzoulis MA, Shore DF. Timing and type of surgery for severe pulmonary regurgitation after repair of tetralogy of Fallot. Int J Cardiol. 2004;97 Suppl 1:91–101.
12. Stephenson EA, Redington AN. Reduction of QRS duration following pulmonary valve replacement in tetralogy of Fallot: implications for arrhythmia reduction? Eur Heart J. 2005;26(9):863–4.
13. Nollert G, Fischlein T, Bouterwek S, Bohmer C, Klinner W, Reichart B. Long-term survival in patients with repair of tetralogy of Fallot: 36-year follow-up of 490 survivors of the first year after surgical repair. J Am Coll Cardiol. 1997;30(5):1374–83.
14. Kugler JD. Predicting sudden death in patients who have undergone tetralogy of fallot repair: is it really as simple as measuring ECG intervals? J Cardiovasc Electrophysiol. 1998;9(1):103–6.
15. Gillette PC, Yeoman MA, Mullins CE, McNamara DG. Sudden death after repair of tetralogy of Fallot. Electrocardiographic and electrophysiologic abnormalities. Circulation. 1977;56(4 Pt 1):566–71.
16. James FW, Kaplan S, Chou TC. Unexpected cardiac arrest in patients after surgical correction of tetralogy of Fallot. Circulation. 1975;52(4):691–5.
17. Marie PY, Marcon F, Brunotte F, Briancon S, Danchin N, Worms AM, Robert J, Pernot C. Right ventricular overload and induced sustained ventricular tachycardia in operatively "repaired" tetralogy of Fallot. Am J Cardiol. 1992;69(8):785–9.
18. Deanfield JE, McKenna WJ, Hallidie-Smith KA. Detection of late arrhythmia and conduction disturbance after correction of tetralogy of Fallot. Br Heart J. 1980;44(3):248–53.
19. Wolff GS, Rowland TW, Ellison RC. Surgically induced right bundle-branch block with left anterior hemiblock. An ominous sign in postoperative tetralogy of Fallot. Circulation. 1972;46(3):587–94.
20. Nakazawa M, Shinohara T, Sasaki A, Echigo S, Kado H, Niwa K, Oyama K, Yokota M, Iwamoto M, Fukushima N and others. Arrhythmias late after repair of tetralogy of fallot: a Japanese Multicenter Study. Circ J. 2004;68(2):126–30.
21. Hokanson JS, Moller JH. Significance of early transient complete heart block as a predictor of sudden death late after operative correction of tetralogy of Fallot. Am J Cardiol. 2001;87(11):1271–7.
22. Downar E, Harris L, Kimber S, Mickleborough L, Williams W, Sevaptsidis E, Masse S, Chen TC, Chan A, Genga A and others. Ventricular tachycardia after surgical repair of tetralogy of Fallot: results of intraoperative mapping studies. J Am Coll Cardiol. 1992;20(3):648–55.
23. Harrison DA, Harris L, Siu SC, MacLoghlin CJ, Connelly MS, Webb GD, Downar E, McLaughlin PR, Williams WG.

Sustained ventricular tachycardia in adult patients late after repair of tetralogy of Fallot. J Am Coll Cardiol. 1997;30(5):1368–73.

24. Kugler JD, Pinsky WW, Cheatham JP, Hofshire PJ, Mooring PK, Fleming WH. Sustained ventricular tachycardia after repair of tetralogy of Fallot: new electrophysiologic findings. Am J Cardiol. 1983;51(7):1137–43.

25. Horowitz LN, Vetter VL, Harken AH, Josephson ME. Electro-physiologic characteristics of sustained ventricular tachycardia occurring after repair of tetralogy of fallot. Am J Cardiol. 1980;46(3):446–52.

26. Kremers MS, Wells PJ, Black WH, Solodyna MA. Entrainment of ventricular tachycardia in postoperative tetralogy of Fallot. Pacing Clin Electrophysiol. 1988;11(9):1310–4.

27. Harken AH, Horowitz LN, Josephson ME. Surgical correction of recurrent sustained ventricular tachycardia following complete repair of tetralogy of Fallot. J Thorac Cardiovasc Surg. 1980;80(5):779–81.

28. Chowdhury UK, Sathia S, Ray R, Singh R, Pradeep KK, Venugopal P. Histopathology of the right ventricular outflow tract and its relationship to clinical outcomes and arrhythmias in patients with tetralogy of Fallot. J Thorac Cardiovasc Surg. 2006;132(2):270–7.

29. Deanfield JE, Ho SY, Anderson RH, McKenna WJ, Allwork SP, Hallidie-Smith KA. Late sudden death after repair of tetralogy of Fallot: a clinicopathologic study. Circulation. 1983;67(3):626–31.

30. Deanfield J, McKenna W, Rowland E. Local abnormalities of right ventricular depolarization after repair of tetralogy of Fallot: a basis for ventricular arrhythmia. Am J Cardiol. 1985;55(5):522–5.

31. Babu-Narayan SV, Kilner PJ, Li W, Moon JC, Goktekin O, Davlouros PA, Khan M, Ho SY, Pennell DJ, Gatzoulis MA. Ventricular fibrosis suggested by cardiovascular magnetic resonance in adults with repaired tetralogy of fallot and its relationship to adverse markers of clinical outcome. Circulation. 2006;113(3):405–13.

32. Moss AJ, Zareba W, Hall WJ, Klein H, Wilber DJ, Cannom DS, Daubert JP, Higgins SL, Brown MW, Andrews ML. Prophylactic implantation of a defibrillator in patients with myocardial infarction and reduced ejection fraction. N Engl J Med. 2002;346(12):877–83.

33. Kadish A, Dyer A, Daubert JP, Quigg R, Estes NA, Anderson KP, Calkins H, Hoch D, Goldberger J, Shalaby A and others. Prophylactic defibrillator implantation in patients with nonischemic dilated cardiomyopathy. N Engl J Med. 2004;350(21):2151–8.

34. Chow T, Kereiakes DJ, Bartone C, Booth T, Schloss EJ, Waller T, Chung ES, Menon S, Nallamothu BK, Chan PS. Prognostic utility of microvolt T-wave alternans in risk stratification of patients with ischemic cardiomyopathy. J Am Coll Cardiol. 2006;47(9):1820–7.

35. Gatzoulis MA, Balaji S, Webber SA, Siu SC, Hokanson JS, Poile C, Rosenthal M, Nakazawa M, Moller JH, Gillette PC and others. Risk factors for arrhythmia and sudden cardiac death late after repair of tetralogy of Fallot: a multicentre study. Lancet. 2000;356(9234):975–81.

36. Steeds RP, Oakley D. Predicting late sudden death from ventricular arrhythmia in adults following surgical repair of tetralogy of Fallot. Qjm. 2004;97(1):7–13.

37. Nollert GD, Dabritz SH, Schmoeckel M, Vicol C, Reichart B. Risk factors for sudden death after repair of tetralogy of Fallot. Ann Thorac Surg. 2003;76(6):1901–5.

38. Gladman G, McCrindle BW, Williams WG, Freedom RM, Benson LN. The modified Blalock-Taussig shunt: clinical impact and morbidity in Fallot's tetralogy in the current era. J Thorac Cardiovasc Surg. 1997;114(1):25–30.

39. d'Udekem Y, Ovaert C, Grandjean F, Gerin V, Cailteux M, Shango-Lody P, Vliers A, Sluysmans T, Robert A, Rubay J. Tetralogy of Fallot: transannular and right ventricular patching equally affect late functional status. Circulation. 2000;102(19 Suppl 3):III116–22.

40. Deanfield JE, McKenna WJ, Presbitero P, England D, Graham GR, Hallidie-Smith K. Ventricular arrhythmia in unrepaired and repaired tetralogy of Fallot. Relation to age, timing of repair, and haemodynamic status. Br Heart J. 1984;52(1):77–81.

41. Chandar JS, Wolff GS, Garson A, Jr., Bell TJ, Beder SD, Bink-Boelkens M, Byrum CJ, Campbell RM, Deal BJ, Dick M, 2nd and others. Ventricular arrhythmias in postoperative tetralogy of Fallot. Am J Cardiol. 1990;65(9):655–61.

42. Khairy P, Landzberg MJ, Gatzoulis MA, Lucron H, Lambert J, Marcon F, Alexander ME, Walsh EP. Value of programmed ventricular stimulation after tetralogy of fallot repair: a multicenter study. Circulation. 2004;109(16):1994–2000.

43. Dietl CA, Cazzaniga ME, Dubner SJ, Perez-Balino NA, Torres AR, Favaloro RG. Life-threatening arrhythmias and RV dysfunction after surgical repair of tetralogy of Fallot. Comparison between transventricular and transatrial approaches. Circulation. 1994;90(5 Pt 2):II7–12.

44. Stellin G, Milanesi O, Rubino M, Michielon G, Bianco R, Moreolo GS, Boneva R, Sorbara C, Casarotto D. Repair of tetralogy of Fallot in the first six months of life: transatrial versus transventricular approach. Ann Thorac Surg. 1995;60 Suppl 6:S588–91.

45. Friedli B, Bolens M, Taktak M. Conduction disturbances after correction of tetralogy of Fallot: are electrophysiologic studies of prognostic value? J Am Coll Cardiol. 1988;11(1):162–5.

46. Quattlebaum TG, Varghese J, Neill CA, Donahoo JS. Sudden death among postoperative patients with tetralogy of Fallot: a follow-up study of 243 patients for an average of twelve years. Circulation. 1976;54(2):289–93.

47. Bharati S, Lev M. Sequelae of atriotomy and ventriculotomy on the endocardium, conduction system and coronary arteries. Am J Cardiol. 1982;50(3):580–7.

48. Geva T, Sandweiss BM, Gauvreau K, Lock JE, Powell AJ. Factors associated with impaired clinical status in long-term survivors of tetralogy of Fallot repair evaluated by magnetic resonance imaging. J Am Coll Cardiol. 2004;43(6):1068–74.

49. van Huysduynen BH, van Straten A, Swenne CA, Maan AC, van Eck HJ, Schalij MJ, van der Wall EE, de Roos A, Hazekamp MG, Vliegen HW. Reduction of QRS duration after pulmonary valve replacement in adult Fallot patients is related to reduction of right ventricular volume. Eur Heart J. 2005;26(9):928–32.

50. Therrien J, Siu SC, Harris L, Dore A, Niwa K, Janousek J, Williams WG, Webb G, Gatzoulis MA. Impact of pulmonary valve replacement on arrhythmia propensity late after repair of tetralogy of Fallot. Circulation. 2001;103(20):2489–94.

51. Gatzoulis MA, Till JA, Redington AN. Depolarization-repolarization inhomogeneity after repair of tetralogy of Fallot. The substrate for malignant ventricular tachycardia? Circulation. 1997;95(2):401–4.

52. Daliento L, Rizzoli G, Menti L, Baratella MC, Turrini P, Nava A, Dalla Volta S. Accuracy of electrocardiographic and echocardiographic indices in predicting life threatening ventricular arrhythmias in patients operated for tetralogy of Fallot. Heart. 1999;81(6):650–5.

53. Russo G, Folino AF, Mazzotti E, Rebellato L, Daliento L. Comparison between QRS duration at standard ECG and signal-averaging ECG for arrhythmic risk stratification after surgical repair of tetralogy of fallot. J Cardiovasc Electrophysiol. 2005;16(3):288–92.

54. McLeod KA, Hillis WS, Houston AB, Wilson N, Trainer A, Neilson J, Doig WB. Reduced heart rate variability following repair of tetralogy of Fallot. Heart. 1999;81(6):656–60.

55. Davos CH, Davlouros PA, Wensel R, Francis D, Davies LC, Kilner PJ, Coats AJ, Piepoli M, Gatzoulis MA. Global impairment of cardiac autonomic nervous activity late after repair of tetralogy of Fallot. Circulation. 2002;106 12 Suppl 1:I69–75.

56. Cheung MM, Weintraub RG, Cohen RJ, Karl TR, Wilkinson JL, Davis AM. T wave alternans threshold late after repair of tetralogy of Fallot. J Cardiovasc Electrophysiol. 2002;13(7):657–61.

57. Zimmermann M, Friedli B, Adamec R, Oberhansli I. Ventricular late potentials and induced ventricular arrhythmias after surgical repair of tetralogy of Fallot. Am J Cardiol. 1991;67(9):873–8.

58. Cullen S, Celermajer DS, Franklin RC, Hallidie-Smith KA, Deanfield JE. Prognostic significance of ventricular arrhythmia after repair of tetralogy of Fallot: a 12-year prospective study. J Am Coll Cardiol. 1994;23(5):1151–5.

59. Wessel HU, Bastanier CK, Paul MH, Berry TE, Cole RB, Muster AJ. Prognostic significance of arrhythmia in tetralogy of Fallot after intracardiac repair. Am J Cardiol. 1980;46(5):843–8.

60. Roos-Hesselink J, Perlroth MG, McGhie J, Spitaels S. Atrial arrhythmias in adults after repair of tetralogy of Fallot. Correlations with clinical, exercise, and echocardiographic findings. Circulation. 1995;91(8):2214–9.

61. Harrison DA, Siu SC, Hussain F, MacLoghlin CJ, Webb GD, Harris L. Sustained atrial arrhythmias in adults late after repair of tetralogy of fallot. Am J Cardiol. 2001;87(5):584–8.

62. Balaji S, Lau YR, Case CL, Gillette PC. QRS prolongation is associated with inducible ventricular tachycardia after repair of tetralogy of Fallot. Am J Cardiol. 1997;80(2):160–3.

63. Lucron H, Marcon F, Bosser G, Lethor JP, Marie PY, Brembilla-Perrot B. Induction of sustained ventricular tachycardia after surgical repair of tetralogy of Fallot. Am J Cardiol. 1999;83(9):1369–73.

64. Bouzas B, Kilner PJ, Gatzoulis MA. Pulmonary regurgitation: not a benign lesion. Eur Heart J. 2005;26(5):433–9.

65. Khambadkone S, Coats L, Taylor A, Boudjemline Y, Derrick G, Tsang V, Cooper J, Muthurangu V, Hegde SR, Razavi RS and others. Percutaneous pulmonary valve implantation in humans: results in 59 consecutive patients. Circulation. 2005;112(8):1189–97.

66. Ghai A, Silversides C, Harris L, Webb GD, Siu SC, Therrien J. Left ventricular dysfunction is a risk factor for sudden cardiac death in adults late after repair of tetralogy of Fallot. J Am Coll Cardiol. 2002;40(9):1675–80.

67. Abd El Rahman MY, Hui W, Yigitbasi M, Dsebissowa F, Schubert S, Hetzer R, Lange PE, Abdul-Khaliq H. Detection of left ventricular asynchrony in patients with right bundle branch block after repair of tetralogy of Fallot using tissue-Doppler imaging-derived strain. J Am Coll Cardiol. 2005;45(6):915–21.

68. Therrien J, Provost Y, Merchant N, Williams W, Colman J, Webb G. Optimal timing for pulmonary valve replacement in adults after tetralogy of Fallot repair. Am J Cardiol. 2005;95(6):779–82.

69. Therrien J, Siu SC, McLaughlin PR, Liu PP, Williams WG, Webb GD. Pulmonary valve replacement in adults late after repair of tetralogy of fallot: are we operating too late? J Am Coll Cardiol. 2000;36(5):1670–5.

70. Connolly SJ, Hallstrom AP, Cappato R, Schron EB, Kuck KH, Zipes DP, Greene HL, Boczor S, Domanski M, Follmann D and others. Meta-analysis of the implantable cardioverter defibrillator secondary prevention trials. AVID, CASH and CIDS studies. Antiarrhythmics vs Implantable Defibrillator study. Cardiac Arrest Study Hamburg. Canadian Implantable Defibrillator Study. Eur Heart J. 2000;21(24):2071–8.

71. Kirsh JA, Stephenson EA, Redington AN. Images in cardiovascular medicine. Recovery of left ventricular systolic function after biventricular resynchronization pacing in a child with repaired tetralogy of Fallot and severe biventricular dysfunction. Circulation. 2006;113(14):e691–2.

32.1 Effect of Chronic PR on the RV

The physiological role of the pulmonary valve (PV) is to allow one-way flow of blood from the right ventricle (RV) to the pulmonary vasculature. An incompetent PV results in varying degrees of pulmonary regurgitation (PR). Isolated trace or mild PR is considered physiologically normal, and has no long-term consequences. Isolated moderate or severe PR is considered pathological and over time results in volume overloading of the RV. Chronic volume overloading leads to RV dilatation and systolic dysfunction, and right-sided congestive heart failure.

Tetralogy of Fallot (TOF) is the most common form of cyanotic congenital heart disease with a prevalence of 0.18–0.26 per 1000 live births [1, 2]. If left untreated, it carries 33% mortality in the first year of life; and a 50% mortality in the first 3 years of life [3]. Primary repair of TOF in the neonate and young infant began in the early 1970s and consisted of ventricular septal defect patch repair and relief of the right ventricular outflow tract (RVOT) obstruction via a transannular patch, valvectomy, and/or valvotomy [4]. Surgical repair is currently considered the standard of care for patients born with TOF. It has an operative mortality below 2% [5, 6], and a 5-year and 36-year survival of 93% and 85%, respectively [7, 8]. Although, the long-term outcome of patients with repaired TOF is favorable, the initial repair to relieve the RV outflow tract obstruction often results in significant PR. PR in the repaired TOF patient is usually well tolerated for long periods of time. The low-resistance, high-capacitance reservoir of the pulmonary circulation minimizes the actual regurgitant volume in the face of free PR. However, over time, chronic PR results in volume overloading of the RV. Volume overloading of the RV eventually leads to an increase in right ventricular end-diastolic volume (RV-EDV), right ventricular end-systolic volume (RV-ESV), and RV systolic dysfunction. The ensuing RV dilatation and dysfunction predisposes the patient to exercise intolerance, congestive heart failure, atrial and ventricular arrhythmias, and may contribute to sudden cardiac death (SCD) [9, 10].

There is a direct relationship between poor exercise capacity and the severity of pulmonary insufficiency and its effects on RV. Carvalho et al. [11], demonstrated that residual PR after complete repair of TOF correlated with impaired exercise capacity. They prospectively evaluated 10 asymptomatic patients more than 5 years after TOF repair. There was a significant negative correlation between the severity of PR and exercise duration. Patients with an abnormal maximal oxygen uptake were statistically more likely to have more severe residual PR. Wessel et al. [12], also demonstrated that in repaired TOF a statistically significant relationship exists between reduced work performance and residual disease.

Rhythm disturbances in patients with repaired TOF are relatively common and it is related to surgical scar and RV enlargement. Chronic PR leads to RV enlargement, which in turn leads to tricuspid annular dilatation and subsequent tricuspid regurgitation. Right atrial enlargement ensues, which predisposes the patient to atrial flutter/fibrillation. Atrial tachyarrhythmias, including atrial fibrillation and atrial flutter occurs in up to one-third of all patients postrepair and contributes significantly to patient morbidity. Right ventricular dilatation results in delayed right ventricular depolarization (wide QRS complex on ECG) and inhomogeneous repolarization patterns, which may serve as a trigger for ventricular reentry tachycardias. There is a mechanico-electrical relationship described in these patients where the degree of RV dilatation corresponds to the width of QRS duration on surface ECG and patients with QRS width > 180 ms are at greater risk of syncope and SCD. The incidence of SCD (presumably from VT) is reported to be between 0.5% and 6%. [9, 13, 14, 15]

G. Martucci (✉)
MAUDE Unit, McGill University, Montreal, QC, Canada

A.N. Redington et al. (eds.), *Congenital Diseases in the Right Heart*, DOI 10.1007/978-1-84800-378-1_32,
© Springer-Verlag London Limited 2009

32.2 Methods of Assessing RV Volume and Function

Until recently echocardiography and radionuclide angiography (RNA) were considered the standard of care when it came to quantifying both PR, and RV size and function. Echocardiography and RNA have largely been replaced by the new gold standard, cardiovascular MRI (CMRI). CMRI has clear advantages over both echocardiography and radio nuclide angiography. CMRI can assess ventricular size and function without making assumptions about ventricular geometry. Moreover, CMRI is able to view the cardiovascular system from many different angles thereby providing the clinician with unprecedented accuracy and three-dimensional detail about surrounding cardiac structures. In addition to providing unParaleled detail about complex cardiac anatomy, CMRI can also address questions about cardiac physiology, such as, the location and severity of a stenosis, the severity of regurgitation, the size and function of the ventricle, and shunt calculations. CMRI has proven to be an invaluable tool for repeat noninvasive assessment of the TOF patient postsurgical repair. In particular, CMRI is unrivalled in its assessment of RV size and function, outflow tract aneurysm formation, severity of pulmonary stenosis and regurgitation, and conduit visualization [16].

32.3 Effect of Surgical Pulmonary Valve Replacement

Surgical pulmonary valve replacement in patients with significant PR can be done safely with low mortality [17, 18]. Symptomatic improvement occurs with objective improvement in exercise capacity [19]. RV volume, for most part, regresses by approximately 30% when pulmonary valve replacement is performed in a timely manner. Bove et al. [20] in 1985 were the first to report an improvement in RV ejection fraction and reduction in RV volumes after pulmonary valve replacement in 11 patients. The patients' mean age at the original repair was 6.6 years, and the mean age at pulmonary valve replacement was 14.6 years. RV volume and RV ejection fraction were assessed before and after pulmonary valve replacement with M-mode echocardiography and RNA. The indications for pulmonary valve replacement were conduit stenosis in three patients, symptoms in two patients, progressive cardiomegally in three patients, and new onset tricuspid regurgitation in three patients. An improvement, defined as a greater than 5% increase in RV ejection fraction, was seen in seven patients, whereas four patients demonstrated no change. The seven patients who demonstrated an improvement in RV ejection fraction also had a subjective improvement in exercise tolerance, and there was a statistically significant reduction in the RV end-diastolic dimension indexed to the LV end-

diastolic dimension. Warner et al. [21], also demonstrated a decrease in RV-ED dimension using M-mode echocardiography. They evaluated 16 patients with severe PR and RV dilatation before and after pulmonary valve replacement. The mean age at initial TOF repair was 2 years, and the mean age at pulmonary valve replacement was 12 years. All 16 patients complained of diminished exercise tolerance, and 10 of the 16 had abnormal exercise tolerance tests. After surgery, all 16 patients reported symptomatic improvement. Twelve of the 16 patients had trace or mild PR after pulmonary valve replacement, and four of the 16 patients had moderate PR after pulmonary valve replacement. The patients with moderate PR after pulmonary valve replacement were more likely to have pulmonary artery diameters and cross-sectional areas that were smaller than those patients who had only trace or mild PR after pulmonary valve replacement. The RV end-diastolic diameter as assessed by M-mode echocardiography decreased in all but one patient. The reduction in RV-end diastolic dimension was greater in those patients who had trace or mild PR after pulmonary valve replacement; as compared to those patients with moderate PR after pulmonary valve replacement. In contrast, both d'Udekem et al. [22] and Discigil et al. [23] could not demonstrate a significant reduction in RV size after surgical pulmonary valve replacement. Also, a study reported by Therrien et al. [24] failed to demonstrate a reduction in RV volumes after pulmonary valve replacement using RNA as the imaging modality in a group of adults with a mean age of 33.9 years. The authors acknowledged the potential limitation of transthoracic echocardiography and/or RNA in assessing RV size.

Vliegen et al. [25], reported the first adult study to show improved RV systolic function using CMRI while significantly reducing RV-EDV and RV-ESV after pulmonary valve replacement. Pulmonary valve replacement was performed late after total repair for TOF in patients with moderate–severe PR and RV dilatation. They evaluated 26 consecutive adult patients who underwent pulmonary valve replacement with a cryo-perserved pulmonary homograft for PR late after correction of TOF. The patients were all evaluated by CMRI approximately 5 months pre-pulmonary valve replacement and 6–12 months post-pulmonary valve replacement. The mean age at the initial TOF repair was 5.0 ± 4.2 years; and the mean age at pulmonary valve replacement was 29.2 ± 9.0 years. All the patients had either moderate or severe PR and 13 of the 26 patients had severe RV dilatation, defined as RV-EDV greater than twice LV-EDV. Ten of the 26 patients were in New York Heart Association (NYHA) functional Class II or greater. After surgery there was a reduction in mean NYHA functional class from 2.0 ± 0.6 to 1.3 ± 0.5; 25 of the 26 patients had no PR or mild PR, and there was a 30% reduction in both RV systolic and diastolic volumes. Before pulmonary valve replacement the mean indexed RV-EDV and RV-ESV were 167 ± 40 ml/m^2 and 99 ± 36 ml/m^2, respectively. After pulmonary valve replacement the indexed RV-EDV and the indexed RV-ESV decreased to 114 ± 35 ml/m^2 and 66 ± 35 ml/m^2, respectively. The RV ejection fraction corrected for regurgitation and shunting increased from $25\% \pm 8\%$ to $43\% \pm 14\%$.

32.4 Timing of Pulmonary Valve Replacement

The perioperative surgical mortality for pulmonary valve replacement is low; however, homograft and/or valved conduits have a finite life expectancy related to calcification, stenosis, intimal hyperproliferation, and graft degeneration. Wells et al. [26], retrospectively analyzed 40 patients who had undergone homograft conduit replacement of the RVOT and reported that the mean interval to conduit failure was 5.3 years. This would result in multiple surgeries over the lifetime of a patient. Repeat surgeries are characterized by specific technical challenges that can result in increased morbidity and mortality. Proper timing of pulmonary valve replacement in these young adult patients becomes critical.

Therrien et al. [27], and Valsangiacoma et al. [28] independently reported on a threshold of RV enlargement above which irreversible dilatation occurs. Both studies used CMRI to assess RV size. Therrien et al. [27] evaluated 17 adult patients with repaired TOF who underwent pulmonary valve replacement with a xenograft pulmonary valve for RV dilatation and hypokinesis. Each patient was evaluated with CMRI before and after surgery. Seven patients were in NYHA class III or IV. Post-pulmonary valve replacement, there was a statistical significant reduction in both systolic and diastolic RV volumes. The mean indexed pre-pulmonary valve replacement RV-EDV and RV-ESV were 163 ± 34 ml/m^2, and 109 ± 27 ml/m^2, respectively. After pulmonary valve replacement the mean indexed RV-EDV and RV-ESV decreased to 107 ± 26 ml/m^2 and 69 ± 22 ml/m^2, respectively. RV remodeling after pulmonary valve replacement resulted in a 34% and 37% reduction in mean RV-EDV and RV-ESV, respectively. More interestingly, despite having a substantial reduction in RV size, no patients with an indexed RV-EDV greater than 170 ml/m^2 or an indexed RV-ESV greater than 85 ml/m^2 achieved normalization of RV volumes. Valsangiacoma et al. [28] evaluated 20 children with repaired TOF who underwent pulmonary value replacement with a valved conduit (18 xenografts and two homografts ± RV reduction plasty performed in five patients) for severe PR. Each patient was evaluated with CMRI 5.6 ± 1.8 months before surgery and 5.9 ± 0.6 months after surgery. Thirteen patients were in NYHA functional class I and seven patients were in NYHA functional class II. Pulmonary valve replacement was indicated for severe PR with RV dilatation as defined by CMRI as an indexed RV-EDV greater than 150 ml/m^2 and/or RV-EDV that is twice the LV-EDV, independent of clinical status. Six months post-pulmonary valve replacement, there was a significant reduction in both systolic and diastolic RV volumes in all 20 patients and a statistically significant reduction in RV mass in 19 of 20 patients. In 12 patients with presurgical-indexed RV-EDV, less than 200 ml/m^2 normalization of the indexed RV-EDV to less than 105 ml/m^2 occurred in eight patients (two patients had RV reduction plasty). In the eight patients with indexed RV-EDV greater than 200 ml/m^2 normalization of the indexed RV-EDV occurred in only one patient and this patient had a RV reduction plasty. These data suggest that when the indexed RV-EDV exceeds 170–200 ml/m^2 the likelihood of normalization of RV volumes is more limited. Although both Therrien et al. [27] and Valsangiacoma et al. [28] have identified an upper limit of RV size beyond which complete normalization does not occur, neither study has determined whether partial recovery versus complete normalization is necessary to reverse the detrimental effects of RV enlargement.

32.5 Current Indications for Pulmonary Valve Replacement

The timing of pulmonary valve replacement in patients with repaired TOF still remains controversial. Pulmonary valve replacement has traditionally been performed when symptoms of RV systolic dysfunction are present. However, waiting for symptoms to be present before intervening may result in irreversible RV enlargement and limit the benefits of pulmonary valve replacement. Given the correlation between RV enlargement and poor outcome; and the current data demonstrating the reversible effects of pulmonary valve replacement on RV enlargement, the indication for pulmonary valve replacement should strongly consider the asymptomatic patient with severe PR and significant RV dilatation. The present indications for pulmonary valve replacement are as follows:

1. the symptomatic patient with severe PR and RV dilatation with or without RV dysfunction;
2. the asymptomatic patient with severe PR, RV dilatation (170–200 cc/m^2), and RV systolic dysfunction;
3. the asymptomatic patient with severe PR, ventricular arrhythmias and RV dilatation (170–200 c/m^2) with or without RV dysfunction;
4. the asymptomatic patient with severe PR, worsening exercise capacity, and RV dilatation (170–200 c/m^2) with or without RV dysfunction; and
5. patients with moderate to severe PR undergoing cardiac surgery for other hemodynamically significant lesions.

32.6 Conclusion

In conclusion, the long-term effects of RV enlargement resulting from chronic PR are poor. Although, surgery is effective at eliminating PR and reversing RV enlargement up to a point, repeat surgical interventions with its associated morbidity and mortality is a real limitation. The indications for surgical pulmonary valve replacement are based on the current data that demonstrates a poor long-term prognosis associated with RV enlargement, the reversibility of RV dilatation with pulmonary valve replacement, and more importantly, the evidence that a threshold of RV enlargement exists beyond which normalization of RV size does not occur. Whether complete versus partial normalization of RV size will alter long-term outcome remains to be determined. The availability of a low morbidity/mortality percutaneous intervention may make the application of pulmonary valve replacement more palatable to the clinician who takes care of the patient with significant PR and RV enlargement, but in no way should change the indication to intervene at this point in time.

References

1. Ferencz C, Rubin JD, McCarter RJ et al. congenital Heart Disease: prevalence at livebirth. The Baltimore-Washington Infant Study. Am J Epidemiol. 1985;121:31–36.
2. Grabitz RG, Joffres MR, Collins-Nakai RL. Congenital heart disease: incidnce in the first year of life. The Alberta Heritage Pediatric Cardiology Program. Am J Epidemiol. 1988;128: 381–388.
3. Bertranou EG, Blackstone EH, Hazelrig JB, Turner Jr ME, et al. Life expectancy without surgery in tetralogy of Fallot. Am J Cardiol. 1978;42:458–466.
4. Castaneda AR, Freed MD, Williams RG, Norwood WI. Repair of tetralogy of Fallot in infancy. Early and late results. J Thorac Cardiovasc Surg. 1977;74:372–381.
5. Reddy VM, Liddicoat JR, McElhinney DB, Brook MM, et al. Routine primary repair of tetralogy of Fallot in neonates and infants less than three months of age. Ann Thoracic Surg. 1995;60:S592–596.
6. Karl TR, Sano S, Pornviliwan S, Mee RB. Tetralogy of Fallot: favourable outcome of nonneonatal transatrial, transpulmonary repair. Ann Thorac Surg. 1992;54:903–907.
7. Hirsch JC, Mosca RS, Bove EL. Complete repair of tetralogy of Fallot in the neonate: results in the modern era. Ann Surg 2000; 232: 508–514.
8. Nollert G, Frischlein T, Bouterwek S, et al. Long-term survival in patients with repair of tetralogy of Fallot: 36-year follow-up of 490 survivors of the first year after surgical repair. J Am Coll Cardiol. 1997;30:1374–1383.
9. Gatzoulis MA, Balaji S, Webber SA et al. Risk factors for arrhythmia and sudden death in repaired tetralogy of Fallot: a multi-centre study. Lancet. 2000;356:975–981.
10. Marie PY, Marcon F, Brunotte F et al. Right ventricular overload and induced sustained ventricular tachycardia in operatively 'repaired' tetralogy of Fallot. Am J Cardiol. 1992;69:785–789.
11. Carvalho JS, Shinebourne EA, Busst C et al. Exercise capacity after complete repair of tetralogy of Fallot: deleterious effects of residula pulmonary regurgitation. Br Heart J. 1992;67: 470–473.
12. Wessel HU, Cunningham WJ, Paul MH et al. Exercise performance in tetralogy of Fallot after intracardiac repair. J Thorac Cardiovasc Surg. 1980;80:582–593.
13. Gatzoulis MA, Till JA, Somerville J et al. Mechanoelectrical interaction in tetralogy of Fallot. QRS prolongation relates to right ventricular size and predicts malignant ventricular arrythmias and sudden death. Circulation. 1995;92:231–237.
14. Gatzoulis MA, Till JA, Redington AN. Depolarisation-repolarisation inhomogeneity after repair of tetralogy of Fallot. Circulation. 1997;95:401–404.
15. Harrison DA, Harris L, Siu SC et al. Sustained ventricular tachycardia in adult patients late after repair of tetralogy of Fallot. J Am Coll Cardiol. 1997;30;1368–1373.
16. Niezen RA, Helbing WA, van der Wall EE, van der Geest RJ, et al. Biventricular systolic function and mass studied with MR imaging in children with pulmonary regurgitation after repair for tetralogy of Fallot. Radiology. 1996;201:135–140.
17. Misbach GA, Turley K, Ebert PA. Pulmonary valve replacement for regurgitation after repair of tetralogy of Fallot. Ann Thorac Surg. 1983;36:684–691.
18. Ebert PA. Second operations for Pulmonary stenosis or insufficiency after repair of tetralogy of Fallot. Am J Cardiol. 1982;50:637–640.
19. Eyskens B, Reybrouck T, Bogaert J, et al. Homograft insertion for pulmonary regurgitation after repair of tetralogy of Fallot improves cardiorespiratory exercise performance. Am J Cardiol. 2000;85:221–225.
20. Bove EL, Kavey RE, Byrum CJ, Sondheimer HM, et al. Improved right ventricular function following late pulmonary valve replacement for residual pulmonary insufficiency or stenosis. J Thorac Cardiovasc Surg. 1985;90:50–55.
21. Warner KG, Anderson JE, Fulton DR, Payne DD, et al. Restoration of the pulmonary valve reduces right ventricular volume overload after previous repair of tetralogy of Fallot. Circulation. 1993;88(II):189–197.
22. D'Udekem Y, Rubay J, Shango-Lody P, et al. Late homograft valve insertion after transannular patch repair of tetralogy of Fallot. J Heart Valve Disease. 1998;7:450–454.
23. Discigil B, Dearani JA, Puga FJ, et al. Late pulmonary valve replacement after repair of tetralogy of Fallot. J Thorac Cardiovasc Surg. 2001;121:344–351.
24. Therrien J, Siu SC, McLaughlin PR, Liu PP, et al. Pulmonary valve replacement in adults late after repair of tetralogy of Fallot: are we operating too late? J Am Coll Cardiol. 2000; 36:1670–1675.
25. Vliegen HW, van Straten A, de Ross A, Roest AA, et al. Magnetic resonance imaging to assess the hemodynamic effects of pulmonary valve replacement in adults late after repair of tetralogy of Fallot. Circulation. 2002;106:1703–1707.
26. Wells WJ, Arroyo H Jr, Bremner RM, et al. Homograft conduit failure in infants is not due to somatic outgrowth. J Thorac Cardiovasc Surg. 2002;124(1):88–96.
27. Therrien J, Provost Y, Merchant N, Williams W, Colman J, Webb G. Optimal timing for pulmonary valve replacement in adults after tetralogy of Fallot repair. Am J Cardiol. 2005;95:779–782.
28. Valsangiacomo Buechel ER, Dave HH, Kellenberger CJ, Dodge-Khatami A, et al. Remodeling of the right ventricle after early pulmonary valve replacement in children with repaired tetralogy of Fallot: assessment by cardiovascular magnetic resonance. Eur Heart J. 2005;26:2721–2727.

Nonsurgical Replacement of the Pulmonary Valve

33

Lee Benson, Claudia Almedia, Kjong-Jin Lee, and Rajiv Chaturvedi

33.1 Introduction

Over the last three decades, transcatheter techniques and devices have evolved to allow effective therapies for coronary artery disease, congenital valve, and great artery stenosis, atrial and ventricular septal defects and obstructive hypertrophic cardiomyopathy. Nonsurgical cardiac valve replacement is the latest and most exciting development in the field of interventional cardiology [1–4]. In this regard, while transcatheter treatment of valvular stenosis has been well established [2], approaches to address regurgitation have remained solely surgical. As such, the prospect of a nonsurgical transcatheter technique to address valvular regurgitation holds considerable promise, considering the inherent advantages to patients, enhancing treatment strategies.

The current techniques for percutaneous transcatheter semilunar valve replacement all involve use of a tissue valve prosthesis mounted within a stent (Table 33.1). Anderson [3] was the first to report in 1992 the implantation of a stent-mounted heart valve. This implant was constructed by suturing a porcine aortic valve into a custom-made stainless steel stent. Measuring 12 mm in diameter when crimped onto a delivery balloon, it was expanded to 32 mm in diameter when deployed. Nine such prostheses were implanted in heterotrophic or orthotropic positions in pigs. However, the requirement of 41 French sheath damped enthusiasm for this technology. The peak systolic gradient was 16 mmHg or less and there was trivial regurgitation seen in only two implants. Despite the technical challenges, this work provided the proof of concept that justified ongoing investigation in transcatheter valve implantation therapies.

33.2 Application in Congenital Heart Disorders

In the management of complex congenital heart disease, right ventricular outflow track reconstruction is a significant component of many surgical repairs. However, despite successful surgery, many patients are left with residual lesions. In this regard, pulmonary regurgitation is increasingly recognized as a factor in risk stratification for long-term morbidity and mortality [1, 5, 6]. Indeed, right ventricular outflow track dysfunction forms the primary indication for reoperation in the adult congenital heart disease population, and multiple operations are often frequent [6, 7]. Surgical management of many forms of pulmonary atresia requires the use of a conduit to create continuity between the ventricular mass and the pulmonary circulation. As such, conduit dysfunction represents a unique anatomic situation for the application of existing technologies for valve implantation. Management of obstructive conduit lesions has been accessible with application of interventional catheterization and bare metal stent implantation [8, 9] with good early and midterm relief of obstruction, prolonging conduit life span. This approach is particularly applicable in addressing obstructive lesions which do not involve the conduit valve leaflets.

The implantation of a valve-stent may address both the obstructive and regurgitant components of such conduit dysfunction. The first percutaneous implantation of a cardiac valve-stent in a human was reported by Bonhoeffer and colleagues in 2000 [10], having been preceded by a series of animal studies [11]. The procedure took place in a 12-year-old boy with pulmonary atresia and ventricular septal defect, placed into a right ventricular to pulmonary conduit. After the implant, the systolic pressure gradient across the conduit fell from 50 mmHg to 25 mmHg and Doppler echocardiography demonstrated no significant valve insufficiency. Subsequently, over 160 patients have undergone similar implantations in Europe and Great

L. Benson (✉)
Department of Paediatrics, The Hospital for Sick Children, 555 University Ave., Toronto, Ontario, Canada, M5G1X8
e-mail: benson@sickkids.ca

A.N. Redington et al. (eds.), *Congenital Diseases and the Right Heart*, DOI 10.1007/978-1-84800-378-1_33,
© Springer-Verlag London Limited 2009

Table 33.1 Percutaneous stent-valves for semi-lunar valve replacement

Device	Tissue valve	Stent
Medtronic Melody Transcatheter Pulmonary Valve (Medtronic, Minneapolis MN, USA)	Bovine jugular vein	Platinum–iridium; balloon expandable
Cribier-Edwards Percutaneous Aortic Bioprosthesis (Edwards Lifesciences, Irving, Calif, USA)	Equine pericardial valve	Stainless steel; balloon expandable
Corevalve Percutaneous Revalving System (Corevalve, Irvine, Calif.)	Porcine pericardial valve	Nitinol, self-expanding

Britain with this valve as have 17 children at the Hospital for Sick Children in Toronto.

33.3 The Implant

The pulmonary valve implant (Melody™, Medtronic Inc., Minneapolis, MN), developed by Bonhoeffer and colleagues is a biological valve, harvested from the jugular vein of fresh bovine cadavers and sutured into a preexpanded stent (CP Stent™ NuMED, Hopkinton, NY). Bovine jugular venous valves can have well-formed bicuspid and tricuspid arrangements (Fig. 33.1). Surgical implantation of such valve conduits (Contegra, Medtronic) has been successfully performed in the primary surgical reconstruction of the right ventricular outflow track in congenital heart lesions [12]. The stent is made of platinum–iridium wire welded together with gold (CP Stent™ NuMED). The valve itself is durable and can be expanded and compressed upon itself multiple times, without loss of integrity. The valve-stent assembly is crimped onto a custom-made 20 French delivery system with a balloon-in-balloon (BIB™, NuMED) configuration (Fig. 33.2), available with 18, 20, and 22 mm diameter outer balloons. The

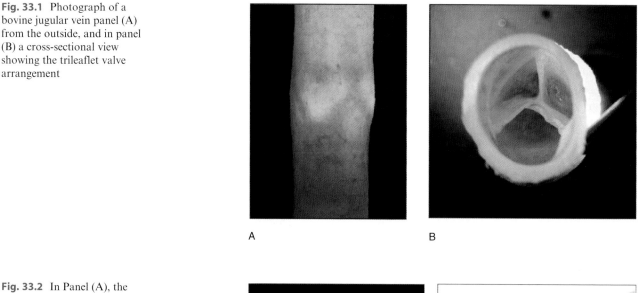

Fig. 33.1 Photograph of a bovine jugular vein panel (A) from the outside, and in panel (B) a cross-sectional view showing the trileaflet valve arrangement

A   B

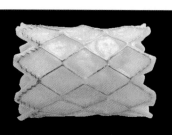 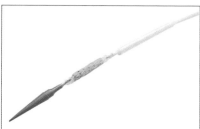

Fig. 33.2 In Panel (A), the expanded stent with the bovine vein graft sewn on the inside. Panel (B), the crimped valve stent on the 20 French balloon-in-balloon delivery system (Ensemble™ Medtronic, Minneapolis MN. USA)

A   B

stent is magnetic resonance imaging compatible, although it will induce an imaging artifact.

33.4 Patient Selection

Presently, patients considered candidates for valve implantation are those who had previously undergone surgery on the right ventricular outflow track for repair of a congenital lesion. It should be noted, however, that optimal timing for such intervention is not well defined and no one investigation gives a reliable guide. Right ventricular dysfunction, tricuspid regurgitation, and worsening symptoms may mark a situation of diminished reversibility and, therefore, are not good indicators for the timing of intervention. Yet, if timed appropriately, valve replacement can improve right ventricular function, control arrhythmias, and improve exercise performance [13, 14]. Symptoms and clinical findings at present, however, should be of a degree that warrant surgical valve replacement [6, 7], although the optimal timing of establishing pulmonary competence before irreversible right ventricular dysfunction has yet to be determined [15]. Conventional practice guidelines presently would include right ventricular hypertension ($> 2/3$ systemic pressure in the clinically symptomatic, or 3/4 systemic pressure in the asymptomatic individual), and in those without outflow tract obstruction: significant pulmonary insufficiency, right ventricular dilation and or failure, the onset of symptoms, effort intolerance, and arrhythmias.

For the valve implant procedure, presently excluded are individuals < 5 years of age or weighing < 20 kg. Other exclusion criteria include pregnancy, occluded central veins, an active infection, outflow tracts of unfavorable morphology (i.e., > 22 mm in diameter) or conduits < 16 mm in diameter at the time of surgical insertion. Additional limitations include outflow tracts of native tissue which may dilate after the prosthetic valve implantation and result in embolization of the implant

and coronary anatomy, which could be compromised by an expanded implant in the right ventricular outflow tract. Conduit calcification is not a counter-indication, indeed, its presence may encourage stability of the potential implant.

33.5 Investigations

All candidates require detailed clinical examination, electrocardiogram, chest radiograph, and echocardiogram including colour and flow Doppler studies. A magnetic resonance imaging scan can be invaluable in assessing the morphology of the right ventricular outflow tract, right ventricular volumes, function, and quantitate pulmonary regurgitation. Cardiopulmonary exercise testing will allow analysis of peak oxygen uptake, anaerobic threshold, and other variables allowing an objective measure of exercise performance and cardiopulmonary reserve.

33.6 The Procedure

The implant procedure is performed under general anesthesia with strict sterile technique. Vascular access for the implantation is generally obtained from the femoral veins (either) but can be achieved as well from the right internal jugular vein. Access from the liver has not been reported. A right heart hemodynamic study is performed and angiography obtained in the right ventricular outflow tract in the $90°$ lateral and $20°$- to $35°$ cranial-$10°$ LAO projections. Technically, a right coronary artery catheter can be used for the hemodynamic study, with its placement into the distal left pulmonary artery. While either branch pulmonary artery can be used, the delivery catheter tends to follow the arc toward the left pulmonary artery and is much more reliable, than if the guide wire is

Fig. 33.3 Panel (A), a lateral angiogram in a right ventricular outflow tract conduit, demonstrating the outflow topology where the valve-stent implant will be implanted. Postimplantation, panel (B) showing the competent valve *in situ*

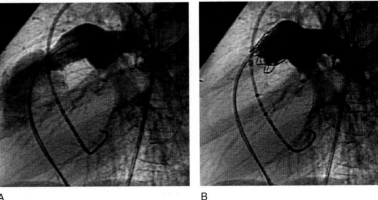

A   B

placed into the right pulmonary artery. An ultra-extra stiff guide wire (Amplatzer-type Ultra Extra Stiff, Cook Inc., Bloomington, IN) is then positioned through the right coronary artery catheter and a MultiTrack™ catheter (6 Fr., NuMED) used for angiography. If the anatomy appears suitable (Fig. 33.3), the device can be crimped onto a delivery system of appropriate balloon diameter and deployed. Prior to crimping the stent-valve onto the balloon system it is washed in a series of saline solutions to remove the gluteraldahyde fixative (generally 5 min in each of three saline solutions). The groin should be pre-dilated with a 22 Fr. dilator before insertion of the delivery system. A bleed-back coaxial sheath which is on the delivery catheter can be used to control groin bleeding around the catheter. After deployment of the stent in the target lesion, high-pressure balloon dilation maybe performed to further seat the stent-valve complex in place (Mullins™ high-pressure balloon, NuMED). If there is any concern about potential coronary artery compression, a coronary angiogram can be performed during balloon dilation of the conduit. All conduits and prosthetic pulmonary valves so implanted should allow at least an 18 mm diameter implant. Prior to stent-valve implantation, a bare metal stent implant can be used to reinforce the conduit if potential sternal compression is a concern (Fig. 33.4). Hemodynamic and angiographic assessment is then repeated after placement. Antibiotics and heparin are administered during the procedure.

33.7 Results

Between January 2000 and September 2004, Khambadkone et al. reported the accumulated experience with the Melody™ Medtronic valve in 59 patients [16]. The median age was 16 years (range 9–43 years) and weight 56 kg (25–110 kg), and mean follow-up 10 months. The majority had a variant of Fallot's tetralogy ($n = 36$), or transposition of the great arteries, ventricular septal defect with pulmonary stenosis ($n = 8$). Acutely, the right ventricular pressure fell (64 ± 17 to 50 ± 14 mm Hg, $p < 0.001$), outflow gradient was reduced (33 ± 24 to 19 ± 15 mm Hg, $p < 0.001$), and pulmonary regurgitation improved (grade 2 or greater before, none greater than grade 2 after, $p < 0.001$) stent-valve implantation. Follow-up magnetic imaging studies documented a significant reduction in regurgitant fraction ($21 \pm 13\%$ versus $3 \pm 4\%$, $p < 0.001$), right ventricular end-diastolic volume (94 ± 28 versus 82 ± 24 ml/beat/m^2, $p < 0.001$), a significant increase in left ventricular end-diastolic volume (64 ± 12 versus 71 ± 13 ml/beat/m^2, $p < 0.005$) and effective right ventricular stroke volume (37 ± 7 versus 42 ± 9 ml/beat/m^2, $p < 0.006$) in 28 patients (age 19 ± 8 years). A further 16 patients had metabolic exercise testing and showed a significant improvement in VO$_2$ max (26 ± 7 versus 29 ± 6 ml/kg/min, $p < 0.001$). There was no mortality, and all patients were discharged the follow morning after the procedure.

The same investigators [17] recently reported additional follow-up studies from 18 individuals (72% male, median age 20 years, from a population of 93 at the time), who had undergone the procedure to relieve right ventricular outflow obstruction, examining the clinical and physiological response to the implantation. All patients had a right ventricular outflow tract gradient of > 50 mm Hg by echocardiography without important pulmonary regurgitation (less than mild) or a regurgitant fraction < 10% on magnetic resonance imaging. Cardiopulmonary exercise testing, tissue Doppler echocardiography, and magnetic resonance imaging were performed before and within 50 days of the stent-valve implant. The procedure reduced the outflow gradient (from 51 to 22 mm Hg, p < 0.001) and right ventricular systolic pressure (from 73 to 47 mm Hg, p < 0.001) at catheterization. Symptoms and aerobic (from

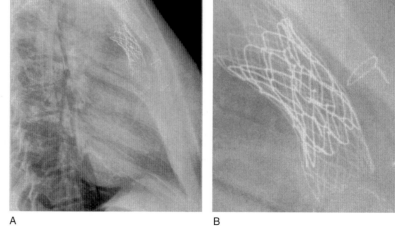

Fig. 33.4 (A) lateral chest radiograph showing an implanted valve-stent. In this child, the conduit was anterior, and parallels the sternum. Panel (B) is a magnified view of the implant, not an additional bare metal stent previously inserted to further strengthen the conduit in an attempt to avoid compression

A   B

25.7 to 28.9 ml/kg/min, $p < 0.002$) and anaerobic (from 14.4 to 16.2 ml/kg/m^2, $p < 0.002$) exercise performance improved. Myocardial systolic velocity improved acutely (tricuspid from 4.8 to 5.3 cm/s, $p < 0.05$; mitral from 4.7 to 5.5 cm/s, $p < 0.01$), whereas isovolumetric acceleration was unchanged. Right ventricular end-diastolic volume (100–90 ml/m^2, $p < 0.001$) fell, whereas effective stroke volume (44–48 ml/m^2, $p < 0.06$) and ejection fraction (48–57%, $p < 0.01$) increased. Left ventricular end-diastolic volume (72–77 ml/m^2, $p < 0.145$), stroke volume (45–51 ml/m^2, $p < 0.02$), and ejection fraction (63–66%, $p < 0.03$) increased. As such, stent-valve replacement relieves outflow tract obstruction, and leads to an early improvement in biventricular performance, reduces symptoms, and improves exercise tolerance.

At the Hospital for Sick Children, Toronto, the Melody™ valve was implanted in 17 patients, eight females, 15.8 ± 2.4 years old (range 13–21 years) and 56.3 ± 8.2 kg (range 42.2–72.3 kg), 5–17 years after surgical right ventricular outflow tract reconstruction between October 2005 and May 2006. Fallot's tetralogy, pulmonary atresia with ventricular septal defect, persistent truncus arteriosus, and Taussig–Bing malformation constituted the underlying cardiac defects. Prior to the procedure, the patients underwent an echocardiogram, heart magnetic resonance scan ($n = 13$), and exercise test ($n = 11$). After the procedure they were seen at 1, 3, and 6 months, with an echocardiogram, electrocardiogram, and chest X-ray. Exercise testing was performed at 3 months and cardiac magnetic resonance scanning repeated at 6 months.

All patients were discharged the day following the procedure. No complications, such as stent dislodgment or fracture, stroke, valve malfunction, or urgent surgery occurred in the 6-month follow-up period. The right ventricular systolic pressure fell from 65 ± 19 to 46 ± 11 mm Hg ($p = 0.01$) right ventricular to aortic pressure ratio fell from 0.75 ± 0.2 to 0.47 ± 0.1 ($p < 0.0005$) right ventricular to pulmonary artery peak pressure gradient fell from 35 ± 20 to 13 ± 8 mm Hg ($p < 0.004$), and pulmonary regurgitation score fell from 3 ± 0.3 to 0.75 ± 0.5 (n = 12, $p < 0.0001$) 1 day after implant. Exercise testing VO$_2$ max (23.95 ± 4.1 to 25.1 ± 3.96 ml/kg/min ($p < 0.35$)) increased significantly, while pre- and postprocedural cardiac output measurements did not change significantly.

33.8 Future Applications and Research.

Clearly, the present implant has a limited application, confined to those patients with a right ventricle to pulmonary artery homograft conduit or heterograft implant. The largest population where pulmonary valve implantations are frequent and presently entirely surgical consists of those patients after Fallot's tetralogy repair [6, 7, 15]. Such patients have patulous outflow tract such that a 22-mm stent-graft would not be secure. A variety of approaches have been considered to address this population. Boudjemline and colleagues recently investigated in an animal model [18], the feasibility of an off-pump hybrid approach in eight ewes were a left thoracotomy was first performed, and the main pulmonary artery was banded by using two radiopaque rings with a diameter of 18 mm. Percutaneous implantation of a valve-stent or through a transventricular approach was performed. The banding allowed the pulmonary diameter to be reduced from 30 to 17 mm and subsequent pulmonary valve replacement through a percutaneous or a transventricular approach was possible without the requirement of extracorporeal circulatory support. This work is intriguing and may lead to strategies where an off-pump

Fig. 33.5 An infundibular reducer design panel (A), constructed to secure the smaller valve-stent a dilated right ventricular outflow tract. Panel (B): a lateral angiogram from an animal study with the reducer in place and valve-stent inserted

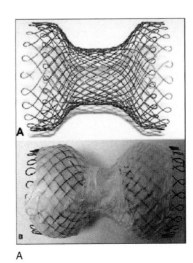

A

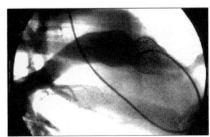

B

main pulmonary artery banding is performed through a limited thoracotomy and the valve-stent implanted through a perventricular right ventricular incision, on a beating heart. Additional work is being done on the design of an infundibular reducer. This percutaneous implant would function as a docking station for the existing valve [19] (Fig. 33.5).

33.9 Summary

While the implant procedure can be technically challenging, due to the morphology of the right ventricular outflow tract, successful implantation rate is high. Valve-stent function appears stable with little pulmonary insufficiency in follow-up. The limitation of this particular implant is the interplay between the 22 mm diameter stent and the conduit. Residual stenosis is frequent, although generally mild to moderate and well tolerated with reverse remodeling of the right ventricle. Future advances to address the patient with a large outflow tract are now being investigated. The technology will have an important impact on a number of treatment algorithms for the patient with congenital heart disease.

References

1. Lutter G, Ardehali R, Cremer J, Bonhoeffer P. Percutaneous valve replacement: current state and future prospects. Ann Thorac Surg. 2004;78(6):2199–206.
2. Hornung TS, Benson LN, McLaughlin PR. Catheter interventions in adult patients with congenital heart disease. Curr Cardiol Rep. 2002;4:54–62.
3. Anderson HR, Knudsen LL, Hasenkam JM. Transluminal implantation of artificial heart valves. Description of a new expandable aortic valve and initial results with implantation by catheter technique in closed chest pigs. Eur Heart J. 1992; 13:704–8.
4. Khambadkone S, Bonhoeffer P. Nonsurgical pulmonary valve replacement: why, when, and how. Catheter Cardiovasc Interv. 2004;62(3):401–8.
5. Bouzas B, Kilner PJ, Gatzoulis MA. Pulmonary regurgitation: not a benign lesion. Eur Heart J. 2005;26:433–9.
6. Karamlou T, McCrindle BW, Williams WG. Surgery insight: late complications following repair of tetralogy of Fallot and related surgical strategies for management. Nat Clin Pract Cardiovasc Med. 2006;3:611–22.
7. Cesnjevar R, Harig F, Raber A, Strecker T, Fischlein T, Koch A, Weyand M, Pfeiffer S. Late pulmonary valve replacement after correction of Fallot's tetralogy. Thorac Cardiovasc Surg. 2004;52:23–8.
8. Sugiyama H, Williams W, Benson LN. Implantation of endovascular stents for the obstructive right ventricular outflow tract. Heart. 2005;91:1058–63.
9. Peng LF, McElhinney DB, Nugent AW, Powell AJ, Marshall AC, Bache EA, Lock JE. Endovascular stenting of obstructed right ventricle-to-pulmonary artery conduits: a 15-year experience. Circulation. 2006 Jun 6;113(22): 2598–605.
10. Bonhoeffer P, Boudjemline Y, Saliva Z, Merck J, Aground Y, Bonnet D, Acer P, Le Bides J, Side D, Kitchener J. Percutaneous replacement of pulmonary valve in a right-ventricle to pulmonary-artery prosthetic conduit with valve dysfunction. Lancet. 2000;356:1403–1405.
11. Bonhoeffer P, Boudjemline Y, Saliva Z, House AO, Aground Y, Bonnet D, Side D, Kitchener J. Transcatheter implantation of a bovine valve in pulmonary position: a lamb study. Circulation. 2000;102:813–816.
12. Rastan AJ, Walther T, Daehnert I, Hambsch J, Mohr FW, Janousek J, Kostelka M. Bovine jugular vein conduit for right ventricular outflow tract reconstruction: evaluation of risk factors for mid-term outcome. Ann Thorac Surg. 2006;82:1308–15.
13. Terrine J, Provost Y, Merchant N, Williams W, Colman J, Webb G. Optimal timing for pulmonary valve replacement in adults after tetralogy of Fallot repair. Am J Cardiol. 2005; 95:779–82.
14. Eyskens B, Redbrick T, Bogart J, Dymarkowsky S, Daenen W, Dumoulin M, Gewillig M. Homograft insertion for pulmonary regurgitation after repair of tetralogy of fallot improves cardiorespiratory exercise performance. Am J Cardiol. 2000;85: 221–5.
15. Cheung MM, Konstantinov IE, Redington AN. Late complications of repair of tetralogy of Fallot and indications for pulmonary valve replacement. Semin Thorac Cardiovasc Surg. 2005;17(2):155–9.
16. Khambadkone S, Coats L, Taylor A, Boudjemline Y, Derrick G, Tsang V, Cooper J, Muthurangu V, Hegde SR, Razavi RS, Pellerin D, Deanfield J, Bonhoeffer P. Percutaneous pulmonary valve implantation in humans: results in 59 consecutive patients. Circulation. 2005;112:1189–97.
17. Coats L, Khambadkone S, Derrick G, Sridharan S, Schievano S, Mist B, Jones R, Deanfield JE, Pellerin D, Bonhoeffer P, Taylor AM. Physiological and clinical consequences of relief of right ventricular outflow tract obstruction late after repair of congenital heart defects. Circulation. 2006;113:2037–44.
18. Boudjemline Y, Schievano S, Bonnet C, Coats L, Agnoletti G, Khambadkone S, Bonnet D, Deanfield J, Sidi D, Bonhoeffer P. Off-pump replacement of the pulmonary valve in large right ventricular outflow tracts: a hybrid approach. J Thorac Cardiovasc Surg. 2005;129:831–7.
19. Boudjemline Y, Agnoletti G, Bonnet D, Sidi D, Bonhoeffer P. Percutaneous pulmonary valve replacement in a large right ventricular outflow tract: an experimental study. J Am Coll Cardiol. 2004;43:1082–7.

Section 8
Ebsteins Anomaly

34.1 Introduction

Ebstein's malformation is a rare disease, with a prevalence of 114 per million live birth [1]. The index case was described by Willem Ebstein, who was born in Jauer, Austria, in 1836. He was educated in Berlin and Breslau, and became a professor of medicine at the University of Göttingen in 1874, dying there in 1912 [2]. He was the author of over 300 papers before the era of *publish or perish*. Among his most noted works was a section on renal disease in the book *Senile Diseases*, a standard medical text, published with Gustav Albert Schwalbe. Other eponymous diseases or syndromes attributed to him include the Pell–Ebstein phenomenon, an afternoon pyrexia associated with lymphomas, described in 1887, and Ebstein nephropathy, a hyaline degeneration and necrosis of the epithelial cells of the renal tubules, sometimes seen in diabetes mellitus. In 1892, he published the article 'Diagnosis of incipient pericardial effusions'.

During the course of Ebstein's tenure in Göttingen, an 18-year-old laborer, Joseph Prescher, presenting with fatigue, cyanosis, and arrhythmia, died during the course of his admission to hospital [3], Ebstein, himself a pathologist, studying under Virchow, performed the autopsy. He commissioned an etcher to make copies of the specimen, and described and illustrated the tricuspid valvar disorder disease that now bears his name. The plates are exquisite in their detail and accuracy.

The first accounts of Ebstein's malformation based on echocardiographic examination describe the large sail-like antero-superior leaflet, and late systolic prolapse of the valve. Using cross-sectional echocardiography from the apical four-chamber plane view, valvar displacement is clearly displayed [4, 5] (Fig. 34.1). The echocardiographic literature has largely focused on displacement of the septal leaflet of the tricuspid valve as an index of morphological severity, stating that the essence of the disease lies in apical displacement of the septal leaflet at its junction with the inferior or mural leaflet exceeding 20 or 8 mm/m^2 in adults [6–10].

The prerequisites for understanding Ebstein's malformation by echocardiography are appreciation of embryological and fetal development and pathology. Elsewhere in this book, there is consideration given to the fetal presentation of patients with Ebstein's malformation, but several points are immediately necessary for understanding the morphological features. First, malformation of the tricuspid valve is related to the delamination of the valve from the underlying myocardium. If this delamination is incomplete, the malformation is expressed to a variable degree along the tricuspid annulus, varying from complete delamination in the normal heart, to a spectrum of lack of delamination in Ebstein's malformation (Fig. 34.2).

It is important to note that the same process occurs throughout the fetal myocardium. Another expression of this phenomenon may well be persistence of the fetal spongy myocardium represented by noncompaction, now called hypertrabeculation syndrome. In Ebstein's malformation, this disorder occurs in up to one-fifth of patients (Fig. 34.3).

The other important aspect to understanding the development of Ebstein's malformation is the peculiar nature of the fetal physiology [11, 12]. The particular pathophysiology is created by ineffective forward flow across the pulmonary valve caused by the combination of tricuspid regurgitation in the presence of systemic pressure, and systemic arterial pressure applied to the pulmonary valve through the arterial duct. Because form, or morphology, follows function, or flow and pressure in the developing heart, in Ebstein's malformation pathological specimens exhibit these progressive changes in the developing heart [11, 12] (Fig. 34.4). As a consequence of tricuspid

N.H. Silverman (✉)
Professor of Pediatrics, Division of Pediatric Cardiology, The Roma and Marvin Auerback Scholar in Pediatric Cardiology, Director, Pediatric and Echocardiography Laboratory, Lucile Packard Children's Hospital, Stanford University Medical Center, 750 Welch Road – Suite 305, Palo Alto, California 94304
e-mail: norm.silverman@stanford.edu

A.N. Redington et al. (eds.), *Congenital Diseases in the Right Heart*, DOI 10.1007/978-1-84800-378-1_34,
© Springer-Verlag London Limited 2009

(a)   (b)

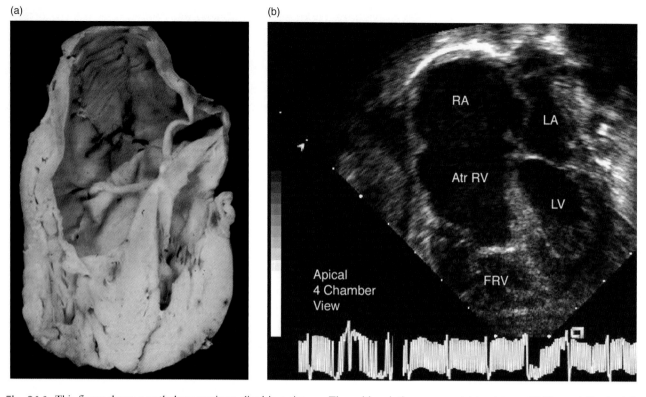

Fig. 34.1 This figure shows a pathology specimen sliced in a simulated apical four-chamber view (courtesy of Robert Anderson), and the corresponding echocardiographic apical four-chamber view, showing the four chambers of the heart in a patient with Ebstein's malformation

The abbreviations are: right atrium (RA), atrialized right ventricle (Atr RV), and functional right ventricle (FRV). The left-sided chambers, left atrium (LA) and left ventricle (LV) are also labeled

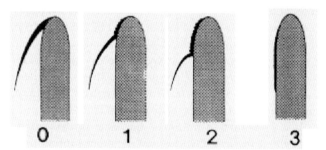

Fig. 34.2 This figure is a diagrammatic representation of the septal leaflet of the tricuspid valve in the normal individual 0, and various degrees of nondelamination in Ebstein's malformation – mild, moderate, and complete, in examples 1, 2, and 3, respectively

thus creating stenosis, or even atresia. As a consequence, the pulmonary annulus does not enlarge, causing an intrinsic lack of valvar, infundibular, and annular development. As fetal blood pressure increases over gestation, wear and tear on the tricuspid valve increases, causing more significant leakage. The right atrium dilates in response to regurgitation and elevated pressure, and may even become thin when overcome by the regurgitant load. Right-to-left shunting at atrial level increases through the oval foramen. The fetus does not accommodate well to the presence of elevated venous pressure. Lymphatic flow is high and the intravascular onchotic pressure from low fetal albumin conspires to produce fetal hydrops, which is a common presentation of this malformation during fetal life.

34.2 Pathology and Findings in Ebstein's Malformation

As an aid to memory, Ebstein's malformation can be encapsulated as consisting of a Dozen D's (Table 34.1). Although some views are intrinsically more valuable in the delineation of Ebstein's malformation, a complete echocardiographic evaluation needs to be performed to

insufficiency, ventricular contraction is associated with ineffective forward flow across the pulmonary valve. As fetal blood pressure rises, the degree of tricuspid regurgitation increases, and the annulus of the tricuspid valve dilates. This prevents coaptation of the valvar leaflets, in turn worsening valvar leakage. An increasing percentage of ductal flow supplies the flow of blood to the lungs while the valvar leaflets are held in the closed position. The pulmonary valve is held in the closed position allowing synecia to develop between the pulmonary valvar leaflets,

(a)   (b)

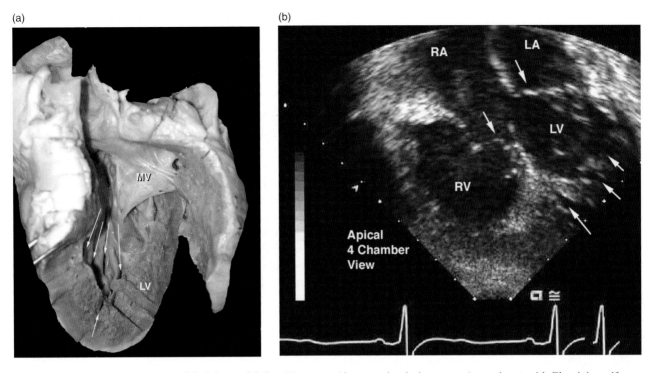

Fig. 34.3 (A) is a view of an explant of the left ventricle in a 50-year-old woman with Ebstein's malformation who also had noncompaction of the right ventricle, a condition perpetuated in her offspring. (B) is an apical four-chamber view from another patient showing clear evidence of tricuspid displacement from the mitral valve (downward pointing arrows), consistent with Ebstein's malformation. The upward-pointing arrows within the left ventricle (LV) demonstrate the well-marked crypts that are characteristic of the condition of noncompaction. Abbreviations: right atrium (RA), left atrium (LA), right ventricle (RV)

(a)   (b)

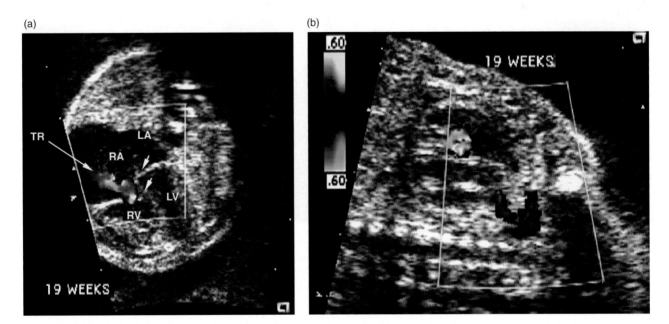

Fig. 34.4 These are two examples taken from a fetus with Ebstein's malformation at 19 weeks gestation. (A) is an apical four-chamber equivalent view showing the four chambers of the heart. Right atrium (RA), right ventricle (RV), left atrium (LA), left ventricle (LV), and the displacement between the septal leaflet of tricuspid and the mitral attachment to the central fibrous body (arrows). A jet of tricuspid regurgitation (TR arrow) is also identified in this early systolic frame. (B) demonstrates the ductus left-to-right shunt (red flow) from the descending aorta (blue flow). The tricuspid regurgitation (TR) is clearly identified proximal to the tricuspid orifice

Table 34.1 The Dozen 'D's'

- • **Displacement of the proximal attachment**
- • **Dysplasia of the valvar leaflets**
- • **Distal abnormalities of attachment**
- • **Dysplasia of the underlying myocardium**
- • **Doppler evidence of tricuspid regurgitation**
- • **Dysrhythmias**
- • **Dilation of the right heart chambers**
- • **Diastolic dysfunctional abnormalities**
- • **Ductal problems**
- • **Deformity of the right ventricular outflow and pulmonary valve**
- • **Defects, other**
- • **Death**

display completely its various features and associated lesions. In older patients, it may be necessary to perform transesophageal echocardiography for appropriate definition.

- • **Displacement of the Proximal Valvar Attachments**

The essence of the malformation is a rotational displacement of the atrioventricular junction so that the inlet of the right ventricle becomes *atrialized*. Displacement

occurs in a spiral. The antero-superior leaflet of the malformed valve is normally attached, and maximal displacement occurs at the junction of the mural and septal leaflets [4] (Fig. 34.5).

- • **Dysplasia of the Valve**

The valvar leaflets are usually dysplastic, being particularly malformed in areas where the tendinous cords are matted together in sheets of valvar tissue. The leaflets themselves may be so malformed that they are hardly recognized as separate from the myocardium, and muscularization of the leaflet is also common. The valvar leaflets may also be thickened, and show verrucous excrescences (Fig. 34.6). Because the septal and mural leaflets do not delaminate from the underlying myocardium, echocardiography becomes a popular means of making a diagnosis.

34.3 Echocardiographic Features

The malformation was first described in a paper using apex echocardiography (Fig. 34.7).

(a)   (b)

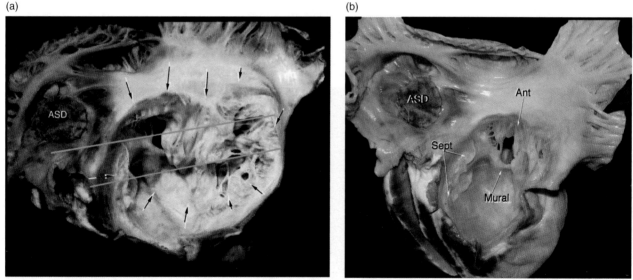

Fig. 34.5 This figure demonstrates two views displaying the tricuspid orifice in an 11-year-old patient with Ebstein's malformation who died subsequently. The atrial septal defect (ASD) was closed, and the tricuspid valve was not repaired. The patient died after the procedure had been completed

In (A) two lines in green are drawn representing the interrogation planes, simulating those found in an apical four-chamber view. The arrows indicate the attachment of the tricuspid valve to the myocardium. Displacement of the mural and septal leaflets is apparent. If the plane had passed anteriorly, no displacement of the septal leaflet would be defined, although displacement is the most severe in the more posterior plane, at the junction between

the septal and mural leaflet (arrow). The septal leaflet moves in an inferior plane, and to define the extent of the displacement the plane must pass through the plane exhibiting the junction of the posterior leaflet. (B) is a more vertical orientation in the same pathology specimen, showing the anterior leaflet with its abnormal caudal and distal attachments, and the septal and the mural leaflet of the tricuspid valve that is completely plastered against the underlying ventricular septum. The spiral displacement of the septal and mural leaflets is well identified. This inlet view defines the difference between the atrialized right ventricle (RV) seen in this example and the functional right ventricle (FVR) observed in later pathological figures

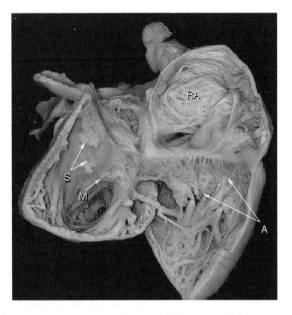

Fig. 34.6 This is an autopsy specimen from a neonate with Ebstein's malformation who succumbed because of his associated valvar pulmonary atresia. (See later figures)
The heart has been opened from the posterior aspect and shows the atrial and ventricular septum with the anterior surface of the heart flapped open in clamshell fashion. The right atrium (RA) is markedly dilated and thinned. The prominent Eustachian and Thebesian valves can be identified within the right atrium. The anterior leaflet

(a)   (b)

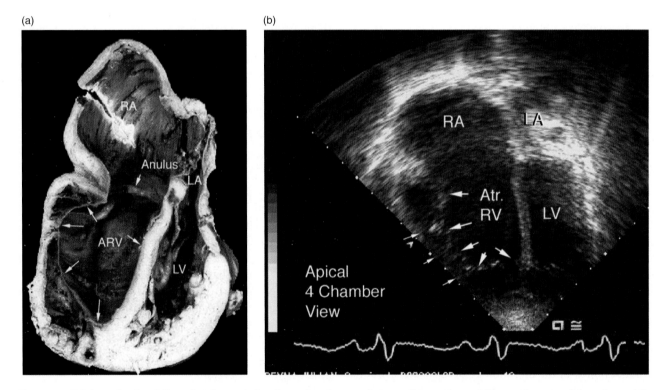

Fig. 34.7 (A) is a simulated four-chamber cut showing a heart reconstituted from standard pathological sectioning. The annulus area of the tricuspid valve is identified, whereas the tricuspid anterior leaflet is clearly applied to the wall of the right ventricle (RV) (arrows) by fine tendinous cords (Arrows), and the septal leaflet is displaced medially on the septum. When viewed from the front this heart shows no visible mural leaflet because of its displacement. The area between the annulus and the annular area of the valve and the inlet portion of this atrioventricular valve defines atrialized right ventricle (ARV) Abbreviations: left atrium (LA) left ventricle (LV) right atrium (RA). (B) is a simulated four-chamber echocardiogram demonstrating the same echocardiographic anatomy as that defined, and demonstrating the cordal attachment to the right ventricular parietal free wall

Ports and colleagues [5] expanded the echocardiographic description, defining an index of displacement as the ratio between the attachment of the mitral valvar leaflet to the septum, and the septal tricuspid leaflet to the apex. As the normal heart has offsetting between these two leaflets, only a ratio of greater than 1.5 to 1 is considered diagnostic of Ebstein's malformation. Recently, measurement of the displacement itself has been performed, and has been shown to be diagnostic if the index is greater than 8 mm/m^2 of body surface area [6, 8, 9]. The potential problem with this measurement is its variability, as it depends on the four-chamber plane. Inspection of Fig. 34.5 will show variable displacement of the septal leaflet of the tricuspid valve as it moves downward from an anterior–superior attachment to a posterior–inferior one. Thus, unless it is possible to define the most postero-inferior attachment, a random four-chamber plane may not define that point accurately. In moderate and severe examples of the malformation, this is not a problem. In patients with milder degrees of malformation, however, the lesion may be missed if the scan plane cuts only through the anterior aspect of the valve. The four-chamber view remains a bastion in the diagnosis of this disorder, and with appropriate postero-inferior angulation, the plane can define a spectrum of severity of displacement from mild to severe (Fig. 34.8).

The apical view is also used to define the severity of the malformation and prognosis of its repair. Initially, Roberson and colleagues [13] described the indexed area of the right atrium and the atrialized portion of the right ventricle in relation to the rest of the heart in the four-chamber view (Fig. 34.9). An index of greater than one to one in fetal life was associated with an adverse outcome. Current reports continue to endorse the value of this index [14, 15]. The four-chamber view is also used to define the attachment of the tendinous chords to the ventricular free wall, providing the surgeon information about the possibility of mobilizing these structures for repair [16–23].

A more definitive evaluation of Ebstein's malformation can be achieved by subcostal imaging in the coronal and subcostal views, as these views provide superior evaluation of displacement of the valve. Subcostal coronal and sagittal imaging also allows appreciation of the mural leaflet, the orientation of the valve, and the relative sizing of the functional right ventricle, the volume of which can be calculated by using Simpson's rule. The view provides an excellent assessment of the morphology of the leaflets, and the degree of their coaptation, as well as the underlying cordal attachments to the myocardium. Images from this projection fit well with the surgical description of the severity of the valvar deformity (Fig. 34.10). From this view, it is possible to show that the essence of the malformation is rotational displacement of the hinge lines of the leaflets so

that part of the right ventricle becomes atrialized. As already discussed, the displacement occurs in spiral fashion, so that the anterosuperior leaflet retains its annular attachments, with maximal displacement occurring at the junction of the mural and septal leaflets on the diaphragmatic surface of the right ventricle. This rotation has the effect of directing tricuspid regurgitation toward the diaphragm, and is well seen from this view [22, 23] (Fig. 34.11). The displacement between the Eustachian valve and the attachment of the mural leaflet to the right ventricle defines more clearly the maximal displacement of the leaflets than does the four-chamber view. In addition, the tricuspid jet is directed toward the diaphragm and the transducer, permitting accurate assessment of the severity of tricuspid regurgitation. Severity of tricuspid regurgitation is one of the most important indicators of the severity of the condition (Fig. 34.12).

- **Distal Abnormalities of Attachment**

The distal attachments of the leaflets, and their pliability, are important factors underlying surgical decisions about how to mobilize the antero-superior leaflet. This leaflet may have a normal distal attachment, be completely adherent to an apical myocardial shelf or be attached via hyphenated cordal attachments. While it may be difficult to appreciate the distal attachments in a severely deformed valve, a multiplanar approach simplifies the situation. As the anterosuperior leaflets, and their attachments to the right ventricular myocardium, are particularly well seen in the parasternal short-axis view, this view is particularly helpful [24] (Fig. 34.13).

- **Dysplasia of the Underlying Myocardium**

Histologists have a specific definition for dysplasia. Dysplasia of the myocardium refers to abnormal muscularity of the right-sided atrium and ventricle, and has been well described. Abnormal ventriculo–ventricular interaction occurs. Thinning of the upper segment of the myocardium in the region of the ventricular septum is frequently noted, which may affect this interaction. In the right ventricle the apical myocardium is often abnormally trabeculated. With regard to the myocardium, the atrial muscle is also abnormal, and the atrial and ventricular response to the regurgitant load is often different from that observed in acquired tricuspid regurgitation, because it begins early in fetal life and is at systemic levels of pressure for the developing fetus (Fig. 34.14).

Dysplasia of the myocardium may relate to the abnormal forces exerted on the right heart in fetal life where the apical trabeculations and papillary muscle architecture are commonly observed, or it may be a fundamental problem of the right ventricle, and be related to the newly discovered association of ventricular noncompaction now found to occur in

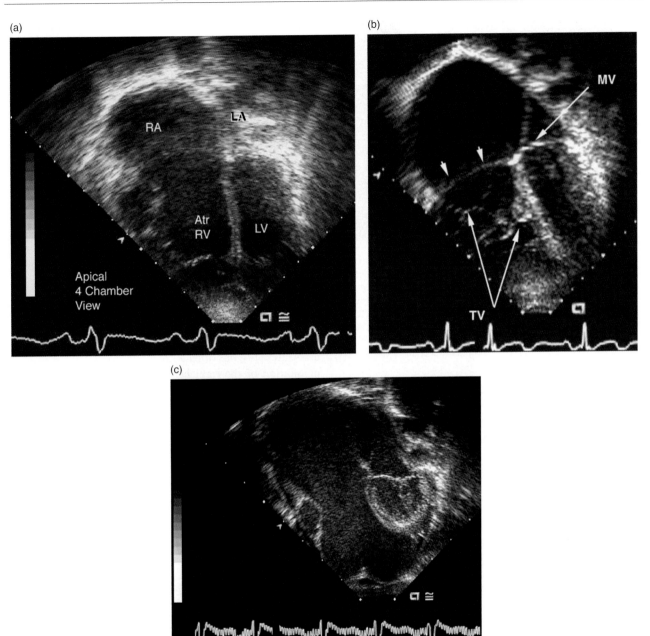

Fig. 34.8 These are three examples showing progressive displacement of the tension apparatus from mild (A) to moderate (B) and severe (C)
The labels indicate (A) the position of the tricuspid annulus opposite the mitral valvar annulus (MV). The tricuspid valve (TV) anterior leaflet and septal leaflet (arrows) can be identified. The middle panel shows a moderate degree of this malformation. The atrialized right ventricle (Atr RV), left atrium (LA), left ventricle (LV), and right atrium (RA) are defined. In the bottom frame the most severe expression shows almost no evidence of tricuspid valve except for a dimple at the apex and the valve surrounding a normally sized left ventricle

about one-fifth of patients with Ebstein's malformation [10, 25–27]. Fibrous replacement of the myocardium has also been described [28].

- **Doppler Evidence of Tricuspid Regurgitation**

The degree of tricuspid regurgitation is an important feature that determines the severity of the disorder.

Although a correlation between the morphologic and functional components often exists, a disparity sometimes occurs when tricuspid valvar regurgitation is less severe than its morphological expression. One of the unique features of tricuspid regurgitation is the direction of the tricuspid jet, which relates to the spiral displacement of the tricuspid valve. Because the valvar plane is rotated

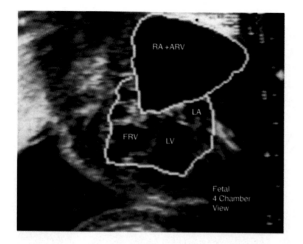

Fig. 34.9 This is a tracing of a 20-week fetus with Ebstein's malformation from the paper of Roberson et al. [13] showing the technique used for measuring the area of the right atrium and atrialized right ventricle, and comparing it to the area seen in the other chambers
In this frame the area right atrium + atrialized right ventricle (RA + Atr R V) is approximately equal to the combined areas of the left atrium (LA), left ventricle (LV), and functional right ventricle (FRV). This index was expanded into four phases by Celermajer and colleagues [14]

anteriorly and superiorly, as seen both pathologically and echocardiographically as noted above, the jet is directed inferiorly and posteriorly. The inferior direction of the jet is not appreciated from the apical or four-chamber views,

but is clearly seen in the subcostal coronal and sagittal views (Fig. 34.15). From this subcostal position of the transducer, Doppler interrogation of the regurgitant jet shows its velocity above the baseline, indicating its diaphragmatic direction. Schreiber and colleagues [23] showed a progressive inferior angulation with increasing degrees of morphological severity, and the direction of the jet appears to correlate, more or less, to this morphological observation, with the more severe degrees of being more vertically oriented (Fig. 34.16).

- **Dysrhythmias**

Arrhythmias are beyond the scope of this presentation. They are related to bypass tracts or result from atrial enlargement and affect cardiac performance.

- **Dilation of the Right Heart Chambers**

Dilation of the right heart chambers, particularly, the right atrium, is a cardinal finding. Indeed, the work of Roberson and colleagues [13], and later Celermajer and associates [14], has done a great deal to define the severity of dilation of the right heart. These data, as well as that from more recent series, suggest that, when the area of the right atrium and atrialized right ventricle exceeds that of the rest of the heart, the prognosis for survival becomes limited [15]. As a consequence of valvar displacement, the

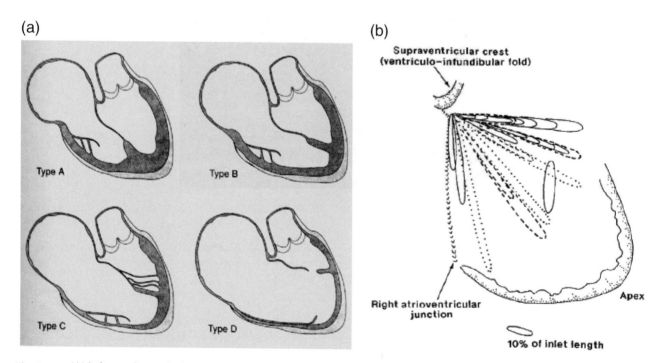

Fig. 34.10 (A) is from reference [16], and the (B) is of the tricuspid valve displacement as described by Schreiber and colleagues [23], and published with permission of the Journal of Thoracic and Cardiovascular Surgery
The panels in (A) are, as described by Chauvaud et al., the varying

degrees of tricuspid pathology displacement and dysplasia of the valve from type A through Type D as can be seen from a subcostal coronal view. In addition, the panels in (B) describe the plane of the valve, the degree of the annulus and the planes of attachment of this valve in a series of patients with Ebstein's malformation.

(a)

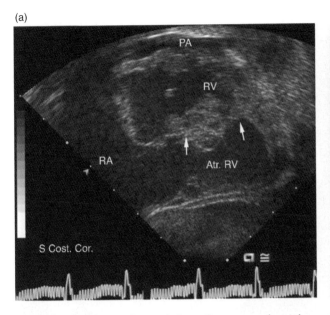

(b)

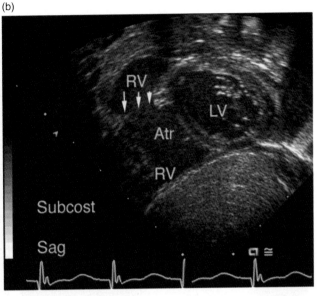

Fig. 34.11 These two orthogonal planes frames are subcostal coronal views, (S Cost Cor) and subcostal sagittal (Subcost Sag) views In (A) the plane of attachment of the valve identifies the area of the atrialized right ventricle. The atrialized right ventricle (Atr RV) is identified proximal to the annulus. The atrium is enlarged; the pulmonary artery (PA) is diminutive, as is the functional right ventricle (RV) proximally. In a corresponding sagittal plane (B), the area of the left ventricle (LV) atrialized right ventricle (Atr RV) and functional right ventricle (RV) can be identified. The arrows mark the plane of attachment of the valve.

(a)

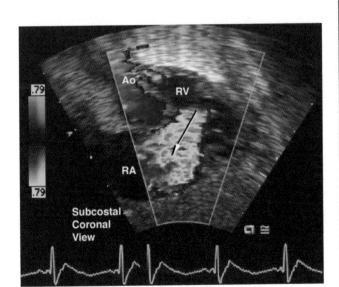

(b)

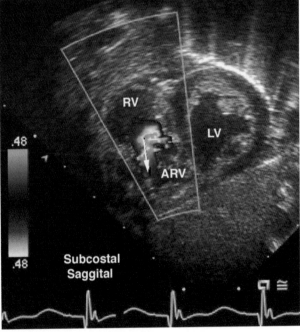

Fig. 34.12 This figure shows a subcostal coronal view (A) and subcostal sagittal view (B) in the same patient with Ebstein's malformation to define the direction of the jet (arrows)
In the left-hand panel the aorta (Ao), the functional right ventricle (RV), and right atrium (RA) are identified. The arrow indicates the direction of the tricuspid regurgitant jet toward the liver. In the right-hand panel the left ventricle (LV), atrialized right ventricle (ARV), and functional right ventricle (RV) are identified. The arrow indicates the inferior position and direction of this jet in the orthogonal plane

(a)   (b)

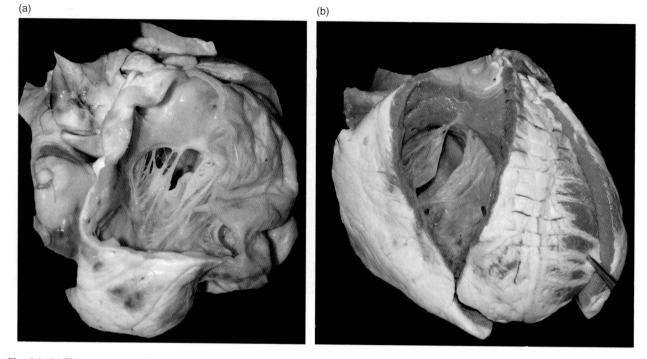

Fig. 34.13 These are two pathologic specimens of Ebstein's malformation viewed from the outlet aspect of the right ventricle showing different forms of attachment of the anterior leaflet of the tricuspid valve to the underlying ventricular septum
(A) shows an example of a hyphenated attachment with few discreet and abnormal septal chords attached to the underlying myocardium. This is the same specimen shown in Fig. 34.6. (B) shows discreet linear attachment of the entire valvar apparatus with the so-called keyhole orifice, identified in that specimen

(a)   (b)

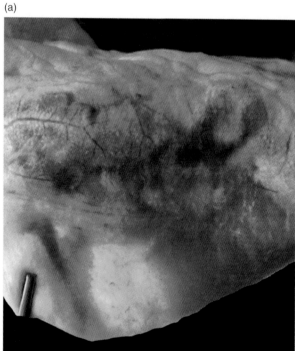

Fig. 34.14 Frame (A) is a pathological specimen illuminated with back lighting to identify the extensive thinning and fibrous tissue replacement of the free wall of the right ventricle as observed from the outside of the heart. (B) is an echocardiographic view demonstrating a fibrous replacement within the upper atrialized right ventricle, causing bulging of the ventricular septum within the left ventricular outflow tract in the subcostal coronal view
Abbreviations: aorta (Ao), right atrium (RA), left ventricle (LV), right ventricle (RV)

(a)

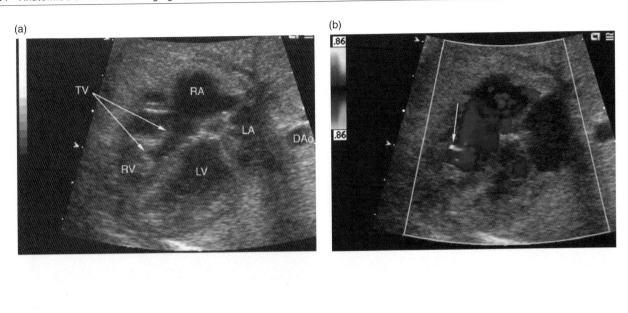

(b)

(c)

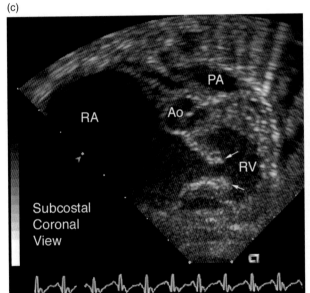

(d)

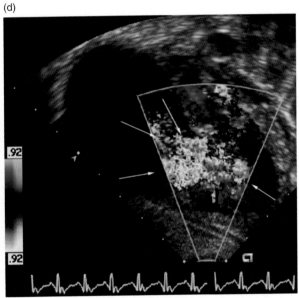

Fig. 34.15 A is an apical four-chamber view of a 30-week fetus with Ebstein's malformation
A(i) shows the typical, A(ii) shows the superimposed Doppler color flow information. The yellow jet (arrow) is the only tricuspid regurgitation noted. This mild regurgitation remained after birth, the fetus had an uneventful neonatal course and was discharged within days of birth.

B is a demonstration in the subcostal coronal view of severe tricuspid regurgitation in a neonate with Ebstein's malformation who failed to survive surgical repair. The valve fails to coapt in systole as judged from the electrocardiographic reference. The tricuspid, anterior, and mural leaflets are thickened and rolled. The pulmonary trunk (PA) is also smaller than the aorta (Ao). Abbreviation (RA) right atrium

size of the functional right ventricle is compromised. The volume of the functional right ventricle may be calculated from subcostal images using the technique of Simpson's biplane rule. Because most surgical procedures obliterate the atrialized right ventricle, it is this functional part of the right ventricle that will remain as the effective ventricle after surgical repair. These data provide a greater degree of specificity in calculating the size of the ventricle than the method of the ratio of areas, providing an estimate of the maximal size of the ventricle. In addition, estimates taken at end systole allow for calculation of the ejection fraction, but overestimate right ventricular performance by the degree of associated tricuspid and pulmonary valvar leakage.

(a)

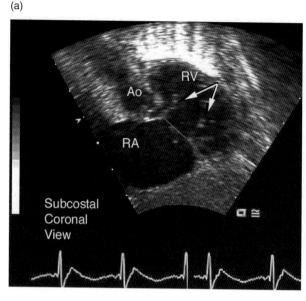

(b)

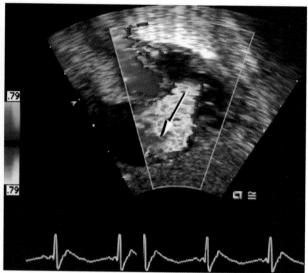

Fig. 34.16 This figure shows two subcostal coronal images in the same patient, demonstrating the valvar plane of the tricuspid valve (A) and valvar insufficiency direction (B)

The arrows in A indicate the anterosuperior and mural leaflet of the valve. The arrow in B indicates the map of the tricuspid regurgitant at right angles to the valve plane

- **Diastolic Dysfunction Abnormalities**

It was not possible to calculate whether the tricuspid orifice is stenotic due to the invariably associated atrial communication, although atrial right-to-left shunting is clearly associated. Tricuspid stenosis is suggested by Rudolph [12]. Tricuspid closure is invariably delayed by more than 50 ms, and was noted on M-mode echocardiography. Celermajer and colleagues [28] also noted an increased distribution of fibrous tissue within the ventricular myocardium in Ebstein's malformation. The upper portion of the left ventricle, and paradoxical septal motion of this segment of the ventricular septum, is associated with the atrialized right ventricle. In neonates and fetuses, the left ventricular Tei index of myocardial performance is noted to be prolonged when compared to normal children and fetuses [29–33]. We have noted that the enlarged right ventricle bulges into the left ventricle, and may reduce left ventricular size, interfering with left ventricular filling as well, explaining in part some of the components of diastolic left ventricular dysfunction (Fig. 34.14).

- **Ductal Problems**

During fetal life, the arterial duct plays an important role in the evolution of Ebstein's malformation, and is particularly important in the transitional circulation. Understanding the physiology is essential to appreciating neonatal presentation. It has been noted that fetal ventricular pressure rises progressively during fetal life. Tricuspid valvar regurgitation becomes more severe as gestation

progresses. As the systemic pressure rises, the pulmonary valve is held in the closed position by the systemic pressure applied to the pulmonary valve via the duct in the face of tricuspid incompetence (Fig. 34.17). As in other conditions where there is fetal left-to-right shunting, the duct is vertical in its orientation [34]. As already emphasized, as the pulmonary valvar leaflets are held in the closed position, synecia tend to develop along their edges, causing them to become stenotic, or even atretic (Fig. 34.18). A number of hemodynamic consequences result from ductal patency. If the right ventricle is incapable of providing sufficient forward flow, ductal flow becomes vital for survival, leading to the surgical option of creation of an aortopulmonary shunt. On the other hand, if the ventricle is capable of forward flow, ductal patency simply transmits systemic pressure in retrograde fashion on to the pulmonary valve, and holds the valve shut, preventing forward flow and causing persistent cyanosis due to right-to-left atrial shunting. If the valve is patent, there may well be some pulmonary regurgitation, setting up a reversed circle of flow under either of the two above-mentioned circumstances.

- **Deformity of the Right Ventricular Outflow and Pulmonary Valve**

The presence of pulmonary regurgitation, not only postnatally but also prenatally, is one of the valuable signs indicating patency of the pulmonary valve (Fig. 34.19). In the fetus with Ebstein's malformation, the presence of retrograde flow in the arterial duct, and

(a)

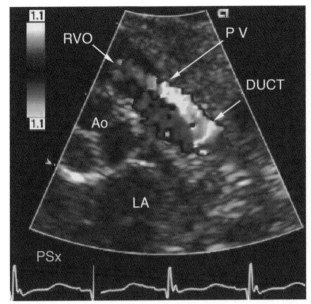

(b)

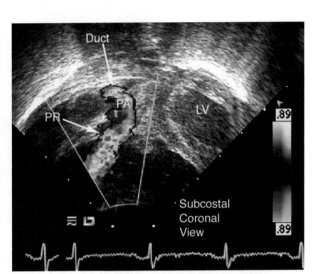

Fig. 34.17 This figure shows two panels demonstrating a patent ductus with left-to-right shunting and pulmonary regurgitation Panel A is a parasternal short-axis view (PSX) and the right-hand panel is a subcostal coronal view. In panel B the flow from the duct is identified (DUCT) passing through the pulmonary valve (PV) and into the right ventricular outflow tract (RVO). The aorta (Ao) is labeled and demonstrates the disparity in size between aorta and the pulmonary artery (LA) left atrium. In B, taken in another patient from a subcostal coronal view, the same physiology, namely, the retrograde circle of flow from the ductus through the pulmonary valve with pulmonary regurgitation (PR) into the right ventricular outflow tract is identified. Abbreviation: LV, left ventricle

diminished forward flow from the right ventricle, can be traced not only by inference, but also directly by echocardiography (Fig. 34.4). The pulmonary trunk and the right ventricular outflow tract tend to be hypoplastic because of altered dynamics of flow. These features are inseparable from the events involving the arterial duct.

- **Defects, Other**

Numerous defects are commonly associated with Ebstein's malformation, including atrial defects, patency of the arterial duct, and ventricular septal defects [25, 27, 32, 35]. Corrected transposition is often associated with Ebstein's malformation, as well as pulmonary stenosis and ventricular septal defect (Figs. 34.20–23). Tricuspid regurgitation in the setting of corrected transposition has to be differentiated from conditions where valvar dysplasia but no displacement of the valve is found. It should be noted that the discordant atrioventricular connections typical for this disorder are usually associated also with mitral regurgitation [25, 32]. Atrial communications, although not invariable, exist in most patients. Defects of the mitral valve, coarctation, and the arterial valves have also been identified.

- **Death**

This is a common occurrence in the fetal period. In our own series, patients with hydrops tended to die. Surgical series with neonatal presentation still exhibit substantial mortality, except for the series reported by Starnes and colleagues [21], which emphasized the advantages of a functionally univentricular repair. The results of repair in older patients are universally better [36, 37].

34.4 Intraoperative and Postoperative Assessment

Transesophageal echocardiography has been a valuable addition to the armamentarium available to the surgeon. It provides an assessment of the extent of tricuspid regurgitation after annuloplasty, and the potential for tricuspid stenosis after vigorous annuloplasty. Repair of the tricuspid valve may be modified by the use of transesophageal evaluation after surgical repair when the patient is prepared for separation from cardiopulmonary bypass. With

(a)

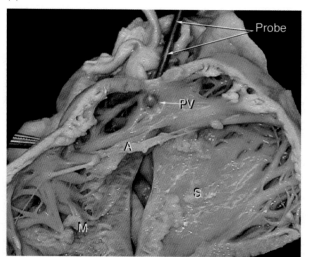

(b)

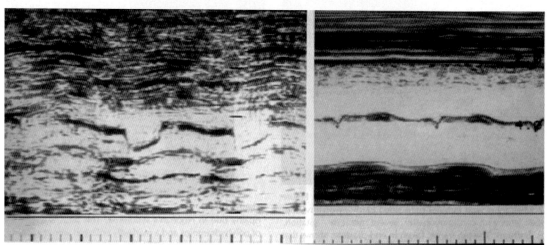

Fig. 34.18 This is a pathological specimen from the same patient as shown in Fig. 34.6. In the view from the right ventricular outflow tract area other portions of the tricuspid valve, showing the septal mural and anterior leaflets: S, M, and A are identified. A probe is passed retrograde into the pulmonary trunk, demonstrating

acquired pulmonary atresia. This specimen of a 20-week fetus, obtained during the M-mode era, shows a normal box-like appearance of the pulmonary valve by M-mode, whereas by 38 weeks, (on the right-hand panel) there is already evidence that the pulmonary valve has no motion

associated lesions, it is equally useful for identifying adequate repair or residual defects (Fig. 34.24).

The intraoperative transesophageal technique provides the surgeon with an additional way of assessing the adequacy of tricuspid annuloplasty and the opportunity to reinstitute cardiopulmonary bypass immediately (Fig. 34.25). In corrected transposition, repair of the valve is not usually possible, but occasionally annuloplasty of the valve is successful and can be assessed echocardiographically (Fig. 34.26). Use of bioprosthetic valves may be evaluated from intraoperative placement and in serial fashion postoperatively (Fig. 34.27). The success of the annuloplasty can

be continually assessed by postoperative echocardiography so as to discover residual regurgitation and stenosis from the annuloplasty.

34.5 Simulation of Ebstein's Malformation

Not all cases of congenital tricuspid incompetence are due to Ebstein's malformation, and distinctive differences are present morphologically [38]. In the condition known as asymmetric short tendinous cords [39], the lack of tricuspid displacement is obvious (Fig. 34.28).

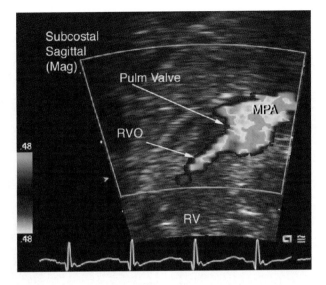

Fig. 34.19 This is a magnified subcostal sagittal view with Doppler color flow imaging in a neonate with pulmonary insuffiency and ductal patency showing the diminutive size of the right ventricular outflow tract (RVO) proximal to the pulmonary trunk (PA) The right ventricular body (RV) and pulmonary trunk (MPA) are also identified

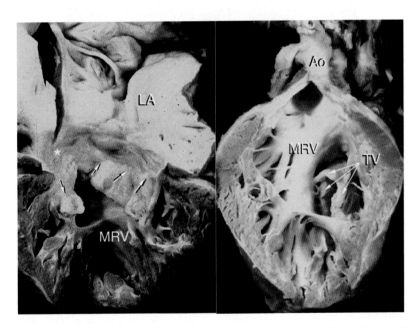

Fig. 34.20 These are two pathological figures of a patient with corrected transposition and Ebstein's malformation
The left-hand panel shows the left atrium (LA) and displaced abnormal tricuspid valve (TV) overriding the morphologically right ventricle (MRV). The second view is open from the right ventricular aspect and shows the abnormal tricuspid valve (TV) from the outflow tract view. The aorta (Ao) is seen with a muscular crest (under the MRV label) separating the aorta from the tricuspid valve (TV). The valvar leaflets of the tricuspid valve are thickened, rolled, and have abnormal tendinous cords associated with them

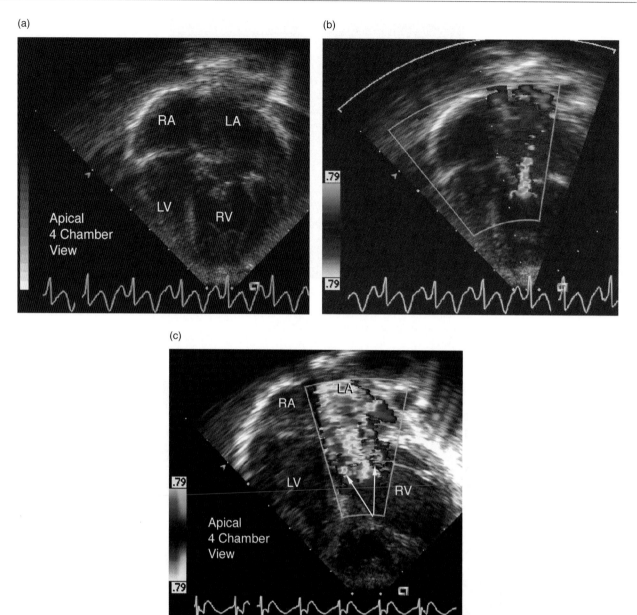

Fig. 34.21 These are three apical four-chamber views in patients with corrected transposition and left-sided Ebstein's malformation A shows the right atrium (RA), left ventricle (LV), left atrium (LA), and right ventricle (RV). The displacement of the tricuspid valve within the morphologically left-sided right ventricle is characteristic of this condition. B demonstrates a systolic frame showing tricuspid regurgitation arising from an apically displaced morphologically right ventricle. C is an apical four-chamber view in a different patient demonstrating a marked degree of tricuspid regurgitation with corrected transposition. In this panel, the right atrium and ventricle are enlarged due to the chronic regurgitant load

(a)

(b)

(c)

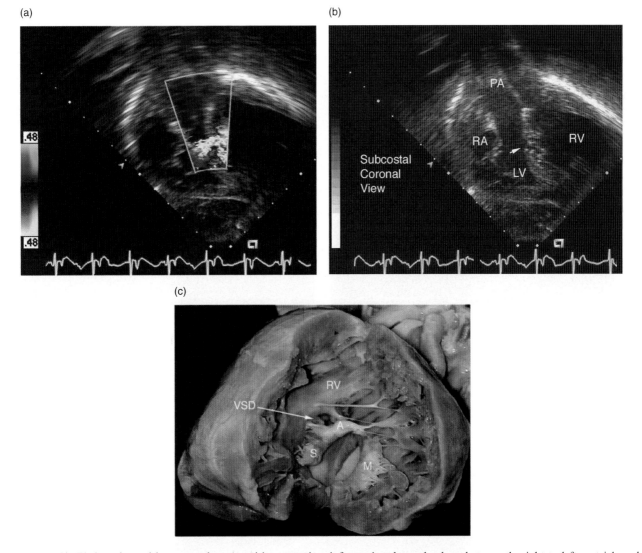

Fig. 34.22 (A, B) A patient with corrected transposition, ventricular septal defect in Ebstein's malformation. A is a subcostal coronal view showing the ventricular septal defect (arrow) between the left-sided morphologically right ventricle and the right-sided morphologically left ventricle. The pulmonary artery is seen arising from the left ventricle. The superimposed Doppler color flow information shows the shunt between the right-to-left ventricle and up into the pulmonary artery. C is a view of the right ventricle from a specimen with corrected transposition and ventricular septal defect (arrow), through which the pulmonary valve can be identified. The anterior (A), septal (S), and mural (M) leaflets can be seen in this ventricle

(a)

(b)

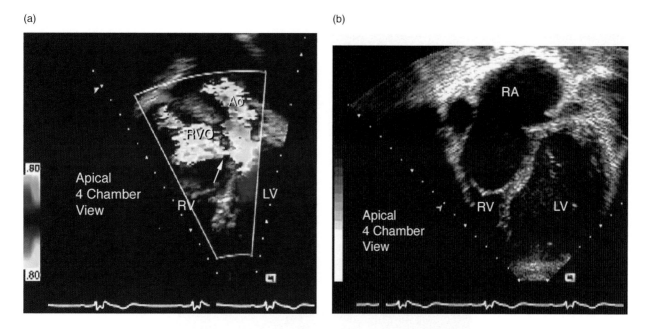

(c)

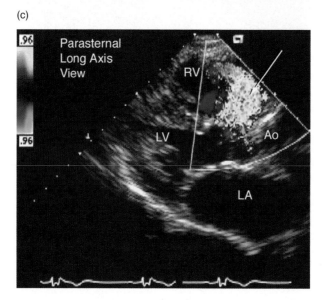

Fig. 34.23 This apical four-chamber view in a teenage patient who had clear displacement of the tricuspid valve consistent with Ebstein's malformation and a ventricular septal defect without any trans-tricuspid flow. Tricuspid atresia of the membranous type is, therefore, also present (A). When viewed from the apical four-chamber view (B) with the superimposition of Doppler color flow information, a ventricular septal defect (VSD) shunt between the left ventricle and the right ventricular outflow tract is identified. Abbreviation: aorta (Ao), left ventricle (LV), right ventricular outflow (RVO), right ventricular body (RV). The arrow indicates the area of the ventricular septal defect. (C) The ventricular septal defect is also identified in the parasternal long-axis view and appears large. The entire pulmonary blood flow is passing through this defect into the pulmonary circulation

(a)

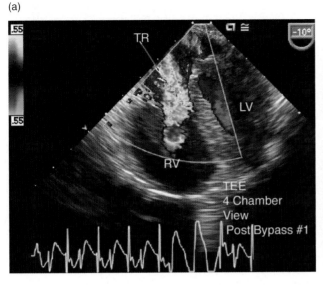

(b)

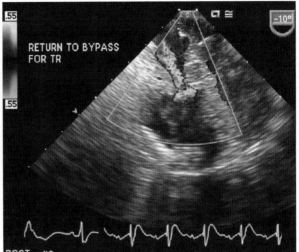

Fig. 34.24 These two transesophageal echocardiograms were taken in an infant who was undergoing an Ebstein's valvoplasty and bidirectional Glenn anastomosis After the first bypass, the transesophageal four-chamber view, panel A demonstrates a substantial amount of residual tricuspid regurgitation. The left ventricle (LV) and right ventricle (RV) are also labeled. The patient was returned to bypass and a more vigorous annuloplasty performed. B shows the marked diminution of the tricuspid regurgitation in the same patient. No tricuspid stenosis could be demonstrated

(a)

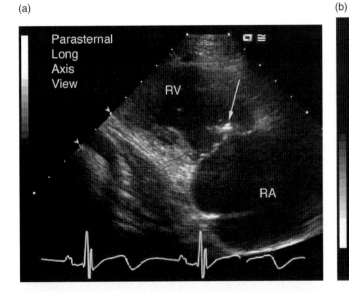

(b)

Fig. 34.25 This postoperative series of transthoracic echocardiograms were taken from a child who had undergone an Ebstein's annuloplasty. Frame A is the apical four-chamber view, frame B is the parasternal long-axis view directed through the right ventricle. Frame C is a subcostal coronal view

In A, the apical four-chamber view demonstrates the area of annuloplasty between the right atrium and the right ventricle (arrows). In B viewed directed through the tricuspid valve, the area of suture between the septal and mural leaflets of the tricuspid valve at that commissure is identified (arrow). In C taken in the subcostal coronal view, a different aspect of the annuloplasty is identified

(c)

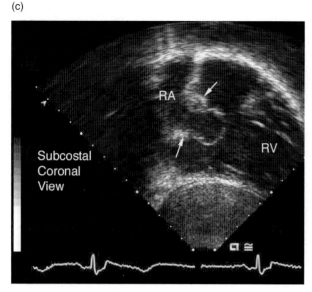

Fig. 34.25 (continued)

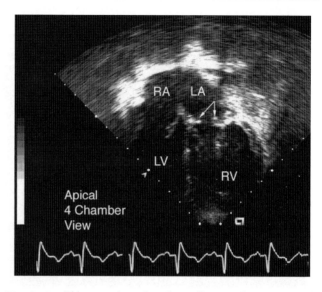

Fig. 34.26 This transthoracic echocardiogram demonstrates an Ebstein's patient who had undergone an annuloplasty of the tricuspid valve (arrows) with corrected transposition

In this patient, the tricuspid valve could not be repaired and, as a consequence, a bioprosthetic valve was inserted in the tricuspid annulus. The two frames are a black and white image on the left-hand frame and a color image on the right, showing the flow passing between the right atrium and right ventricle

(a)

(b)

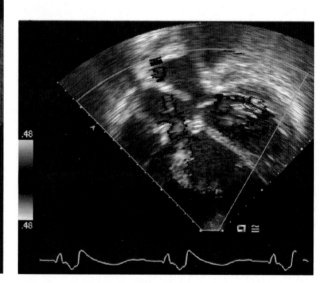

Fig. 34.27 This figure demonstrates a bioprosthetic valve in a patient with Ebstein's malformation

In this patient tricuspid repair could not be affected and a bioprosthetic

valve (V, arrows) had to be inserted between the right atrium (RA) and right ventricle RV). B is the superimposed Doppler color flow information showing a small degree of prosthetic valve regurgitation

(a)

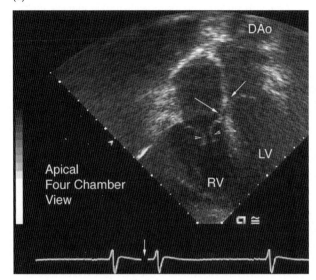

(b)

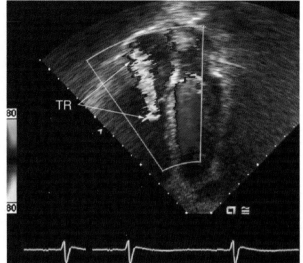

Fig. 34.28 This is a series of apical four-chamber views in a patient with asymmetrically short tendinous chords of the right ventricle-simulating Ebstein's malformation

Note that the area of insertion of the tricuspid and mitral valves to the area of the central fibrous body (arrows) is almost at the same level, and the area of tricuspid insuffiency through these non-coapted tendinous cords and valvar leaflets (small arrowheads) is easily identifiable in this apical four-chamber view series. The morphological information is in the panel A and the superimposed color information is in B. Abbreviations: DAo descending thoracic aorta, LV left ventricle, RV right ventricle, TR tricuspid regurgitation

Although the morphology of such lesions is different, it is clear that long-standing tricuspid regurgitation of whatever cause, particularly when developing during fetal life may present with the same secondary features of tricuspid regurgitation and right-heart dilation. It should also be noted that surgical repair of such lesions is directed at an effective relief of tricuspid regurgitation, cordal reimplantation, and annuloplasty.

References

1. Hoffman and Kaplan, Hoffman, JIE, Kaplan S. The Incidence of Congenital Heart Disease. J Am Coll Cardiol. 2002;39(12): 1890–1900.
2. Mann RJ, Lie JT. The life story of Wilhelm Ebstein (1836–1912) and his almost overlooked description of a congenital disease. Mayo Clin Proc. 54:197–204.
3. Zuberbuhler JR, Anderson RH: Ebstein's malformation of the tricuspid valve. In: Anderson RH, Neches WH, Park SC, Zuberbuhler JR: Perspectives in Paediatric Cardiology. New York: Futura, Mount Kisco; 1988. p 97–112.
4. Silverman NH, Schiller NB: Apex echocardiography: A two-dimensional technique for evaluating congenital heart disease. Circulation. 1978;57:503.
5. Ports TA, Silverman NH, Schiller NB: Two-dimensional assessment of Ebstein's anomaly. Circulation. 1978;58:336.

6. Oechslin E, Buchholz S, Jenni R. Ebstein's anomaly in adults: Doppler-echocardiographic evaluationMimics of Ebstein's anomaly. J Thorac Cardiovasc Surg. 2000;48:209–13.
7. Ammash NM, Warnes CA, Connolly HM, Danielson G K. Seward JB. Mimics of Ebstein's anomaly. Am Heart J. 1997;134:508–13.
8. Shiina A, Seward JB, Edwards WD, Hagler DJ, Tajik AJ. Two-dimensional echocardiographic spectrum of Ebstein's anomaly: detailed anatomic assessment. J Am Coll Cardiol. 1984;3:356–370.
9. Shiina A, Seward JB, Tajik AJ, Hagler DJ, Danielson GK. Two dimensional echocardiographic-surgical correlation in Ebstein's malformation: preoperative determination of patients requiring tricuspid valve application vs. replacement. Circulation. 1983;68:534–544.
10. Attenhofer-Jost C H, Connolly HM, Warnes CA, O'Leary P, Tajik AJ, Pellikka FACC, Seward J B Noncompacted Myocardium in Ebstein's anomaly: Initial Description in Three Patients. J Am Soc Echocardiogr. 2004;17:677–80.
11. Sommerville J. Congenital Heat Disease- Change in form and function Brit Heart J. 1979;41:1–22
12. Rudolph AM. Congenital Diseases of the Heart: Clinical Physiological Considerations. 2nd ed. Futura Publishing Company Armonk, NY. 2001. Chapter 16 p 655–672
13. Roberson DA, Silverman NH: Ebstein's anomaly: echocardiographic and clinical features in the fetus and neonate. J Am Coll Cardiol. 1989;14:1300–1307.
14. Celermajer DS, Bull C, Till JA, Cullen S, Vassillikos VP, Sullivan ID, Allan L, Annopoulos NP, Sommerville J, Deanfield JE. "Ebstein's anomaly: Presentation and Outcome from Fetus to Adult". JACC. 1994:170–6.
15. Arizmendi AF, Pineda FL, Jiménez CQ, Azcárate MJ, Sarachaga IH, Urroz E, Pérez de León J, Moya JL, Jiménez MQ.

The clinical profile of Ebstein's malformation as seen from the fetus to the adult in 52 patients. Cardiol Young. 2004;14:55–63.

16. Chauvaud SM, Mihaileanu SA, Gaer JAR, Carpentier AC. Surgical treatment of Ebstein's malformation – the "Hôpital Broussais" Experience. Cardiol Young. 1996;6:4–11.

17. Dearani JA, Danielson GK. Congenital Heart Surgery Nomenclature and Database Project: Ebstein's malformation and tricuspid valve disease. Ann Thorac Surg. 2000;69: S106–S117.

18. Mair DD. Ebstein's malformation: natural history and management. J Am Coll Cardiol. 1992;19:1047–1048.

19. Knott-Craig CJ, Overholt ED, Ward KE, Ringewald JM, Baker SS, Razook JD. Repair of Ebstein's malformation in the symptomatic neonate: an evolution of technique with 7-year follow-up. Ann Thorac Surg. 2002;73:1786–1792.

20. Chavaud S, Fuzellier JF, Berrebi A, et al. Bi-directional cavopulmonary shunt associated with ventriculo and valvuloplasty in Ebstein's malformation: benefits in high risk patients. Eur J Cardiothoracic Surg. 1998;13:514–519.

21. Starnes VA, Pitlick PT, Bernstein D, Griffin ML, Choy M, Shumway NE. Ebstein's malformation appearing in the neonate. A new surgical approach. J Thorac Cardiovasc Surg. 1991;101:1082–1087.

22. Anderson RH. The surgical treatment of Ebstein's malformation. Cardiol Young. 1996;6:1–3.

23. Schreiber C, Cook A, Ho S-Y, Augustin N, Anderson RH. Morphologic Spectrum of Ebstein's malformation: Revisitation Relative to Surgical Repair. J Thorac Cardiovasc Surg. 1999;117:148–55.

24. Zuberbuhler JR, Anderson RH: Ebstein's malformation of the tricuspid valve. In: Anderson RH, Neches WH, Park SC, Zuberbuhler JR: Perspectives in Paediatric Cardiology. New York: Futura, Mount Kisco. 1988. p 97–112.

25. Attenhofer-Jost CH, Connolly HM, O'Leary PW, Warnes CA, Tajik AJ, Seward JB, Left Heart Lesions in Patients With Ebstein Anomaly Mayo. Clin Proc. 2005;80:361–368.

26. Lee AHS, Moore IE, Nuala LK. Fagg NLK, Cook AC, Kakadekar AP, Allan LD, Keeton BL, Anderson RH. Histological Changes in the Left and Right Ventricle in Hearts with Ebstein's Malformation and Tricuspid Valvar Dysplasia: A Morphometric Study of Patients Dying in the Fetal and Perinatal Periods. Cardiovascular Path.1995;4:19–24.

27. Rudolph AM. Congenital Diseases of the Heart: Clinical Physiological Considerations. 2nd ed. Futura Publishing Company, Armonk, NY. 2001. Chapter 16 p 655–672

28. Celermajer DS, Dodd SM, Greenwald SE, et al. Morbid Anatomy in Neonates with Ebstein's anomaly of the Tricuspid Valve: Pathophysiological and Clinical Implications. J Am Coll Cardiol. 1992;19:1049–53.

29. Eidem BW, Tei C, O'Leary PW, Cetta F, Seward JB. Nongeometric quantitative assessment of right and left ventricular function: myocardial performance index in normal children and patients with Ebstein's anomaly. J Am Soc Echocardiogr. 1998;11:849–856.

30. Inamura N, Taketazu M, Smallhorn JF, Hornberger LK. Left Ventricular Myocardial Performance in the Fetus with Severe Tricuspid Valve Disease and Tricuspid Insufficiency. Am J Perinatol.2005;22:91–7.

31. Tei C, Dujardin KS, Hodge DO, Kyle RA, Tajik AJ, Seward JB. Doppler index combining systolic and diastolic myocardial performance: clinical value in cardiac amyloidosis. J Am Coll Cardiol. 1996;28:658–664.

32. Attenhofer CJ, Connolly HM, Edwards WD, Hayes D, Warnes CA, Danielson GK. Ebstein's Anomaly- review of a multifaceted congenital cardiac lesion. Swiss Med Weekly. 2005;135:269–281.

33. Sharma S, Rajani M, Mukhopadhyay SI, Aggarwal S, Shrivastava S Rajan Tandon R. Angiographic abnormalities of the morphologically left ventricle in the presence of Ebstein's malformation. Int. J Cardiol. 1989;22:109–113.

34. Rudolph AM. Congenital Diseases of the Heart: Clinical Physiological Considerations. 2nd ed. Futura Publishing Company, Armonk, NY. 2001. Chapter 13 p 489–549

35. Silverman NH, Gerlis LM, Horowitz ES, Ho SY, Neches WH, Anderson RH: Pathologic elucidation of the echocardiographic features of Ebstein's malformation of the tricuspid valve in discordant atrioventricular connections. Am J Cardiol. 1995;76:1277–1283.

36. Hornberger LK, Sahn DJ, Kleinman CS, Copel JA, Reed KL. Tricuspid valve disease with significant tricuspid insufficiency in the fetus: diagnosis and outcome. J Am Coll Cardiol. Jan 1991;17:167–73.

37. McElhinney DB, Salvin JA, Colan SD, Thiagarajan R, Crawford EC, Marcus EN, del Nido Pedro J, Tworetzky W, Improving Outcomes in Fetuses and Neonates with Congenital Displacement (Ebstein's Malformation) or Dysplasia of the Tricuspid Valve. Am J Cardiol. 2005;96: 582–586.

38. Ammash NM, Warnes CA, Connolly HM, Danielson GK, Seward JB. Mimics of Ebstein's anomaly. Am Heart J. 1997;134:508–13.

39. McElhinney DB, Silverman NH, Brook MM, Hanley FL, Stanger P: Asymmetrically short tendinous chords causing congenital tricuspid regurgitation: improved understanding of tricuspid valvar dysplasia in the era of color flow echocardiography. Cardiol Young. 1999;9:300–304.

Edgar T. Jaeggi and Tiscar Cavalle-Garido

35.1 Historical Background

In 1866, Wilhelm Ebstein was the first to describe the clinical and pathological–anatomical characteristics of a rare, yet important, developmental anomaly of the right heart and the tricuspid valve apparatus, now bearing his name [1]. The subject of his case report, a 19-year-old laborer named Joseph Preschler, had a long-standing history of dyspnea, palpitations, and pronounced cyanosis. Marked jugular venous pulsations synchronous with the heart beat, cardiomegaly, and a systolic murmur extending in diastole was found prior to Mr. Preschler's death. At the postmortem cardiac dissection, the proximal attachments of the thickened septal and mural or posterior tricuspid valvular leaflets were found displaced from the true atrio-ventricular junction into the right ventricle, while the redundant and fenestrated anterior–superior leaflet retained its normal annular position. The atrialized portion of the right ventricle was thinned and dilated and the foramen ovale was still patent. In early 1950, Ebstein's anomaly of the tricuspid valve (EA) was diagnosed for the first time in a living patient [2] but it took another three decades until major fetal cardiac malformations became detectable by two-dimensional ultrasound imaging [3]. As a result of extensive research on the morphological peculiarities and with advances in noninvasive imaging techniques, the understanding of the underlying pathophysiology and the natural history of EA as an abnormality with multiple facets has evolved considerably since Ebstein's original description [4–8]. Echocardiography has become the method of choice to diagnose EA on its own and in association with other heart defects. In modern countries, the majority of cases with clinically relevant tricuspid valvular pathology is nowadays detected *in utero*. In this chapter we discuss the more common morphological and functional cardiovascular findings associated with EA, and then focus on the distinctiveness of the prenatal physiology as it relates to the outcome of the fetus with this entity.

35.2 Morphological Features of Ebstein's Malformation of the Tricuspid Valve

Irrespective of whether the diagnosis is made before or after birth, EA of the tricuspid valve comprises a wide spectrum of clinical and pathological features, with certain findings being common and essential to the diagnosis. The anatomical hallmark is a rotational displacement of the atrio-ventricular junction into the inlet portion of the right ventricle due to incomplete delamination of the septal and mural tricuspid leaflets from the myocardial surface [4–7]. This is accompanied by varying degrees of valvular dysplasia and abnormal attachments of the distal valvular margins. The result is that part of the ventricular inlet component becomes incorporated into the right atrium, which has been described as the *atrialized* portion of the right ventricle. In mildly affected cases, it may only be the septal leaflet that has a lower attachment. In the four-chamber view, the distal septal displacement should be at least 8 mm/m^2 of body surface area to fulfill the diagnostic criteria of EA. At the severe end of the spectrum, the septal and mural leaflets may be virtually plastered to the right ventricular myocardium or be absent [9]. There is a spectrum between these two extremes. The sail-like antero-superior leaflet typically retains its normal proximal attachments at the AV junction, but its leading edge may be inserted in a linear fashion and partially or completely occlude the right ventricular outflow tract [5, 8, 10]. The atrialized inlet portion of the right ventricle is usually thinned and dilated, and the atrialized ventricular septum bulges toward the left ventricle. The remaining functional right ventricle may be of adequate size,

E.T. Jaeggi (✉)
Fetal Cardiac Program, Division of Paediatrics, The Hospital for Sick Children, Toronto, Canada

diminutive, and hypertrophic, or even thin walled and dilated [10, 11]. Intrinsic myocardial abnormalities may also affect the ventricular performance.

EA can be found in association with a wide variety of more or less common cardiac and extracardiac abnormalities. This includes atrial and ventricular septal defects, pulmonary stenosis and atresia, Wolf–Parkinson–White syndrome, congenitally corrected transposition, coarctation of the aorta, and tetralogy of Fallot, among other defects [10, 12–14]. Moreover, mitral valve abnormalities, paradoxical ventricular septal wall motion, myocardial fibrosis, and noncompaction underlie left ventricular dysfunction in some patients, suggesting that EA is not solely confined to the right side of the heart [15–18]. In the Baltimore Washington Infant Study, including 47 cases with EA, additional cardiac malformations were present in 38.3% and extracardiac lesions in 19.7% [19]. Celermajer and colleagues [13], including those patients with concordant AV connections, found associated cardiac anomalies other than foramen ovale and atrial septal defects in 54%. There is no obvious predilection for extracardiac malformations, but trisomy 13, trisomy 18, trisomy 21, trisomy 9p, duplication at the distal arm of chromosome 15, Noonan's syndrome, Apert syndrome, CHARGE association, and cleft lip and palate have been described in association with EA [20–24]. Lastly, EA may affect several family members and generations, which points to a genetic etiology with an increased recurrence risk for some of the offspring [19, 25–29].

35.3 Fetal Presentation

Reflecting the wide variation of anomalies, it is not surprising that some individuals with mild EA may have no symptoms during life, while the more severely affected babies and those with associated lesions present *in utero* or at birth with clinical findings such as cardiomegaly, fetal hydrops, heart failure, postnatal cyanosis, and murmurs. The perinatal symptomatology is not necessarily a reflection of the severity of the valvular displacement but rather of the morbid function of the tricuspid valve, exacerbated by the physiologically high fetal right ventricular afterload and pathological right ventricular outflow obstruction. In fact, the prenatal hemodynamic consequences of tricuspid valve dysplasia (TVD) with normally or near normally attached leaflets are often strikingly similar to that of EA, which may explain why most larger fetal series report combined outcome data of both entities [21, 22, 30].

Echocardiography is the technique of choice to display the relevant morphological features and functional consequences of EA and TVD. Evidence of cardiomegaly with right atrial enlargement and a leftward rotated heart axis [31] in the cardiac four-chamber view will raise immediate suspicion during the sonographic examination. The attachments of the septal and mural valves are displaced in EA and the leaflets appear thickened, relatively fixed and non-coapting. Usually, there is color Doppler evidence of severe regurgitation at the level of the functional AV junction [21, 22, 30], but in some cases the tricuspid valve is stenotic or even atretic. Significant tricuspid pathology typically affects the diastolic Doppler flow pattern of precordial systemic veins: during atrial contraction, there is increased flow reversal in the vena cava and absent or reversed flow in the venous duct [32, 33]. Progression from mild to severe tricuspid regurgitation with ensuing secondary atrial enlargement may occur during the course of gestation [34]. This may explain why EA is, on average, referred later in gestation to our Fetal Cardiac Program than other congenital cardiac defects (mean gestational age: 28 versus 22 weeks). Typically, there is an atrial communication allowing unrestricted right–left atrial shunting. Antegrade flow through the main pulmonary artery depends on many factors, among which are the severity of tricuspid valve regurgitation, the functional capacity of the remaining right ventricle, the pulmonary arterial pressure, and the presence of subpulmonary and pulmonary obstruction. Functional pulmonary atresia occurs when the pulmonary arterial pressure exceeds the pressure that the right ventricle is able to generate, and the pulmonary valve leaflets fail to open. The same mechanism may underlie progression of anatomical pulmonary stenosis to atresia during fetal life [11, 35, 36]. Relying exclusively on echocardiographic techniques, it may be impossible to differentiate between anatomical and functional fetal pulmonary atresia. In both situations, the pulmonary blood flow is essentially maintained by retrograde flow coming from the arterial duct. In the subset of patients with a patent outflow tract but functional obstruction to the flow of blood to the lungs, time and medical manipulation to improve the compliance of the pulmonary circulation after birth may eventually set the scene for antegrade flow to the lungs, obviating in some patients the need of surgical intervention in the neonatal period [37–40]. These considerations obviously have little relevance when the obstruction to flow is anatomic rather than functional. At last, many patients are compromised due to a combination of biventricular low cardiac output, increased systemic venous pressure, and compressed lung tissue leading to secondary pulmonary arterial and parenchymal hypoplasia [21, 22].

35.4 Outcome After Fetal Diagnosis of Ebstein's Anomaly

The primary task of this review is to assess whether and how morphological and clinical features influence the fate of the fetus with EA. Figure 35.1 summarizes the outcome data of four larger retrospective studies on isolated fetal EA and TVD that were reported between 1991 and 2006 [21, 22, 30, 41]. Following the fetal diagnosis, the overall probability of surviving to infancy was less than 25%, despite minor improvements in the early outcomes in the two more recent publications. There is little doubt that the worst end of the cardiovascular disease spectrum is preferentially detected in the fetus, with most EA cases notable for striking cardiomegaly, significant tricuspid incompetence, and absent antegrade pulmonary blood flow [21, 22, 30, 41, 42]. Fetuses with these ultrasound findings are also the most likely to develop fetal hydrops and/or clinically relevant tachyarrhythmias. Hornberger et al. found concomitant atrial flutter in 20% of fetuses with severe tricuspid regurgitation, while she and others reported an even higher incidence of fetal hydrops, affecting up to 30% of pregnancies [21, 30, 43]. On the other side, cases with mild anomalies and without cardiac enlargement are predominantly detected after birth, accounting for the more favorable life expectancy of the cohort of newborns, children, and adults with this diagnosis [30, 38, 32, 44–50].

Various authors have studied those factors affecting fetal and neonatal outcomes. This includes echocardiographic parameters such as the cardiothoracic ratio and the right atrial (RA) area index, which is based on the ratio of the combined area of the right atrium and the atrialized portion of the right ventricle to that of the combined area of the functional right ventricle, left atrium, and left ventricle measured in a cardiac four-chamber view at end diastole. The RA area index, initially described by Robertson and Silverman [41] and subsequently modified by Celermajer and colleagues [13] with the introduction of a grading system (Grade 1: < 0.5; Grade 2: 0.5–0.99; Grade 3: 1–1.49; Grade 4: ≥ 1.5), reflects the impact of morphological and hemodynamic variables on cardiac geometry and dimension, such as the amount of distal AV valve displacement and tricuspid regurgitation. The echocardiographic grade of severity is a strong, independent predictor of the neonatal outcome of fetuses and newborns with EA and concordant AV connections [13, 30, 41]. Celermajer et al. [13], reporting the outcome of 50 mainly cyanotic neonates diagnosed with this anomaly between 1961 and 1990, found that a Grade 1 RA area ratio (< 0.5) was associated with 0% mortality, whereas a Grade 4 index (≥ 1.5) correlated with no survival [12]. Adjusting for the presence of associated defects, an estimated relative risk of 5.34 was found for each increase in grade.

McElhinney and colleagues [30] reviewed 66 patients with a fetal ($n = 33$) or neonatal ($n = 33$) presentation of EA ($n = 61$) or TVD ($n = 5$) at the Boston Children's Hospital between the years 1984 and 2004. Among 49 live-born patients, fetal diagnosis was associated with the worst neonatal outcome (56% mortality), as were an RA area index > 1 (80% mortality) and the absence of antegrade flow across the pulmonary valve (62% mortality). The cohort of fetuses not born alive, including cases with pregnancy termination as well as spontaneous intrauterine death, were detected earlier than those who were eventually live-born (20 ± 4 weeks vs. 29 ± 6 weeks; $p < 0.001$) and were more likely to present severe (Grade 4) tricuspid regurgitation (59% mortality). By contrast, 32 of 34 (94%) patients with RA area indexes < 1 survived to infancy and thereafter. Interestingly, a functionally biventricular physiology or repair was achieved in all 35 patients by the time of discharge from the Boston Children's Hospital.

In the most recent study, reported by Andrews and colleagues [41] from Guy's Hospital in 2006 [24], cardiothoracic ratio > 70% ($p < 0.001$), RA area index > 1 ($p = 0.001$), reduced antegrade pulmonary flow or retrograde arterial duct flow (p = 0.001), and a right/left ventricular length ratio > 1.5 were significantly associated with increased mortality following the prenatal diagnosis of tricuspid valve pathology. Atrial tachyarrhythmias were seen in three of totally 44 fetuses, who all died. Not associated with an increased risk were the gestational age at diagnosis, left ventricular output, the ratio of foramen ovale diameter/atrial septal length, the ratio of the functional tricuspid valve opening to the annulus, and the degree of tricuspid displacement. Survival was 35% at birth and 23% at 1 month, or 63% and 42%, respectively, on an intention-to-treat basis.

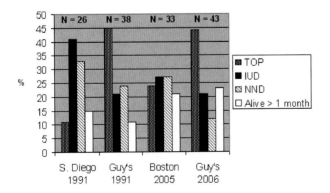

Fig. 35.1 Outcome after prenatal diagnosis of Ebstein's anomaly or tricuspid valve dysplasia in three tertiary care institutions (San Diego 1991 = Ref. 21; Boston 2005 = Ref. 30; Guy's 1991 = Ref. 22; Guy's 2006 = Ref. 41). When compared to London's Guy's Hospital, the two US centers have lower pregnancy termination rates but comparable low 1-month survival

Pavlova et al. [43] examined those factors affecting the outcome of eight fetuses with EA. The RA area index and the cardiothoracic ratio had a significant impact on neonatal but not on intrauterine survival. The smallest ratio of fossa ovalis diameter over atrial septal length was found in two fetuses with fetal hydrops (0.16 and 0.18, respectively). All six fetuses who reached term without difficulties had ratios > 0.3 and higher left cardiac output. A positive linear correlation was found between the z score of left ventricular output and the size of the fossa ovalis. There were no significant differences between the hydropic and nonhydropic fetuses concerning septal leaflet displacement, severity of tricuspid insufficiency, pulmonary valve obstruction, or cardiothoracic ratio, with the limitations that these findings were based on small patient numbers. The authors concluded that the prognosis of EA during fetal life is not influenced by criteria described for postnatal life but may be related to factors that control the volume load of the left ventricle. On the other hand, the high risk of fetal death in the presence of a small and restrictive foramen ovale could explain why in postnatal life EA with persistent right–left shunting is commonly associated with larger and unrestricted atrial septal defects.

After birth, a large atrial communication may be a less beneficial finding, based on the results of a retrospective study by Yetman et al. at the Hospital for Sick Children in Toronto [38]. In this study, risk factors for mortality were identified in 46 cyanotic newborns with a diagnosis of EA between 1954 and 1996. Most of the neonates presented immediately after birth with significant cyanosis (O_2 saturation: $62 \pm 12\%$). An atrial septal defect larger than 4 mm was found in 20, functional pulmonary atresia in 25, and anatomical pulmonary obstruction in 11 cases. Thirteen neonates underwent surgery for severe cyanosis, which included Blalock-Taussig shunts ($n = 8$), pulmonary valvotomies ($n = 3$), and tricuspid valve repair ($n = 2$). Surgical interventions after the neonatal period included tricuspid valve replacements ($n = 4$), bilateral cavopulmonary shunts ($n = 7$) and Fontan operations ($n = 2$). Overall, 32 patients died, predominantly as newborns ($n = 26$), including 19 prior to surgery because of hypoxemia and low cardiac output. One-month, 1-year and 20-year survival rates of the entire cohort of cyanotic neonates with EA were 48%, 38%, and 30%, respectively. Reduced left ventricular function (OR 4.1; $p = 0.002$), the presence of an atrial septal defect of at least 4 mm (OR 2.39; $p = 0.04$), and functional or anatomic pulmonary atresia (OR 2.44; $p = 0.003$ and 5.97; $p = 0.004$, respectively) were independent predictors of mortality. An RA area index of more than one was predictive of 100% mortality.

Due to the relative rarity of the disease and overall poor prognosis, none of the above-mentioned studies specifically addressed the impact on outcome of associated cardiac anomalies other than atrial septal defects and right outflow obstruction.

35.5 The Role of the Fetal Physiology

Nobody concerned with congenital cardiac disease will deny that prenatally diagnosed EA has been associated with a particularly high risk of intrauterine and neonatal demise, even when compared to other severe forms of structural congenital heart disease. To better understand the determinants that decide on prenatal outcome, we will first review some of the fundamental differences that exist between the fetal and postnatal circulation. This includes:

1) The *parallel arrangement* of the right and left ventricular fetal circulation with a predominant contribution of the right ventricle to the combined cardiac output of about 450 ml/kg/min [51]. Both ventricles share the same systemic ejection pressure, which steadily increases with advancing gestation. The parallel disposition of the two fetal circuits is the key element in intrauterine survival of any fetus with severe dysfunction of one side of the heart, including EA with pulmonary obstruction.

2) A physiologically *low fetal cardiac pump reserve*, allowing an increase in combined cardiac output by only about 25% above the baseline. Cardiac output is the product of heart rate and stroke volume, of which the latter is determined by loading conditions and myocardial contractility. The fetus has normally high resting heart rates, which cannot substantially increase during stress. The myocardium is also less compliant and contractile than after birth [52–54]. Related to the reduced compliance, an increment in atrial pressure causes relatively small increases in ventricular end-diastolic volume and in the ejected stroke volume.

3) Additional *constraining effects* exerted by the surrounding fluid-filled lungs and the amniotic fluid limit ventricular preload, expansion, and stroke volumes [54–59];

4) An *increased sensitivity to afterload*. When compared to the left ventricle, right ventricular systolic wall stress is physiologically greater and increases to any rise in afterload by a greater amount. This may explain why the right ventricle responds preferentially with a more rapid decline in stroke volume to increased pulmonary arterial pressure or to obstruction of its outflow [60, 61].

(a)   (b)

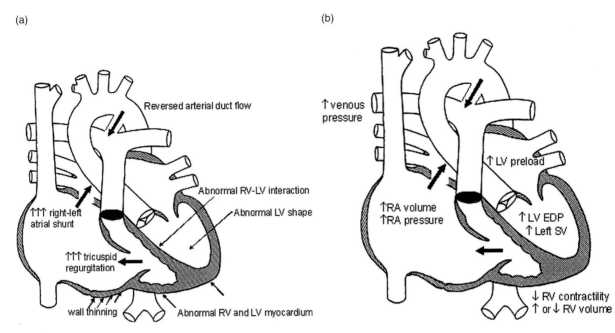

Fig. 35.2 Hemodynamic consequences of severe Ebstein's anomaly of the tricuspid valve. (Panel A) Commonly, the fetus presents with significant tricuspid insufficiency, functional or anatomic right outflow obstruction, and right heart enlargement. (Panel B) Right atrial pressure and volume load rises as a result of the tricuspid regurgitation, favoring right-to-left shunting across the foramen ovale. The increment in left atrial preload is expected to increase left ventricular end-diastolic volume and stroke volume to compensate for the absent right ventricular output. In Ebstein's anomaly, however, systolic and diastolic ventricular function may be adversely influenced by restricted flow across the fossa ovalis, abnormal ventricular–ventricular interaction, intrinsic myocardial disease (fibrosis, con-compaction, and wall thinning), and increased cardiac constraint, for example, due to interstitial fluid accumulation and cardiomegaly EDP = end-diastolic pressure; LV = left ventricular; RA = right atrial; RV = right ventricular; SV = stroke volume

5) A fetal *predisposition to interstitial fluid accumulation and hydrops*, which is related to a lower colloid oncotic plasma pressure, an increased permeability of the capillary membranes for plasma proteins, a more compliant interstitial space that permits retention of more water for any given perivascular hydraulic pressure, and the dependence on increased lymphatic drainage to return the interstitial fluid and proteins to the vascular space [62, 63]. In fetal lambs, the lymphatic flow rate in the thoracic duct reduces substantially if the systemic venous pressure increases above the physiological range of 3–4 mmHg and ceases at only 16 mmHg, which is substantially lower than in adult animals [62, 64, 65].

6) *Ventricular geometry and systolo-diastolic ventricular interaction.* Anatomically and functionally, the two ventricles are interlinked by a common septum, which constitutes part of the load against which each ventricle must work. Increase in contralateral ventricular volume and end-diastolic pressure shifts the ipsilateral pressure–volume ratio to the left, which means that a given filling pressure is less able to fill the ipsilateral ventricle. This effect is similar for both ventricles, but more pronounced in the fetus than after birth [66].

Figure 35.2 illustrates the hemodynamic consequences of a typical case of fetal EA, presenting with severe tricuspid insufficiency, right heart enlargement, pulmonary atresia, and bypass of the pulmonary circulation via the right–left shunt across the foramen ovale. Related to the parallel disposition of the fetal circulation, intrauterine survival is not dependent on adequate pulmonary blood flow, but on the ability of the left ventricle to compensate for the right ventricular dysfunction by increasing its own stroke volume. As mentioned above, fetal cardiac reserve is physiologically impaired due to intrinsic properties of the immature myocardium, the high resting heart rate, and additional constraints on the heart by surrounding fluid-filled tissues. In EA, size, shape, and function of the left ventricle are adversely affected by the enlarged portions of the functional and atrialized right ventricle. The right ventricular dilation may be so marked that the leftward-bulging septum reduces the compressed left ventricular cavity to a small crescent-shaped chamber. Paradoxical wall motion of the thinned and fibrotic interventricular septum further alters ventricular geometry and function. Survival of the fetus with a dysfunctional right ventricle depends on unrestricted blood flow across a wide atrial communication [43, 67, 68] and on an amplified filling pressure to sustain a higher left heart volume flow. In the presence of severe tricuspid regurgitation, right atrial pressure is high, favoring right-left atrial shunting. The amount of blood flow across the foramen ovale is therefore significantly increased, at least in those cases surviving to birth. Restriction of intra-atrial blood flow due to a small communication may not only critically impair left cardiac output, but result in fetal hydrops secondary to high atrial pressure and congestion of the systemic veins. Marked atrial distention and the increased incidence of ventricular pre-excitation are the electrophysiological conditions that underlie the increased prevalence of supraventricular tachyarrhythmias in EA, and may be an additional cause of cardiac failure and fetal hydrops.

35.6 Prenatal Treatment Options

The prenatal management options are very limited if a fetus with EA presents with hydrops in early gestation. Because of the poor prognosis, termination of the pregnancy or expectant acceptance of the intrauterine fetal death is the preferred management. If associated with sustained tachyarrhythmia, transplacental pharmacological treatment with anti-arrhythmic drugs may be successful in controlling the heart rate and improving the hemodynamic consequences. At least theoretically, increasing the size of a restrictive fetal atrial communication by means of an ultrasound-guided atrial balloon septoplasty may be considered to decompress the right atrium and to increase left cardiac output. Indeed, a similar approach has been elected in a small number of fetuses with hypoplastic left heart syndrome and highly restrictive atrial septum [69]. However, while it was possible to successfully perforate and balloon-dilate the atrial septum in six of seven fetuses with a hypoplastic left heart, the iatrogenic defects were in general too small to alleviate atrial hypertension.

The chance of an individual mid-gestational fetus with an apparently less severe EA to reach term without problems is difficult to establish. The risk of progressive right outflow obstruction and tricuspid regurgitation demands careful pregnancy surveillance. For some cases with intrauterine poorly tolerated EA, preterm delivery followed by an aggressive neonatal reanimation may become life saving. Moreover, successful biventricular repair has been possible in a number of severely affected neonates [70]. The survival of neonates with EA and TVD essentially depends on the ability to establish adequate pulmonary flow. Prostaglandin is unequivocal in maintaining pulmonary blood flow via the patent arterial duct, while mechanical ventilation and inhaled nitric oxide are

used to reduce pulmonary vascular resistance. Early discontinuation of the prostaglandin administration, ductal constriction, and subsequent decrease in pulmonary arterial pressure enables the differentiation between functional and anatomic pulmonary atresia. Moreover, it allows the assessment of the functional capability of the small right ventricle, and therefore has important implications on postnatal surgical management (biventricular vs. nonbiventricular repair) [40]. Surgery or catheter intervention is used to relieve anatomic pulmonary atresia. Prolonged patency of the arterial duct in patients without anatomic outflow tract obstruction may have undesirable hemodynamic consequences. If the ductus arteriosus fails to close upon discontinuation of prostaglandin infusion in the presence of pulmonary and tricuspid insufficiency, a *circular shunt physiology* may cause life-threatening hemodynamic instability. In this situation, that usually follows pulmonary balloon valvuloplasty, systemic blood from the aorta streams through the patent arterial duct into the pulmonary artery, the right ventricle, and atrium, then across the foramen ovale to the left side of the heart, resulting in a large ineffective blood flow and rapid deterioration of the affected child until the duct closes spontaneously or is ligated. Tailored neonatal management strategies have yielded a substantial reduction in neonatal loss to less than 7% in the high-risk cohort of newborns with EA and TVD. This improved outcome is also confirmed by our most recent experience (Fig. 35.3; unpublished data). Ninety-two percent of the neonates (*n* = 13) diagnosed with EA or TVD since 2000 at the Hospital for Sick Children survived beyond infancy. The outcome (*n* = 21) of fetuses with the same tricuspid valve pathology has

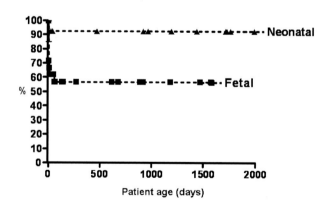

Fig. 35.3 Survival estimates after fetal (*n* = 21) or neonatal (*n* = 13) diagnosis of Ebstein's anomaly (*n* = 22) or tricuspid valve dysplasia (*n* = 12) at the Hospital for Sick Children, Toronto, between the years 2000 and 2005. Of those with a prenatal diagnosis, 71% were live-born (intrauterine demise: 19%; pregnancy termination: 10%) and 58% remained alive at 1 year of age. In the neonatal group, the only demise affected a newborn with trisomy 18

improved when compared to the published fetal series of other centers, with survival rates to birth and infancy of 71% and 57%, respectively.

In summary, the mortality risk of cases with EA is highest during the fetal and neonatal periods. Most studies on infantile EA emphasize the importance of the RA area index > 1, which is related to the severity of tricuspid regurgitation and the presence of functional or structural pulmonary atresia as prognostic markers of poor outcome. Some of the most severely affected babies may demonstrate spectacular clinical improvement with the transition from the fetal to the postnatal circulation coinciding with the fall in pulmonary vascular resistance.

References

1. Ebstein W. Ueber einen sehr seltenen Fall von Insuffizienz der Valvula tricuspidalis, bedingt durch eine angeborene Missbildung derselben. Arch Anat Physiol Wissensch Med. 1866;238–254.
2. Soloff LA, Stauffer HM, Zatuchni J. Ebstein's disease: report of the first case diagnosed during life. Am J Med Sci. 1951;222:554–561.
3. Sharf M, Abinader EG, Shapiro I, Rosenfeld T, Eibschitz I. Prenatal echocardiographic diagnosis of Ebstein's anomaly with pulmonary atresia. Am J Obstet Gynecol. 1983;147:300–303.
4. Anderson KR, Lie JT. Pathologic anatomy of Ebstein's anomaly of the heart revisited. Am J Cardiol. 1978;41:739–745.
5. Zuberbuhler JR, Allwork SP, Anderson RH. The spectrum of Ebstein's anomaly of the tricuspid valve. J Thorac Cardiovasc Surg. 1979;77:202–211.
6. Shiina A, Seward JB, Edwards WD, Hagler DJ, Tajik AJ. Two-dimensional echocardiographic spectrum of Ebstein's anomaly: detailed anatomic assessment. J Am Coll Cardiol. 1984;3:356–370.
7. Gussenhoven EJ, Stewart PA, Becker AE, Essed CE, Ligtvoet KM, De Villeneuve VH. "Offsetting" of the septal tricuspid leaflet in normal hearts and in hearts with Ebstein's anomaly. Anatomic and echographic correlation. Am J Cardiol. 1984;54:172–176.
8. Zuberbuhler JR, Anderson RH. Morphological variations in pulmonary atresia with intact ventricular septum. Br Heart J. 1979;41:281–288.
9. Schreiber C, Cook A, Ho SY, Augustin N, Anderson RH. Morphological spectrum of Ebstein's malformation: revisitation relative to surgical repair. J Thorac Cardiovasc Surg. 1999;117:148–155.
10. Stellin G, Santini F, Thiene G, Bortolotti U, Daliento L, Milanesi O, Sorbara C, Mazzucco A, Casarotto D. Pulmonary atresia, intact ventricular septum, and Ebstein's anomaly of the tricuspid valve. J Thorac Cardiovasc Surg. 1993;106:255–261.
11. Freedom RM, Jaeggi E, Perrin D, Yoo SJ, Anderson RH. The "wall-to-wall" heart in patients with pulmonary atresia and intact ventricular septum. Cardiol Young. 2006;16:18–29.
12. Lang D, Oberhoffer R, Cook A, Sharland G, Allan L, Fagg N, Anderson RH. Pathologic spectrum of malformations of the tricuspid valve in prenatal and neonatal life. J Am Coll Cardiol. 1991;17:1161–1167.
13. Celermajer DS, Cullen S, Sullivan ID, Spiegelhalter DJ, Wyse RK, Deanfield JE. Outcome in neonates with Ebstein's anomaly. J Am Coll Cardiol. 1992;19:1041–1046.
14. Celermajer DS, Dodd SM, Greenwald SE, Wyse RK, Deanfield JE. Morbid anatomy in neonates with Ebstein's anomaly of the tricuspid valve: pathophysiologic and clinical implications. J Am Coll Cardiol. 1992;19:1049–1053.
15. Monibi AA, Neches WH, Lenox CC, Park SC, Mathews RA, Zuberbuhler JR. Left ventricular anomalies associated with Ebstein's malformation of the tricuspid valve. Circulation. 1978;57:303–306.
16. Benson LN, Child JS, Schwaiger M, Perloff JK, Schelbert HR. Left ventricular geometry and function in adults with Ebstein's anomaly of the tricuspid valve. Circulation. 1987;75:353–359.
17. Gerlis LM, Ho SY, Sweeney AE. Mitral valve anomalies associated with Ebstein's malformation of the tricuspid valve. Am J Cardiovasc Pathol. 1993;4:294–301.
18. Attenhofer Jost CH, Connolly HM, O'Leary PW, Warnes CA, Tajik AJ, Seward JB. Left heart lesions in patients with Ebstein anomaly. Mayo Clin Proc. 2005;80:361–368.
19. Correa-Villasenor A, Ferencz C, Neill CA, Wilson PD, Boughman JA. Ebstein's malformation of the tricuspid valve: genetic and environmental factors. Teratology. 1994;50:137–147.
20. Freedom RM, Yoo SJ. Ebstein malformation of the tricuspid valve. In: Freedom RM, Yoo SJ, Mikailian H, Williams WG, editors. The natural and modified history of congenital heart disease. New York: Blackwell Publishing; USA. 2004. p 91–96.
21. Hornberger LK, Sahn DJ, Kleinman CS, Copel JA, Reed KL. Tricuspid valve disease with significant insufficiency in the fetus: diagnosis and outcome. J Am Coll Cardiol. 1991;17:167–173
22. Sharland GK, Chita SK, Allan LD. Tricuspid valve dysplasia or displacement in intrauterine life. J Am Coll Cardiol. 1991;17:944–949.
23. Miller MS, Rao PN, Dudovitz RN, Falk RE. Ebstein anomaly and duplication of the distal arm of chromosome 15: report of two patients. Am J Med Genet A. 2005;139:141–145.
24. Nakagawa M, Kato H, Aotani H, Kondo M. Ebstein's anomaly associated with trisomy 9p. Clin Genet. 1999;55:383–385.
25. Attenhofer Jost CH, Connolly HM, Warnes CA, O'Leary P, Tajik AJ, Pelikka SA, Seward JB. Noncompacted myocardium in Ebstein's anomaly: initial description in three patients. J Am Soc Echocardiography. 2004;17:677–680.
26. McIntosh N, Chitayat D, Bardanis M, Fouron JC. Ebstein anomaly: report of a familial occurrence and prenatal diagnosis. Am J Med Genet. 1992;42:307–309.
27. Balaji S, Dennis NR, Keeton BR. Familial Ebstein's anomaly: a report of six cases in two generations associated with mild skeletal abnormalities. Br Heart J. 1991;66:28–28.
28. Rosenmann A, Arad I, Simcha A, Schaap T. Familial Ebstein's anomaly. J Med Genet. 1976;13:532–535.
29. Donegon CC, Jr., Moore MM, Wiley TM, Jr., Hernandez FA, Green JR, Jr., Schiebler GL. Familial Ebstein's anomaly of the tricuspid valve. Am Heart J. 1968;75:375–379.
30. McElhinney DB, Salvin JW, Colan SD, Thiagarajan R, Crawford EC, Marcus EN, del Nido PJ, Tworetzky W. Improved outcomes in fetuses and neonates with congenital displacement (Ebstein's malformation) or dysplasia of the tricuspid valve. Am J Cardiol. 2005;96:582–586.
31. Shipp TD, Bromley B, Hornberger LK, Nadel A, Benacerraf BR. Levorotation of the fetal cardiac axis: a clue for the presence of congenital heart disease. Obstet Gynecol. 1995;85:97–102.

32. Berning RA, Silverman NH, Villegas M, Sahn DJ, Martin GR, Rice MJ. Reversed shunting across the ductus arteriosus or atrial septum in utero heralds severe congenital heart disease. J Am Coll Cardiol. 1996;27:481–486.

33. Berg C, Kremer C, Geipel A, Kohl T, Germer U, Gembruch U. Ductus venosus blood flow alterations in fetuses with obstructive lesions of the right heart. Ultrasound Obstet Gynecol. 2006;28:137–1342.

34. Schwartz ML. Fetal progression of Ebstein's anomaly. Circulation. 2003;108:c86–c87.

35. Todros T, Paladini D, Chiappa E, Russo MG, Gaglioti P, Pacileo G, Cau MA, Martinelli P. Pulmonary stenosis and atresia with intact ventricular septum during prenatal life. Ultrasound Obstet Gynecol. 2003; 21:228–233.

36. Roman KS, Fouron JC, Nii M, Smallhorn JF, Chaturvedi R, Jaeggi ET. Determinants of outcome in pulmonary valve stenosis or atresia with intact ventricular septum. Am J Cardiol. 2007; In Press.

37. Haworth SG, Shinebourne EA, Miller GA. Right-to-left interatrial shunting with normal right ventricular pressure. A puzzling haemodynamic picture associated with some rare congenital malformations of the right ventricle and tricuspid valve. Br Heart J. 1975;37:386–391.

38. Yetman AT, Freedom RM, McCrindle BW. Outcome in cyanotic neonates with Ebstein's anomaly. Am J Cardiol. 1998;81:749–754.

39. Atz AM, Munoz RA, Adatia I, Wessel DL. Diagnostic and therapeutic uses of inhaled nitric oxide in neonatal Ebstein's anomaly. Am J Cardiol. 2003;91:906–908.

40. Wald RM, Adatia I, Van Arsdell GS, Hornberger LK. Relation of limiting ductal patency to survival in neonatal Ebstein's anomaly. Am J Cardiol. 2005;96:851–856.

41. Andrews RE, Tibby SM, Sharland G, Simpson JM. Outcome following diagnosis of isolated tricuspid valve malformations in the fetus. Cardiol Young. 2006;16 Suppl 2:6–19.

42. Celermajer DS, Bull C, Till JA, Cullen S, Vassillikos VP, Sullivan ID, Allan L, Nihoyannopoulos P, Somerville J, Deanfield JE. Ebstein's anomaly: presentation and outcome from fetus to adult. J Am Coll Cardiol. 1994;23:170–176.

43. Robertson DA, Silverman NH. Ebstein's anomaly: echocardiographic and clinical features in the fetus and neonate. J Am Coll Cardiol. 1989;14:1300–1307.

44. Pavlova M, Fouron JC, Drblik SP, van Doesburg NH, Bigras JL, Smallhorn J, Harder J, Robertson M. Factors influencing the prognosis of Ebstein's anomaly during fetal life. Am Heart J. 1998;135:1081–1085.

45. Watson H. The natural history of Ebstein's anomaly in childhood and adolescence. A preliminary report on the first 100 cases. Proc Assoc Eur Cardiol. 1970;6:35–39.

46. Watson H. Natural history of Ebstein's anomaly of the tricuspid valve in childhood and adolescence: an international cooperative study of 505 cases. Br Heart J. 1974;36:417–427.

47. Giuliani ER, Fuster V, Brandenburg RO, Mair DD. Ebstein's anomaly: the clinical features and natural history of Ebstein's anomaly of the tricuspid valve. Mayo Clin Proc. 1979;54:163–173.

48. Radford DJ, Graff RF, Neilson GH. Diagnosis and natural history of Ebstein's anomaly. Br Heart J. 1985;36:517–522.

49. Kumar AE, Fyler DC, Miettinen OS, Nadas AS. Ebstein's anomaly: clinical profile and natural history. Am J Cardiol. 1971;28:84–95.

50. Hong YM, Moller JH. Ebstein's anomaly: a long term study of survival. Am Heart J. 1993;125:1419–1424.

51. Arduini D, Rizzo G, Romanini C. Fetal cardiac output measurements in normal and pathological states. In: Copel JA, Reed KL, editors. Doppler ultrasound in obstetrics and gynecology. New York: Raven Press; USA. 1995. p. 271–290.

52. Friedman WF. The intrinsic physiologic properties of the developing heart. Prog Cardiovasc Dis. 1972;15:87–111.

53. Kaufman TM, Horton JW, White DJ, Mahoney L. Age-related changes in myocardial relaxation and sarcoplasmatic reticulum function. Am J Physiol. 1990;259:H309–H316.

54. Rudolph AM. Fetal circulation. In: Yagel S, Silverman NH, Gembruch U, editors. Fetal Cardiology. London: Martin Dunits; UK. 2003. p.107–120.

55. Morton MJ, Thornburg KL. The pericardium and cardiac transmural filling pressure in the fetal sheep. J Dev Physiol. 1987;9:159–168.

56. Grant DA, Maloney JE, Tyberg JV, Walker AM. Effects of external constraint on the fetal left ventricular function curve. Am Heart J. 1992;123:1601–1609.

57. Grant DA, Kondo CS, Maloney JE, Walker AM, Tyberg V. Changes in pericardial pressure during the perinatal period. Circulation. 1992;86:1615–1621.

58. Grant DA, Walker AM. Pleural and pericardial pressures limit fetal right ventricular output. Circulation. 1996;94:555–561.

59. Grant DA, Fauchère JC, Eede KJ, Tyberg JV, Walker AM. Left ventricular stroke volume in the fetal sheep is limited by extracardiac constraint and arterial pressure. J Physiol. 2001;535:231–239.

60. Gilbert RD. Effects of afterload and baroreceptors on cardiac function in fetal sheep. J Dev Physiol. 1982;4:299–309.

61. Reller MD, Morton MJ, Reid DL, Thornberg KL. Fetal lamb ventricles respond differently to filling and arterial pressures and to in utero ventilation. Pediatr Res. 1987;22:621–626.

62. Gold PS, Brace RA. Fetal whole-body interstitial compliance and capillary filtration coefficient. Am J Physiol. 1984;247:R800–R805.

63. Johnson SA, Vander Straten MC, Parellada JA, Schnakenberg W, Gest AL. Thoracic duct function in fetal, newborn and adult sheep. Lymphology. 1996;29:50–56.

64. Gest AL, Blair DK, Vander Straten MC. The effect of outflow pressure upon thoracic duct lymph flow rate in fetal sheep. Pediatr Res. 1992;32:585–588.

65. Gest AL, Bair DK, Vander Straten MC. Thoracic duct lymph flow in fetal sheep with increased venous pressure from electrically induced tachycardia. Biol Neonate. 1993;64:325–330.

66. Pinson CW, Morton MJ, Thornburg KL. An anatomic basis for fetal right ventricular dominance and arterial pressure sensitivity. J Dev Physiol. 1987;9:253–269.

67. Atkins DL, Clark EB, Marvin WJ, Jr. Foramen ovale/atrial septum area ratio: a marker of transatrial blood flow. Circulation. 1982;66:281–283.

68. Feit LR, Copel JA, Kleinman CS. Foramen ovale size in the normal and abnormal human fetal heart: an indicator of transatrial flow physiology Ultrasound Obstet Gynecol. 1991;1:313–319.

69. Marshall AC, van der Velde ME, Tworetzky W, Gomez CA, Wilkins-Haug L, Benson CB, Jennings RW, Lock JE. Creation of an atrial septal defect in utero for fetuses with hypoplastic left heart syndrome and intact or highly restrictive atrial septum. Circulation. 2004;110:253–258.

70. Knott-Craig CJ, Overholt ED, Ward KE, Ringewald JM, Baker SS, Razook JD. Repair of Ebstein's anomaly in the symptomatic neonate: an evolution of technique with 7-year follow-up. Ann Thorac Surg. 2002;73:1786–1792.

Nicholas Collins and Eric Horlick

Ebstein's anomaly is an uncommon condition, classically considered an abnormality of tricuspid valve morphology. It is typically characterized by apical and inferior displacement of the septal and posterior leaflets of the tricuspid valve. The subsequent atrialization of the ventricle leads to a hypoplastic functional right ventricular chamber. The marked spectrum of tricuspid valve deformity and heterogeneity seen in right ventricular size and function is reflected in the remarkable variability in the prognosis of those with Ebstein's anomaly. In the past, deterioration in functional status has required treatment with medical therapy and surgical intervention. With the advent of transcatheter treatment for intracardiac defects, an additional method of therapy can now be utilized to improve the functional status of a select group of patients with Ebstein's anomaly.

Important considerations in identifying appropriate candidates for transcatheter closure requires an understanding of the spectrum of the disease, results and outcomes after surgical repair, and the physiologic effect of device closure on the remaining unrepaired structural abnormalities.

Ebstein's anomaly may present at any age, with disease severity at presentation closely linked to prognosis. Presentation in the neonatal period is typically associated with unfavorable anatomical characteristics and poor survival. Anatomical factors associated with poor prognosis include tethering of the superior tricuspid valve leaflet, right ventricular dysplasia, and left ventricular compression by the dilated right heart [1]. It has been suggested that those patients presenting as adults have a milder form of the disease. Using M-mode echocardiography to assess right ventricular function through movement of the tricuspid valve annulus and right ventricular apex, children with Ebstein's anomaly have decreased

right ventricular systolic excursion and decreased peak lengthening compared to age-matched controls. Interestingly, patients who presented later did not manifest any differences in these indices compared to controls [2].

With improved understanding of the anatomical abnormalities associated with Ebstein's anomaly, it is clear that it is not a condition limited to the tricuspid valve. In addition to the clearly defined tricuspid valve abnormalities, 80% of patients will have an interatrial communication [3]. Furthermore, echocardiographic series have documented a higher-than-expected incidence of bicuspid aortic valve, ventricular septal defect, and mitral valve dysplasia [4]. Abnormal left ventricular function has also been described, complicating distortion of left ventricular geometry [5] and left ventricular noncompaction [4].

36.1 Interatrial Communication in Ebstein's Anomaly

The importance of an associated atrial septal defect is reflected in the natural history of Ebstein's anomaly. There is clearly a spectrum of disease severity, which, as mentioned, has important prognostic implications. Failure of leaflet coaptation leads to variable degrees of tricuspid regurgitation due to adherence of the leaflets to the right ventricular endocardium. The presence of redundant tricuspid valve leaflets and associated leaflet prolapse coexists with dilatation of the tricuspid valve annulus [6, 7]. Patients with an absent or dysplastic septal leaflet are also more likely to have greater degrees of tricuspid incompetence [8]. Progressive tricuspid valve dysfunction and reduced right ventricular compliance leads to elevated right atrial pressure, which in turn promotes right to left shunting at the atrial level with concomitant systemic hypoxemia [9]. In addition to atrial septal defects, the presence of a patent foramen ovale is

N. Collins (✉)
Toronto General Cardiac Centre for Adults, University Health Network, Toronto, ON, Canada

A.N. Redington et al. (eds.), *Congenital Diseases in the Right Heart*, DOI 10.1007/978-1-84800-378-1_36,
© Springer-Verlag London Limited 2009

similarly relevant as a source of intracardiac shunting. The right atrium, the atrialized right ventricle and the functional right ventricle may be dilated, with mural thrombus on the surface of the right atrium described [7]. This clearly has implications in terms of paradoxical embolization in those patients with interatrial defects. Furthermore, not all patients manifest shunting as a result of a pressure imbalance between the atria. Streaming of tricuspid insufficiency or inferior vena cava flow across the septum because of counterclockwise cardiac rotation may also play a role.

36.2 Guidelines for Intervention

The recommended indications for surgical intervention in Ebstein's anomaly in the adult are based on recommendations from the Canadian and European guidelines [10, 11] and include deteriorating functional class, increasing heart size as manifested by an increase in the cardiothoracic ratio to $> 60\%$ on chest X-ray, important cyanosis ($SaO_2 < 90\%$), severe symptomatic tricuspid insufficiency, sustained atrial flutter or fibrillation, or arrhythmia secondary to an accessory pathway. The present guidelines do not offer catheter-based interatrial defect closure a place in the management of these patients. This omission reflects that present guidelines fail to take into account recent relevant literature regarding interatrial defect closure in this patient population.

36.3 Current Surgical Strategies

Previously published surgical results for Ebstein's anomaly have demonstrated excellent short- and medium-term results [7, 12, 13]. Surgical repair offers the possibility of valve repair or replacement, as well as closure of any interatrial defects and anti-arrhythmic surgery as appropriate. The nature of surgical repair, however, is markedly variable in the published series.

The Mayo Clinic experience of over 500 cases has been notable for a 35% valve repair rate and a 65% rate of prosthetic valve implantation. There was an extremely low rate ($< 10\%$) of bidirectional cavopulmonary anastamosis, which may be advantageous in unloading the right ventricle after valvular surgery. In this series, the preferred operative technique was transverse plication with a monocusp repair in conjunction with aggressive antiarrhythmic surgery. Their experience which extends from the early 1970s, and has yielded a 5.4% early mortality and 7.6% late mortality up to a maximum of 25 years of

follow-up (mean 7 years), with a need for reoperation in 16.7%.

Chauvaud et al. have reported results from over 200 patients and have emphasized a strategy of valve repair, which has reportedly been successful in over 95% of patients [14]. They favor a high rate of valve repair, augmented with a cavopulmonary anastamosis. Their repair strategy includes the mobilization and detachment of the anterior leaflet to facilitate repair and a longitudinal plication. This groups' early mortality rate was 9% early with a late actuarial mortality of 9%. The reoperation rate during follow-up was somewhat lower than the Mayo clinic data, at 11%.

While excellent results from these published series have been achieved, it is clear that even in experienced centers, there remains a risk of morbidity and mortality associated with surgical repair. Caution is drawn to the possibility of an amplification of surgical mortality in centers without such vast experience.

Despite the heterogeneity in surgical strategy, similar results in terms of mortality mean the optimal strategy for treatment of this group remains elusive. Additional considerations, therefore, to evaluate the results of surgical repair include the influence of surgery on ventricular size and function, as well as exercise capacity.

36.4 Effect of Surgery on Cardiac Chamber Size and Function

While there is a beneficial effect on tricuspid valve function following surgery, recent data suggests that the effect of surgery on right ventricular status is potentially adverse, as demonstrated in a recent study [15] assessing right ventricular volumes before and after tricuspid valve surgery. Right ventricular volumes were evaluated pre- and postoperatively by multislice computed tomography (CT) scanning in 26 consecutive adult patients. Patients had a mean age of 30 years and underwent this group's usual type of repair with mobilization of the anterior leaflet and plication of the atrialized right ventricle with a reduction of the tricuspid annulus. A bidirectional cavopulmonary shunt was used in 14 patients. The systolic and diastolic volume index of the right ventricle, left ventricle, and atrialized right ventricle were determined.

Several interesting findings came to light. First, the atrialized right ventricle, which was routinely plicated, had a stroke volume index of 36 ml/m² preoperatively, before obliteration at surgery. This led to the authors' questioning the routine practice of effectively resecting functional tissue. The effective stroke volume index and ejection fraction of the right ventricle both fell postoperatively from 100 cc/m^2 to 52 cc/m^2 and from 56% to 41%, respectively. This was in contrast to the small increase in left ventricle stroke volume index and ejection fraction 33 cc/m^2 to 37 cc/m^2, and 56 to 68%, respectively. The authors concluded that routine plication of the atrialized right ventricle was not always advantageous and that resection should potentially be limited only to dyskinetic or akinetic segments. The reduction in right ventricle function was related to poor myocardial preservation and possibly myocardial stunning (CT scans were performed between 7 and 10 days postoperatively). Although these changes were said to have little clinical impact, they raise the issue of the rather uncertain benefit and potentially harmful effects of surgery in this population. Acknowledged limitations of this study included the difficulty in assessing the thin-walled atrialized right ventricle by this method, and the unconventional choice of CT with its attendant radiation burden versus magnetic resonance imaging (MRI).

36.5 Cardiopulmonary Exercise Testing

Progressive impairment of exercise capacity is typical in unoperated patients with Ebstein's anomaly [16]. Cardiopulmonary stress testing has demonstrated a reduction in exercise performance, reduced peak oxygen uptake, impaired chronotropic response to exercise, and lower peak systolic blood pressure in these patients. These functional abnormalities correlate with the echocardiographic severity of the Ebstein's malformation of the tricuspid valve. Reduced exercise capacity has been attributed to reduced cardiac output complicating both tricuspid regurgitation and impaired right ventricular systolic function and diastolic filling. Displacement of the ventricular septum during systole may also produce a reduction in left ventricular size and systolic function. Importantly, however, impaired exercise tolerance in patients with Ebstein's anomaly may also reflect interatrial shunting [17] and exercise-induced hypoxemia [9]. The hypoplastic right ventricle may not tolerate increased venous return with exercise, leading to increased right-to-left shunting in that large proportion of patients with an interatrial defect.

The contribution of interatrial shunting to exercise intolerance in Ebstein's anomaly is supported by previously published data by MacLellan-Tobert et al. In this series of 117 patients, results of 124 exercise tests performed between 1980 and 1994 were reviewed [18]. The exercise tests were performed in 76 preoperative patients, 23 postoperative patients, with 7 patients undergoing testing both before and after surgical repair. An additional 18 patients underwent exercise testing, but did not proceed to operative repair. In the preoperative group, patients with an interatrial communication ($n = 67$) had significantly lower saturations at rest than those without ($n = 9$) (SaO$_2$ 85% vs. 96%), with lower saturations during exercise (SaO$_2$ 72% vs. 93%). A strong correlation was noted between exercise tolerance and resting saturation. No significant difference was noted between postoperative patients and preoperative patients without an interatrial communication. This suggests that the major factor contributing to exercise intolerance in unrepaired Ebstein's anomaly was the presence and magnitude of the interatrial shunt, with associated valve repair or replacement not shown to influence subsequent exercise capacity. This important study confirms the importance of the interatrial communication in these patients, and demonstrates that defect closure may be beneficial in symptom relief.

With the possibility of deleterious effects on the right ventricle through surgical intervention and the majority of benefit seemingly related to atrial defect closure, a more appropriate course of therapy for many patients, especially those adults with a milder form of the disease who present late, is device closure for symptom management.

36.6 Percutaneous Closure of Interatrial Defects

The use of percutaneous closure devices to ameliorate systemic hypoxemia complicating right-to-left shunting through an interatrial defect has been safely performed in a number of clinical settings. Such examples include hypoxia-complicating atrial shunting in right ventricular infarction, prior to and following pneumonectomy, with use of high positive-pressure ventilation, following left ventricular assist device insertion, and in the platypnoea–orthodoexia syndrome [19–23].

Percutaneous device closure of both atrial septal defects, up to 40 mm in diameter [24], and patent foramen ovale have been demonstrated to be safe, with excellent procedural outcomes [25]. In addition, they offer acceptable procedural success compared to surgical intervention, with reduced incidence of major procedural complications, reduced length of stay, and reduced risk of postprocedure arrhythmia [26]. It is unlikely that the benefits in right ventricular function seen in atrial septal defect closure can be extrapolated to patients with Ebstein's anomaly, given the nature of the hypoplastic right ventricle and the tendency to right-to-left shunting, compared to the volume-overloaded right ventricle seen

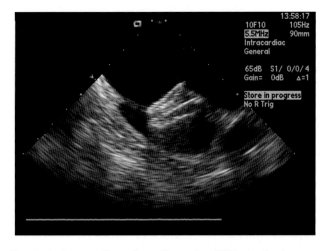

Fig. 36.1 Intracardiac echocardiography (ICE) confirming successful device placement and interatrial defect closure in a patient with Ebstein's anomaly. ICE provides excellent images of the interatrial septum to confirm device position and exclude residual shunting following the procedure

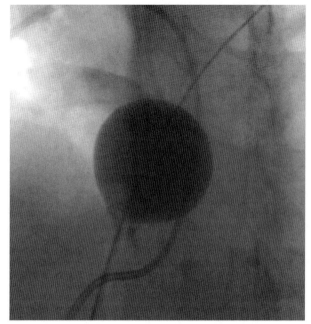

Fig. 36.2 Cineangiogram obtained during test balloon occlusion in a 49-year-old male with Ebstein's anomaly and systemic hypoxemia complicating right-to-left shunting at the atrial level. The interatrial defect is occluded with a Meditech Sizing Balloon (Boston Scientific Corporation, Watertown, Massachusetts, USA) with an 8 Fr. Genseni catheter (Cordis/Johnson and Johnson, Warren, New Jersey, USA) positioned initially in the pulmonary artery and then the right atrium to assess any change in pressure during test occlusion

with left-to-right shunting. However, the benefit of avoiding right ventricular injury at the time of surgical repair cannot be understated.

Despite the anatomical distortion associated with Ebstein's anomaly, no significant additional procedural difficulty should be anticipated associated with transcatheter closure of these defects [9]. In our experience, we have noted that the interatrial defect in Ebstein's anomaly tends to be more superior and posterior in the anteroposterior projection than in the usual secundum atrial septal defect or patent foramen ovale. This is not, however, a significant impediment to crossing the defect using standard equipment.

Transesophageal or intracardiac echocardiography can be successfully utilized to define atrial septal anatomy, localize the defect, guide closure, and interrogate the septum to exclude residual shunts, additional lesions and adequate device positioning. Intracardiac echocardiography can reduce fluoroscopy exposure, obviates the need for general anesthesia and improves patient tolerability [27]. When positioned in the right atrium, intracardiac echocardiography also permits excellent visualization and assessment of tricuspid valve structure and function. (Fig. 36.1)

36.7 Importance of Test Occlusion

Temporary test occlusion of an interatrial defect plays an important role in the invasive assessment of these patients. We obtain access for two catheters in the right

femoral vein and place an arterial cannula for invasive hemodynamic monitoring. We have used a Meditech (Boston Scientific Corporation, Watertown, Massachusetts, USA) sizing balloon to occlude the intratrial defect over a period of 15–20 min while monitoring right atrial pressure and saturation, left atrial pressure, and systemic arterial pressure and saturation (Fig. 36.2). Use of suture-mediated vascular closure devices have been demonstrated to be effective in obtaining hemostasis in patients requiring large diameter venous sheaths [28], such as those required for intracardiac echocardiography and atrial septal defect closure device delivery. We use this strategy routinely in our institution. Documentation of normal pulmonary vascular resistance is performed invasively and compliments a noninvasive assessment.

One of the major concerns regarding percutaneous device closure of interatrial defects in those patients with a hypoplastic right ventricle, characteristic of Ebstein's anomaly, is the precipitation of right heart failure. This reflects the possibility that the right ventricle may not be able to tolerate the additional volume loading that inevitably complicates interatrial defect closure in the setting of right-to-left shunting. It has been suggested that transcatheter closure of an interatrial defect in patients with Ebstein's anomaly may also contribute to right atrial dilatation [9]; further follow-up is required to determine if this predisposes to atrial arrhythmia.

In the pediatric population, atrial septal defect closure for treatment of hypoxia complicating right-to-left shunting in patients with a hypoplastic right ventricle has been safely performed by the Toronto group [29]. Patients were eligible for closure if they had unobstructed flow to confluent pulmonary arteries, a resting oxygen saturation (SaO_2) > 90%, and the absence of right heart failure. In this published series, patients underwent initial test occlusion to exclude a decrease in systemic blood pressure, an elevation in mean right atrial pressure (< 20%), or a decrease in right atrial saturation (< 10%). In these patients, closure was demonstrated to improve systemic oxygen saturation (91% at baseline to 98% postclosure), with no change in right ventricular or right atrial area. Right ventricular volume and tricuspid insufficiency were unchanged. Patients with systemic oxygen saturation less than 91% were excluded as they were considered to be unlikely to have adequate right ventricular function to tolerate device closure.

A more aggressive approach to catheter-based treatment of patients with lower saturations has also recently been reported [8], with four patients with Ebstein's anomaly included as part of this group. Patients were aged 8–29 years with a mean resting saturation of 88% (two patients had saturations < 86%). Exercise tests were performed before and after closure in this series adding an important piece to the previous work from Toronto. A significant improvement in peak exercise oximetry was noted following device closure (baseline SaO_2 83% improving to 94% postclosure). When a single patient with a large residual leak postclosure was excluded, mean exercise saturation was 98%. There was a significant increase in the baseline external work that could be performed following closure (5.4 to 7 Metabolic equivalents).

36.8 Additional Considerations

An assessment designed to exclude anatomical characteristics associated with Ebstein's anomaly is important before proceeding to percutaneous device closure. In particular, the presence of confluent pulmonary arteries and low pulmonary artery pressure is essential. Patients presenting early in life are more likely to have associated cardiac lesions, typically right ventricular outflow tract obstruction, which may contraindicate catheter-based device closure [30]. In addition, those diagnosed in the perinatal period are more likely to have increased ventricular fibrosis and wall thinning, which in turn is associated with poor outcome and hemodynamic compromise

[31]. These observations are important, as the variable prognosis of this condition has implications for the applicability of transcatheter treatment. Patients presenting before adolescence are more likely to represent the more severe spectrum of Ebstein's anomaly, and are less likely to tolerate device closure. In this setting, surgical intervention may be more appropriate, as device closure to limit right-to-left shunting is unlikely to significantly improve functional capacity or delay the need for surgery. Young adults and older patients who present with mild hypoxemia at rest or with desaturation with exercise are likely to have more favorable anatomy to support closure of an interatrial defect. Identification of patients at an earlier stage of disease progression by utilizing stress testing to identify desaturation during exercise may permit transcatheter closure before the development of significant right ventricular dysfunction and subsequent hypoxemia at rest. Indeed, measurement of pulse oximetry during exercise has been recommended as part of the diagnostic evaluation for patients with Ebstein's anomaly [6]. It is clear based upon our current limited experience that any patient undergoing interatrial defect closure requires intensive follow-up following device closure for clinical evidence of right heart failure or atrial arrhythmia.

Another potential benefit of closure of the interatrial defect in these patients may also be a reduction in future stroke risk. This may be achieved by prevention of paradoxical emboli, but also by reduction in cyanosis. Chronic hypoxemia results in impaired tissue oxygenation, with a consequent increase in erythropoietin production. This leads to secondary erythrocytosis and associated hyperviscosity syndrome. Secondary erythrocytosis may predispose to stroke in the context of iron deficiency or dehydration [32].

The exclusion of the presence of Wolff–Parkinson–White syndrome, which is seen in between 14% and 21% of patients with Ebstein's anomaly is another important consideration [13, 33]. Accessory pathways in Ebstein's anomaly are almost universally right sided and typically difficult to treat using catheter-based therapy. However, left atrial access through an atrial septal defect or patent foramen ovale obviates the need for a transeptal puncture, and its attendant risks, in the treatment of uncommon left-sided pathways.

Surgery represents an important and essential therapeutic tool in those cases where right heart failure may complicate closure of interatrial defect. As such, assessment of surgical candidacy, including coronary angiography where appropriate, should be included as part of the assessment preceding device closure. Tricuspid valve surgery may not only correct the tricuspid valve abnormality, but in patients with unfavorable anatomy, the creation of a bidirectional Glenn shunt may further reduce the volume load on the hypoplastic right ventricle [34].

Given the heterogeneity in right ventricular size and function in this population, it is difficult to apply such transcatheter treatment for all patients. Development of MRI technology has significantly improved the ability to assess right ventricular size and function, as well as give a clearer definition of tricuspid valve anatomy [35]. Advances in the management of Ebstein's anomaly may include MR imaging to identify those right ventricular parameters that may predict those patients more likely to tolerate transcatheter interatrial defect closure.

Future investigation into the role of interatrial defect closure will focus upon assessment and patient selection, with an emphasis on the need for careful follow-up to assess for the development of right heart failure and the need for tricuspid valve surgery. In particular, those clinical and imaging characteristics that will determine which patients will derive most benefit from intervention require definition. While attractive as a therapeutic measure in Ebstein's anomaly, experience in the use of transcatheter closure of interatrial defects in these patients remains limited. It is a potentially valuable treatment tool with improvements in exercise capacity, reduction in systemic hypoxemia, and diminution of future stroke risk. Confirmation that interatrial defect closure leads to sustained clinical benefit, with delay, or prevention, of future tricuspid valve surgery is also critical.

References

1. Roberson DA, Silverman NH. Ebstein's anomaly: echocardiographic and clinical features in the fetus and neonate. J Am Coll Cardiol. 1989;14:1300–7.
2. Therrien J, Henein MY, Li W, Somerville J, Rigby M. Right ventricular long axis function in adults and children with Ebstein's malformation. Int J Cardiol. 2000;73:243–9.
3. Brickner ME, Hillis LD, Lange RA. Congenital heart disease in adults. Second of two parts. N Engl J Med. 2000;342:334–42.
4. Attenhofer Jost CH, Connolly HM, O'Leary PW, Warnes CA, Tajik AJ, Seward JB. Left heart lesions in patients with Ebstein anomaly. Mayo Clin Proc. 2005;80:361–8.
5. Benson LN, Child JS, Schwaiger M, Perloff JK, Schelbert HR. Left ventricular geometry and function in adults with Ebstein's anomaly of the tricuspid valve. Circulation. 1987;75:353–9.
6. Bonow RO, Carabello B, de Leon AC, et al. ACC/AHA guidelines for the management of patients with valvular heart disease. Executive summary. A report of the American college of cardiology/American heart association task force on practice guidelines (committee on management of patients with valvular heart disease). J Heart Valve Dis. 1998;7:672–707.
7. Dearani JA, Danielson GK. Surgical management of Ebstein's anomaly in the adult. Semin Thorac Cardiovasc Surg. 2005;17:148–54.
8. Shiina A, Seward JB, Tajik AJ, Hagler DJ, Danielson GK. Two-dimensional echocardiographic–surgical correlation in Ebstein's anomaly: preoperative determination of patients requiring tricuspid valve plication vs replacement. Circulation. 1983;68:534–44.
9. Agnoletti G, Boudjemline Y, Ou P, Bonnet D, Sidi D. Right to left shunt through interatrial septal defects in patients with congenital heart disease: results of interventional closure. Heart. 2006;92:827–31.
10. Therrien J, Gatzoulis M, Graham T, et al. Canadian cardiovascular society consensus conference 2001 update: Recommendations for the management of adults with congenital heart disease–Part II. Can J Cardiol. 2001;17:1029–50.
11. Deanfield J, Thaulow E, Warnes C, et al. Management of grown up congenital heart disease. Eur Heart J. 2003;24:1035–84.
12. Chen JM, Mosca RS, Altmann K, et al. Early and medium-term results for repair of Ebstein anomaly. J Thorac Cardiovasc Surg. 2004;127:990–8; Discussion 998–9.
13. Oh JK, Holmes DR, Jr., Hayes DL, Porter CB, Danielson GK. Cardiac arrhythmias in patients with surgical repair of Ebstein's anomaly. J Am Coll Cardiol. 1985;6:1351–7.
14. Chauvaud S, Berrebi A, d'Attellis N, Mousseaux E, Hernigou A, Carpentier A. Ebstein's anomaly: repair based on functional analysis. Eur J Cardiothorac Surg. 2003;23:525–31.
15. Chauvaud SM, Hernigou AC, Mousseaux ER, Sidi D, Hebert JL. Ventricular volumes in Ebstein's anomaly: x-ray multislice computed tomography before and after repair. Ann Thorac Surg. 2006;81:1443–9.
16. Trojnarska O, Szyszka A, Gwizdala A, et al. Adults with Ebstein's anomaly-cardiopulmonary exercise testing and BNP levels exercise capacity and BNP in adults with Ebstein's anomaly. Int J Cardiol. 2005.
17. Mair DD. Ebstein's anomaly: natural history and management. J Am Coll Cardiol. 1992;19:1047–8.
18. MacLellan-Tobert SG, Driscoll DJ, Mottram CD, Mahoney DW, Wollan PC, Danielson GK. Exercise tolerance in patients with Ebstein's anomaly. J Am Coll Cardiol. 1997;29:1615–22.
19. Yalonetsky S, Nun AB, Shwartz Y, Lorber A. Transcatheter closure of a patent foramen ovale prior to a pneumonectomy to prevent platypnea syndrome. Eur J Cardiothorac Surg. 2006;29:622–4.
20. Godart F, Rey C, Prat A, et al. Atrial right-to-left shunting causing severe hypoxaemia despite normal right-sided pressures. Report of 11 consecutive cases corrected by percutaneous closure. Eur Heart J. 2000;21:483–9.
21. Ilkhanoff L, Naidu SS, Rohatgi S, Ross MJ, Silvestry FE, Herrmann HC. Transcatheter device closure of interatrial septal defects in patients with hypoxia. J Interv Cardiol. 2005;18:227–32.
22. Nguyen DQ, Das GS, Grubbs BC, Bolman RM, 3rd, Park SJ. Transcatheter closure of patent foramen ovale for hypoxemia during left ventricular assist device support. J Heart Lung Transplant. 1999;18:1021–3.
23. Kubler P, Gibbs H, Garrahy P. Platypnoea-orthodeoxia syndrome. Heart. 2000;83:221–3.
24. Lopez K, Dalvi BV, Balzer D, et al. Transcatheter closure of large secundum atrial septal defects using the 40 mm Amplatzer septal occluder: results of an international registry. Catheter Cardiovasc Interv. 2005;66:580–4.
25. Butera G, De Rosa G, Chessa M, et al. Transcatheter closure of atrial septal defect in young children: results and follow-up. J Am Coll Cardiol. 2003;42:241–5.

26. Du ZD, Hijazi ZM, Kleinman CS, Silverman NH, Larntz K. Comparison between transcatheter and surgical closure of secundum atrial septal defect in children and adults: results of a multicenter nonrandomized trial. J Am Coll Cardiol. 2002;39:1836–44.

27. Jongbloed MR, Schalij MJ, Zeppenfeld K, Oemrawsingh PV, van der Wall EE, Bax JJ. Clinical applications of intracardiac echocardiography in interventional procedures. Heart. 2005;91:981–90.

28. Shaw JA, Dewire E, Nugent A, Eisenhauer AC. Use of suture-mediated vascular closure devices for the management of femoral vein access after transcatheter procedures. Catheter Cardiovasc Interv. 2004;63:439–43.

29. Atiq M, Lai L, Lee KJ, Benson LN. Transcatheter closure of atrial septal defects in children with a hypoplastic right ventricle. Catheter Cardiovasc Interv. 2005;64:112–6.

30. Celermajer DS, Bull C, Till JA, et al. Ebstein's anomaly: presentation and outcome from fetus to adult. J Am Coll Cardiol. 1994;23:170–6.

31. Celermajer DS, Dodd SM, Greenwald SE, Wyse RK, Deanfield JE. Morbid anatomy in neonates with Ebstein's anomaly of the tricuspid valve: pathophysiologic and clinical implications. J Am Coll Cardiol. 1992;19:1049–53.

32. Oechslin E. Hematological management of the cyanotic adult with congenital heart disease. Int J Cardiol. 2004;97 Suppl 1:109–15.

33. Khositseth A, Danielson GK, Dearani JA, Munger TM, Porter CJ. Supraventricular tachyarrhythmias in Ebstein anomaly: management and outcome. J Thorac Cardiovasc Surg. 2004;128:826–33.

34. Chauvaud S, Fuzellier JF, Berrebi A, et al. Bi-directional cavopulmonary shunt associated with ventriculo and valvuloplasty in Ebstein's anomaly: benefits in high risk patients. Eur J Cardiothorac Surg. 1998;13:514–9.

35. Davlouros PA, Niwa K, Webb G, Gatzoulis MA. The right ventricle in congenital heart disease. Heart. 2006;92 Suppl 1:i27–i38.

Jennifer C. Hirsch and Edward L. Bove

37.1 Introduction

Ebstein's malformation was first described by Wilhelm Ebstein in 1866 as a constellation of clinical findings resulting from an abnormality of the tricuspid valve [1]. It has become evident over time that the malformation is a disease of the entire right ventricle and the development of the tricuspid valve. It involves a spectrum of anatomical abnormalities of variable severity, including apical displacement of the septal and mural leaflets of the tricuspid valve, which have failed to delaminate from the underlying myocardium; thinning or atrialization of the inlet component of the right ventricle, with variable dilation; and malformation of the antero-superior leaflet, with anomalous attachments, redundancy, and fenestrations. Several other cardiac anomalies are often associated with the right ventricular changes, such as atrial and ventricular septal defects, obstruction of the outlet from the right ventricle, and Wolff–Parkinson–White syndrome. Ebstein's malformation can also afflict the left-sided systemic atrioventricular valve in the setting of congenitally corrected transposition [2].

37.2 Clinical Presentation

The malformation is rare, accounting for no more than 1% of all congenital cardiac anomalies. Due to the significant anatomic variability in the abnormalities of the tricuspid valve and right ventricle, the age at presentation and severity of symptoms can also be highly variable. Patients who present in infancy have the poorest prognosis. There is a high rate of fetal death, hydrops, and pulmonary hypoplasia when the diagnosis is made during fetal life. Cyanosis is the most common presentation in infancy. These patients have severe tricuspid regurgitation with a poorly functioning right ventricle in the face of elevated pulmonary arterial resistance. The result is a state of low cardiac output dependent upon right-to-left shunting across the oval fossa.

With less severe derangements of the tricuspid valve, and preserved ventricular function, patients tend to present later in adolescence or early adulthood. Many patients are asymptomatic, and present with a murmur, noted on physical examination. In symptomatic patients, a common presentation involves the new onset of atrial arrhythmias or reentrant tachycardia. Exercise tolerance may be diminished, with cyanosis during extreme exertion if an atrial septal defect is present. Those patients with an intact atrial septum will often progress to congestive heart failure with increasing cardiomegaly.

37.3 Diagnosis

Echocardiography is usually sufficient for accurate diagnosis and anatomic evaluation. The degree of displacement, tethering, and dysplasia of the valvar leaflets can be determined, as well as the amount of regurgitation. Ventricular function, and the extent of atrialization of the right ventricle, can also be evaluated. Additional abnormalities, including the presence and direction of a shunt at the atrial level, can be assessed. Electrocardiographic findings include incomplete right bundle branch block, right-axis deviation, ventricular preexcitation, and atrial arrhythmias. The chest radiograph can vary from normal, in patients with mild anatomic abnormalities, to the classic *wall-to-wall* heart. Cardiac catheterization is rarely necessary.

E.L. Bove (✉)
F7830, Mott Children's Hospital, 1500 East Medical Center Drive, Ann Arbor, MI 48109, USA
e-mail: elbove@umich.edu

A.N. Redington et al. (eds.), *Congenital Diseases in the Right Heart*, DOI 10.1007/978-1-84800-378-1_37,
© Springer-Verlag London Limited 2009

37.4 Management in Neonates

As noted previously, neonates often present with profound cyanosis, and may require prostaglandins to maintain adequate flow of blood to the lungs during the early neonatal period when pulmonary resistance is high. It is important to distinguish functional from anatomic pulmonary atresia. In those with functional atresia, it may be possible to wean from the infusion of prostaglandins while maintaining adequate saturations of oxygen as pulmonary resistance falls. These patients can then be followed for development of further symptoms.

In neonates who cannot be weaned from prostaglandins due to unacceptable levels of hypoxemia, or in those with anatomic pulmonary atresia, it is necessary to construct a systemic-to-pulmonary shunt to maintain adequate pulmonary blood flow. For those neonates who also develop significant symptoms of congestive heart failure while on prostaglandin, it is necessary to address the underlying valvar pathology. The options include closure of the tricuspid valve, with or without fenestration, along with construction of a modified Blalock-Taussig shunt, repair of the tricuspid valve if ventricular function is reasonable, or cardiac transplantation.

In the older patient with progressive symptoms, a variety of surgical options exist to address the malformed tricuspid valve. Most are based on techniques designed to mobilize the leading edge of the antero-superior leaflet, aiming to create a competent monocusp valve with or without plication of the atrialized portion of the right ventricle. There is ongoing debate as to the necessity of obliterating the atrialized portion of the right ventricle. Historically, plication of this portion of the ventricle has been an integral part of most repairs, albeit that no clear physiologic benefit with regard to improved ventricular function has been demonstrated. In addition, the potential exists for injury to the right coronary artery as a result of the plication, which may adversely impact on late outcomes and contribute to ventricular arrhythmias.

The technique reported by Danielson and colleagues involves the horizontal plication of the atrialized portion of the right ventricle, mobilization of the antero-superior leaflet to create a monocusp valve, and closure of the atrial septal defect if the oval fossa is patent [3]. The modified technique developed by Carpentier [4] involves the mobilization of the antero-superior leaflet, followed by the detachment of that leaflet from the annulus. The atrialized ventricle is then plicated longitudinally, the antero-superior leaflet is reattached at the true annulus, and the atrial septal defect, if present, is closed. The technique promoted by Ullmann and associates [5] does not involve exclusion of the atrialized ventricle. With this technique, the septal leaflet is mobilized and reattached to the true annulus. The secondary attachments of the antero-superior leaflet are also mobilized to allow the free edge to coapt with the newly liberated septal leaflet. The valvoplasty technique pioneered by Sebening [6] also does not involve the exclusion of the atrialized ventricle. The repair creates a monocusp valve using a single-mattress suture reinforced with a pledget placed from the midportion of the free edge of the antero-superior leaflet to the atrialized wall of the right ventricle directly opposite. The antero-inferior commissure is closed, and a De Vega [7] annuloplasty is performed as necessary to achieve valvar competence.

Replacement of the tricuspid valve is a final option, and has been performed with late survival free from reoperation equivalent to valvar repair. If replacement is required, heterografts are preferred over mechanical valves due to risks of thrombosis. Other options using tissue valves include the insertion of pulmonary autografts, mitral valvar homografts, and *top-hat* mounted pulmonary or aortic homografts. When replacing the valve, the sutures should be brought around the coronary sinus, leaving it to drain into the right ventricle so as to minimize potential injury to the atrioventricular node [8].

Many issues remain regarding the surgical management of this complex and variable anomaly. For symptomatic neonates, a trial of prostaglandins can differentiate those who can simply be shunted versus those that require valvar intervention and possible closure. The role of repair of the tricuspid valve in the neonate and infant as opposed to closure using a patch is controversial. In the severely symptomatic neonate, symptoms are as much from ventricular as valvar problems. In older patients, surgery is usually reserved for those with progressive or severe symptoms. In general, repair is preferred, if possible, over replacement. Some argue that early repair may improve right ventricular function by reconditioning. This may be of benefit for patients with severe anatomy and early onset of symptoms.

As stated previously, the question of early *elective* repair to preserve and possibly improve ventricular function, and reduce the risk of late arrhthymias in relatively asymptomatic children, continues to be debated. Plication of the atrialized ventricle has largely fallen out of favor, but remains a mainstay of surgical therapy in many institutions. Some surgeons construct a bidirectional Glenn anastomosis to decrease the volume load placed on the ventricle. Finally, the conversion to functionally univentricular palliation with a Fontan connection can be performed for the severely symptomatic patient.

37.5 Summary

Ebstein's malformation is a rare but challenging congenital cardiac defect. The high degree of anatomic variability makes it difficult to have a standardized approach to these children. The symptomatic neonate carries a very grave prognosis. The presence of associated cardiac, and other congenital, anomalies often make survival impossible. Surgical options are limited at this age, and often still result in a poor outcome. Medical management, if possible, is the best, as surgical success improves with age. If surgery is required, conversion to functional tricuspid atresia often offers the best survival, as the ventricle in the severely symptomatic neonate functions poorly. Transplantation remains an option, but the availability of organs limits its utility.

Patients who are not symptomatic in the neonatal period will often remain free from symptoms well into adolescence. Electrophysiologic symptoms usually precede symptoms of congestive heart failure. Indications for repair at these ages include symptoms, cyanosis, and progressive cardiomegaly.

References

1. Ebstein W. Ueber einen sehr seltenen Fall von Insufficienz der valvula tricuspidalis, bedingt durch eine angeborene hochgradige Missbildung derselben, Arch Anat Physiol Wiss Med. 1866;238.
2. Anderson KR, Danielson GK, McGoon DC, et al. Ebstein's anomaly of the left-sided tricuspid valve: pathological anatomy of the valvular malformation. Circulation. 1978;58 Suppl:I87–I91.
3. Danielson GK, Driscoll DJ, Mair DD, et al. Operative treatment of Ebstein's anomaly. J Thorac Cardiovasc Surg. 1992;104:1195–2002.
4. Carpentier A, Cahuvaud S, Mace L, et al. A new reconstructive operation for Ebstein's anomaly of the tricuspid valve. J Thorac Cardiovasc Surg. 1988;96:92–101.
5. Ullmann MV, Born S, Sebening C, et al. Ventricularization of the atrialized chamber: a concept of Ebstein's anomaly repair. Ann Thorac Surg. 2004;78:918–25.
6. Augustin N, Scmidt-Habelmann P, Wottke M, et al. Results after surgical repair of Ebstein's anomaly. Ann Thorac Surg. 1997;63:1650–6.
7. De Vega NG. [Selective, adjustable and permanent annuloplasty. An original technic for the treatment of tricuspid insufficiency]. Rev Exp Cardiol. 1972;25:555–6.
8. Dearani JA and Danielson GK. Tricuspid valve repair for Ebstein's anomaly. Operative techniques in thorac cardiovasc surgery. 2004;8:188–92.

Section 9
Special Topics

The Role of Resynchronization Therapy in Congenital Heart Disease: Right–Left Heart Interactions

38

Elizabeth A. Stephenson

Key Words Tetralogy of Fallot • abnormalities of cardiac rhythm • cardiac resynchronization • heart failure

Heart failure can be seen in a variety of clinical scenarios, and frequently these patients also demonstrate an associated delay in intraventricular electrical conduction. A lack of synchrony in the cardiac contraction can contribute to a lower cardiac output due to shorter filling times, inefficient contraction, as well as increased atrioventricular valve regurgitation. Cardiac resynchronization therapy (CRT) is a pacing technique through which multiple areas of the heart are stimulated to trigger a cardiac contraction that minimizes dyssynchrony and maximizes cardiac output. CRT developed initially in the adult population in patients with a left bundle branch block due to postmyocardial infarction, [1, 2] and has since been shown to also be effective with patients with dilated cardiomyopathy as well [2, 3]. The patients who comprised the majority of the early work had both electrical dyssynchrony, represented by prolonged QRS, as well as mechanical dyssynchrony, which can been described with a variety of imaging techniques. Initial studies of CRT showed an improvement in quality of life, but not a mortality reduction. [1] As the patient population became better defined, and the study groups became larger, it was possible to demonstrate a benefit in mortality as well [4, 5].

The congenital heart disease population is also affected by cardiac dysfunction, but is a more difficult one to study due to heterogeneity as well as fewer patients overall. Similar to those in the earlier ischemic cardiomyopathy studies, these patients frequently have abnormal QRS duration, but usually with a right bundle branch block due to surgical repair. This first step in considering whether CRT would be a useful therapy in this population is determining if indeed dyssynchrony does exist, mechanical as well as electrical. Vogel et al. examined a large group of patients late following tetralogy of Fallot repair, and found that right ventricular wall motion abnormalities were common, and that they correlated with repolarization–depolarization abnormalities [6]. Another study in tetralogy of Fallot patients similarly demonstrated that in those patients with right bundle branch block there were also clear right ventricular motion abnormalities, that is, electrical *and* mechanical dyssynchrony [7]. A study by Abd El Rahman et al. showed that ventriculo–ventricular dyssynchrony, secondary to repaired tetralogy of Fallot could be identified in these patients with right bundle branch block [8]. The patients who had undergone repair of tetralogy of Fallot demonstrated increased left ventricular delay when compared with healthy controls. This supports the model that disadvantageous ventriculo–ventricular interaction due to right bundle branch block can impair left ventricular function. It has also been shown that the subset of patients who have marked ventricular electrical dyssynchrony, again based on primarily right ventricular conduction delays, also have increased left ventricular dysfunction, and higher risk of death [9]. Ghai et al. showed that sudden cardiac death and ventricular tachycardia were more common in tetralogy of Fallot patients who had moderate or severe left ventricular dysfunction [10]. This is similar to the pattern seen in the general adult population, with increasing dysfunction leading to increasing risk of death, both sudden arrhythmic deaths and those from congestive heart failure [4].

CRT has been explored in the congenital heart disease population in both children and adults. One of the first studies was done by Janousek et al. in acute postoperative patients [11]. They looked at 20 children, approximately half of whom had tetralogy of Fallot, and tested both atrioventricular optimization as well as ventriculo–ventricular optimization. They were able to demonstrate shortened QRS duration in the majority of these patients as well as increased blood pressure. As expected, this

E.A. Stephenson (✉)
Paediatric Cardiology, The Hospital for Sick Children, 555 University Avenue, Toronto, Ontario, Canada, M5G 1X8
e-mail: elizabeth.stephenson@sickkids.ca

group of patients had predominantly right bundle branch block (and thus likely predominantly right ventricular dyssynchrony) rather than left bundle branch block. Zimmerman et al. similarly examined patients immediately following repair of congenital heart disease, and was able to show a decrease in QRS duration, increase in cardiac output, and increase in systolic blood pressure for almost all of the patients with multisite pacing within the right ventricle [12]. They also found that acute multisite pacing was able to facilitate weaning from cardiopulmonary bypass following surgical repair. Included in this group were some patients with single ventricles, and multisite pacing was performed via two sites within the same ventricle, in an attempt to synchronize the contraction of the ventricle. Dubin et al. looked at seven patients in the catheterization laboratory with right ventricular dysfunction and right bundle branch block and paced in three right ventricular sites: the apex, outflow tract, and septum [13]. They were able to show improved cardiac index and dP/dt in these patients, as well as decreased QRS duration in many. Interestingly, the site of right ventricular pacing which produced the narrowest QRS duration correlated with the increases in cardiac output, but not with dP/dt. Another study looked at the feasibility of accomplishing right ventricular resychronization using traditional transvenous pacing sites. A population of approximately 25 patients with tetralogy of Fallot who had ICDs placed and typical RV apical-pacing sites was examined, to see if via atrioventricular optimization the QRS could be shortened. All of these patients had intact ventricular conduction, and resynchronization was attempted via fusion of the native conduction along with pacing in the right ventricle. In this group, AV optimization could lead to a narrower, more normal QRS duration, suggestive of possible correction of some of the electrical dyssynchrony [14]. Clearly, the focus of many of these studies has been resynchronization of the right, rather than the left ventricle, as that is the origin of the dyssynchrony. As ventricular dysfunction progresses, the left ventricle can become more dyssynchronous, either due to conduction delay in the left ventricle itself, or due to ventriculo–ventricular interactions (Fig. 38.1).

CRT has also been evaluated on a chronic basis in this population, with the first case studies published in 2003 and 2004. In 2003, Roofthooft et al. and Blom et al. both described case studies of children (one infant, one 6-yearold) with cardiac dysfunction following congenital heart disease repair [15, 16]. Both patients demonstrated improvement following placement of the pacemaker, both in terms of symptoms and echo measurements of cardiac function and synchrony. Janousek et al. described two patients with cardiomyopathy, one with repaired congenital heart disease and another with congenital heart

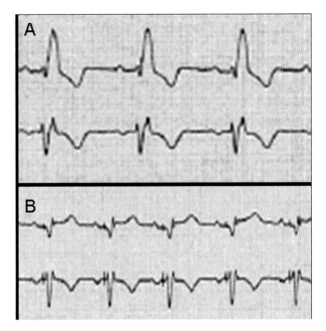

Fig. 38.1 QRS duration of a patient with tetralogy of Fallot, before (A) and after (B) resynchronization

block and a pacemaker [17]. The first improved with CRT, and the second with cessation of pacing and return to narrow QRS escape rhythm. In both patients, cardiac function improved when dyssynchrony was reduced. In a case series, Strieper et al. describe seven patients with implantation of a CRT device. These patients were initially considered for possible transplantation, and following institution of CRT 5 were clinically improved enough to be removed from transplantation consideration [18]. CRT has also been shown to be effective in the systemic morphological right ventricle, when right ventricular conduction delay and dysfunction are present [19, 20]. One large, multicenter study was recently published by Dubin et al. [21]. This was a retrospective study of children with cardiac dysfunction and congenital heart disease or congenital AV block who underwent CRT. There were a total of 103 patients, 73 with congenital heart disease, and the group overall showed an improvement of approximately 12% in ejection fraction. There were 11 patients who were considered to be nonresponders, with either no change, or a decline in ejection fraction. There was no clear difference in response rate between the etiologic and anatomic subtypes, but it was a very heterogeneous population. Kirsh et al. described a patient with complete heart block, tetralogy of Fallot, and marked abnormal septal movement [22]. Prior to resynchronization, the patient had marked left ventricular dilation, and after approximately 3 months there was a dramatic reduction in left ventricular volumes due to reverse remodeling, and the child went from being symptomatic during his activities of daily life to being essentially asymptomatic (Fig. 38.2).

Fig. 38.2 Echo before and after resynchronization, demonstrating volume reduction and reverse remodeling

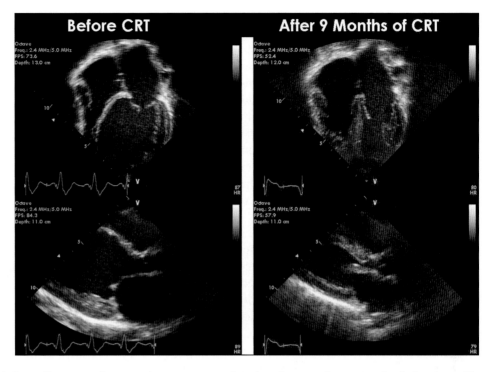

It is very clear from the adult cardiomyopathy experience that not all patients with myocardial dysfunction will respond to CRT. Response rates in the adult ischemic population range, but overall approximately 80% of patients are likely to respond to CRT, and similar rates were seen in the large series of pediatric CRT described above [21]. These differences in response are likely due to individual differences in etiology and location of dysfunction and dyssynchrony. Patients will vary in terms of location of both septal and ventriculotomy scars, as well as whether they encountered any ischemic damage around the time of the repair. All of these factors and more will lead to differences in interventricular and intraventricular conduction, and a tremendous amount of research is underway to attempt to identify imaging and measurement techniques to better understand these differences. One more recent study utilized tissue Doppler imaging in this congenital heart disease population, and was able to demonstrate a reduction in mechanical dyssynchrony, in addition to increased cardiac index with initiation of CRT [23]. Predictors of this type of response are growing in the ischemic heart disease population, although they remain to be tested in the congenital heart disease population.

The technical aspects of CRT in the pediatric and congenital heart disease population can be particularly challenging, due to cardiac anatomy, venous capacitance, overall body size, and possible intracardiac shunts. CRT devices can be implanted either via epicardial or transvenous routes. Children have to be fairly large to tolerate the transvenous method as the systems require three leads, one atrial and two ventricular. The pacemaker generator is also larger than standard bradycardia devices, and may not be tolerated in a pectoral pocket in smaller children. Due to these issues, epicardial devices are used more frequently in the pediatric and congenital heart disease population than in the ischemic heart disease population. (Fig. 38.3) Another concern in CRT is

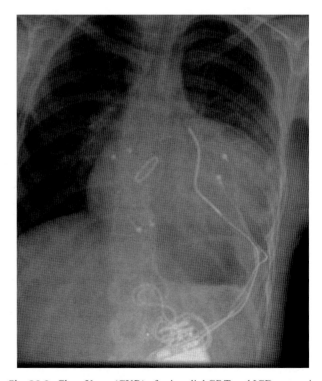

Fig. 38.3 Chest X-ray (CXR) of epicardial CRT and ICD system in child with congenital heart disease

the possibility of proarrhythmia. The large series by Dubin et al. noted three patients with new onset of arrhythmic events, and although this is a population already at risk for arrhythmias, the onset following initiation of CRT was concerning [21]. Fish et al. have also described similar events in the adult (primarily ischemic) adult CRT population, thought to be secondary to prolongation the QT interval. The shift in activation through the myocardium may prolong repolarization, and place patients at increased risk of arrhythmias. This clearly only appears in a small number of patients, and further study is required to anticipate which patients might be at risk [24].

As congenital heart disease patients are surviving longer and longer, issues of chronic heart function protection and heart failure management become paramount. Dyssynchrony is clearly present in the congenital heart disease population, affects both the right and the left ventricle, and correlates with arrhythmias and cardiac dysfunction. Acute resynchronization can increase cardiac output via right or left ventricular resynchronization. The next challenges of CRT are identification of the ideal population and alternative techniques of resynchronization of the nonresponders.

References

1. Abraham WT, Fisher WG, Smith AL, Delurgio DB, Leon AR, Loh E, Kocovic DZ, Packer M, Clavell AL, Hayes DL, Ellestad M, Trupp RJ, Underwood J, Pickering F, Truex C, McAtee P, Messenger J, Evaluation MSGMIRC. Cardiac resynchronization in chronic heart failure.[see comment]. New England J Med. 2002;346(24):1845–1853.

2. Bristow MR, Feldman AM, Saxon LA. Heart failure management using implantable devices for ventricular resynchronization: Comparison of Medical Therapy, Pacing, and Defibrillation in Chronic Heart Failure (COMPANION) trial. COMPANION Steering Committee and COMPANION Clinical Investigators. J Card Fail. 2000;6(3):276–285.

3. Carson P, Anand I, O'Connor C, Jaski B, Steinberg J, Lwin A, Lindenfeld J, Ghali J, Barnet JH, Feldman AM, Bristow MR. Mode of death in advanced heart failure: the Comparison of Medical, Pacing, and Defibrillation Therapies in Heart Failure (COMPANION) trial. J Am Coll Cardiol. 2005;46(12): 2329–2334.

4. Bristow MR, Saxon LA, Boehmer J, Krueger S, Kass DA, De Marco T, Carson P, DiCarlo L, DeMets D, White BG, DeVries DW, Feldman AM, Comparison of Medical Therapy PaDiHFI. Cardiac-resynchronization therapy with or without an implantable defibrillator in advanced chronic heart failure. [see comment]. New England J Med. 2004;350(21):2140–2150.

5. Cleland JG, Daubert JC, Erdmann E, Freemantle N, Gras D, Kappenberger L, Tavazzi L, Cardiac Resynchronization-Heart Failure Study I. The effect of cardiac resynchronization on morbidity and mortality in heart failure.[see comment]. New England J Med. 2005;352(15):1539–1549.

6. Vogel M, Sponring J, Cullen S, Deanfield JE, Redington AN. Regional wall motion and abnormalities of electrical depolarization and repolarization in patients after surgical repair of tetralogy of Fallot. Circulation. 2001;103(12):1669–1673.

7. D'Andrea A, Caso P, Sarubbi B, D'Alto M, Giovanna Russo M, Scherillo M, Cotrufo M, Calabro R. Right ventricular myocardial activation delay in adult patients with right bundle branch block late after repair of Tetralogy of Fallot. Eur J Echocardiogr. Mar 2004;5(2):123–131.

8. Abd El Rahman MY, Hui W, Yigitbasi M, Dsebissowa F, Schubert S, Hetzer R, Lange PE, Abdul-Khaliq H. Detection of left ventricular asynchrony in patients with right bundle branch block after repair of tetralogy of Fallot using tissue-Doppler imaging-derived strain. J Am Coll Cardiol. Mar 15 2005;45(6):915–921.

9. Gatzoulis MA, Till JA, Somerville J, Redington AN. Mechanoelectrical interaction in tetralogy of Fallot. QRS prolongation relates to right ventricular size and predicts malignant ventricular arrhythmias and sudden death.[see comment]. Circulation. 1995;92(2):231–237.

10. Ghai A, Silversides C, Harris L, Webb GD, Siu SC, Therrien J. Left ventricular dysfunction is a risk factor for sudden cardiac death in adults late after repair of tetralogy of Fallot. J Am Coll Cardiol. Nov 6 2002;40(9):1675–1680.

11. Janousek J, Vojtovic P, Hucin B, Tlaskal T, Gebauer RA, Gebauer R, Matejka T, Marek J, Reich O. Resynchronization pacing is a useful adjunct to the management of acute heart failure after surgery for congenital heart defects. Am J Cardiol. 2001;88(2):145–152.

12. Zimmerman FJ, Starr JP, Koenig PR, Smith P, Hijazi ZM, Bacha EA. Acute hemodynamic benefit of multisite ventricular pacing after congenital heart surgery. Ann of Thorac Surg. 2003;75(6):1775–1780.

13. Dubin AM, Feinstein JA, Reddy VM, Hanley FL, Van Hare GF, Rosenthal DN. Electrical resynchronization: a novel therapy for the failing right ventricle.[see comment]. Circulation. 2003;107(18):2287–2289.

14. Stephenson EA, Cecchin F, Alexander ME, Triedman JK, Walsh EP, Berul CI. Relation of right ventricular pacing in tetralogy of Fallot to electrical resynchronization. Am J Cardiol. 2004;93(11):1449–1452.

15. Roofthooft MT, Blom NA, Rijlaarsdam ME, Bokenkamp R, Ottenkamp J, Schalij MJ, Bax JJ, Hazekamp MG. Resynchronization therapy after congenital heart surgery to improve left ventricular function. Pacing & Clin Electrophysiol. 2003;26(10): 2042–2044.

16. Blom NA, Bax JJ, Ottenkamp J, Schalij MJ. Transvenous biventricular pacing in a child after congenital heart surgery as an alternative therapy for congestive heart failure. J Cardiovasc Electrophysiol. Oct 2003;14(10):1110–1112.

17. Janousek J, Tomek V, Chaloupecky V, Gebauer RA. Dilated cardiomyopathy associated with dual-chamber pacing in infants: improvement through either left ventricular cardiac resynchronization or programming the pacemaker off allowing intrinsic normal conduction. J Cardiovasc Electrophysiol. 2004;15(4):470–474.

18. Strieper M, Karpawich P, Frias P, Gooden K, Ketchum D, Fyfe D, Campbell R. Initial experience with cardiac resynchronization therapy for ventricular dysfunction in young patients with surgically operated congenital heart disease. Am J Cardiol. 2004;94(10):1352–1354.

19. Janousek J, Tomek V, Chaloupecky VA, Reich O, Gebauer RA, Kautzner J, Hucin B. Cardiac resynchronization therapy: a novel adjunct to the treatment and prevention of systemic right ventricular failure. J Am Coll Cardiol. Nov 2 2004;44(9):1927–1931.

20. Khairy P, Fournier A, Thibault B, Dubuc M, Therien J, Vobecky SJ. Cardiac resynchronization therapy in congenital heart disease. Int J Cardiol. Aug 8 2005.

21. Dubin AM, Janousek J, Rhee E, Strieper MJ, Cecchin F, Law IH, Shannon KM, Temple J, Rosenthal E, Zimmerman FJ, Davis A, Karpawich PP, Al Ahmad A, Vetter VL, Kertesz NJ, Shah M, Snyder C, Stephenson E, Emmel M, Sanatani S, Kanter R, Batra A, Collins KK. Resynchronization therapy in pediatric and congenital heart disease patients: an international multicenter study. J Am Coll Cardiol. 2005;46(12):2277–2283.

22. Kirsh JA, Stephenson EA, Redington AN. Images in cardiovascular medicine. Recovery of left ventricular systolic function after biventricular resynchronization pacing in a child with repaired tetralogy of Fallot and severe biventricular dysfunction. Circulation. Apr 11 2006;113(14):e691–692.

23. Pham PP, Balaji S, Shen I, Ungerleider R, Li X, Sahn DJ. Impact of conventional versus biventricular pacing on hemodynamics and tissue Doppler imaging indexes of resynchronization postoperatively in children with congenital heart disease.[see comment]. J Am Coll Cardiol. 2005;46(12):2284–2289.

24. Fish JM, Brugada J, Antzelevitch C. Potential proarrhythmic effects of biventricular pacing. J Am Coll Cardiol. Dec 20 2005;46(12):2340–2347.

Philip J. Kilner

39.1 Introduction

The palliative surgical reconstruction which has become known as the Fontan operation is performed mainly in children who have hearts with only one adequately formed ventricle, or two that cannot be separated functionally. Fontan operations have undergone several modifications and refinements in the decades since Fontan and Baudet published their initial results in humans in 1971[1] (Figs. 39.1, 39.2 and 39.3). The procedure entails a radical rearrangement of the circulation. Such patients would have been born with mixing and shunting of blood at ventricular and possibly other levels. They may have undergone preliminary palliative surgery to limit or supplement blood flow to the lungs, in many cases with a bidirectional superior vena cava (SVC)–pulmonary artery (Glenn) anastomosis. Completion of the Fontan reconstruction aims to eliminate shunting and the consequent volume loading of the dominant ventricle with desaturation of the arterial blood. The procedure involves connection of the pulmonary arteries downstream of and in series with the systemic veins so that the single effective ventricle delivers flow through the systemic then the pulmonary resistances, in series rather than in parallel, as would have been the case before operation. In effect, Fontan surgery creates a *pulmonary portal circulation*, and, from the gastrointestinal organs, a *hepato–pulmonary porto–portal circulation*. Elevated systemic venous and hepatic portal pressure is needed to propel the blood forward through the relatively low resistance of the pulmonary vessels. The delivery of flow through the pulmonary as well as the systemic resistance adds only about 10% to the ventricle's workload when maintaining a given output—less strenuous for the myocardium than the volume loading that would have been present prior to surgery. The

most critical and unavoidable pathophysiological consequence of Fontan surgery, however, is the height of the systemic venous pressure and its effects on the microvessels upstream.

The indications for Fontan surgery, pathophysiology, complications, and management have been summarized by Marc Gewillig [2, 3] and the late complications clearly

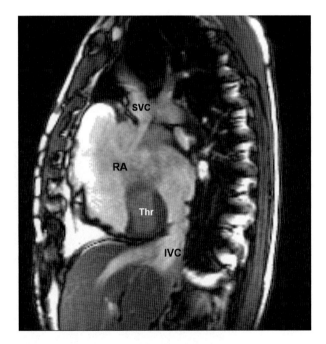

Fig. 39.1 Complications of an early atriopulmonary Fontan operation that incorporated atrial inflow valves. The sagittal cinemagnetic resonance image shows the dilated right atrium (RA) with a large thrombus attached to its floor (Thr). The solidified, ineffective leaflets of the homograft valves can be seen, mildly restricting inflow from the SVC and IVC. There is no capacitant atrial chamber upstream of these valves so, if they did close, flow would be interrupted in the distended caval veins. This contrasts with the closure and apical displacement of a normal ventricular inflow valve, which allows continued atrial filling. Fontan right atrial inflow valves tended to solidify in a half-open position, as seen here, and were not included in later variants of the operation

P.J. Kilner (✉)
Cardiovascular Magnetic Resonance Unit, Royal Brompton Hospital, London, UK

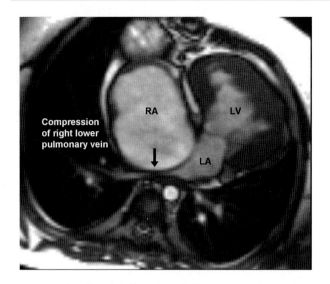

Fig. 39.2 The dilated right atrium (RA) upstream of an atriopulmonary Fontan connection causing compression of the right lower pulmonary vein (arrow), which will then slightly exacerbate the right atrial distension

summarized by Robert Freedom and colleagues.[4] This chapter owes much to these and other publications.

Fontan reconstruction should achieve nearly normal arterial saturation and avoids chronic volume overload, but at the cost of significant elevation of the systemic venous and hepatic portal pressure, typically to about 12–15 mm Hg at rest. There is usually decreased cardiac output at rest, and limited capacity to increase output on

exercise. The author is not aware that the feedback mechanisms which limit exercise capacity are adequately understood, but they are likely to relate to the critical elevation of systemic venous pressure with the increased flow, predominantly from the lower body, during exercise.

39.2 The Development of Fontan Surgery and CavoPulmonary Streamlining

Until the end of the 1980s, the right atrium was routinely included between the caval veins and the pulmonary arteries. Initially, atrial inflow and outflow valves were inserted, but they were not found to function satisfactorily. This may have been due to inadequate right atrial compared with left ventricular stroke volume, and due to the distended caval veins which lack capacitant *atrial* function upstream of the contractile chamber (Fig. 39.1). In patients with atriopulmonary Fontan connections, the right atrium, which tends to become dilated and subject to arrhythmias, superimposes pulsatility on the underlying cavopulmonary flow that is maintained indirectly by the work of the systemic ventricle. The peaks of pressure caused by the contraction of a right atrium included in a Fontan circulation are propagated, detrimentally, upstream to the systemic and hepatic veins as well as beneficially downstream to pulmonary arteries. The

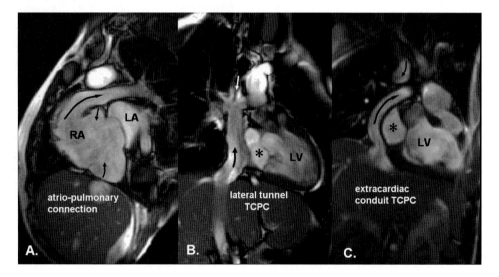

Fig. 39.3 Three types of Fontan connection illustrated by MRI. (A): atriopulmonary connection, (B): lateral tunnel, and (C): extracardiac conduit. B and C are variants of total cavopulmonary connection (TCPC) As a transitional stage to Fontan physiology, a limited residual shunt may be left in the form of a fenestration between the IVC pathway and the low-pressure atrial cavity to slightly alleviate systemic venous pressure. The TCPC avoids the

progressive right atrial distension which can predispose to atrial arrhythmias, stagnation, and thrombosis, and the coronary sinus drains to the low-pressure part of the right atrium, which is marked *. The TCPC gives almost nonpulsatile pulmonary arterial flow, which may in itself be a disadvantage, but at the same time, it avoids detrimental atrial systolic peaks of back-pressure to the hepatic and other systemic veins work put into this part of the circulation by right atrial contraction not only fails to contribute usefully, the extra energy being largely dissipated in turbulent flow, but also the turbulence itself slightly increases the local resistance to flow through the cavity and adjacent vessels. This was part of the rationale put forward by Marc de Leval and colleagues, this author included, for total cavopulmonary connection (TCPC) [5], a surgical approach which had previously been implemented by Kawashima in patients with anomalous systemic venous returns [6]. This type of procedure also excludes part or all of the right atrial cavity from the elevated pressure of the cavopulmonary flow path, which may help to avoid the atrial distension which predisposes to arrhythmias, stagnation, and thrombosis. It also allows the coronary sinus to drain to the low-pressure part of the right atrium and then to the left atrium via an atrial septal defect. Fenestration of a TCPC was a further modification introduced in 1990 as a transitional stage, slightly alleviating systemic venous congestion and augmenting filling of the systemic ventricle [7]. A small fenestration may close spontaneously, or be closed by an occlusion device in the months following surgery.

Marc de Leval and colleagues as well as other groups have gone on to apply computational fluid dynamic modeling to studies of the geometries and fluid dynamics of TCPC, either by lateral tunnel or extracardiac conduit [8]. There is little doubt that the dimensions and shapes of the connections matter. From the author's own observations and measurements of flow in models, and from magnetic resonance studies in patients, the factors likely to optimize cavopulmonary flow and minimize systemic venous congestion are these:

1) **Avoidance of stenosis.** Each flow path (IVC and SVC to RPA and LPA) and the junctions between them must have adequate cross-sectional area for the flow carried. On exercise, flow normally increases mainly from the lower body, so it is questionable whether the lower part of a transected SVC, which has sometimes been used to form the upper part of the IVC flow path after lateral tunnel TCPC, has adequate diameter for the exercising state.

2) **Avoidance of sharp angulation** at the suture lines of the cavopulmonary anastomoses. Abrupt changes of direction predispose to flow separation and turbulence.[8] This means that the inevitable changes of direction between the caval pathways and the pulmonary arteries should be gradual and rounded off by means of appropriate tailoring or patching. There may be a case for prefabricating appropriately sized and shaped interposition grafts.[9]

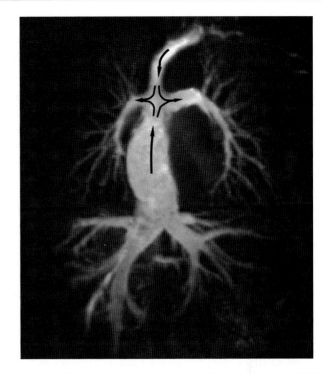

Fig. 39.4 The hepato–cavo–pulmonary flow paths after TCPC Fontan connection illustrated by a magnetic resonance contrast angiogram. It is important that hepatic venous blood flows via the IVC pathway to both lungs as it carries a factor which prevents the formation of pulmonary arteriovenous malformations, a potential cause of desaturation (see Fig. 39.8B)

3) **Avoidance of opposing or competing streams** from the upward-flowing IVC and the downward-flowing SVC. In other words, they should not collide head on, but be slightly offset relative to one another. It is important, however, that hepatic venous blood contributes, via the IVC pathway, to both lungs (Fig. 39.4) as it carries a factor which prevents the formation of pulmonary arteriovenous malformations, a potential cause of progressive desaturation.

4) **Minimization of flow separation**, flow disturbance, and regions of stagnation that might predispose to thrombosis by maintaining uniform diameters and smooth contours through the cavopulmonary flow paths.

The minimization of energy dissipation is important, and so is the avoidance of potentially arrhythmogenic and thrombogenic atrial scarring and distension. When these are included in the reckoning, it is not surprising that total cavopulmonary connection, particularly using an extracardiac conduit, has become the most widely practiced form of Fontan connection. But the procedure remains far from ideal. It is a radical palliation leaving the patient with abnormal circulatory physiology which can lead, after years or decades, to a series of possible complications.

39.3 Causes of Failure in a Fontan Circulation

There are several factors that may contribute to failure of a Fontan circulation. They include:

(1) **elevated resistance of the cavo(atrio)pulmonary vasculature**, including stenosis at surgical connections, hypoplasia or stenosis of pulmonary arteries, thrombo-embolic obstruction, and pulmonary vein compression due to right atrial distension after atriopulmonary connection (Fig. 39.2);

(2) **atrial arrhythmias** (sinus node dysfunction or atrial reentry tachycardia) particularly late after atriopulmonary connection.

(3) **thrombo-embolism** [10];

(4) **dysfunction of the dominant ventricle**, its inflow valve and outflow tract;

(5) **systemic venous and hepatic portal congestion** and complications following from these;

(6) **protein-losing enteropathy**,[11] lymphatic congestion, plastic bronchitis [3]; and

(7) **shunts** due to leaks from the Fontan pathway, aortopulmonary or systemic vein–pulmonary vein or other collaterals [4].

As illustrated in Fig. 39.5, these can be progressively and mutually detrimental, with several possible feedback pathways causing exacerbation of one factor by another. This underlines the importance of avoidance of complications in the first place by appropriate selection for surgery, and optimal surgical preparation [3], timing, and technique. And following surgery, careful follow-up is needed to detect and, if possible, correct potential problems before the onset of symptoms. As Marc Gewillig has emphasized, the management of arrhythmia and/or heart failure after Fontan surgery is challenging [3]. Several factors need to be considered, investigated, and treated appropriately. There are a particular group of problems associated with progressive right atrial dilatation following atriopulmonary connection, but the prevalence of complications in this patient group may be partly related to an earlier era of surgery, and more years of follow-up. In such patients, conversion from atriopulmonary to the potentially slightly more streamlined total cavopulmonary connection is an option to consider, combined with a right atrial maze procedure [12]. Such surgery is relatively high risk in most hands, however. It is therefore crucial to establish to what extent pathophysiology is present, which is likely to be alleviated by reoperation, as opposed to pathology that would not be alleviated but might exacerbate the risk.

39.4 Elevation of Cavo(Atrio)Pulmonary Resistance

Elevation of pulmonary vascular resistance due to hypoplasia of the pulmonary arteries or pulmonary vascular disease is a contraindication to Fontan surgery in the first place,[13, 14] as it would result in excessive systemic venous congestion. After a Fontan operation, resistance to flow through the cavopulmonary connections may be elevated due to suboptimal surgery, as discussed above, particularly if there is residual stenosis at a suture line. In the long term, thrombo-embolic disease particularly due to thrombus formation in a dilated right atrium (Fig. 39.1) may cause gradual elevation of pulmonary resistance. This is one of several possible self-perpetuating cycles. Elevated resistance may cause right atrial dilatation and arrhythmia, which in turn predisposes to thrombosis, possible embolization, and further elevation of resistance. Another deteriorating cycle is the compression of one or more pulmonary vein, usually the right lower, between the dilated right atrium and the spine (Fig. 39.2).

Fig. 39.5 Factors that may contribute to the failure of a Fontan circulation, and their possible interactions. Those marked with asterisks (*) mainly affect patients with atriopulmonary Fontan connections. These may be alleviated by conversion to TCPC, but other factors may not be, and could increase the risk of reoperation

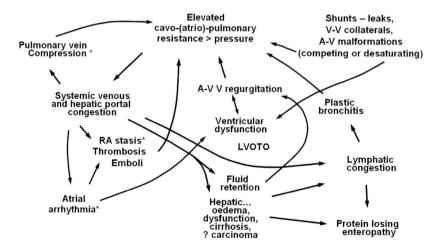

This may elevate pulmonary vascular resistance, increasing the atrial distension, and so on.

39.5 Arrhythmias and Thrombo-embolism

The most common type of arrhythmia is probably atrial reentry tachycardia or atrial flutter. It may occur through dilatation and/or previous scarring of the right atrium, particularly after atriopulmonary Fontan connection. It can lead to marked deterioration of circulatory function, not necessarily because the atrium was contributing useful hemodynamic work, but because of the right atrium's role in initiating left atrioventricular coordination. Right atrial flutter results in irregular filling and contraction of the systemic ventricle, and it usually requires resynchronization therapy as soon as possible before there is further deterioration due to left heart failure, elevation of pulmonary resistance, atrial thrombus formation, embolization, and so on. At the same time, it is essential to establish whether there is any treatable hemodynamic lesion, such as anastomotic or pulmonary arterial stenosis, which may exacerbate atrial distension. Anticoagulation may be needed, [10] arguably in all Fontan circulations known to have complex, low-velocity cavo(atrio)pulmonary flow, visible as right atrial *smoke* on echocardiography.

39.6 Systemic and Hepatic Portal Venous Congestion and Sequelae

Elevation of systemic venous pressure to near-critical levels seems to be an inevitable consequence of Fontan surgery. Further elevation through the factors outlined above can have damaging consequences for the microvessels and tissues of the organs upstream, notably the liver and, upstream of the liver, the intestines. [11] Even greater elevation of systemic venous flow and, therefore, pressure during exercise is a factor to take into account. Ascites and hepatic edema, and less commonly, cirrhosis and hepatic carcinoma have been reported as sequelae [15, 16]. Protein-losing enteropathy is a further, fortunately relatively uncommon, complication related to portal and lymphatic congestion. Plastic bronchitis, probably due to pulmonary lymphatic congestion and exudates is an uncommon but potentially fatal complication. The liver is vulnerable to increased venous and portal venous pressure. Experiments in rats have shown that local elevation of hepatic vascular flow and presumably pressure through partial hepatectomy leads remarkably quickly to gaping of the fenestrae in the endothelial walls of the

intrahepatic sinusoids, and so potential damage through leakage blood cells and larger molecules between the hepaticytes [17]. There is normally respiratory variation of hepatic portal flow through the emptying and refilling of the portal venous reservoir as the diaphragm moves down and up again. In some Fontan patients, abnormal reversal of hepatic portal flow has been shown during expiration, implying abnormally wide sinusoidal communications [18]. It seems likely that the post-Fontan pathology of hepatic and intestinal microvessels, lymphatics, and tissues is an area that needs further research and understanding.

39.7 Ventricular Dysfunction

The underlying congenital malformation, volume loading of the systemic ventricle prior to completion of Fontan reconstruction, the surgical procedure itself, particularly if performed with prolonged bypass, and possibly the abnormal pre- and afterloading of the ventricle following Fontan surgery may all contribute to ongoing ventricular dysfunction. This may cause and be exacerbated by regurgitation of the inflow valve (Fig. 39.6). Outflow to the aorta via a ventricular septal defect/or an infundibulum can be subject to progressive obstruction (Fig. 39.7).

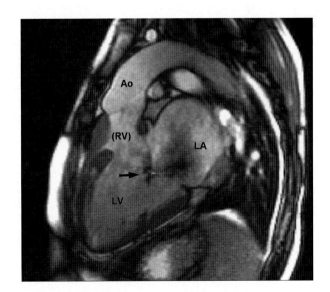

Fig. 39.6 Mitral regurgitation (arrow) in a patient with Fontan operation contributes to back pressure into the pulmonary and hence the systemic veins. In this particular patient, who also had a pleural effusion, treatment of fluid retention alleviated the regurgitation

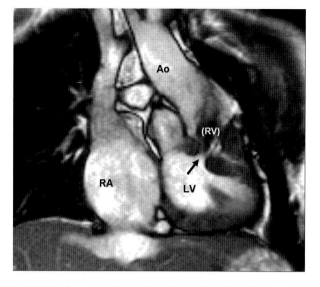

Fig. 39.7 Left ventricular outflow obstruction after Fontan operation caused by a moderately restrictive VSD and the hypertrophied infundibulum of the rudimentary, subaortic right ventricle

39.8 Shunts: Desaturating or Congesting

The Fontan circulation should achieve a transcutaneous oxygen saturation of at least 94%, assuming there is no significant residual shunting. A limited desaturating shunt may have been created deliberately as a fenestration between the cavopulmonary flow path and the low-pressure atrial compartment(s). Unwanted shunts may occur, however, through a patch of baffle leak (Fig. 39.8A) or through the development of pulmonary arteriovenous malformations (Fig. 39.8B) or systemic vein to pulmonary vein collaterals (Figs. 39.8C and D)[19]. Shunts that exacerbate pulmonary congestion, rather than causing systemic arterial desaturation, include ventricular to right atrial leaks, for example, at a patch intended to close a right atrioventricular valve, or a residual or acquired systemic-to-pulmonary arterial shunt.

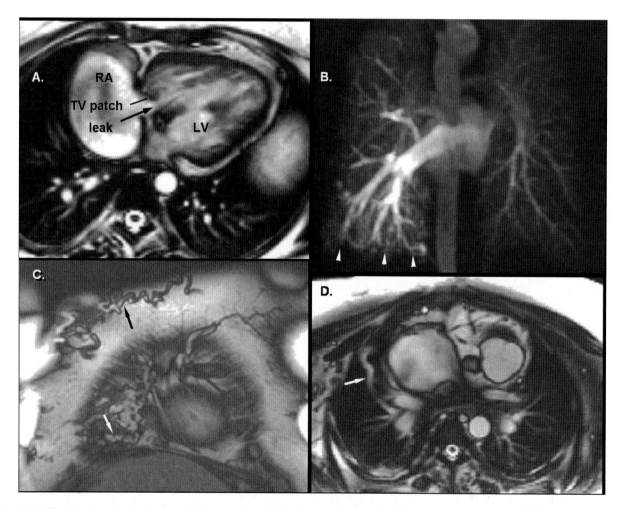

Fig. 39.8. Desaturating shunts in three different patients. (A) A diastolic leak through the detachment of a patch placed across the right atrioventricular valve of a patient with double-inlet left ventricle and an atriopulmonary Fontan connection. (B) Magnetic resonance contrast angiogram showing evidence of right pulmonary arteriovenous malformations (arrows) in a patient after Kawashima operation, in whom hepatic venous return was flowing to the left lung, but not the right. (C and D) Subcutaneous (black arrow) and intrathoracic (white arrows) branches of systemic venous to pulmonary venous collateral veins

39.9 Conclusion

The range of procedures known as Fontan operations are radical palliative procedures, not corrections, and there is no such thing a *perfect* Fontan operation. Fontan surgery should, as far as possible, be undertaken only by experienced congenital cardiac surgical teams. Follow-up needs to be life-long, by cardiologists with specific knowledge of the peculiarities of Fontan pathophysiology. Expert imaging, including cardiovascular magnetic resonance, is an important aspect of follow-up. The progressive cascade of possible complications (Fig. 39.5) underlines the importance of excellent pre-Fontan management and decision making, careful selection and planning for surgery, excellent surgical technique, and from then on, appropriate diagnostic follow-up and management.

References

1. Fontan F, Baudet E. Surgical repair of tricuspid atresia. Thorax. 1971;26(3):240–8.
2. Gewillig M, Kalis N. Pathophysiological aspects after cavopulmonary anastomosis. Thorac Cardiovasc Surg. 2000 Dec;48(6):336–41.
3. Gewillig M. The Fontan circulation. Heart. 2005;91(6):839–46.
4. Freedom RM, Li J, Yoo S-J. Late complications following the Fontan operation. In Gatzoulis MA, Webb GD, Daubeney PEF editors. 'Diagnosis and management of adult congenital heart disease', Churchill Livingstone, Edinburgh, 2003.
5. de Leval MR, Kilner P, Gewillig M, Bull C. Total cavopulmonary connection. J Thorac Cardiovasc Surg. 1989;97(4):636.
6. Kawashima Y, Kitamura S, Matsuda H, Shimazaki Y, Nakano S, Hirose H. Total cavopulmonary shunt operation in complex cardiac anomalies. A new operation. J Thorac Cardiovasc Surg. 1984;87(1):74–81.
7. Bridges ND, Lock JE, Castaneda AR. Baffle fenestration with subsequent transcatheter closure. Modification of the Fontan operation for patients at increased risk. Circulation. 1990; 82:1681–9
8. Hsia TY, Migliavacca F, Pittaccio S, Radaelli A, Dubini G, Pennati G, de Leval M. Computational fluid dynamic study of flow optimization in realistic models of the total cavopulmonary connections. J Surg Res. 2004;116(2):305–13.
9. Soerensen D, Pekkan K, Sundareswaran K, Yoganathan A. New power loss optimized Fontan connection evaluated by calculation of power loss using high resolution PC-MRI and CFD. Conf Proc IEEE Eng Med Biol Soc. 2004;2:1144–7.
10. Monagle P, Karl TR. Thromboembolic problems after the Fontan operation. Semin Thorac Cardiovasc Surg Pediatr Card Surg Annu 2002;5:36–47.
11. Mertens L, Hagler D, Sommerville J, et al. Protein losing enteropathy after the Fontan operation: an international multicenter evaluation. J Thorac and Cardiovasc Surg. 1998; 115:1063–73.
12. Mavroudis C, Deal BJ, Backer CL. The beneficial effects of total cavopulmonary conversion and arrhythmia surgery for the failed Fontan. Semin Thorac Cardiovasc Surg Pediatr Card Surg Annu. 2002;5:12–24.
13. Choussat A, Fontan F, Besse F, et al. Selection criteria for Fontan's procedure. In: Anderson R, Shinebourne E, editors. Paediatric cardiology. Edinburgh: Churchill Livingstone; 1978. p 559–66.
14. Knott-Craig CJ, Danielson GK, Schaff HV, et al. The modified Fontan operation. An analysis of risk factors for early postoperative death or takedown in 702 consecutive patients from one institution. J Thorac Cardiovasc Surg 1995;109:1237–43.
15. Ghaferi AA, Hutchins GM. Progression of liver pathology in patients undergoing the Fontan procedure: Chronic passive congestion, cardiac cirrhosis, hepatic adenoma, and hepatocellular carcinoma. J Thorac Cardiovasc Surg. 2005; 129(6):1348–52.
16. Kiesewetter C, Sheron N, Vettukattill J, Hacking N, Stedman B, Millward-Sadler H, Haw M, Cope R, Salmon A, Sivaprakasam M, Kendall T, Keeton B, Iredale J, Veldtman G. Hepatic changes in the failing Fontan circulation. Heart. Sep 27 2006. [Epub ahead of print]
17. Braet F, Shleper M, Paizi M, Brodsky S, Kopeiko N, Resnick N, Spira G. Liver sinusoidal endothelial cell modulation upon resection and shear stress in vitro. Comp Hepatol. 2004;3(1):7.
18. Hsia TY, Khambadkone S, Redington AN, Migliavacca F, Deanfield JE, de Leval MR. Effects of respiration and gravity on infradiaphragmatic venous flow in normal and Fontan patients. Circulation. 2000;102 19 Suppl 3:III148–53.
19. Magee AG, McCrindle BW, Mawson J, Benson LN, Williams WG, Freedom RM. Systemic venous collateral development after the bidirectional cavopulmonary anastomosis. Prevalence and predictors. J Am Coll Cardiol. 1998;32(2):502–8.

Index

Printed in the United States of America